GALANIN:
BASIC RESEARCH
DISCOVERIES AND
THERAPEUTIC
IMPLICATIONS

ANNALS OF THE NEW YORK ACADEMY OF SCIENCES

Volume 863

GALANIN: BASIC RESEARCH DISCOVERIES AND THERAPEUTIC IMPLICATIONS

Edited by Tomas Hökfelt, Tamas Bartfai, and Jacqueline Crawley

The New York Academy of Sciences
New York, New York
1998

Copying fees: For each copy of an article made beyond the free copying permitted under Section 107 or 108 of the 1976 Copyright Act, fee should be paid through the Copyright Clearance Center, Inc., 222 Rosewood Drive, Danvers, MA 01923. The fee for copying an article is $3.00 for non-academic use; for use in the classroom it is $0.07 per page.

♾The paper used in this publication meets the minimum requirements of American National Standard for Information Sciences—Permanence of Paper for Printed Library Materials, ANSI Z39.48-1984.

Cover: This illustration is a composite of a double immunofluorescence micrograph and a schematic drawing of the galanin R1 receptor. The immunofluorescence staining shows galanin (in green) and dopamine β-hydroxylase (in red) positive fibers in the hippocampal formation. There are many yellow fibers indicating the presence of galanin in noradrenergic terminals, but there are also many galanin-alone fibers as well as noradrenaline fibers without galanin (from Xu et al., unpublished data). A major advance in the galanin field was the first cloning of the human galanin receptor by Habert-Ortoli et al. (Proc. Natl. Acad. Sci. USA **91**: 9780–9783, 1994) followed by the rat counterpart (Burgevin et al. J. Mol. Neurosci. **6**: 1–8, 1995; Parker et al. Mol. Brain Res. **34**: 179–189, 1995). Kask et al. (EMBO J. **15**: 236–244, 1996) have delineated the peptide binding site of the human galanin receptor, and the amino acid residues involved in binding are indicated by red (modified from Berthold et al. Eur. J. Biochem. **249**: 601–606, 1997). This cover illustration was made by Zhi-Qing David Xu.

Library of Congress Cataloging-in-Publication Data

Galanin : basic research discoveries and therapeutic implications /
    edited by Tomas Hökfelt, Tamas Bartfai, and Jacqueline Crawley.
        p.   cm. — (Annals of the New York Academy of Sciences ; v. 863)
    Includes bibliographical references and index.
    ISBN 1-57331-174-X (cloth : alk. paper). — ISBN 1-57331-175-8
(pbk. : alk. paper)
        1. Galanin—Congresses. 2. Galanin—Therapeutic use—Testing—
Congresses. I. Hökfelt, Tomas. II. Bartfai, Tamas. III. Crawley,
Jacqueline N. IV. Series.
Q11.N5   no. 863
[QP552.G25]
500 s–dc21
[572'.65]   98-53496
                                                                              CIP

E-Media/PCP
Printed in the United States of America
ISBN 1-57331-174-X (cloth)
ISBN 1-57331-175-8 (paper)
ISSN 0077-8923

ANNALS OF THE NEW YORK ACADEMY OF SCIENCES

Volume 863
December 21, 1998

GALANIN: BASIC RESEARCH DISCOVERIES AND THERAPEUTIC IMPLICATIONS[a]

Editors
TOMAS HÖKFELT, TAMAS BARTFAI, AND JACQUELINE CRAWLEY

CONTENTS

[a]This volume is the result of a conference entitled **Galanin: Basic Research Discoveries and Therapeutic Implications** sponsored by the Wenner-Gren Foundations and held on May 3-5, 1998 in Stockholm, Sweden.

Part 6. Galanin in Ascending Systems

Part 7. Learning, Memory, Aging, and Disease

Financial assistance was received from:

• Wenner-Gren Foundations

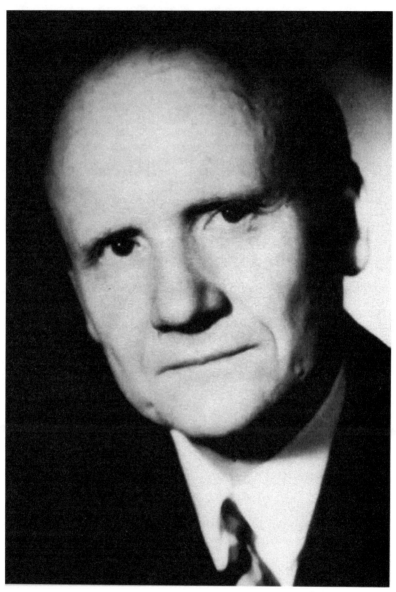

Viktor Mutt 1923–1998

In Memoriam

At the Wenner-Gren Symposium on "Galanin: Basic Research Discoveries and Therapeutic Implications," which was held in Stockholm in the beginning of May 1998, the participants honored Viktor Mutt, the discoverer of galanin. Mutt had then worked in peptide research for 50 years, it was 15 years since he had published the first paper on galanin, and he was going to celebrate his 75th birthday at the end of the year. We, who were present at the symposium are glad that we at that time could express our appreciation. Viktor Mutt died on September 9 after an active day and after attending a meeting at the Royal Swedish Academy of Sciences.

Viktor Mutt came to Sweden from Estonia during the Second World War. He was employed as a technician by Professor Erik Jorpes at the Karolinska Institute in 1944. After a few years' work on heparin he was asked by Jorpes to purify secretin for clinical use. To this was later added the purification of cholecystokinin and pancreozymin, which Mutt showed to be two activities of the same peptide. It was painstaking work; each step of purification could take years and each fraction had to be assayed on living cats. As a fellow graduate student in the same department during the 1950s it was with admiration that I followed Mutt's work. It would take him close to 20 years to isolate the pure peptides and to determine their structures. A graduate student of today will hardly accept that it takes 15 years of full-time work to get material for a doctoral thesis, which was the time it took Viktor Mutt. The work could never have been finished without his working capacity, tenacity, and patience.

The success with secretin and cholecystokinin merited for Mutt a chair in Biochemistry at the Karolinska Institute, which he held for two decades, and thereafter he worked as an emeritus. During this period he designed methods to search for new active intestinal peptides, and a large number with important functions were discovered in his laboratory. One of them was galanin. Viktor Mutt was devoted to science. He was always meticulous in his work and scrupulous in his judgments. By his work he laid the foundation for modern neuropeptide research. He received honors but he never liked to be in the limelight. He has always been unobtrusive and humble, and it has sometimes been difficult to imagine that he held the eminent position that he did in the scientific community. He was a great man and a great scientist.

TORVARD C LAURENT
Science Secretary
Wenner-Gren Foundation

Preface

TOMAS HÖKFELT,[a] TAMAS BARTFAI,[b] AND JACQUELINE CRAWLEY[c]

[a]Department of Neuroscience, Karolinska Institutet, S-171 77 Stockholm, Sweden

[b]Department of Neurochemistry and Neurotoxicology, Stockholms Universitet, S-106 91 Stockholm, Sweden

[c]Section on Behavioral Neuropharmacology, National Institute of Mental Health, Bethesda, Maryland 20892-1375, USA

Galanin is a neuropeptide that was discovered in 1983 by Professor Viktor Mutt at Karolinska Institutet in Stockholm. Over the last 15 years, major biological actions of galanin have been elucidated by prominent scientists throughout the international biomedical and pharmaceutical research community. Genes for the galanin peptide have been cloned for a wide variety of species, demonstrating a remarkable homology at the NH_2-terminal for this unique neuropeptide. cDNAs have been identified for three distinct galanin receptors in rat and man. Considerable insight has been gained into the anatomic distribution of galanin and its receptor subtypes, regulation of galanin expression, and the amino acids that are critical for galanin binding. Expression of galanin and its receptors is widespread in the mammalian nervous system, including coexistence with several monoamines and with gonadotropin-releasing hormone in sexually dimorphic forebrain nuclei. Dramatic upregulation of galanin mRNA is seen in sensory neurons after neuronal injury, and overexpression of galanin fibers and terminals is prominent in the basal forebrain in Alzheimer's disease. Central administration of galanin in rats induces analgesia, stimulates feeding, impairs learning and memory, stimulates sexual behavior, inhibits neuronal firing rates, and inhibits the release of several neurotransmitters as well as adenylate cyclase activity. Peripheral administration of galanin induces the release of several pituitary hormones, inhibits glucose-stimulated pancreatic insulin release in some species, and modulates smooth muscle contraction and relaxation in the gastrointestinal tract and sphincters.

The present volume is designed to highlight the major findings in the galanin field and their potential clinical applications. These papers represent the proceedings of the *International Symposium on Galanin: Basic Research Discoveries and Therapeutic Implications,* held in Stockholm, Sweden, May 3–5, 1998, as well as several invited contributions not presented at the meeting. This conference focused on the advances in galanin research made since the first symposium on galanin, *Galanin: A New Multifunctional Peptide in the Neuro-endocrine System,* June 14–16, 1990, which was also held at the Wenner-Gren Center in Stockholm and its proceedings published in 1991. Research tools developed since the 1990 meeting, including high affinity peptidergic ligands of galanin receptors, the first nonpeptide ligands selective for galanin receptor subtypes, and a galanin knockout mouse, have further advanced our understanding of the role of endogenous galanin in major physiologic and behavioral functions. Current data suggest that galanin antagonists may contribute to the treatment of Alzheimer's disease and obesity and that a galanin agonist may be useful as an analgesic in the treatment of neuropathic pain.

As conference co-organizers, we are pleased to present this important collection of articles by the premiere galanin researchers. Our appreciation is extended to these outstanding authors for their excellent contributions. We are particularly grateful to Professor Torvard Laurent, Science Secretary of the Wenner-Gren Foundations, for his warm welcome and kind introduction to the conference, and to the Wenner-Gren Foundations, whose generous support promoted the highest quality of presentations and informal discussions at the beautiful venue in Stockholm. We thank Gun Lennerstrand and Karin Lagerman for most efficient and valuable help with the organization and administration of the meeting. We thank Bill Boland and Angela Fink of the New York Academy of Sciences' Editorial Office for their superb work on the publication of this volume in the prestigious *Annals of the New York Academy of Sciences*. Most importantly, we dedicate this book with our warmest gratitude to Viktor Mutt, the father of galanin research.

Transcriptional Control of the Galanin Gene

Tissue-Specific Expression and Induction by NGF, Protein Kinase C, and Estrogen[a]

ÅKE RÖKAEUS,[b,c] KAI JIANG,[b] GIANNIS SPYROU,[d] AND JAMES A. WASCHEK[e]

[b]Department of Medical Biochemistry and Biophysics (MBB), Karolinska Institutet, S-171 77 Stockholm, Sweden

[d]Department of Biosciences, Center for Biotechnology, Karolinska Institutet, NOVUM, S-141 57 Huddinge, Sweden

[e]Department of Psychiatry, Neurobiochemistry Research Group, Mental Retardation Research Center, University of California, Los Angeles, California 90024-1759, USA

ABSTRACT: Galanin is a neuropeptide widely expressed in the central and peripheral nervous system where it acts as a neurotransmitter/neuromodulator and possibly an immunoregulator and growth factor. Galanin gene expression is highly regulated during development and by certain hormones and injury situations. We have examined transcriptional control mechanisms for this gene using chimeric bovine galanin/luciferase reporter genes. These were analyzed in cultured cells and in transgenic mice. The studies reveal that enhancer and silencer sequences are involved in conferring cell- and tissue-specific expression, and that specific elements close to the promoter are responsible for nerve growth factor and protein kinase C induction. So far, the studies have not revealed sequences on the bovine gene that mediate the action of estrogen.

Galanin (GAL)[1] is a 29/30 amino acid residue neuroendocrine peptide that is present in specific neuronal systems in the brain and spinal cord. It is also found in neurons and neuroendocrine cells in a variety of peripheral tissues, including the gastrointestinal tract, pancreas, adrenal gland, and urogenital tract (for a review, see refs. 2 and 3). GAL has been implicated in diseases such as diabetes (for a review, see refs. 3 and 4) and dementia of the Alzheimer's type (for a review, see ref. 5). In addition, GAL potently induces plasma growth hormone and prolactin levels, plays a role in nociception, regulates gastrointestinal motility,[2,6,7] and influences food intake.[8,9]

To accomplish these diverse biologic functions on demand, GAL gene expression (peptide and/or mRNA) is highly plastic. It is dramatically upregulated in the rat anterior pituitary by estrogen,[10,11] in the rat basal forebrain by nerve growth factor (NGF),[12] in the adrenal medulla by sympathetic activation,[13] and in the dorsal root and trigeminal ganglia following denervation and injury[14–16] as well as following herpes simplex virus 1 infection.[17,18] The expression of GAL is upregulated by several factors in cultured cells. For

[a]Åke Rökaeus and Giannis Spyrou as well as this study were supported by grants from The Swedish Medical Research Council (Project No: 7906 and 8997 to Å.R. and project No. 10370 to G.S.), Magnus Bergvall's Foundation, Karolinska Institutet, Novo Nordisk Foundation, and ASTRA Pharmaceutical. This work was also supported by National Institutes of Health Grants HD04612 and HD06576, the nonprofit group SHARE, Inc., and the American Paralysis Association.

[c]To whom correspondence should be addressed. Phone, SWE-46-8-728 6993; fax, SWE-46-8-319497; e-mail, Ake.Rokaeus@mbb.ki.se

example, GAL expression is increased by NGF in rat pheochromocytoma (PC12) cells and phorbol 12-myristate-13-acetate (PMA) in both primary cultures of bovine adrenal chromaffin cells and neural crest-derived human neuroblastoma (SK-N-SH subclone SH-SY5Y) cells.[19,20] Induction by PMA suggests that a signaling pathway involving protein kinase C (PKC) may be involved in GAL gene regulation.[19-21]

In view of the foregoing data and the possible physiologic and pathophysiologic implications of GAL, we thought it of great interest to obtain information on the processes governing GAL gene regulation and mRNA processing. Hence, the partial organization and sequence of the bovine GAL gene were determined, that is, the promoter region and the first three exons and introns.[20,21] Our further analysis[20] of the bovine GAL promoter in human neuroblastoma SH-SY5Y cells demonstrated that 0.1 kb of the promoter conferred high basal expression and that apparent silencer-like elements (up to 16-fold repression[20]) were located further upstream between 5 and 0.1 kb from the transcriptional start site.

During the last 4–5 years we have tried to elucidate mechanisms whereby PMA, NGF, and estrogen regulate GAL expression and the mechanisms responsible for tissue-specific GAL expression. In this paper, our findings during these years are presented and discussed.

PHORBOL ESTER RESPONSE ELEMENT

The bovine GAL gene promoter contains several consensus-binding-sequences that typically mediate phorbol ester (PMA) induction and other responses (FIG. 1A). Thus, plasmids containing different lengths of the bovine GAL promoter fused to luciferase (FIG. 1B) were transfected into human neuroblastoma SH-SY5Y cells, and the induction of expression was determined. In initial studies, none of our GAL constructs, which contained up to 5 kb and 131 bp of the promoter and the first exon, could clearly be *trans*activated by PMA.[20] This suggested to us that such a PMA-responsive element(s) may reside elsewhere on the GAL gene or may not have been clearly revealed in the SH-SY5Y cells under the conditions used. However, when we used a modified transfection protocol compared with our previous study, that is, letting the cells recover for 48 hours (instead of 24 hours) after plating before they were transfected, a PMA-responsive element could indeed be identified (FIG. 2). This was located in the promoter region –68 to –46 bp.[22] This is in agreement with findings by Anouar and coworker[21] who analyzed this region in bovine chromaffin cells. Moreover, when we performed cotransfection experiments with plasmids expressing cJun and cFos (AP1), we found that the Fos/Jun combination could transactivate bovine promoters containing these sequences in the absence of PMA, although PMA caused further induction (FIG. 3). Similar inductions, albeit approximately threefold higher, were obtained with a control plasmid PK3-tk-CAT that contained three consensus binding elements for AP1 in front of a thymidine kinase promoter driving the expression of the enzyme chloramphenicol acetyltransferase. Electrical mobility shift assays (EMSAs), using a ^{32}P-labeled double-stranded oligonucleotide corresponding to the promoter between –66 and –44 bp, revealed that a highly conserved (FIG. 4; human, mice, and rat[23-25]) cyclic AMP response element (CRE)-like sequence (TGACGCGG; –59 to – 52 bp) bound PMA-inducible nuclear proteins present in SH-SY5Y cells in two complexes (FIG. 5). Immunologic characterization of these proteins and competition experiments revealed that these complexes appear to consist mainly of CRE-binding-protein/ activating-transcription-factor (CREB/ATF) and Jun/ATF heterodimers. In addition, an apparent PMA-inducible protein(s) not recognized by CREB/ATF and Jun antibodies also bound to the CRE-like containing probe.[22] Further experiments are needed to determine whether or not PKC activation in SH-SY5Y cells also involves Fos and Jun heterodimerization as it does in some cells.

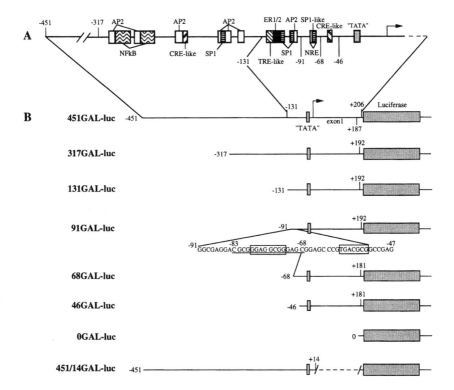

FIGURE 1. Schematic drawing of **(A)** the bovine GAL promoter and the localization of consensus binding sites for *trans*activating proteins. **(B)** Schematic drawing of the different chimeric bovine GAL promoter-luciferase (luc) constructs used in this study for which the exact sizes are known: 451GAL-luc, 131GAL-luc, 91GAL-luc, 68GAL-luc, and 46GAL-luc as well as an exon deletion-construct, 451/14GAL-luc. Numbers in the figure indicate base pairs (bp) in the promoter upstream from the transcriptional start site or downstream thereof; the first exon extends from the transcriptional start site down to +187 bp.[20] The naming of all these constructs followed the principle of putting the size of the 5'-end in front of GAL-luc except, for example, 451GAL-luc (*top construct*). In naming the deletion construct 451/14GAL-luc (*bottom*), we also wanted to indicate the presence of the remaining 14-bp portion of exon 1 in this construct. The promoterless pXP2-luc reporter plasmid is marked "0". The approximate location of the "TATA-box" is also indicated in all constructs. The two boxed nucleotide sequences shown under 91GAL-luc are completely conserved in the bovine, human, mouse, and rat GAL promoters,[20,23–25] and an NGF response element (NRE) functionally identified is underlined. In addition, two other constructs for which only the approximate sizes of the 5'-ends are known (5 and 0.9 kb)[20] were also used in these studies, but are not shown.

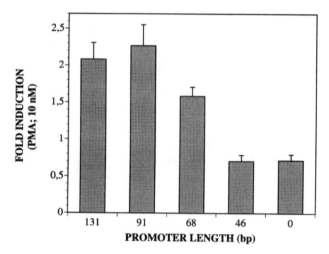

FIGURE 2. Mapping of a phorbol ester (PMA) region within the GAL promoter using human neuroblastoma (SK-N-SH-SY5Y) cells. Luciferase activity (fold induction corrected for transfection efficiency using β-galactosidase; mean ± SD) after treatment with PMA (10 nM) for 18 hours versus promoter length using a subset of the constructs indicated in FIGURE 1B. Data and methods of transfection were previously described by Jiang and coworkers.[22]

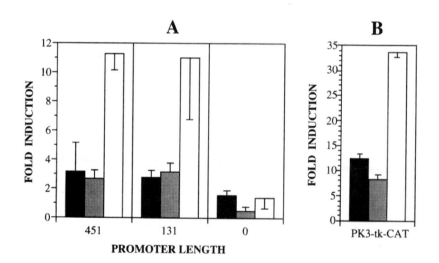

FIGURE 3. Mapping of an AP1-responsive region within the GAL promoter using human neuroblastoma (SK-N-SH-SY5Y) cells. **(A)** Luciferase activity (fold induction corrected for transfection efficiency using β-galactosidase; mean ± SD) obtained after (a) cotransfection with plasmids expressing AP1 proteins (cJun/cFos; *bold bars*), (b) treatment with PMA (10 nM; *hatched bars*), or (c) a combination of the two procedures (*open bars*) for 18 hours. There were three independent experiments, and each experiment was performed in triplicate or duplicate. **(B)** Corrected chloramphenicol acetyltransferase (CAT) reporter activity (fold induction; mean ± SD) for the PK3-tk-CAT-promoter plasmid (control) from one representative experiment. Graph modified from ref. 22.

```
                            NRE                    CRE-like
          -91        -83            -68      -59    -52       -46
Bovine: GGC GAGGA CGCGGGAGGCGGGAGC GGAGCCCG TGACGCGG CCGAG CGGCT
Human:  GGC GAGGG TGCAGGAGGCGGGCGC TGAGCCGG TGACGCGA CTCCG GGCGG
Mouse:  TTG GGACT CGCAGGAGGCGG-CGC TGAGCCGG TGACGCGG CAGCT CCCAC
Rat:    TTG GGACT CGCAGGAGGCGG-CGC TGAGCGGG TGACGCGG CAGCT CCCAC

SP1-consensus:        GAGGCGGGAC
```

FIGURE 4. Comparison of the bovine,[20] human,[23] mouse,[24] and rat[25] GAL nucleotide sequences in the promoter region to which functional NGF and PMA responses were mapped in these studies. *Bold characters* indicate a species-conserved NGF response element (NRE) with a completely conserved SP1-like 8 bp core and a species conserved (in 7 out of 8 bp) cAMP response element (CRE)-like element. *Underlined* are nucleotides in the human, mouse, and rat GAL promoters that are different from the bovine sequence. For comparison an SP1-consensus sequence is also indicated.[29]

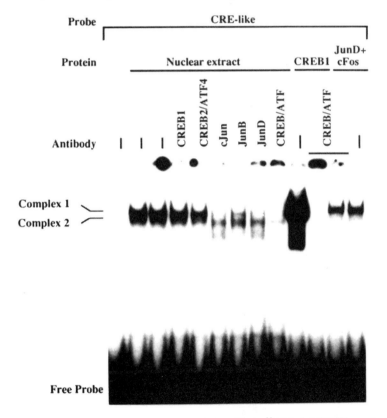

FIGURE 5. Identification of protein-forming complexes with the ^{32}P-labeled CRE-like probe. Electrical mobility shift assay was performed using human neuroblastoma (SK-N-SH-SY5Y) nuclear extracts prepared after treatment with 10 nM PMA for 18 hours. Equal amounts of nuclear extracts (4 μg), recombinantly produced CREB1 (0.2μg), and *in vitro* translated JunD/cFos (2 μl) were incubated with ^{32}P-labeled CRE-like probe. Proteins were immunologically identified by the disrupted binding in the complexes using antibodies (4–10 μl) specifically recognizing cJun, JunB, and JunD, CREB1 and CREB2/ATF4 as well as a general CREB/ATF antibody recognizing all tested members in the CREB/ATF families. Figure adapted from ref. 22.

NERVE GROWTH FACTOR RESPONSE ELEMENT

As just discussed, GAL expression is elevated by PMA treatment, suggesting that PKC activation could be involved in signaling cascades that regulate GAL expression.[19–22] Nerve growth factor (NGF) in some cases activates PKC and several immediate early genes such as cJun, JunB, and cFos.[26,27] NGF was recently shown to elevate GAL mRNA in the rat basal forebrain.[12] The latter might have relevance to elevation of the GAL expression observed in the basal forebrain of Alzheimer's patients (for a review, see ref. 5). It was therefore of interest to see if NGF could *trans*activate the bovine GAL gene. Rat pheochromocytoma PC12 cells were selected to study this because NGF had been suggested to increase levels of GAL mRNA in these cells,[28] similar to the *in vivo* findings.[12] Plasmids containing different lengths of the bovine GAL promoter fused to luciferase (FIG. 1B) were transiently transfected into this cell line. Cells were treated with NGF (10 ng/ml) for 16 hours. Using this protocol, we identified an NGF-responsive region in the GAL promoter between 91 and 68 bp upstream of the transcriptional start site (manuscript in preparation). EMSAs revealed that PC12 nuclear extracts cells contain NGF-inducible factors that bind to a deoxyoligonucleotide that corresponds to a sequence (−83 to −68 bp; denoted NGF-response element [NRE]) (FIG. 4) conserved in the GAL promoter of several species. This includes an 8-bp completely conserved core (GGAGGCGG) with similarities to an SP1-consensus element (GAGGCGGGAC[29]). Two complexes were routinely formed with this deoxyoligonucleotide. PC12 nuclear extracts also bound to a second deoxyoligonucleotide corresponding to sequences −66 to −43 bp. This contained the CRE-like element and also mediated the PMA response in SH-SY5Y cells (see above). Three apparent complexes were routinely formed with this deoxyoligonucleotide. The middle-shifted complex contained more then 80% of the total bound deoxyoligonucleotide. Protein binding to either or both elements may mediate the functional NGF response. We propose that the NGF-responsive elements identified here in PC12 cells might also mediate the NGF-induced increase in GAL expression observed in the rat basal forebrain *in vivo*.[12]

BASAL REGULATION

Identification of a Promoter Region of Importance for Apparent Maximal Basal Activity

We found earlier that 131 bp of the bovine GAL promoter is sufficient for high basal activity in SH-SY5Y cells.[20] To more precisely specify the promoter region of importance for basal GAL gene expression, a set of plasmids (FIG. 1B) containing different lengths of the GAL promoter with the first exon were transfected into the human SH-SY5Y and rat PC12 cell lines. In doing so, we could functionally identify apparent regulatory regions (TABLE 1) in the GAL promoter and/or exon 1. Two regions of importance were localized to gene segments between −91 and −69 bp and between −68 and −47 bp. Noteworthy, this is in agreement with the localization of the NGF- and PMA-responsive regions, respectively (see above). The latter region contains the TATA-box, that is, the primary binding element for the general basal transcription machinery. Thus, it appears that NGF and PMA confer their action on the same GAL promoter sequences that are used to control basal expression.

TABLE 1. Basal Luciferase Activity in Human Neuroblastoma (SK-N-SH-SY5Y) Cells and Rat Pheocromocytoma (PC12) Cells Transfected with a Set of Chimeric Galanin/Luciferase Plasmids.[a]

	Basal Activity (arbitrary units)	
	SH-SY5Y Cells	PC12 Cells
Galanin/luciferase		
131	459 ± 90	1,079 ± 418
91	345 ± 192	1,239 ± 425
68	179 ± 91	392 ± 122
46	14 ± 14	321 ± 310
Control		
0 (promoterless parent; pXP2)	2.4 ± 1.4	2.6 ± 1.5

[a]Basal luciferase activity (arbitrary units) for the various bovine GAL-promoter plasmids corrected for transfection efficiency using β-galactosidase activity. Numbers for the various promoters indicate base pairs upstream from the transcriptional start site. Data represent mean ± SD for 4–6 independent experiments performed in duplicate or triplicate using at least two batches of plasmids for each construct. Basal data in SH-SY5Y cells are obtained from ref. 22.

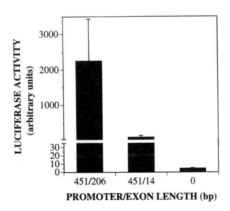

FIGURE 6. Identification of a GAL gene region in the first exon of importance for maximal basal activity in human neuroblastoma (SK-N-SH-SY5Y) cells. Basal luciferase activities (arbitrary units corrected for transfection efficiency using β-galactosidase activity; mean ± SD) after 18 hours of transgene expression versus promoter/exon length using a limited set of the constructs indicated in FIGURE 1B are illustrated. The exon-deleted construct 451/14 GAL-luc as well as two control plasmids, 451/206GAL-luc and 0GAL-luc, were used in these experiments. There were two independent experiments, and each was performed in triplicate or duplicate.

Functional Identification of a Region in Exon 1 of the
Bovine GAL Gene Important for Basal Activity

To further delineate important elements for basal GAL expression we separately explored the role of exon 1. To do this, we removed almost the entire first exon from the 451GAL-luc construct, using the restriction enzyme TaqI. This reduced the size of the exon from 206 to 14 bp (the new construct was denoted 451/14GAL-luc; FIG. 1B). The activity of this construct was significantly reduced from that of the 451GAL-luc (FIG. 6), that is, from >2,000 to <100 (arbitrary units), and in fact the activity was also significantly lower than that observed with the 46GAL-luc construct, which harbored mainly the TATA-box and exon 1 (data not shown). This suggests that elements in the first exon may also be of importance for controlling basal expression.

TISSUE-SPECIFIC ENHANCERS AND SILENCERS

Identification of an Apparent Tissue-Specific Silencer in the Upstream Promoter Region

As previously mentioned, we earlier found that basal GAL-promoter driven luciferase activity in the human SH-SY5Y cells was reduced $\geq$16-fold when the promoter length was increased from 451 bp to 5 kb, suggesting the presence of one or more upstream silencers.[20] We have recently explored these findings further and found that similar repression was observed when the corresponding constructs were transfected into PC12 and JEG-3 human choriocarcinoma cells (FIG. 7). In preliminary experiments, the latter was also found to

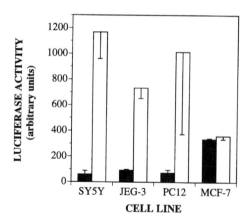

FIGURE 7. Identification of one or more apparent cell-specific silencers in the upstream region of the bovine GAL promoter functional in human neuroblastoma (SK-N-SH-SY5Y) cells, human choriocarcinoma (JEG-3) cells, rat pheochromocytoma (PC12) cells, but not in human breast cancer (MCF-7) cells. Basal luciferase activities (arbitrary units corrected for transfection effecency using β-galactosidase activity; mean $\pm$ SEM) after 18 hours of transgene expression versus promoter length are illustrated. The number of independent experiments was one to four, and each was performed in triplicate or duplicate. The maximal length 5-kb promoter construct, the minimal 131-bp promoter construct (131GAl-luc), and the promoterless plasmid pXP2 plasmid (0) were tested.

endogenously express GAL. However, the apparent silencer element/s was found to be inactive in the human breast (MCF-7) cell line. This suggests that one or more repressor elements indeed are present in the upstream GAL promoter region and that these elements act in an apparent tissue-specific manner.

Transgenic Animals

To test whether or not apparent silencer and other regulator regions identified in the different cell culture systems were also functional *in vivo*, we created several lines of transgenic mouse harboring 5 kb or 131 bp of the GAL promoter (including the first exon) fused to the luciferase reporter (FIG. 1B). Our analysis of these animals[30] revealed that these and/or other silencers appear to function *in vivo* in tissues such as heart, kidney, and liver and in certain regions of the CNS such as the cerebellum. However, the 5-kb fragment appeared to contain enhancer activity that functioned in other regions (for example, hypothalamus) of the CNS. Thus, we concluded that 5 kb of flanking sequence contains elements that mediate basal transcriptional activity in certain parts of the CNS, but also contains sequences that restrict expression in many tissues. However, because the larger transgene was expressed at very low levels in some peripheral sites of high endogenous GAL expression such as the intestine, it was concluded that sequences on the 5-kb transgene are not sufficient for direct expression to all peripheral tissues in mice.

ESTROGEN

Neuropeptides act within the pituitary as autocrine or paracrine factors modulating the synthesis and release of pituitary hormones. Manipulation of the endocrine status of rats using estrogen produces dramatic long-term changes in the pituitary expression of GAL.[10,11] A preliminary report indicated that an estrogen-responsive element (ERE) is present in the rat GAL promoter within 1.8 kb of the transcriptional start site.[31] A half ERE is present in the bovine GAL promoter between 104 and 100 bp upstream from the transcriptional start site.[20] Half EREs in the correct promoter context and/or several half EREs are reported to be sufficient to mediate cell-specific estrogen responsiveness.[32,33] Thus, to determine if this half ERE and/or other EREs not yet identified in the bovine GAL promoter could mediate an estrogen response, we transiently transfected our chimeric GAL promoter-luc constructs into the estrogen receptor (ER) expressing human MCF-7 cell line. A control luc-plasmid carrying an ERE under the control of a thymidine kinase (tk) promoter (ERE-tk-luc) was also transfected into these cells. The latter plasmid responded with a roughly 80-fold induction of reporter activity following estrogen treatment (100 nM for 40 hours), whereas all GAL-luc constructs up to 5 kb did not show any response (FIG. 8). This may indicate that species-specific regulatory features are present in the GAL gene or that the relevant elements are located elsewhere on the bovine GAL gene. Alternatively, an ER may need additional factors to bind tightly to the ERE in the GAL promoter, and such factors might only present in tissues such as the anterior pituitary,[10,11] hypothalamus,[34] and uterus.[35] These are the main tissues in the rat where the GAL gene was demonstrated to be activated by estrogen.

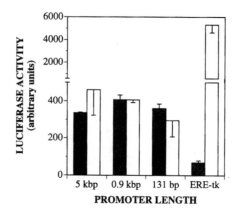

FIGURE 8. Comparison of basal and estrogen-induced transgene activity in human breast cancer (MCF-7) cells using a set of different bovine GAL promoter-luciferase constructs (FIG. 1B) and a control thymidine kinase (tk)-luciferase construct harboring an estrogen-responsive element (ERE). Luciferase activity (arbitrary units corrected for transfection efficiency using β-galactosidase activity; mean ± SEM) after control (*filled bars*) and estrogen treatment (100 nM, 40 hours; *open bars*). Plasmids containing different GAL promoter length are illustrated together with the positive control plasmid ERE-tk-luc. The number of independent experiments was two, and each experiment was performed in triplicate or duplicate.

To test the latter hypothesis, we transiently transfected the GH_12C_1 (mainly growth hormone expressing; data not shown) and GH_3 (equally growth hormone and prolactin expressing; FIG. 9) rat pituitary tumor cell lines[36] with the 5-kb GAL-luc and 131GAL-luc constructs (FIG. 1B), ERE-tk-luc, and investigated their ability to respond to estrogen. The

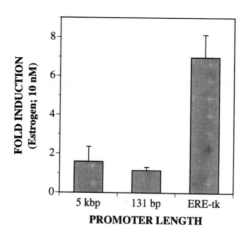

FIGURE 9. Comparison of estrogen-induced transgene activity in rat pituitary (GH_3) cells using a limited set of different bovine GAL promoter-luciferase constructs (FIG. 1B) and a control thymidine kinase (tk)-luciferase construct harboring an estrogen-responsive element (ERE). Luciferase activities (fold induction; mean ± SEM) after estrogen (10 nM) treatment for 48–72 hours of transgene expression versus promoter length are illustrated. The number of independent experiments was ≥4, and each experiment was performed in triplicate or duplicate.

control plasmid ERE-tk-luc, but none of the GAL constructs responded to estrogen treatment despite the use of phenol-free medium containing charcoal-stripped serum as well as extended estrogen (10 nM for 48–72 hours) treatment periods. These latter findings may indicate that the bovine GAL gene does not respond to estrogen. Species differences on the gene or in transcription proteins may be relevant, because a lack of estrogen-induced increase in GAL expression was reported in the mice pituitary *in vivo.*[37] However, it is also possible that a functional ERE in the bovine GAL gene may reside elsewhere on the gene, that is, not present in our chimeric GAL promoter luciferase constructs.

CONCLUSIONS

The present work has specifically demonstrated that the AP1 proteins cJun/cFos as well as the phorbol ester PMA, can *trans*activate the bovine GAL gene in human neuroblastoma SK-N-SH-SY5Y cells. The functional response to PMA was mapped to the GAL promoter region between 68 and 46 bp upstream from the transcriptional start site. Moreover, the studies identified a CRE-like element in the bovine GAL promoter region −59 to −52 bp. Seven of these eight nucleotides are completely conserved in different species including the human GAL promoter. This CRE-like element appears to bind PMA-inducible human proteins mainly in the form of Jun/ATF and CREB/ATF heterodimers and possibly also CREB/CREB and ATF/ATF homodimers. In addition, this CRE-like element may also bind a hitherto unknown PMA-inducible protein(s) present in the human SH-SY5Y cells.

In addition, the studies demonstrated that NGF can induce *trans*activation of the bovine GAL gene in rat adrenal pheochromocytoma-derived PC12 cells. The functional response to NGF was mapped to the GAL promoter region between 91 and 68 bp upstream from the transcriptional start site. This contains a highly species-conserved sequence (−83 to −68 bp CGCGGGAGGCGGGAGC; denoted NGF response element [NRE], with an 8-bp completely conserved core that is similar to an SP1 binding element [GGAGGCGG, between −79 and −72 bp; denoted SP1-like; FIG. 1A]). The NRE appears to bind NGF-inducible proteins in PC12 cells and may hence play a crucial role in the ability of NGF to *trans*activate the bovine GAL gene. In addition, the CRE-like element located between −59 and −52 bp also bound NGF-inducible proteins and may thus also be involved in the NGF *trans*activation of the GAL gene, possibly in a cooperative manner.

Bovine GAL promoter sequences up to −91 bp as well as sequences within the first exon appear to be needed for maximal basal gene expression in both human SH-SY5Y cells and PC12 cells. Because the NGF response element and CRE-like element are also localized in this promoter region, and both of them bind proteins during unstimulated basal conditions, it may be speculated that they are also involved in the regulation of basal GAL expression. In addition, *in vitro* as well as *in vivo* findings in transgenic mice indicate that apparent silencers and enhancers are present in the promoter regions between 5 kb and 131 bp.

In terms of estrogen-induced regulation we suggest that species differences may occur and that the bovine GAL gene may not be responsive to estrogen or that such an element is located elsewhere on the gene not studied by us.

Moreover, the present work has laid the foundation for future studies of GAL gene regulation and for further characterization of GAL gene *cis-* and *trans*acting elements and factors, especially in terms of NGF induction, silencers, and enhancers, but also for identification of the apparently GAL-gene specific CRE-like binding activity.

REFERENCES

1. TATEMOTO, K., Å. RÖKAEUS, H. JÖRNVALL, T.J. McDONALD & V. MUTT. 1983. Galanin, a novel biologically active peptide isolated form porcine intestine. FEBS Lett. **164:** 124–128.
2. RÖKAEUS, Å. 1987. Galanin: A newly isolated biologically active neuropeptide. Trends Neurosci. **10:** 158–164.
3. CRAWLEY, J.N. 1995. Biological actions of galanin. Regul. Pept. **59:** 1–16.
4. DUPRÉ, J. 1988. Galanin: a selective inhibitor of insulin secretion? Pancreas **3:** 119–121.
5. CRAWLEY, J.N. 1996. Minireview. Galanin-acetylcholine interactions: Relevance to memory and Alzheimer's disease. Life Sci. **58:** 2185–2199.
6. RATTAN, S. 1991. Role of galanin in the gut. Gastroenterology **100:** 1762–1768.
7. HÖKFELT, T., X. ZHANG & Z. WIESENFELD-HALLIN. 1994. Messenger plasticity in primary sensory neurons following axotomy and its functional implications. Trends Neurosci. **17:** 22–30.
8. CRAWLEY, J.N., M.C. AUSTIN, S.M. FISKE, B. MARTIN, S. CONSOLO, M. BERTHOLD, U. LANGEL, G. FISONE & T. BARTFAI. 1990. Activity of centrally administered galanin fragments on stimulation of feeding behavior and on galanin receptor binding in the rat hypothalamus. J. Neurosci. **10:** 3695–3700.
9. SCHICK, R.R., S. SAMSAMI, J.P. ZIMMERMANN, T. EBERL, C. ENDRES, V. SCHUSDZIARRA & M. CLASSEN. 1993. Effect of galanin on food intake in rats: Involvement of lateral and ventromedial hypothalamic sites. Am. J. Physiol. **264:** R355–R361.
10. VRONTAKIS, M.E., L.M. PEDEN, M.C. DUCKWORTH & H.G. FRIESEN. 1987. Isolation and characterization of a complementary DNA (galanin) clone from estrogen induced pituitary tumour messenger RNA. J. Biol. Chem. **35:** 16755–16757.
11. KAPLAN, L.M., S.M. GABRIEL, J.I. KOENIG, M.E. SUNDAY, E.R. SPINDEL, J.B. MARTIN & W.W. CHIN. 1988. Galanin is an estrogen-inducible, secretory product of the rat anterior pituitary. Proc. Natl. Acad. Sci. USA **85:** 7408–7412.
12. PLANAS, B., P.E. KOLB, M.A. RASKIND & M.A. MILLER. 1997. Nerve growth factor induces galanin gene expression in the rat basal forebrain: Implications for the treatment of cholinergic dysfunction. J. Comp. Neurol. **379:** 563–570.
13. PELTO-HUIKKO, M. & M. SCHALLING. 1990. Rapid changes in peptide and enzyme mRNA levels in rat adrenal gland following capsaicin treatment. *In* In situ hybridization studies on regulatory molecules in neural and endocrine tissues with special reference to expression of coexisting peptides. Ph.D. thesis by M. Schalling, Karolinska Institutet, Stockholm, Sweden.
14. HÖKFELT, T., Z. WIESENFELD-HALLIN, M. VILLAR & T. MELANDER. 1987. Increase of galanin-like immunoreactivity in rat dorsal root ganglion cells after peripheral axotomy. Neurosci. Lett. **83:** 217–220.
15. MEISTER, B., M.J. VILLAR, S. CECCATELLI & T. HÖKFELT. 1990. Localization of chemical messengers in magnocellular neurons of the hypothalamic supraoptic and paraventricular nuclei: An immunohistochemical study using experimental manipulations. Neuroscience **37:** 603–633.
16. KASHIBA, H., E. SENBA, Y. UEDA & M. TOHYAMA. 1992. Co-localized but target-unrelated expression of vasoactive intestinal polypeptide and galanin in rat dorsal root ganglion neurons after peripheral nerve crush injury. Brain Res. **582:** 47–57.
17. HENKEN, D.B. & J.R. MARTIN. 1991. Effects of herpes simplex virus (HSV) infection on the neuropeptides calcitonin gene-related peptide (CGRP) and galanin (GAL) in mouse dorsal root ganglia (DRG) [abstr. 165.2]. Soc. Neurosci. **17:** 397.
18. HENKEN, D.B. & J.R. MARTIN. 1992. The proportion of galanin-immunoreactive neurons in mouse trigeminal ganglia is transiently increased following corneal inoculation of herpes simplex virus type-1. Neurosci. Lett. **140:** 177–180.

19. Rökaeus, Å., R.M. Pruss & L.E. Eiden. 1990. Galanin gene expression in chromaffin cells is controlled by calcium and protein kinase signaling pathways. Endocrinology 127: 3096–3102.

20. Rökaeus, Å. & J.A. Waschek. 1994. Primary sequence and functional analysis of the bovine galanin gene promoter in human neuroblastoma cells. DNA Cell Biol. 13: 845–855.

21. Anouar, Y., L. MacArthur, J. Cohen, A.L. Iacangelo & L.E. Eiden. 1994. Identification of a TPA-responsive element mediating preferential transactivation of the galanin gene promoter in chromaffin cells. J. Biol. Chem. 269: 6823–6831.

22. Jiang, K., G. Spyrou & Å. Rökaeus. 1998. Phorbolester and AP1 induces transcriptional activation of the galanin gene in human neuroblastoma cells. Biochem. Biophys. Res. Commun. 246: 192–198.

23. Kofler, B., H.F. Evans, M.L. Liu, V. Falls, T.P. Iismaa, J. Shine & H. Herzog. 1995. Characterization of the 5′-flanking region of the human preprogalanin gene. DNA Cell Biol. 14: 321–329.

24. Kofler, B., M.L. Liu, A.S. Jacoby, J. Shine & T.P. Iismaa. 1996. Molecular cloning and characterisation of the mouse preprogalanin gene. Gene 182: 71–75.

25. Corness, J.D., J.P. Burbach & T. Hökfelt. 1997. The rat galanin-gene promoter: Response to members of the nuclear hormone receptor family, phorbol ester and forskolin. Mol. Brain Res. 47: 11–23.

26. Cavalié, A., B. Berninger, C.A. Haas, D.E. Garc'a, D. Lindholm & H.D. Lux. 1994. Constitutive upregulation of calcium channel currents in rat phaeochromocytoma cells: Role of *c-fos* and *c-jun*. J. Physiol. 479.1: 11–27.

27. Luc, P.V. & J.A. Wagner. 1997. Regulation of the neural-specific gene VGF in PC12 cells. Identification of transcription factors interacting with NGF-responsive elements. J. Mol. Neurosci. 8: 223–241.

28. Kaplan, L.M., S.C. Hooi, D.R. Abraczinskas, R.M. Strauss, M.B. Davidson, D.W. Hsu & J.I. Koenig. 1991. Neuroendocrine regulation of galanin gene expression. *In* Galanin: A New Multifunctional Peptide in the Neuroendocrine System. T. Hökfelt, T. Bartfai, D. Jacobowitz & D. Ottoson, Eds. Wenner-Gren Center International Symposium Series. 58: 43–65. The Macmillan Press Ltd. New York.

29. Briggs, M.R., J.T. Kadonaga, S.P. Bell & R. Tjian. 1986. Purification and biochemical characterization of the promoter-specific transcription factor, Sp1. Science 234: 47–52.

30. Rökaeus, Å. & J.A. Washek. 1998. Tissue-specific enhancement and restriction of galanin gene expression in transgenic mice by 5′ flanking sequences. Mol. Brain Res. In press.

31. Kaplan, L.M., D. Abraczinskas, M. Davidson & W.W. Chin. 1989. Estrogen regulation of rat galanin transcription is mediated by sequences in the 5′-flanking region of the galanin gene [abstr. 261.9]. Soc. Neurosci. 15: 646.

32. Tora, L., M.-P. Gaub, S. Mader, A. Dierich, M. Bellard & P. Chambon. 1988. Cell-specific activity of GGTCA half-palindromic oestrogen-responsive element in the chicken ovalbumin gene promoter. EMBO J. 7: 3771–3778.

33. Nardulli, A.M., L.E. Romine, C. Carpo, G.L. Greene & B. Rainish. 1996. Estrogen receptor affinity and location of consensus and imperfect estrogen response elements influence transcriptional activation of simplified promoters. Mol. Endocrinol. 10: 694–704.

34. Levin, M.C. & P.E. Sawchenko. 1993. Neuropeptide co-expression in the magnocellular neurosecretory system of the female rat: Evidence for differential modulation by estrogen. Neuroscience 54: 1001–1018.

35. Vrontakis, M., I. Schroedter, V. Leite & H.G. Friesen. 1993. Estrogen regulation and localization of galanin gene expression in the rat uterus. Biol. Reprod. 49: 1245–1250.

36. Tashjian, A.H.J., F.C. Bancroft & L. Levine. 1970. Production of both prolactin and growth hormone by clonal strains of rat pituitary tumor cells: Differential effects of hydrocortisone and tissue extracts. J. Cell Biol. 47: 61–70.

37. Lundkvist, J., T. Land, U. Kahl, K. Bedecs & T. Bartfai. 1995. cDNA sequence, ligand biding, and regulation of galanin/GMAP in mouse brain. Neurosci. Lett. 200: 121–124.

Analysis of Selected Regulatory Pathways for Rat Galanin Gene Transcription and Their Suitability As Putative Models for Negative Regulation by NGF[a]

JACQUELINE CORNESS[b] AND TOMAS HÖKFELT

Department of Neuroscience, Karolinska Institutet, 171 77 Stockholm, Sweden

ABSTRACT: Nerve growth factor (NGF) is known to negatively regulate the transcription of the rat galanin gene both *in vivo* and *in vitro* in dorsal root ganglion neurons, yet it is unclear how this regulation actually occurs. We propose here several possible pathways whereby NGF could interact to exert negative control on galanin regulation. These include: (1) repression of AP1-mediated transcription, (2) repression of nuclear binding protein-mediated transcription, and (3) repression of cytokine-mediated transcription. Although not enough data are available for speculation on which, if any, of these pathways is most relevant for NGF repression of galanin transcription, the mechanisms we describe can provide putative models for regulatory pathways. From here we can carry out further experiments that may help to elucidate the possible mechanisms of NGF repression *in vivo*.

Axotomy has a complex effect on the expression of neuronal genes, resulting in differential changes in the levels of proteins involved in structure and regeneration.[1–3] In the dorsal root ganglion (DRG), axotomy of the sciatic nerve leads to downregulation of expression for peptides, such as CGRP, and substance P,[4–8] whereas other neuropeptides, specifically galanin, neuropeptide (NPY) and vasoactive intestinal peptide (VIP) are simultaneously upregulated.[5,8–13]

Although the effects of axotomy in primary sensory neurons were extensively described at a histochemical level, the nature of the molecular interactions taking place inside an axotomized neuron is still far from understood. It is believed that the axotomy-induced changes may be due, at least in part, to altered availability of growth factors in the neuronal cell bodies. Indeed, it has been possible to essentially mimic the physiologic state of axotomy by using colchicine[14] or vinblastine treatment[15] as a model of axonal transport blockade. In addition, cultured sensory neurons deprived of growth factors show a similar peptide regulation profile to that of an axotomized neuron, an effect that, for some peptides, has been reversible through the addition of nerve growth factor (NGF).[16–19] As an example of galanin regulation by NGF in culture, Kerekes *et al.*[20] demonstrated that the number of galanin-immunoreactive neurons can be reduced by 30% after 3 days of 100 ng/ml NGF treatment of adult primary DRG cultures. Attempts have also been made to alleviate the axotomy-induced changes within the *in vivo* system through replacement of

[a]This work was supported by grants from the Swedish Medical Research Council (04X-2887, 14XC-11976), the European Commission (BMH4-CT95-0172), Astra Pain Control AB, and Marianne och Marcus Wallenbergs Stiftelse.

[b]Author to whom correspondence should be addressed. Phone, +(468) 728-7060; fax, +(468) 331692; e-mail, Jacquie.Corness@neuro.ki.se

14

NGF. *In situ* hybridization has been used by Verge *et al.*[21] to demonstrate a reverse of the axotomy-induced peptide upregulation in DRGs by NGF. In this experiment it was shown that the number of galanin-positive neurons seen in DRG sections 2 weeks after axotomy can be reduced to 50% by intrathecal administration of NGF for 7 days. Availability of growth factor, specifically NGF, may consequently be at least partially involved in affecting the changes that occur in this state.

The transcription factor c-Jun is also upregulated in the DRG neurons after axotomy,[22] and it has been found that this regulation correlates with that of galanin. Indeed, 85% of all galanin-positive neurons after axotomy show upregulation of c-Jun immunoreactivity.[23] Gold *et al.*[24] reported that c-Jun could be both upregulated in DRGs by injections of NGF antiserum into the hindlimb as well as subsequently downregulated after axotomy by intrathecal NGF infusion. In JEG-3 cells, the rat galanin promoter responded positively to 12-*O*-tetradecanoyl phorbol-13-acetate (TPA) treatment, a potent stimulator of AP1 proteins.[25] The bovine galanin gene, as well, can be upregulated by phorbol esters *in vitro*.[26,27] This suggests that the interaction of c-Jun with the galanin promoter might be one possible mechanism by which the peptide's expression is regulated via NGF. To test this possibility we looked at the interaction of whole cell DRG proteins with parts of the galanin promoter and compared these interactions with those seen on a consensus AP1 site.[28] In addition, we tested the effects of axotomy on the binding of AP1 proteins to assess how NGF replacement can affect the degree of protein-DNA binding.

Work in our laboratory with a cloned section of the rat galanin gene promoter has included studies on galanin regulation by steroid hormones. Our results show a strong positive regulatory effect of ELP1 on this galanin regulation.[25] We suggest here a role for NGF in the modulation of nuclear orphan receptor control of galanin transcription, possibly through negative interaction of the NGF-inducible factor NGFI-B (otherwise known as nur77) with positive regulatory elements.

Lastly, we described recent results involving the regulation of galanin mRNA in embryonic DRG cultures by a combination of NGF and leukemia inhibitory factor (LIF).[29] We saw that NGF and LIF can interact through an unknown mechanism which results in an apparently inhibitory effect of NGF on LIF-inducible galanin transcription. We suggest that the blocking effects of NGF on LIF-mediated control of galanin transcription provide another possible model to explain the negative regulatory effects of the growth factor on galanin transcription.

AP1-MEDIATED TRANSCRIPTION

Using a cloned fragment of the rat galanin gene to study the control of galanin promoter-driven reporter-gene activity *in vitro* (FIG. 1), we looked at possible sites of action for c-Jun and related proteins on galanin gene transcription. Results from our laboratory and others show that the galanin gene promoter contains a partial AP1-protein consensus sequence that is necessary for the induction of galanin by phorbol esters.[25–27] Indeed Jiang *et al.*[27] showed that cotransfection of a c-jun expression vector along with a galanin promoter-driven reporter gene can confer induction of reporter-gene expression through this site. We looked at the binding of nuclear extracts from JEG-3 cells to a double-stranded probe that matched the sequence for the putative galanin AP1 site and found that the protein c-Fos was able to bind to this element.[30] However, the protein with which this

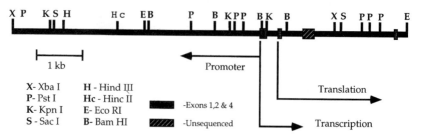

FIGURE 1. The restriction endonuclease map of the rat genomic clone that we used for *in vitro* studies in heterologous cell lines. In addition to the 9 kb of sequence, we obtained an additional fragment containing 3.5 kb of sequence which is distal to the 5′ Xba I site shown here. The subcloned fragments that are available for our studies total 12.5 kb in length, 9 kb of which lies 5′ of the transcriptional start site.

factor presumably dimerizes was not assessed in this study. In light of the studies by Herdegen *et al.*,[23] which suggest a role of c-Jun in galanin regulation within the DRG neurons, we used whole cell extracts of DRG cells and compared the DNA binding of an AP1 consensus sequence to that of the partial galanin AP1 site. Weak binding to the galanin probe was observed at the level of AP1 binding. As expected, the binding of factors to the AP1 consensus sequence was strongly upregulated in extracts taken from 3-day post-axotomy DRG cells. Moreover, the intensity of binding to the AP1 probe was reduced to pre-axotomy levels when NGF was added to the severed end of the axotomized nerve and allowed to be transported to the neuronal cell nuclei during the 3-day axotomy (in preparation).[28] This is in agreement with the results previously published by Gold *et al.*[24] which suggest that NGF can negatively regulate AP1 protein binding in DRG neurons. Although binding at the level of the AP1 proteins on the galanin probe was weak, specific binding to the galanin probe by an as yet unidentified protein was observed, and this binding was also significantly affected by NGF treatment. Thus, there is reason to believe that NGF may exert negative regulatory effects through the partial AP1 site in the proximal promoter region of the galanin gene; however, the identity of the proteins involved has not been established. The NGF-regulated protein c-Jun seems to be the most likely candidate for this action, but this remains to be confirmed.

STEROID HORMONE-MEDIATED TRANSCRIPTION

As previously reported by Corness *et al.*,[25] a strong regulatory effect is seen when 374 bp of the galanin-gene promoter driving a luciferase reporter gene is cotransfected along with an expression vector for the ELP1 orphan receptor. Cotransfection resulted in a 35-fold increase in promoter-driven luciferase expression (FIG. 2). The significance of this result is that the ELP1 receptor can bind to a cis element on the promoter which is identical to the binding site for nur77.[31,32] Kendall *et al.*[33] showed that nur77 is upregulated in DRG neurons after NGF treatment. In addition, it was previously shown by Wu *et al.*[34] that nur77 can interact with other orphan receptors, namely COUP-TF, to interfere with its regulation of gene transcription (see also ref. 35). Although we have not been able to show

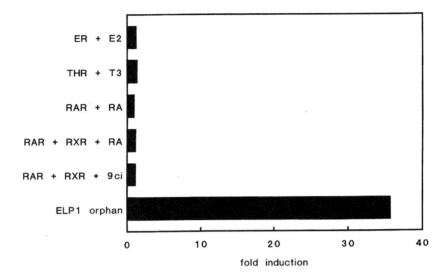

FIGURE 2. Galanin reporter gene construct expression in response to treatment with steroid hormones. The construct rGAL374 (-374 bp) was transiently transfected into Neuro 2A neuroblastoma cells together with one of the following hormone receptors: estrogen (ER), thyroid hormone (THR), or retinoic acid (RAR/RXR), then treated with estrogen, thyroid hormone, retinoic acid, or 9-cis-retinoic acid, respectively. Cotransfection of the orphan receptor ELP1 was also carried out with no subsequent treatment.

any interaction between nur77 and ELP1, we propose that after upregulation of nur77 by NGF in DRGs, it is possible that nur77 could interfere with the positive regulation by ELP1 or other orphan receptors of galanin gene expression.

CYTOKINE-MEDIATED TRANSCRIPTION

It was previously reported by others and by us that LIF knockout mice show a diminished ability to upregulate galanin after peripheral nerve injury[36,37] and that LIF may be able to stimulate galanin expression.[38] We recently looked at the effect of LIF on galanin-gene expression and found that NGF plays an important role in the cytokine response by acting as a repressor of cytokine-mediated transcription.[29] In the presence of 50 ng/ml NGF, LIF treatment was not able to significantly affect galanin expression in 2-week-old DRG cultures taken from E13.5 mouse embryos. Conversely, these results show that NGF deprivation from these neuronally enriched cultures results in an approximately 4.5-fold upregulation of galanin mRNA after either 3 or 4 days of withdrawal. However, we were not able to sustain these samples in an NGF-withdrawal state with the added treatment of an LIF-neutralizing antibody due to the effects of antibody treatment on cell survival (although NGF withdrawal alone did not have any effect on cell survival[39]). We cannot then rule out that this NGF withdrawal response was taking place in the presence of endogenous LIF, which is known to be produced by non-neuronal cells in a mixed DRG culture.[40,41] Furthermore, the NGF withdrawal state was able to provide a favorable condition for additional induction through exogenous LIF treatment. In the absence of NGF, 10 ng/ml of LIF over 3 days stimulated mRNA levels 18-fold over those of controls, which is a 9-fold increase in mRNA levels over those of cultures treated with 10 ng/ml LIF in the presence of NGF (FIG. 3). Results were similar, although not as dramatic, over 2 days, where an 11-fold increase was seen for mRNA levels in the LIF-treated, NGF-deprived samples over NGF-containing controls, and this upregulation corresponded to a fourfold increase over that seen by LIF in the presence of NGF. It therefore seems that 50 ng/ml NGF in the culture media could be acting as a potent inhibitor of the LIF response. By removing this inhibition, as is the case with NGF withdrawal from the culture media, we may allow for basal LIF levels to stimulate galanin gene transcription as well as for excess LIF to have a more pronounced effect than it would alone. This would explain the "synergistic" phenomenon that appears in this experiment between the two factors. It may also explain the previously reported "inhibitory" NGF effects on the postaxotomy upregulation of galanin described by Verge et al.[21] If this hypothesis for the indirect mechanism of NGF action were true, experiments carried out in culture would show an effect of NGF depen-

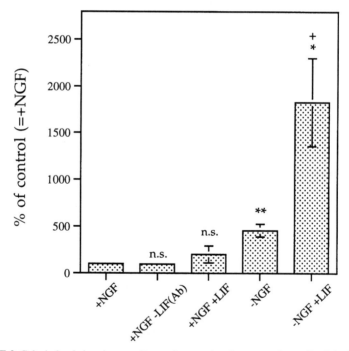

FIGURE 3. Galanin levels in primary cultures of mouse dorsal root ganglion cells. Galanin mRNA was quantified using the Image Quantifier program and corrected for levels of neuron-specific enolase (NSE) in each sample. ($n = 3 \pm 3$ SEM). Treatment conditions were: 50 ng/ml nerve growth factor (NGF), 4 days; 10 ng/ml leukemia inhibitory factor (LIF), 3 days. (*$p \leq 0.05$; **$p \leq 0.01$ in comparison with +NGF treatment. $^{+}p \leq 0.05$ in comparison with –NGF treatment).

dent on the amount of endogenous LIF in the cultures. In addition, the time of NGF application would be important in these models, as the levels of endogenous cytokine are not expected to remain stable after establishing culture conditions. Although we are aware that measurement by RT-PCR is semiquantitative at best, we propose that these differences in cytokine content may provide another explanation for the differences between the effects of NGF in the experiment just described and that carried out by Kerekes et al.,[20] in which NGF is added to adult DRG cultures within 4 hours of plating. To test this theory, it would be useful to measure endogenous LIF levels for each experiment in which NGF effects are being studied and to assess whether the cytokine levels are important in dictating the potency of NGF in each experimental condition. It is possible that NGF levels merely act to alter the efficacy of LIF, which would imply direct and specific interaction. Recent work by Shadiack et al.[42] has also shown interaction between NGF and LIF in vivo in sympathetic ganglia. At this stage it is not possible to determine at what level this interaction might take place, but it is hoped that further studies will help us to understand the mechanisms behind these results.

CONCLUSIONS

In summary, we hypothesize that several different mechanisms exist through which NGF may act indirectly to bring about changes in transcriptional regulation of the galanin gene in DRG neurons. As was already shown in previous work, the role of NGF in this tissue is to downregulate galanin gene transcription; however, it is unclear how inhibition by NGF is mediated. We propose here three different mechanisms that serve only as models and have yet to be substantiated: (1) NGF inhibition of c-Jun may lead to downregulation of a positive AP1-mediated effect on galanin gene transcription; (2) NGF upregulation of nur77 may lead to inhibition of a positive transcriptional regulation by a hormone receptor such as ELP1 or a related orphan receptor; and (3) NGF inhibition of the cytokine response, through an unknown mechanism, may serve to mask the effects of cytokines such as LIF.

ACKNOWLEDGMENTS

We gratefully acknowledge productive collaborations with Doug Fields, Beth Stevens, Peter Burbach, Aviva Symes, and John Quinn.

REFERENCES

1. Wong, J. & M.M. Oblinger. 1987. Changes in neurofilament gene expression occur after axotomy of dorsal root ganglion neurons: An in situ hybridization study. Metab. Brain Dis. **2:** 291–303.
2. Oblinger, M.M. & R.J. Lasek. 1988. Axotomy-induced alterations in the synthesis and transport of neurofilaments and microtubules in dorsal root ganglion cells. J. Neurosci. **8:** 1747–1758.
3. Woolf, C.J., M.L. Reynolds, C. Molander, C. O'Brian, R.M. Lindsay & L.I. Benowitz. 1990. The growth-associated protein GAP-43 appears in dorsal root ganglion cells and in the dorsal horn of the rat spinal cord following peripheral nerve injury. Neuroscience **34:** 465–478.

4. NIELSCH, V., M.A. BISBY & P. KEEN. 1987. Effect of cutting or crushing the rat sciatic nerve on synthesis of substance P by isolated L5 dorsal root ganglia. Neuropeptides 10: 137–145.
5. NIELSCH, V. & P. KEEN. 1989. Reciprocal regulation of tachykinin- and vasoactive intestinal peptide-gene expression in rat sensory neurones following cut and crush injury. Brain Res. 481: 25–30.
6. NOGUCHI, K., E. SENBA, Y. MORITA, M. SATO & M. TOHYAMA. 1990. α-CGRP and β-CGRP mRNAs are differentially regulated in the rat spinal cord and dorsal root ganglion. Mol. Brain Res. 7: 299–304.
7. DUMOULIN, F.L., G. RAIVICH, W.J. STREIT & G.W. KREUTZBERG. 1991. Differential regulation of calcitonin gene-related peptide (CGRP) in regenerating rat facial nucleus and dorsal root ganglion. Eur. J. Neurosci. 3: 338–342.
8. ZHANG, X., G. JU, R. ELDE & T. HÖKFELT. 1993. Effect of peripheral nerve cut on neuropeptides in dorsal root ganglia and the spinal cord of monkey with special reference to galanin. J. Neurocytol. 22: 342–381.
9. SHEHAB, S.A.S. & M.E. ATKINSON. 1986. Vasoactive intestinal polypeptide (VIP) increases in the spinal cord after peripheral axotomy of the sciatic nerve originate from primary afferent neurons. Brain Res. 372: 37–44.
10. HÖKFELT, T., Z. WIESENFELD-HALLIN, M.J. VILLAR & T. MELANDER. 1987. Increase of galanin-like immunoreactivity in the rat dorsal root ganglion cells after peripheral axotomy. Neurosci. Lett. 83: 217–220.
11. NOGUCHI, K., E. SENBA, Y. MORITA, M. SATO & M. TOHYAMA. 1989. Prepro-VIP and preprotachykinin mRNAs in the rat dorsal root ganglion cells following peripheral axotomy. Mol. Brain Res. 6: 327–330.
12. VILLAR, M.J., R. CORTES, E. THEODORSSON, Z. WIESENFELD-HALLIN, M. SCHALLING, J. FAHRENKRUG, P.C. EMSON & T. T. HÖKFELT. 1989. Neuropeptide expression in rat dorsal root ganglion cells and spinal cord after peripheral nerve injury with special reference to galanin. Neuroscience 33: 587–604.
13. WAKISAKA, S., K.C. KAJANDER & G.J. BENNETT. 1991. Increased neuropeptide (NPY)-like immunoreactivity in rat sensory neurons following peripheral axotomy. Neurosci. Lett. 124: 200–203.
14. LEAH, J.D., T. HERDEGEN & R. BRAVO. 1991. Selective expression of Jun proteins following axotomy and axonal transport block in peripheral nerves in the rat: Evidence for a role in the regeneration process. Brain Res. 566: 198–207.
15. KASHIBA, H., E. SENBA, Y. KAWAI, Y. UEDA & M. TOHYAMA. 1992. Axonal blockade induces the expression of vasoactive intestinal polypeptide and galanin in the dorsal root ganglion neurons. Brain Res. 577: 19–28.
16. LINDSAY, R.M. & A.J. HARMAR. 1989. Nerve growth factor regulates expression of neuropeptide genes in adult sensory neurons. Nature 337: 362–364.
17. LINDSAY, R.M., C. LOCKETT, J. STERNBERG & J. WINTER. 1989. Neuropeptide expression in cultures of adult sensory neurons: Modulation of substance P and calcitonin gene-related peptide levels by nerve growth factor. Neuroscience 33: 53–65.
18. MULDERRY, P.K. 1994. Neuropeptide expression by newborn and adult rat sensory neurons in culture: Effects of nerve growth factor and other neurotrophic factors. Neuroscience 59: 673–88.
19. WATSON, A., E. ENSOR, A. SYMES, J. WINTER, G. KENDALL & D. LATCHMAN. 1995. A minimal CGRP gene promoter is inducible by nerve growth factor in adult rat dorsal root ganglion neurons but not in PC12 phaeochromocytoma cells. Eur. J. Neurosci. 7: 394–400.
20 KEREKES, N., M. LANDRY, M. RYDH-RINDER & T. HÖKFELT. 1997. The effect of NGF, BDNF and bFGF on expression of galanin in cultured rat dorsal root ganglia. Brain Res. 754: 131–141.
21 VERGE, V.M.K., P.M. RICHARDSON, Z. WIESENFELD-HALLIN & T. HÖKFELT. 1994. Differential influence of nerve growth factor on neuropeptide expression in vivo: A novel role in peptide suppression in adult sensory neurons. J. Neurosci. 15: 2081–2096.
22. HERDEGEN, T., C.E. FIALLOS-ESTRADA, W. SCHMID, R. BRAVO & M. ZIMMERMANN. 1992. The transcription factors c-JUN, JUN D and CREB, but not FOS and KROX-24, are differentially regulated in axotomized neurons following transection of rat sciatic nerve. Mol. Brain Res. 14: 155–165.

23. HERDEGEN, T., C.E. FIALLOS-ESTRADA, R. BRAVO & M. ZIMMERMAN. 1993. Colocalisation and covariation of c-jun transcription factor with galanin in primary afferent neurons and with CGRP in spinal motoneurons following transection of rat sciatic nerve. Mol. Brain Res. **17:** 147–154.
24. GOLD, B.G., T. STORM-DICKERSON & D.R. AUSTIN. 1993. Regulation of the transcription factor c-JUN by nerve growth factor in adult sensory neurons. Neurosci. Lett. **154:** 129–133.
25. CORNESS, J.D., J.P.H. BURBACH & T. HÖKFELT. 1997. The rat galanin-gene promoter: Response to members of the nuclear hormone receptor family, phorbol ester and forskolin. Mol. Brain Res. **47:** 11–23.
26. ANOUAR, Y., L. MACARTHUR, J. COHEN, A.L. IACANGELO & L.E. EIDEN. 1994. Identification of a TPA-responsive element mediating preferential transactivation of the galanin gene promoter in chromaffin cells. J. Biol. Chem. **269:** 6823–6831.
27. JIANG, K., G. SPYROU & Å. RÖKAEUS. 1998. Characterization of phorbolester-inducible human neuronal factors involved in trans-activation of the galanin gene. Biochem. Biophys. Res. Commun. **246:** 192–198.
28. CORNESS, J.D., T.-J. SHI & T.HÖKFELT 1996. Quantitative changes in the binding of transcription factors to response elements in axotomized and NGF-treated dorsal root ganglion neurons. Soc. Neurosci. Abstr. **225.5.**
29. CORNESS, J., B. STEVENS, R.D. FIELDS & T. HÖKFELT 1998. NGF and LIF both regulate galanin gene expression in primary DRG cultures. NeuroReport **9:** 1533–1536.
30. CORNESS, J.D., P.H. BURBACH, A. PRAMANIK & T. HÖKFELT 1995. Identification of a phorbol ester response element in the rat galanin gene promoter. Soc. Neurosci. Abstr. **332.12.**
31. WILSON, T.E., T.J. FAHRNER, M JOHNSTON & J. MILBRANDT. 1991. Identification of the DNA binding site for NGFI-B by genetic selection in yeast. Science **252:** 1296–1300.
32. LOPES DA SILVA, S. & P. BURBACH. 1993. The nuclear hormone receptor family in the brain: Classics and orphans. Trends Neurosci. **18:** 542–548.
33. KENDALL, G., E. ENSOR, A. BRAR-RAI, J. WINTER & D.S. LATCHMAN. 1994. Nerve growth factor induces expression of immediate early genes NGFI-A (Egr1) and NGFI-B (nur77) in adult rat dorsal root ganglion neurons. Mol. Brain Res. **25:** 73–79.
34. WU, Q., Y. LI, R. LIU, A. AGADIR, M.-O. LEE, Y. LIU & X. ZHANG 1997. Modulation of retinoic acid sensitivity in lung cancer cells through dynamic balance of orphan receptors nur77 and COUP-TF and their heterodimerization. EMBO J. **16:** 1656–1669.
35. KOTOMURA, N., Y. NINOMIYA, K. UMESONO & O. NIWA. 1997. Transcriptional regulation by competition between ELP isoforms and nuclear receptors. Biochem. Biophys. Res. Commun. **230:** 407–412.
36. RAO, M.S., Y. SUN, J.L. ESCARY, J. PERREAU, S. TRESSER, P.H. PATTERSON, R.E. ZIGMOND, P. BRULET & S.C. LANDIS. 1993. Leukemia inhibitory factor mediates an injury response but not a target-directed developmental transmitter switch in sympathetic neurons. Neuron **11:** 1175–1185.
37. CORNESS, J., T.-J. SHI, Z.-Q. XU, P. BRULET & T. HÖKFELT 1996. Influence of leukemia inhibitory factor on galanin/GMAP and neuropeptide Y expression in mouse primary sensory neurons after axotomy. Exp. Brain Res. **112:** 79–88.
38. SUN, Y. & R. ZIGMOND. 1996. Leukemia inhibitory factor induced in the sciatic nerve after axotomy is involved in the induction of galanin in sensory neurons. Eur. J. Neurosci. **8:** 2213–2220.
39. ITOH, K., M. OZAKI, B. STEVENS & R.D. FIELDS. 1997. Activity-dependent regulation of N-cadherin in DRG neurons: Differential regulation of N-cadherin, NCAM and L1 by distinct patterns of action potentials. J. Neurobiol. **22:** 735–748.
40. SUN, Y., M.S. RAO, R.E. ZIGMOND & S.C. LANDIS. 1994. Regulation of vasoactive intestinal peptide expression in sympathetic neurons in culture and after axotomy: The role of cholinergic differentiation factor/leukemia inhibitory factor. J. Neurobiol. **25:** 415–430.
41. BANNER, L.R. & P.H. PATTERSON. 1994. Major changes in the expression of the mRNAs for cholinergic differentiation factor/leukemia inhibitory factor and its receptor after injury to adult peripheral nerves and ganglia. Proc. Natl. Acad. Sci. USA **91:** 7109–7113.
42. SHADIACK, A.M., S.A. VACCARIELLO, Y. SUN & R. ZIGMOND. 1998. Nerve growth factor inhibits sympathetic neurons' response to an injury cytokine. Proc. Natl. Acad. Sci. USA **95:** 7727–7730.

Targeted Disruption of the Murine Galanin Gene[a]

DAVID WYNICK,[b,c] CAROLINE J. SMALL,[c] STEPHEN R. BLOOM,[c]
AND VASSILIS PACHNIS[d]

[b]Department of Medicine, Bristol University, Marlborough Street, Bristol BS2 8HW, UK

[c]Imperial School of Science Technology and Medicine, Endocrine Unit, Hammersmith Hospital, DuCane Road, London W12 0NN, UK

[d]Developmental Neurobiology, National Institute for Medical Research, The Ridgeway, London NW7 1AA, UK

ABSTRACT: The 29 amino acid neuropeptide galanin is widely distributed in the nervous and endocrine systems; highest levels of galanin synthesis and storage occur within the hypothalamus in the median eminence, but it is also abundantly expressed in the basal forebrain, the peripheral nervous system, and gut. To further define the role played by galanin in the peripheral nervous and endocrine systems, a mouse strain carrying a loss-of-function germ-line mutation of the galanin locus, engineered by targeted mutagenesis in embryonic stem cells, has been generated. The mutation removes the first five exons containing the entire coding region for the galanin peptide. Germ-line transmission of the disrupted galanin locus has been obtained, and the mutation has been bred to homozygosity on the inbred 129O1aHsd background. Phenotypic analysis of mice lacking a functional galanin gene demonstrate that these animals are viable, grow normally, and can reproduce. A marked reduction in both the anterior pituitary prolactin content and in circulating plasma levels of the hormone is evident. Lactation is abolished along with abrogation of the proliferative response of the lactotroph to estrogen. The responses of sensory neurons to injury in the mutants are markedly impaired. Peripheral nerve regeneration is reduced with associated long-term functional deficits. There is a striking reduction in the development of chronic neuropathic pain. These two phenotypic changes may be explained, in part, by the observation that a subset of dorsal root ganglion neurons is lost in the mutant animals, implying a role for galanin as a trophic cell survival factor. These initial findings have important implications for our understanding and potential therapeutic treatment of (a) sensory nerve regeneration and neuropathic pain and (b) disordered pituitary proliferation and the development of prolactinoma.

G alinin is a 29 amino acid peptide discovered in extracts of porcine intestine in 1983 by Mutt and colleagues[1] at the Karolinska Institute in Stockholm, Sweden. The name galanin derives from the first and last amino acids of the porcine sequence glycine and alanine. Porcine galanin is cleaved from a 123 amino acid precursor prepropeptide along with a 59 amino acid sequence known as galanin message-associated peptide (GMAP). The galanin gene was independently cloned in 1987 by two groups. Vrontakis et al.[2] isolated a 700 bp mRNA from a rat anterior pituitary library, demonstrating that its expression was

[a]This work was supported by the MRC and Wellcome Trust.

[b]Address for cprrespondence: Dr. David Wynick, Department of Medicine, Bristol University, Marlborough Street, Bristol BS2 8HW, UK. Phone, 44 (0)117 9283396; fax, 44 (0)117 9283976, e-mail, wynick@bris.ac.uk

induced by the addition of estrogens. Kaplan *et al.*[3] isolated and published the same sequence a few months later from rat hypothalamus. Nucleotide and amino acid sequence analysis suggest that galanin and GMAP are unrelated to any of the other known families of neuropeptides. Galanin remains the only member of its family. Galanin has been isolated and sequenced from 11 species to date. The human galanin sequence is unique, in that it consists of 30 amino acids, with no amidation at the NH_2-terminus.[4] Species homologies indicate that the NH_2 terminal 1-15 amino acids are highly conserved (TABLE 1), and galanin 1-16 shows full agonistic activity on several functional assays.[5,6]

In the central nervous system galanin is widely, but by no means ubiquitously, distributed with moderate to high concentrations in the cerebral cortex, nucleus accumbens, striatum, hippocampus, dentate gyrus, hypothalamus, cerebellum, medulla, and dorsal horn of the spinal cord.[7–10] In the periphery galanin is present in high concentrations in the pituitary, adrenal gland, pancreas, urogenital tract, and ganglia innervating the heart, kidney, and gut.[11–13]

The physiologic actions of galanin at these anatomic sites on feeding, cognition, and memory, modulation of the hypothalamo-pituitary axis, analgesia, insulin release, and smooth muscle contraction have been extensively studied over the 15 years since galanin was first discovered. There are currently over 1,300 references to galanin in the Medline and BIDS databases.

I do not intend in this brief introduction to provide an exhaustive survey of the literature relating to the actions of galanin in every tissue studied. Rather, I will concentrate on its actions in the central and peripheral nervous systems because these are where its main biologic roles are thought to reside. Before the actions of galanin are described, the signaling systems that mediate these effects and the characterization of antagonists to these receptors will first be reviewed.

GALANIN RECEPTORS

The rat pancreatic galanin receptor was the first to be characterized.[14] Using radioiodinated ^{125}I-galanin, interaction of the peptide with pancreatic membranes was shown to be saturable, reversible, and time, temperature, membrane protein concentration, pH, and ionic strength dependent. In optimized equilibrium conditions of binding, native galanin competitively inhibited the binding of ^{125}I-galanin in a dose-dependent manner (from 10^{-11}–10^{-8} M); half-maximal inhibition is induced by 1 nM peptide. Scatchard analysis indicated the existence of a single population of sites of high affinity (kD of 1.5 nM) and low capacity (44 fmol/mg protein). The monophasic dissociation process confirmed the homogeneity of galanin-binding sites. Galanin-binding sites were highly specific; none of the numerous biologically active peptides tested competed with ^{125}I-galanin for binding to pancreatic membranes. Cross-linking of ^{125}I-galanin to beta-cell membranes indicated a single band of 57 kilodalton (kD). Labeling of this 57-kD component was abolished only by native galanin. Assuming one molecule of ^{125}I-galanin is bound per molecule of protein, a 54-kD G-protein coupled glycoprotein was identified as the pancreatic galanin receptor. These studies were then extended to a number of brain areas confirming the foregoing results.[15]

In various tissues, galanin binding has been associated with pertussis toxin sensitive G proteins, which are probably G_i subtypes.[16,17] These may be coupled to opening of potas-

TABLE 1. Alignment of Mature Galanin Peptide from 11 Species Characterized to Date[a]

Species	1				5					10					15					20					25					30
Human	G	W	T	L	N	S	A	G	Y	L	L	G	P	H	A	V	G	N	H	R	S	F	S	D	K	N	G	L	T	S
Cow	G	W	T	L	N	S	A	G	Y	L	L	G	P	H	A	L	D	S	H	R	S	F	Q	D	K	H	G	L	A	
Sheep	G	W	T	L	N	S	A	G	Y	L	L	G	P	H	A	L	D	S	H	R	S	F	Q	D	K	H	G	L	A	
Pig	G	W	T	L	N	S	A	G	Y	L	L	G	P	H	A	I	D	N	H	R	S	F	H	D	K	Y	G	L	A	
Dog	G	W	T	L	N	S	A	G	Y	L	L	G	P	H	A	I	D	N	H	R	S	F	H	E	K	P	G	L	T	
Chicken	G	W	T	L	N	S	A	G	Y	L	L	G	P	H	A	V	D	N	H	R	S	F	N	D	K	H	G	F	T	
Rat	G	W	T	L	N	S	A	G	Y	L	L	G	P	H	A	I	D	N	H	R	S	F	S	D	K	H	G	L	T	
Alligator	G	W	T	L	N	S	A	G	Y	L	L	G	P	H	A	I	D	N	H	R	S	F	N	E	K	H	G	I	X	
Frog	G	W	T	L	N	S	A	G	Y	L	L	G	P	H	A	L	D	S	H	R	S	F	N	D	K	H	G	L	A	
Trout	G	W	T	L	N	S	A	G	Y	L	L	G	P	H	G	I	D	G	H	R	T	L	S	D	K	H	G	L	A	
Bowfin	G	W	T	N	L	S	A	G	Y	L	L	G	P	H	A	V	D	N	H	R	S	L	N	D	K	H	G	L	A	

[a]Human galanin sequence is unique, consisting of 30 amino acids, with no amidation at the NH$_2$-terminus. The NH$_2$-terminal 15 amino acids are identical in all species with the exception of the trout.

sium channels,[18,19] closure of voltage-sensitive calcium channels,[20,21] or inhibition of basal and/or forskolin-stimulated adenylate cyclase.[22–24]

The distribution of galanin binding sites closely matches that of the galanin immunoreactive rat and human nerve terminals in the central and peripheral nervous systems.[25–27] One notable exception is the anterior pituitary where no galanin binding sites have been demonstrated[28,29] despite a considerable body of data demonstrating direct effects of galanin on pituitary hormone release (see below). Our own data resolved this apparent contradiction with the characterization of an apparently novel galanin receptor subtype.[30] The regions 3-10 and amino acid 25 appear to be crucial for membrane binding and biologic activity, in contrast to the known gut/brain galanin receptor. A number of tissues known to bind or respond to galanin were screened; the novel receptor subtype would only appear to be expressed in the anterior pituitary and hypothalamus.

GALANIN ANTAGONISTS

Further evidence for other receptor subtypes came from the discovery of a number of galanin antagonists by Bartfai's group at the Karolinska Institute.[31–34] These are all chimeric peptides, based on the conserved NH_2-terminus of galanin. All are composed of galanin 1-12 or 1-13 and use a proline residue to form a bridge to various COOH-terminal sequences. M15 is a chimera with substance P (5-11), M35 with bradykinin(2-9)-amide, C7 with spantide, and M40 with 7 amino-acids (PALALAA)-amide which are not homologous to any known peptide. These compounds block a number of the biologic actions of galanin.[31–33,35–40] Functional subtypes are suggested by the use of M40 which blocks the actions of galanin in the hypothalamus and hippocampus but not in the spinal cord or pancreas.[37,41] None of the antagonists thus far described block galanin induced prolactin release in dispersed pituitary cells.[30]

There is increasing evidence that the chimeric peptide galanin antagonists may act as full or partial agonists in some tissues[42] and at high dose bind and nonspecifically activate other receptor systems.[43]

CLONING OF GALANIN RECEPTOR SUBTYPES

The whole field of galanin receptor subtypes has been simplified with the recent cloning of at least three novel and distinct seven transmembrane spanning domain G-protein coupled receptors.[44–46] These receptors, like their ligand, have little homology (less than 30%) to any of the other neuropeptide G-protein coupled receptors. The first receptor subtype (GALR1) was cloned from a Bowes melanoma cell line cDNA expression library by using a radioligand binding strategy.[46] The nucleotide sequence of the cloned receptor reveals an open reading frame encoding a 349 amino acid protein with seven putative hydrophobic transmembrane domains and significant homology with members of the guanine nucleotide binding protein-coupled neuropeptide receptor family. The cloned receptor expressed in COS cells specifically binds human, porcine, and rat galanin with high affinity (kD in the nanomolar range) and mediates the galanin inhibition of adenylate cyclase. A 2.7-kb galanin receptor transcript was identified in several human tissues including the intestine and fetal brain. The rat homolog of GALR1 has 346 amino acids and is 91% homologous to the human receptor.[47,48] Distribution of the rat cDNA has been localized by Northern blotting and *in situ* hybridization to hippocampus, thalamus, amygdala, dorsal horn of the spinal cord, intestine, and pancreas, but not the anterior pituitary.[47,49]

Recently, two further novel G-protein coupled galanin receptor subtypes were independently cloned by a number of groups, designated GALR2[44,50,51] and GALR3,[52] with 38% and 36% homology, respectively, to the previously cloned GALR1. The GALR2 is expressed at high levels in a subset of adult DRG neurons with much less expression in the spinal cord.[53] In contrast, GALR1 is expressed in a differing and almost mutually exclusive population of DRG neurons[54] and at high levels in the dorsal spinal cord.[48] The GALR2 is also expressed in the anterior pituitary, although which cell types express the receptor is not known.[50] Little is yet known about the distribution of GALR3.

PHYSIOLOGIC ACTIONS OF GALANIN

Feeding

Galanin was first demonstrated to affect feeding behavior in 1986.[55] This and much of the subsequent work on galanin effects on feeding has come from the Leibowitz group at the Rockefeller University. Acute icv injection of galanin potently stimulates feeding in fed or fasted rats, with a twofold increase in food intake.[31,56–59] Unlike neuropeptide Y (NPY), the effect is short lived, and tachyphylaxis rapidly occurs after multiple injections or continuous infusion.[60] Alterations in macronutrient selection after galanin injection, with a preference for fat, have been reported by Leibowitz *et al.*, but a number of other groups have had some difficulty in fully reproducing the published data.[59,61,62] Furthermore, while the feeding effects of galanin are no doubt antagonized by M40 and M35, controversy exists as to their effects when infused alone.[31,38] It is still unclear whether blockade of endogenous galanin secretion using the antagonists has significant effects on feeding and weight gain.[31,37,38,41] In summary, there is little evidence to date to indicate that galanin is a major regulator of feeding. Furthermore, given the absence of a major demonstrable phenotype in NPY knockout mice,[63] there is doubt that the long-term modulation of a single factor or neuropeptide will perturb feeding in a sustained manner.

Memory and Cognition

Galanin colocalizes with choline acetyltransferase (ChAT), the synthetic enzyme for acetylcholine, in the basal forebrain cell bodies of most lower mammalian species.[64–67] It is only the higher primates (gorilla, chimpanzee, and human) that fail to demonstrate colocalization.[68] Mufson and colleagues[68] speculate that an evolutionary change occurred in the galanin-acetylcholine neurons of the forebrain at the branch point between monkeys and apes, but the reason for this remains unclear. Although galanin does not coexist with acetylcholine in apes and humans, small galaninergic interneurons are localized near the large cholinergic cell bodies.[68–70] Galaninergic fibers are both widespread and dense in the nucleus basalis and probably originate in the locus coeruleus cell bodies.[71,72]

The most consistent marker of neuronal loss in Alzheimer's disease is the decline in the number of cholinergic neurons in the nucleus basalis.[73] Dramatic reductions in ChAT are routinely seen in postmortem brain samples of the basal forebrain compared to those of age-matched controls. Cholinergic deficits are highly correlated with loss of memory, cognition, and the development of dementia.[74] Postmortem studies of the basal forebrain of Alzheimer's patients reveal a twofold increase in galanin expression with a concomitant decline in ChAT activity of 50–75%. Expression of other neuropeptides including substance P and NPY are unchanged.[75] The galaninergic fibers in the forebrain hyperinnervate the remaining large cholinergic cell bodies.[69,76] The axons of the galanin-positive neurons are enlarged and show varicosities wrapping around the cholinergic neurons and dendrites.[69] The increased galanin expression appears to correlate with the severity of the Alzheimer's disease.[69,70]

The mechanism and reason for this hyperinnervation are not known. In particular, the location of the cell bodies that hyperinnervate the cholinergic neurons is unknown. Assays of cerebrospinal fluid of Alzheimer's patients show no increase in galanin levels.[77] Similarly, the number of galanin binding sites is normal in the hippocampus despite the loss of cholinergic fibers.[78]

One possible explanation for increased galanin expression in Alzheimer's disease may be related to the general phenomenon of plasticity in galanin expression following injury.[79] Some studies have demonstrated a profound and long-lived upregulation of galanin levels after injury in many areas of the central and peripheral nervous systems.[80–87] It is therefore tempting to speculate that progressive neuronal damage and death by amyloid deposition cause a secondary increase in galanin expression. An alternative hypothesis is that galanin is playing a cell survival or trophic role to the cholinergic neurons, explaining its upregulation in Alzheimer's disease.

The consequences of increased galanin expression (and presumably increased release) in Alzheimer's disease are unknown. To address the role played by galanin in acetylcholine release and, by extension, on cognition, a number of groups have administered pharmacologic doses of galanin into the hippocampus or third ventricle (icv). Galanin inhibits scopolamine-induced acetylcholine release in a dose-dependent manner,[6,88] which is reversed by the galanin antagonists M15 and M40.[33,37] By contrast, in the rat striatum, galanin stimulates the release of acetylcholine,[39,89] an effect again inhibited by M15.[90]

The consequences of a change in acetylcholine release have major effects on cognition. Centrally administered galanin has inhibitory effects on several tests of learning and memory such as the Morris water maze and tests involving conditioning.[91–94] These effects are reversed by M35 and have been shown to be specific to the ventral hippocampus.[95,96]

Neither antagonist has an effect on acetylcholine release or on cognition, in the absence of added galanin, casting doubt on the role played by galanin in the normal tonic regulation of acetylcholine release and cognitive processes.[33,37]

Release of Pituitary Hormones

Galanin is synthesized and secreted in the rodent anterior pituitary principally by the lactotrophs but also by the growth hormone and thyrotropin-secreting cell types[97] (somatotrophs and thyrotrophs) while in man its principal site of production is the ACTH-secreting cell, the corticotroph.[98,99] Electron microscopy has shown that galanin is co-stored in prolactin secretory granules.[100] The anterior pituitary is also exposed to a second source of galanin originating from the hypothalamus. Galanin-containing neurons are predominantly found in the arcuate, paraventricular, and supraoptic nuclei and medial preoptic area, and they project to other hypothalamic nuclei, the median eminence and the posterior pituitary.[101–103] Almost 70% of galaninergic neurons in the median eminence have cell bodies in the arcuate nucleus.[7] Galanin controls its own release from these neurons via an ultra-short loop feedback.[104]

Growth Hormone

A subset of galaninergic neurons in the arcuate nucleus contains growth hormone-releasing hormone (GHRH),[105] and in the periventricular nucleus, galaninergic neurons projecting from other hypothalamic nuclei synapse on neurons containing somatostatin.[106] This anatomic localization implicates galanin in the control of somatostatin and GHRH release, and this is probably the mechanism underlying galanin's proposed role as a physiologic regulator of growth hormone secretion in rat and man.[107,108] Direct effects of galanin on the somatotroph have been reported, but they are variable and modest compared to its role in the hypothalamus.[28,109–111]

Gonadotropin-Releasing Hormone

Estrogen-concentrating neurons in the medial preoptic area contain galanin,[112] and exposure to 17β estradiol for 7 days results in a two- to threefold increase in galanin mRNA in both the paraventricular nucleus and medial preoptic area.[113] This induction of synthesis by estrogen results in an elevation in galanin concentrations at the onset of puberty,[113] which is more pronounced in females.[114] In these hypothalamic nuclei galanin colocalizes to gonadotropin-releasing hormone (GnRH) neurons[115–117] and may be co-secreted with GnRH.[118] In the rat, immunoneutralization of galanin co-secreted into the portal circulation blunts the gonadotropin response to GnRH,[118] and intravenous administration of galanin antisera attenuates the proestrus gonadotropin surge.[119] Thus, galanin appears to have an important role in regulating reproductive function.

Prolactin

Galanin stimulates prolactin release when injected icv[120–122] by stimulating adrenergic[123,124] and opioidergic[123] mechanisms. In the rat, in vivo studies using intravenous infusion of galanin antisera[119,125] demonstrated a reduction in circulating prolactin levels, with attenuation of the proestrus surge. Although hypothalamic galanin may influence prolactin secretion, its most important physiologic role appears to be as an paracrine regulator of prolactin release.

The exogenous administration of estrogen in pharmacologic doses to primates or rodents of either sex potently induces prolactin gene transcription and secretion.[126–131] Chronic hyperestrogenization first stimulates lactotroph proliferation, inducing hyperplasia, followed by adenoma formation and finally the development of prolactinomas.[132–134] The mechanism by which tumor formation occurs is currently unknown, but the addition of estrogens to anterior pituitary cultures stimulates the production of neuropeptides, most potently galanin.[135] Galanin, like prolactin, is extremely sensitive to the estrogen status of the animal (but not progesterone); a marked elevation occurs during pregnancy and lactation.[136] Exogenous 17β estradiol can cause a 3,000-fold increase in anterior pituitary galanin mRNA, while the peptide content rises 500-fold.[137]

We previously demonstrated that galanin stimulates prolactin release in dispersed rat pituitary cells and in the 235-1 clonal lactotroph cell line.[138,139] Hyperestrogenization increases both the number of galanin-secreting cells to about 40% of all lactotrophs and the total number of lactotrophs to 70% of all pituitary cells. Immunoneutralization of locally secreted galanin profoundly inhibits prolactin release, particularly in the hyperestrogenized state, suggesting a paracrine role in regulating lactotroph function.[138]

Hyperestrogenization for 2 weeks has a strong mitogenic effect on pituitary size and cell number and markedly increases pituitary prolactin content. Estradiol also quadruples the percentage of lactotrophs that secrete galanin.[138] Furthermore, we were able to show that galanin is also a mitogen for the 235-1 lactotroph cell line, increasing the incorporation of ^{3}H-thymidine by 170%, and that these effects are abolished by the coadministration of galanin-neutralizing antisera.[138,139]

Galanin may thus be involved in the induction of prolactin-secreting adenomas and subsequent prolactinoma formation. A number of groups have analyzed galanin expression in human prolactinoma tissue and failed to demonstrate increased levels in either the tumors themselves or the surrounding normal pituitary tissue.[98,99,140] The possibility that an activating mutation in the pituitary galanin receptor results in oncogenesis and prolactinoma formation is now a testable hypothesis, because the pituitary galanin receptor was recently cloned.

Pain and Regeneration

The disconnection of nerve fibers from their normal peripheral targets results in a loss of sensory and motor function. Damage to a peripheral nerve causes changes within the cell body that promote neuronal survival, axonal regeneration, and functional recovery. Under favorable conditions, for instance following a crush injury, most nerve fibers successfully regenerate. However, in most clinically relevant circumstances, traumatic or disease-induced nerve injury has a poor outcome, with only limited return of function and often with considerable delay. The factors controlling the degree and rate of peripheral nerve regeneration remain important scientific issues. Damage to peripheral nerves can also result in chronic pain. The incidence of such states is typically low following traumatic nerve injury but, conversely, pain is a common complaint in diabetic neuropathy. Neuropathic pain is frequently persistent and resistant to conventional analgesic therapies. The mechanisms that regulate both the regenerative process and the development of neuropathic pain are currently largely unknown.

Peripheral nerve injury in mammals induces major and long-lasting changes in the expression patterns of neuropeptides and their receptors in primary sensory neurons, the most potent being the upregulation of galanin.[80] In the developing rat dorsal root ganglia

(DRG), galanin is expressed at high levels from day 16 of gestation (E16), but downregulates after birth.[141] In the adult, it is expressed at low levels in only 2–3% of DRG cells;[142] higher levels are detected in the dorsal horn (lamina II) of the spinal cord and in the second order neurons in the spinothalamic tracts.[143] The plasticity in galanin expression after nerve section (axotomy) is striking; DRG mRNA and peptide levels rise by up to 120-fold and remain elevated while the neuron is regenerating.[80] The increase in expression is no longer confined to a small percentage of small fiber neurons, but it is now abundantly expressed in 30–40% of all neurons.[79] Similar changes in galanin expression and distribution in the DRG are seen after treatment with resiniferatoxin, a potent analog of the nerve toxin capsaicin.[144] The rise in galanin expression in the dorsal horn following axotomy is modest compared to that of the DRG,[145] and it may reflect a decrease in galanin transport from the cell body to the dorsal horn as anterograde movement along the nerve increases. Sectioning the nerve between the DRG and the dorsal horn[146,147] (rhizotomy) or neonatal treatment with capsaicin[143,148] (which destroys small fiber neuropeptidergic neurons) reduces galanin expression in the dorsal horn of the spinal cord by at least 75%, indicating that much of the lamina II expression originates in the primary afferent cell body and is then transported to, and stored in, the dorsal horn.

The published data on the effects of galanin on spinal cord transmission and nociception are contradictory, and the functional correlates of the plasticity in galanin expression following nerve injury are unclear. The work of Hokfelt and Wiesenfeld-Hallin would indicate a biphasic, dose-dependent change in spinal cord excitability following the administration of galanin intrathecally.[149] Galanin at high dose has an analgesic effect in mice on tail-flick and hot-plate tests.[150] In contrast, Kuraishi et al.[151] showed that high doses of galanin facilitated mechanical nociceptive transmission. These data are also consistent with those of Henry Cridland and who showed that galanin in the nanomolar range also induced mechanical and thermal hyperalgesia.[152] High dose galanin potentiates the spinal analgesic effects of morphine in a naloxone-reversible fashion in both the hot-plate and flexor reflex models; these effects are reversed using the antagonists M15 or M35.[35] The Swedish group also demonstrated that after axotomy chronic intrathical infusion of M35 greatly potentiates spinal cord excitability and is associated with an increase in the severity of autotomy.[40]

To date there is little evidence that galanin is important for cell survival or regeneration of sensory neurons following injury, but studies have shown that two other neuropeptides (NPY and VIP), whose expression is also upregulated following nerve injury, increase neuritic outgrowth in dispersed DRG or neuroblast cultures.[153,154] Furthermore, we previously demonstrated that galanin is a growth factor to the prolactin-secreting cells of the pituitary gland,[139] acting via a novel pituitary-specific receptor[30] as just discussed.

While in vitro techniques and cell lines (which are not available for the DRG) have an important place in integrated studies of biologic systems, homeostatic mechanisms are best studied within the intact organism. The generation and analysis of transgenic animals provide a bridge between molecular studies and experiments that seek to understand physiologic function and mechanism within the context of the intact organism. To further define the role of galanin in the nervous and endocrine systems, we have generated a mouse mutant lacking a functional galanin gene (galanin knockout). Analysis of these mutant mice has allowed the function of galanin to be studied in a manner not previously possible.

RESULTS AND DISCUSSION

A mouse 129sv cosmic genomic library (a generous gift of Dr. A.M. Frischauf, ICRF, London) was screened using the full-length rat galanin cDNA as a probe under high stringency. A positive/negative selection targeting vector was constructed (FIG. 1A) in which a PGK-*Neo* cassette in reverse orientation was used to replace exons one to five of the galanin gene, removing the signal peptide, the coding region for galanin, and most of the galanin-associated peptide. A 1.9-kb *EcoRI/BamHI* fragment, 5′ to the gene (the *BamHI* is 13-bp downstream of the transcriptional start site), was cloned in between the thymidine kinase and *Neo* cassettes. A further 7.8–kb of 3′ homology was added as a *BglII* fragment, removing a total of 3.7 kb of the galanin locus (containing the first five exons of the gene). The vector was linearized and electroporated into the previously described E14-embryonic stem-cell (ES) line.[155] Double selection was performed over a 10-day period; G418/gancyclovir-resistant clones were screened by Southern blotting. Restriction mapping of the wild-type locus with *BglII* generates a 9.3-kb fragment when probed with a 5′ external probe (marked A, FIG. 1A), while the correctly targeted locus generates a 4.4-kb fragment. In total, nine clones were identified in which one allele of the galanin gene was correctly targeted by homologous recombination among 209 double-resistant colonies, yielding a targeting frequency of 4.3%. These nine clones were karyotyped, confirming euploidy, and injected into 3.5-day-old blastocysts from C57BL/6 mice. Germ-line transmission of the disrupted galanin locus was obtained from three separate ES cell clones. Subsequent to germ-line transmission, animals were genotyped by both Southern blotting and polymerase chain reaction (PCR). FIGURE 1B demonstrates identical results obtained by Southern blotting and PCR screening on the same litter derived from a mating of two heterozygotes. Two sets of primers were utilized in the same PCR reaction. The first set of primers corresponds to exons 4 and 5, respectively, of the deleted galanin gene and generate a 350-bp fragment. The second set correspond to the 5′ end of the *Neo* gene and generate a 600-bp fragment.

The galanin loss-of-function mutation has been bred to homozygosity on the in-bred 129/OlaHsd mouse strain, and all data presented are from mice on this background. Galanin levels were measured in a number of brain regions, stomach, and small intestine by RIA.[156] Levels in heterozygotes were 50% of wild-type controls, while levels in the homozygotes were below the limit of detectability in all cases (TABLE 2). Results of genotype analysis of live births were in the expected ratio predicted by Mendelian genetics, and the sex ratio of homozygote offspring was 1:1.

Prolactin message levels and protein content (FIGS. 2 and 3A) were reduced by 30% and 40%, respectively, in randomly cycling adult female mutants when compared to wild-type controls. Immunocytochemistry confirmed that the number of lactotrophs remained unchanged (46 ± 4% vs. 44 ± 5% adult female wild-type vs. mutants, $n = 5$), as was the distribution of lactotrophs within the gland. Plasma prolactin was unchanged in randomly cycling adult female mutants compared to wild-type controls (10 ± 2.7 vs. 11 ± 2.6 ng/ml prolactin, respectively; $n = 10$). The disparity between the decrease in pituitary prolactin synthesis and content and the unchanged circulating levels may reflect rapid changes in prolactin secretion during the estrous cycle since we studied randomly cycling adult females. The expression of other factors known to regulate prolactin storage and release were studied. Anterior pituitary content of the neuropeptide vasoactive intestinal polypeptide, previously demonstrated to be a prolactin secretagog,[9] was unchanged in mutant

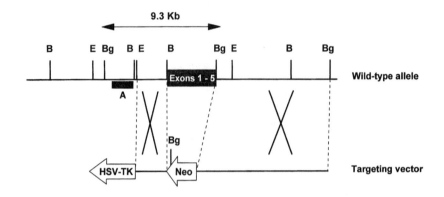

(A)

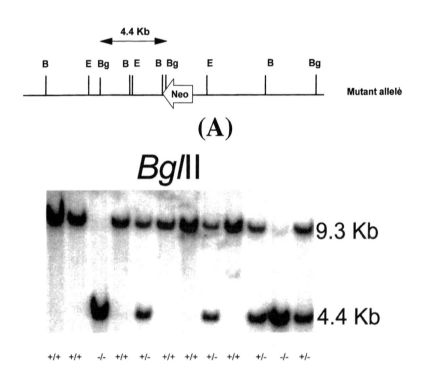

*Bg*II

9.3 Kb

4.4 Kb

+/+ +/+ -/- +/+ +/- +/+ +/+ +/- +/+ +/- -/- +/-

PCR

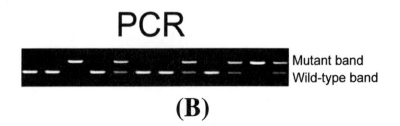

Mutant band
Wild-type band

(B)

FIGURE 1. (**A**) Targeted disruption of the murine galanin gene. The targeting vector replaces the first five exons of the galanin gene with a *Neo* cassette in reverse orientation. HSV-TK denotes the herpes simplex thymidine kinase and *Neo* the neomycin resistance gene. (**A**) The 5′ external probe. Abbreviations: B, *BamH*I; Bg, *Bgl*II; E, *EcoR*I. (**B**) Identical results obtained by Southern blotting (genomic DNA digested with *Bgl*II and probed with the 5′ external probe) and PCR screening on the same litter derived from a mating of two heterozygotes.

TABLE 2. Galanin Content in Various Brain and Peripheral Tissues Measured by RIA[a]

Genotype	Cortex	Hypothalamus	Stomach	Duodenum	Ileum
+/+	5.8 ± 0.3	110.3 ± 7.8	27.5 ± 1.9	122.9 ± 11.6	267.4 ± 13.5
+/−	2.9 ± 0.2	53.8 ± 3.8	13.8 ± 0.8	68.4 ± 5.7	125.9 ± 7.6
−/−	UD	UD	UD	UD	UD

[a]All values are mean galanin-LI pmol/g of wet tissue $\pm$ SEM, $n = 10$ for all groups. Levels in the mutant animals were below the detection limit of the radioimmunoassay in all cases (UD).

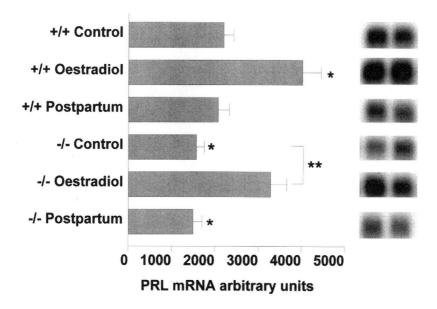

FIGURE 2. Pituitary prolactin message levels in arbitrary units, measured by Northern blotting of randomly cycling wild-type and mutant females (denoted control), a second group of randomly cycling wild-type and mutant females treated for 3 weeks with 17β estradiol treatment (estradiol), and thirdly, another group of wild-type and mutant females 7 days postpartum. Values were determined relative to GAPDH as a control probe. $n = 5$ for all groups, *$p < 0.05$, denotes levels of significance compared to the wild-type control group. Two representative pituitary samples are illustrated for each group.

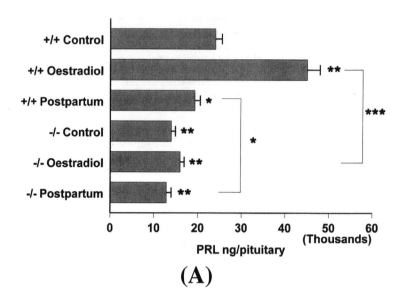

(A)

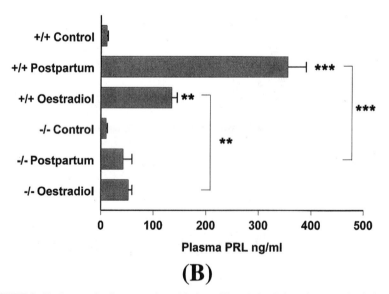

(B)

FIGURE 3. Pituitary prolactin content in ng/pituitary (**A**) and circulating plasma prolactin in ng/ml (**B**) of randomly cycling wild-type and mutant females (denoted control), a second group of randomly cycling wild-type and mutant females treated for 3 weeks with 17β estradiol treatment (estradiol), and thirdly, another group of wild-type and mutant females 7 days postpartum. $n = 10$ for all groups, *$p < 0.05$, **$p < 0.01$, ***$p < 0.001$, denote levels of significance compared to the wild-type control group.

TABLE 3. Pituitary Content of GH, TSH, FSH, and LH and Hypothalamic Neuropeptide Content of Male and Female Mice of Each Genotype[a]

Sex/Genotype	GH	TSH	LH	FSH	GnRH	SRIF	TRH	NPY	GLP-1	AVP
Male +/+	51781 ± 517	141 ± 8	1,794 ± 98	855 ± 44	55 ± 7	888 ± 85	447 ± 52	510 ± 71	4.4 ± 0.6	544 ± 69
Male +/−	52161 ± 623	136 ± 8	1,830 ± 119	897 ± 40	62 ± 20	1,111 ± 100	553 ± 52	463 ± 95	4.7 ± 0.7	590 ± 78
Male −/−	50975 ± 619	154 ± 9	1,980 ± 102	834 ± 38	44 ± 13	1,153 ± 200	472 ± 56	577 ± 82	6.0 ± 1.0	574 ± 82
Female +/+	30719 ± 380	133 ± 12	334 ± 18	287 ± 13	51 ± 19	500 ± 47	490 ± 40	550 ± 47	6.2 ± 1.2	490 ± 53
Female +/−	31162 ± 356	145 ± 7	360 ± 16	324 ± 11	62 ± 24	624 ± 50	575 ± 50	614 ± 50	6.7 ± 0.8	516 ± 66
Female −/−	30883 ± 310	136 ± 9	386 ± 21	315 ± 17	44 ± 14	472 ± 20	467 ± 31	482 ± 20	5.6 ± 0.6	483 ± 71

[a]All hormones are expressed as mean ng hormone/pituitary ± SEM, while hypothalamic neuropeptides are expressed as mean neuropeptide-LI fmol/mg of wet weight tissue ± SEM. $n = 10$ for all groups.

females (65 ± 9 vs. 71 ± 10 fmol/gland, mutant and wild-type, respectively; $n = 8$). Hypothalamic thyroid releasing hormone content (TABLE 3) was also unaffected by the mutation. No phenotypic changes have thus far been delineated in animals heterozygote for the mutation.

Mutant females were unable to lactate, and all pups died of dehydration/starvation within 48 hours unless fostered by wild-type mothers. This apparent failure of lactation was absolute during the first two pregnancies. In subsequent pregnancies, approximately 80% of pups died, but on some occasions one or two survived to the weaning period. Such pups, once weaned, were indistinguishable in every respect from mutant pups born to heterozygote mothers. Pituitary prolactin message levels (FIG. 2), protein content (FIG. 3A), and serum levels (FIG. 3B) were significantly reduced 1.4-, 1.5-, and 8-fold, respectively, in 7-day postpartum (first pregnancy) mutant females when compared to lactating age-matched wild-type controls. It is likely that an eightfold decrease in circulating prolactin levels in the mutants is sufficient to account for the complete abolition of lactation. Previous human and rat data would indicate that a 50% reduction in circulating prolactin levels using dopamine agonists halves or in some cases abolishes milk production.[157–159] The relation between the levels of prolactin and the production of breast milk is probably nonlinear; once prolactin levels fall below a particular threshold, milk production ceases.

The initial failure of lactation in the first two pregnancies may also be explained by a delay in the maturation of the mammary gland due to low levels of circulating prolactin in the postpartum mutant females. The observation of an almost identical phenotype in mice carrying a heterozygous null mutation in the prolactin receptor[160] adds weight to the hypothesis that the actions of galanin on lactation are mediated, in part, via the effects of prolactin on the mammary gland. It is also of interest that studies have identified both prolactin[161,162] and galanin[163] in rat and human mammary tissue and, most recently, an estrogen-inducible increase in galanin mRNA in a number of breast cancer cell lines.[164]

To study galanin-estrogenic interactions and their effects on prolactin expression and lactotroph growth, adult randomly cycling female mice were injected subcutaneously with 0.5 mg 17β estradiol dissolved in safflower oil given once a week for a 3-week period. This dose regimen was previously demonstrated to induce prolactin gene transcription and secretion in both rats and mice, but the increase is less robust in the mouse than in the rat.[165] Pituitary prolactin message levels and protein content (FIGS. 2 and 3A) rose two fold in wild-type females after chronic hyperestrogenization, with a 13-fold increase in plasma prolactin levels (FIG. 3B). In parallel, galanin content rose sixfold (7.5 ± 0.5 vs. 1.2 ± 0.1 pmol/gland, $p < 0.001$, $n = 10$, hyperestrogenized vs. control). Mutant females demonstrated a similar rise in prolactin message levels (FIG. 2) but not in protein content (FIG. 3A). Consistent with these findings was a marked attenuation in the rise in plasma prolactin levels (FIG. 3B). The proliferative effect of estradiol on dispersed pituitary cell number[138] was also studied, demonstrating an almost complete abolition of the increase in cell number observed in the wild-type animals (FIG. 4). The percentage of lactotrophs, as determined by immunocytochemistry, was also significantly lower in mutant animals than in wild-type estrogen-treated controls ($51 \pm 4\%$ vs. $62 \pm 7\%$ mutant vs. wild-type, $p < 0.01$, $n = 5$).

Recent data by Borrelli and colleagues[166] elegantly demonstrate that prolactin itself acts as an autocrine growth factor to the lactotroph through the activation of pituitary prolactin receptors. Signal transduction of the prolactin receptor occurs primarily through JAK2, a tyrosine kinase whose major phosphorylation targets are the STAT5 transcription

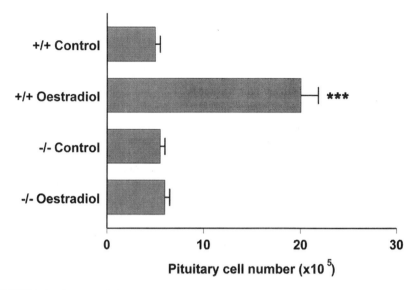

FIGURE 4. Dispersed pituitary cell number in randomly cycling wild-type and mutant females (control) and following 3 weeks of 17β estradiol treatment (estradiol). $n = 10$ for all groups, $**p < 0.01$, $***p < 0.001$ denotes levels of significance compared to wild-type control values.

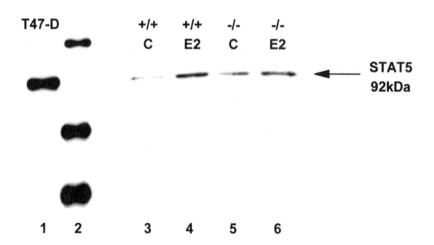

FIGURE 5. Representative Western blot of activated STATS. *Lane 1*, positive control using lysate of T47-D breast cancer cell line; *lane 2*, size marker; *lanes 3 and 4*, wild-type anterior pituitary lysates with and without 17β estradiol (E2); *lanes 5 and 6*, mutant anterior pituitary lysates with and without 17β estradiol. $n = 3$.

factors.[167] Phosphorylated STAT5 transcription factors are translocated to the nucleus where they are thought to modulate cell cycle and proliferation. We therefore studied the expression by Western blotting of activated STAT5 in wild-type and mutant animals before and after chronic hyperestrogenization. Results demonstrate that the fourfold increase in STAT5 expression following estradiol administration in wild-type females fails to occur in mutant animals (FIG. 5). These data are therefore compatible with the hypothesis that galanin may in part regulate lactotroph growth by tonically modulating prolactin release and the activation of the prolactin receptor signaling pathway.

As described in the introduction, galanin has been demonstrated, under various physiologic circumstances, to modulate the release of growth hormone (GH),[107] the gonadotropins[118] (luteinizing [LH] and follicle-stimulating hormone [FSH]), and vasopressin[168] as well as playing a role in food intake and the regulation of body weight.[31] Despite these studies, we were unable to demonstrate changes in the time to enter puberty or gestation period in mutant or heterozygote animals compared to wild-type littermate controls. These normal physiologic parameters were paralleled by a lack of change in the pituitary content of GH, TSH, LH, and FSH in the mutants (TABLE 3). Furthermore, the hypothalamic content of many of the major releasing factors known to control the secretion of these hormones was also unchanged (TABLE 3). The growth rates and final adult size of the mutant mice was not different from those of their wild-type littermates (FIG. 6). Consistent with this observation, the hypothalamic content of neuropeptide Y and glucagon-like peptide-1, two neuropeptides known to modulate food intake were unchanged in

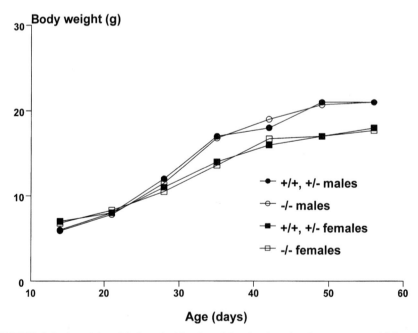

FIGURE 6. Body weights of 2–8-week-old male and female mice of each genotype; $n = 10$ for all groups.

the mutant animals (TABLE 3). Similarly, hypothalamic content of vasopressin (TABLE 3) and water intake were also unaltered by the mutation.

The forgoing data provide good evidence for a causal role for galanin as a prolactin-releasing and growth factor to the lactotroph, especially in states of high estrogen exposure. Galanin would appear to principally regulate circulating prolactin levels at the level of storage and release rather than by the regulation of gene transcription, although whether these effects are mediated at the level of the pituitary and/or hypothalamus is, as yet, unknown. Further support for a role for galanin as a growth factor to the pituitary comes from recent data (Hyde and Vrontakis, this volume), indicating that targeted overexpression of galanin to the lactotrophs and/or somatotroph of transgenic mice induces pituitary hyperplasia and adenoma formation. Our recent observation in galanin mutant animals (this volume) of (a) a long-term impairment in peripheral nerve regeneration following injury and (b) deficits in LTP and tests of cognitive function also indicate a trophic role for galanin in regenerating sensory neurons and the hippocampus. Galanin is expressed at relatively low levels under normal physiologic conditions in both the lactotroph and dorsal root ganglion. It is only after pathophysiologic stimuli (injury to primary sensory neurons and states of high estrogen exposure to the lactotroph) that a marked plasticity in the expression pattern of galanin occurs. Galanin may thus be acting as a trophic factor in a number of tissues in response to injury or pathologic charge. Recent data indicate that galanin also has proliferative effects on endocrine small cell lung cancer cells acting by the activation of the p42 isoform of the mitogen-activated protein kinase pathway.[169]

REFERENCES

1. TATEMOTO, K., A. ROKAEUS, H. JORNVALL, T.J. MCDONALD & V. MUTT. 1983. Galanin, a novel biologically active peptide from porcine intestine. FEBS Lett. **164:** 124–128.
2. VRONTAKIS, M.E., L.M. PEDEN, M.L. DUCKWORTH & H.G. FRIESEN. 1987. Isolation and characterization of a complementary DNA (galanin) clone from estrogen-induced pituitary tumor messenger RNA. J. Biol. Chem. **262:** 16755–16758.
3. KAPLAN, L.M., E.R. SPINDEL, K.J. ISSELBACHER & W.W. CHIN. 1988. Tissue-specific expression of the rat galanin gene. Proc. Natl. Acad. Sci. USA **85:** 1065–1069.
4. EVANS, H.F. & J. SHINE. 1991. Human galanin: Molecular cloning reveals a unique structure. Endocrinology **129:** 1682–1684.
5. HEDLUND, P.B., N. YANAIHARA & K. FUXE. 1992. Evidence for specific N-terminal galanin fragment binding sites in the rat brain. Eur. J. Pharmacol. **224:** 203–205.
6. FISONE, G., M. BERTHOLD, K. BEDECS, A. UNDEN, T. BARTFAI, R. BERTORELLI, S. CONSOLO, J. CRAWLEY, B. MARTIN, S. NILSSON *et al.* 1989. N-terminal galanin-(1-16) fragment is an agonist at the hippocampal galanin receptor. Proc. Natl. Acad. Sci. USA **186:** 9588–9591.
7. MERCHENTHALER, I., F.J. LOPEZ & A. NEGRO-VILAR. 1993. Anatomy and physiology of central galanin-containing pathways. Prog. Neurobiol. **40:** 711–769.
8. HOKFELT, T., T. BARTFAI, T. CECCATELLI, S. CORTES, G. FISONE, A.L. HULTING, U. LANGEL, B. MEISTER, T. MELANDER, V. PIERIBONE, M. SCHALLING, V. VERGE, M. VILLAR, Z. WIESENFELD-HALLIN, Z. XU & X.J. XU. 1992. Central and sensory galanin neurons and functional-aspects. Biomed. Res. **13:** 311–317.
9. SKOFITSCH, G. & D.M. JACOBOWITZ. 1986. Quantitative distribution of galanin-like immunoreactivity in the rat central nervous system. Peptides **7:** 609–613.
10. MELANDER, T., W.A. STAINES, T. HOKFELT, A. ROKAEUS, F. ECKENSTEIN, P.M. SALVATERRA & B.H. WAINER. 1985. Galanin-like immunoreactivity in cholinergic neurons of the septum-basal forebrain complex projecting to the hippocampus of the rat. Brain Res. **360:** 130–138.
11. MCDONALD, T.J., B.D. BROOKS, A. ROKAEUS, B. TINNER & W.A. STAINES. 1992. Pancreatic galanin: Molecular forms and anatomical locations. Pancreas **7:** 624–635.

12. EKBLAD, E., A. ROKAEUS, R. HAKANSON & F. SUNDLER. 1985. Galanin nerve fibers in the rat gut: Distribution, origin and projections. Neuroscience **16:** 355–363.
13. MELANDER, T., T. HOKFELT, A. ROKAEUS, J. FAHRENKRUG, K. TATEMOTO & V. MUTT. 1985. Distribution of galanin-like immunoreactivity in the gastro-intestinal tract of several mammalian species. Cell Tissue Res. **239:** 253–270.
14. AMIRANOFF, B., A.L. SERVIN, C. ROUYER-FESSARD, A. COUVINEAU, K. TATEMOTO & M. LABURTHE. 1987. Galanin receptors in a hamster pancreatic beta-cell tumor: Identification and molecular characterization. Endocrinology **121:** 284–289.
15. SERVIN, A.L., B. AMIRANOFF, C. ROUYER-FESSARD, K. TATEMOTO & M. LABURTHE. 1987. Identification and molecular characterization of galanin receptor sites in rat brain. Biochem. Biophys. Res. Commun. **144:** 298–306.
16. GILLISON, S.L. & G.W.G. SHARP. 1994. ADP ribosylation by cholera toxin identifies three G-proteins that are activated by the galanin receptor. Diabetes **43:** 24–32.
17. FISONE, G., U. LANGEL, M. CARLQUIST, T. BERGMAN, S. CONSOLO, T. HOKFELT, A. UNDEN, S. ANDELL & T. BARTFAI. 1989. Galanin receptor and its ligands in the rat hippocampus. Eur. J. Biochem. **181:** 269–276.
18 DUNNE, M.J., M.J. BULLETT, G.D. LI, C.B. WOLLHEIM & O.H. PETERSEN. 1989. Galanin activates nucleotide-dependent K+ channels in insulin-secreting cells via a pertussis toxin-sensitive G-protein. EMBO J. **8:** 413–420.
19. DE WEILLE, J., H. SCHMID ANTOMARCHI, M. FOSSET & M. LAZDUNSKI. 1988. ATP-sensitive K+ channels that are blocked by hypoglycemia-inducing sulfonylureas in insulin-secreting cells are activated by galanin, a hyperglycemia-inducing hormone, Proc. Natl. Acad. Sci. USA **85:** 1312–1316.
20. NILSSON, T., P. ARKHAMMAR, P. RORSMAN & P.O. BERGGREN. 1989. Suppression of insulin release by galanin and somatostatin is mediated by a G-protein. An effect involving repolarization and reduction in cytoplasmic free Ca2+ concentration. J. Biol. Chem. **264:** 973–980.
21. SHARP, G.W., Y. LE-MARCHAND-BRUSTEL, T. YADA, L.L. RUSSO, C.R. BLISS, M. CORMONT, L. MONGE & E. VAN-OBBERGHEN. 1989. Galanin can inhibit insulin release by a mechanism other than membrane hyperpolarization or inhibition of adenylate cyclase. J. Biol. Chem. **264:** 7302–7309.
22. CHEN, Y., M. LABURTHE & B. AMIRANOFF. 1992. Galanin inhibits adenylate cyclase of rat brain membranes. Peptides **13:** 339–341.
23. FEHMANN, H.C. & J.F. HABENER. 1992. Galanin inhibits proinsulin gene expression stimulated by the insulinotropic hormone glucagon-like peptide-I(7-37) in mouse insulinoma beta TC-1 cells. Endocrinology **130:** 2890–2896.
24. AMIRANOFF, B., A.M. LORINET, I. LAGNY POURMIR & M. LABURTHE. 1988. Mechanism of galanin-inhibited insulin release. Occurrence of a pertussis-toxin-sensitive inhibition of adenylate cyclase. Eur. J. Biochem. **177:** 147–152.
25. KOHLER, C. & V. CHAN-PALAY. 1990. Galanin receptors in the post-mortem human brain. Regional distribution of ^{125}I-galanin binding sites using the method of in vitro receptor autoradiography Neurosci. Lett. **120:** 179–182.
26. KOHLER, C., A. PERSSON, T. MELANDER, E. THEODORSSON, G. SEDVALL & T. HOKFELT. 1989. Distribution of galanin-binding sites in the monkey and human telencephalon: Preliminary observations. Exp. Brain Res. **75:** 375–380.
27. SKOFITSCH, G., M.A. SILLS & D.M. JACOBOWITZ. 1986. Autoradiographic distribution of ^{125}I-galanin binding sites in the rat central nervous system. Peptides **7:** 1029–1042.
28. HULTING, A.L., B. MEISTER, L. CARLSSON, A. HILDING & O. ISAKSSON. 1991. On the role of the peptide galanin in regulation of growth hormone secretion. Acta Endocrinol. Copenh. **125:** 518–525.
29. GAYMANN, W. & N. FALKE. 1990. Galanin lacks binding sites in the porcine pituitary and has no detectable effect on oxytocin and vasopressin release from rat neurosecretory endings. Neurosci. Lett. **112:** 114–119.
30. WYNICK, D., D.M. SMITH, M. GHATEI, K. AKINSANYA, R. BHOGAL, P. PURKISS, P. BYFIELD, N. YANAIHARA & S.R. BLOOM. 1993. Characterization of a high-affinity galanin receptor in the rat anterior pituitary: Absence of biological effect and reduced membrane binding of the antagonist M15 differentiate it from the brain/gut receptor. Proc. Natl. Acad. Sci. USA **90:** 4231–4235.

31. LEIBOWITZ, S.F. & T. KIM. 1992. Impact of a galanin antagonist on exogenous galanin and natural patterns of fat ingestion. Brain Res. **599:** 148–152.
32. WIESENFELD-HALLIN, Z., X.J. XU, U. LANGEL, K. BEDECS, T. HOKFELT & T. BARTFAI. 1992. Galanin-mediated control of pain: Enhanced role after nerve injury. Proc. Natl. Acad. Sci. USA **89:** 3334–3337.
33. BARTFAI, T., K. BEDECS, T. LAND, U. LANGEL, R. BERTORELLI, P. GIROTTI, S. CONSOLO, X.J. XU, Z. WIESENFELD-HALLIN, S. NILSSON *et al.* 1991. M-15: High-affinity chimeric peptide that blocks the neuronal actions of galanin in the hippocampus, locus coeruleus, and spinal cord. Proc. Natl. Acad. Sci. USA **188:** 10961–10965.
34. XU, X.J., Z. WIESENFELD-HALLIN, U. LANGEL, K. BEDECS & T. BARTFAI. 1995. New high affinity peptide antagonists to the spinal galanin receptor. Br. J. Pharmacol. **116:** 2076–2080.
35. REIMANN, W., W. ENGLBERGER, E. FRIDERICHS, N. SELVE & B. WILFFERT. 1994. Spinal antinociception by morphine in rats is antagonised by galanin receptor antagonists. Naunyn-Schmiedebergs Arch. Pharmakol. **350:** 380–386.
36. ULMAN. L.G., E.K. POTTER & D.I. MCCLOSKEY. 1994. Functional effects of a family of galanin antagonists on the cardiovascular system in anaesthetised cats. Regul. Pept. **51:** 17–23.
37. BARTFAI, T., U. LANGEL, K. BEDECS, S. ANDELL, T. LAND, S. GREGERSEN, B. AHREN, P. GIROTTI, S. CONSOLO, R. CORWIN *et al.* 1993. Galanin-receptor ligand M40 peptide distinguishes between putative galanin-receptor subtypes. Proc. Natl. Acad. Sci. USA **90:** 11287–11291.
38. CRAWLEY, J.N., J.K. ROBINSON, U. LANGEL & T. BARTFAI. 1993. Galanin receptor antagonists M40 and C7 block galanin-induced feeding. Brain Res. **600:** 268–272.
39. PRAMANIK, A. & S.O. OGREN. 1993. Galanin stimulates striatal acetylcholine release via a mechanism unrelated to cholinergic receptor stimulation. Regul. Pept. **45:** 353–362.
40. VERGE, V.M., X.J. XU, U. LANGEL, T. HOKFELT, Z. WIESENFELD-HALLIN & T. BARTFAI. 1993. Evidence for endogenous inhibition of autotomy by galanin in the rat after sciatic nerve section: Demonstrated by chronic intrathecal infusion of a high affinity galanin receptor antagonist Neurosci. Lett. **149:** 193–197.
41 CORWIN, R.L., J.K. ROBINSON & J.N. CRAWLEY. 1993. Galanin antagonists block galanin-induced feeding in the hypothalamus and amygdala of the rat. Eur. J. Neurosci. **5:** 1528–1533.
42. GU, Z.F., W.J. ROSSOWSKI, D.H. COY, T.K. PRADHAN & R.T. JENSEN. 1993. Chimeric galanin analogs that function as antagonists in the CNS are full agonists in gastrointestinal smooth muscle J. Pharmacol. Exp. Ther. **266:** 912–918.
43. KOROLKIEWICZ, R., W. SLIWINSKI, P. REKOWSKI, A. HALAMA, P. MUCHA, A. SZCZUROWICZ, P. GUZOWSKI & K.Z. KOROLKIEWICZ. 1996. Contractile action of galanin analogues on rat isolated gastric fundus strips is modified by tachyphylaxis to substance P. Pharmacol. Res. **33:** 361–365.
44. HOWARD, A.D., C. TAN, L.L. SHIAO, O.C. PALYHA, K.K. MCKEE, D.H. WEINBERG, S.D. FEIGHNER, M.A. CASCIERI, R.G. SMITH, L.H. VAN DER PLOEG & K.A. SULLIVAN. 1997. Molecular cloning and characterization of a new receptor for galanin. FEBS Lett. **405:** 285–290.
45. AHMAD, S., S.H. SHEN, P. WALKER & C. WAHLESTEDT. 1996. Soc. Neurosci. **661.10** (Abstr).
46. HABERT ORTOLI, E., B. AMIRANOFF, I. LOQUET, M. LABURTHE & J.F. MAYAUX. 1994. Molecular cloning of a functional human galanin receptor. Proc ,Natl. Acad. Sci. USA **91:** 9780–9783.
47. BURGEVIN, M.C., I. LOQUET, D. QUARTERONET & E. HABERT ORTOLI. 1995. Cloning, pharmacological characterization, and anatomical distribution of a rat cDNA encoding for a galanin receptor. J. Mol. Neurosci. **6:** 33–41.
48. PARKER, E.M., D.G. IZZARELLI, H.P. NOWAK, C.D. MAHLE, L.G. IBEN, J. WANG & M.E. GOLDSTEIN. 1995. Cloning and characterization of the rat GALR1 galanin receptor from RINl4B insulinoma cells. Brain Res. Mol. Brain Res. **34:** 179–189.
49. PARKER, E.M., D.G. IZZARELLI, H.P. NOWAK, C.D. MAHLE, L.G. IBEN, J.C. WANG & M.E. GOLDSTEIN. 1995. Cloning and characterization of the rat galr1 galanin receptor from RIN14b insulinoma cells. Mol. Brain Res. **34:** 179–189.
50. FATHI, Z., A.M. CUNNINGHAM, L.G. IBEN, P.B. BATTAGLINO, S.A. WARD, K.A. NICHOL, K.A. PINE, J.C. WANG, M.E. GOLDSTEIN, T.P. IISMAA & I.A. ZIMANYI. 1997. Cloning, pharmacological characterization and distribution of a novel galanin receptor, Mol. Brain Res. **51:** 49–59.
51. WANG, S., T. HASHEMI, C. HE, C. STRADER & M. BAYNE. 1997. Molecular cloning and pharmacological characterization of a new galanin receptor subtype. Mol. Pharmacol. **52:** 337–343.

52. WANG, S.K., C.G. HE, T. HASHEMI & M. BAYNE. 1997. Cloning and expressional characterization of a novel galanin receptor: Identification of different pharmacophores within galanin for the three galanin receptor subtypes. J. Biol. Chem. **272**: 31949–31952.

53. O'DONNELL, D., S. AHMAD, P. WALKER & C. WAHLESTEDT. 1996. Soc. Neurosci. **517.9** (Abstr).

54 XU, Z.Q., T.J. SHI, M. LANDRY & T. HOKFELT. 1996. Evidence for galanin receptors in primary sensory neurones and effect of axotomy and inflammation. Neuroreport **8**: 237–242.

55 KYRKOULI, S.E., B.G. STANLEY & S.F. LEIBOWITZ. 1986. Galanin: Stimulation of feeding induced by medial hypothalamic injection of this novel peptide. Eur. J. Pharmacol. **122**: 159–160.

56. DUBE, M.G., T.L. HORVATH, C. LERANTH, P.S. KALRA & S.P. KALRA. 1994. Naloxone reduces the feeding evoked by intracerebroventricular galanin injection. Physiol. Behav. **56**: 811–813.

57. CRAWLEY, J.N., M.C. AUSTIN, S.M. FISKE, B. MARTIN, S. CONSOLO, M. BERTHOLD, U. LANGEL, G. FISONE & T. BARTFAI. 1990. Activity of centrally administered galanin fragments on stimulation of feeding behavior and on galanin receptor binding in the rat hypothalamus. J. Neurosci. **10**: 3695–3700.

58. KYRKOULI, S.E., B.G. STANLEY, R.D. SEIRAFI & S.F. LEIBOWITZ. 1990. Stimulation of feeding by galanin: Anatomical localization and behavioral specificity of this peptide's effects in the brain. Peptides **11**: 995–1001.

59. TEMPEL, D.L., K.J. LEIBOWITZ & S.F. LEIBOWITZ. 1988. Effects of PVN galanin on macronutrient selection. Peptides **9**: 309–314.

60. SMITH, B.K., D.A. YORK & G.A. BRAY. 1994. Chronic cerebroventricular galanin does not induce sustained hyperphagia or obesity. Peptides **15**: 1267–1272.

61. Bray, G.A. 1992. Peptides affect the intake of specific nutrients and the sympathetic nervous system, Am. J. Clin. Nutr. **55**: 265S–271S.

62. SMITH, B.K., H.R. BERTHOUD, D.A. YORK & G.A. BRAY. 1997. Differential effects of baseline macronutrient preferences on macronutrient selection after galanin, NPY, and an overnight fast. Peptides **18**: 207–211.

63. ERICKSON, J.C., K.E. CLEGG & R.D. PALMITER. 1996. Sensitivity to leptin and susceptibility to seizures of mice lacking neuropeptide Y [see comments] Nature **381**: 415–421.

64. KORDOWER, J.H., H.K. LE & E.J. MUFSON. 1992. Galanin immunoreactivity in the primate central nervous system. J. Comp. Neurol. **319**: 479–500.

65. MELANDER, T., T. BARTFAI, N. BRYNNE, S. CONSOLO, G. FISONE, T. HOKFELT, C. KOHLER, O. NORDSTROM, E. NORHEIM THEODORSSON, A. PERSSON et al. 1989. Galanin in the cholinergic basal forebrain: Histochemical, autoradiographic and in vivo studies. Prog. Brain Res. **79**: 85–91.

66. MELANDER, T. & W.A. STAINES. 1986. A galanin-like peptide coexists in putative cholinergic somata of the septum-basal forebrain complex and in acetylcholinesterase containing fibers and varicosities within the hippocampus in the owl monkey (Aotus trivirgatus). Neurosci. Lett. **68**: 17–22.

67. MELANDER, T., W.A. STAINES & A. ROKAEUS. 1986. Galanin-like immunoreactivity in hippocampal afferents in the rat, with special reference to cholinergic and noradrenergic inputs. Neuroscience **19**: 223–240.

68. BENZING, W.C., M.D. IKONOMOVIC, D.R. BRADY, E.J. MUFSON & D.M. ARMSTRONG. 1993. Evidence that transmitter-containing dystrophic neurites precede paired helical filament and Alz-50 formation within senile plaques in the amygdala of nondemented elderly and patients with Alzheimer's disease. J. Comp. Neurol. **334**: 176–191.

69. MUFSON, E.J., E. COCHRAN, W. BENZING & J.H. KORDOWER. 1993. Galaninergic innervation of the cholinergic vertical limb of the diagonal band (Ch2) and bed nucleus of the strict terminalis in aging, Alzheimer's disease and Down's syndrome. Dementia **4**: 237–250.

70. GENTLEMAN, S.M., P. FALKAI, B. BOGERTS, M.T. HERRERO, J.M. POLAK & G.W. ROBERTS. 1989. Distribution of galanin-like immunoreactivity in the human brain. Brain Res. **505**: 311–315.

71. CHAN PALAY, V. 1991. Alterations in the locus coeruleus in dementias of Alzheimer's and Parkinson's disease. Prog. Brain Res. **88**: 625–630.

72. HOLETS, V.R., T. HOKFELT, A. ROKAEUS, L. TERENIUS & M. GOLDSTEIN. 1988. Locus coeruleus neurons in the rat containing neuropeptide Y, tyrosine hydroxylase or galanin and their efferent projections to the spinal cord, cerebral cortex and hypothalamus. Neuroscience **24**: 893–906.

73. COYLE, J.T., D.L. PRICE & M.R. DELONG. 1983. Alzheimer's disease: A disorder of cortical cholinergic innervation. Science **219**: 1184–1190.

74. BIERER, L.M., V. HAROUTUNIAN, S. GABRIEL, P.J. KNOTT, L.S. CARLIN, D.P. PUROHIT, D.P. PERL, J. SCHMEIDLER, P. KANOF & K.L. DAVIS. 1995. Neurochemical correlates of dementia severity in Alzheimer's disease: Relative importance of the cholinergic deficits. J. Neurochem. **64:** 749–760.

75. BEAL, M.F., U. MACGARVEY & K.J. SWARTZ. 1990. Galanin immunoreactivity is increased in the nucleus basalis of Meynert in Alzheimer's disease. Ann. Neurol. **28:** 157–161.

76. CHAN-PALAY, V. 1988. Galanin hyperinnervates surviving neurons of the human basal nucleus of Meynert in dementias of Alzheimer's and Parkinson's disease: A hypothesis for the role of galanin in accentuating cholinergic dysfunction in dementia. J. Comp. Neurol. **273:** 543–557.

77. EDVINSSON, L., L. MINTHON, R. EKMAN & L. GUSTAFSON. 1993. Neuropeptides in cerebrospinal fluid of patients with Alzheimer's disease and dementia with frontotemporal lobe degeneration. Dementia **4:** 167–171.

78. IKEDA, M., D. DEWAR & J. MCCULLOCH. 1991. Preservation of [^{125}I]galanin binding sites despite loss of cholinergic neurones to the hippocampus in Alzheimer's disease. Brain Res. **568:** 303–306.

79. HOKFELT, T., X. ZHANG & Z. WIESENFELD-HALLIN. 1994. Messenger plasticity in primary sensory neurons following axotomy and its functional implications. Trends Neurosci. **17:** 22–30.

80. HOKFELT, T., Z. WIESENFELD-HALLIN, M. VILLAR & T. MELANDER. 1987. Increase of galanin-like immunoreactivity in rat dorsal root ganglion cells after peripheral axotomy. Neurosci. Lett. **83:** 217–220.

81. AGOSTON, D.V., S. KOMOLY & M. PALKOVITS. 1994. Selective up-regulation of neuropeptide synthesis by blocking the neuronal activity: Galanin expression in septohippocampal neurons. Exp. Neurol. **126:** 247–255.

82. MOHNEY, R.P., R.E. SIEGEL & R.E. ZIGMOND. 1994. Galanin and vasoactive intestinal peptide messenger RNAs increase following axotomy of adult sympathetic neurons. J, Neurobiol. **25:** 108–118.

83. NAHIN, R.L., K. REN, M. DELEON & M. RUDA. 1994. Primary sensory neurons exhibit altered gene expression in a rat model of neuropathic pain. Pain **58:** 95–108.

84. OHNO, K., N. TAKEDA, H. KIYAMA, T. KUBO & M. TOHYAMA. 1994. Occurrence of galanin-like immunoreactivity in vestibular and cochlear efferent neurons after labyrinthectomy in the rat. Brain Res. **644:** 135–143.

85. WHITE, F.A., B.F. HOEFLINGER, N.L. CHIAIA, C.A. BENNETTCLARKE, R.S. CRISSMAN & R.W. RHOADES. 1994. Evidence for survival of the central arbors of trigeminal primary afferents after peripheral neonatal axotomy: Experiments with galanin immunocytochemistry and Di-I labelling. J. Comp. Neurol. **350:** 397–411.

86. ZHANG, X., G. JU, R. ELDE & T. HOKFELT. 1993. Effect of peripheral nerve cut on neuropeptides in dorsal root ganglia and the spinal cord of monkey with special reference to galanin. J. Neurocytol. **22:** 342–381.

87. HENKEN, D.B. & J.R. MARTIN. 1992. The proportion of galanin-immunoreactive neurons in mouse trigeminal ganglia is transiently increased following corneal inoculation of herpes simplex virus type-I. Neurosci. Lett. **140:** 177–180.

88. ORGEN, S.O., J. KEHR & P.A. SCHOTT. 1996. Effects of ventral hippocampal galanin on spatial learning and on in vivo acetylcholine release in the rat. Neuroscience **75:** 1127–1140.

89. AMOROSO, D., P. GIROTTI, G. FISONE, T. BARTFAI & S. CONSOLO. 1992. Mechanism of the galanin induced increase in acetylcholine release in vivo from striate of freely moving rats. Brain Res. **589:** 33–38.

90. PRAMANIK, A. & S.O. OGREN. 1992. Galanin-evoked acetylcholine release in the rat striatum is blocked by the putative galanin antagonist M15. Brain Res. **574:** 317–319.

91. MCDONALD, M.P., G.L. WENK & J.N. CRAWLEY. 1997. Analysis of galanin and the galanin antagonist M40 on delayed non-matching-to-position performance in rats lesioned with the cholinergic immunotoxin 192 IgG-saporin. Behav. Neurosci. **111:** 552–563.

92. MCDONALD, M.P. & J.N. CRAWLEY. 1996. Galanin receptor antagonist M40 blocks galanin-induced choice accuracy deficits on a delayed-nonmatching-to-position task. Behav. Neurosci. **110:** 1025–1032.

93. GIVENS, B.S., D.S. OLTON & J.N. CRAWLEY. 1992. Galanin in the medial septal area impairs working memory. Brain Res. **582:** 71–77.

94. MASTROPAOLO, J., N.S. NADI, N.L. OSTROWSKI & J.N. CRAWLEY. 1988. Galanin antagonizes acetylcholine on a memory task in basal forebrain-lesioned rats. Proc. Natl. Acad. Sci. USA **85:** 9841–9845.

95. ROBINSON, J.K. & J.N. CRAWLEY. 1994. Analysis of anatomical sites at which galanin impairs delayed nonmatching to sample in rats. Behav. Neurosci. **108:** 941–950.

96. ROBINSON, J.K. & J.N. CRAWLEY. 1993. Intraventricular galanin impairs delayed nonmatching-to-sample performance in rats. Behav. Neurosci. **107:** 458–467.

97. KAPILOFF, M.S., Y. FARKASH, M. WEGNER & M.G. ROSENFELD. 1991. Variable effects of phosphorylation of Pit-1 dictated by the DNA response elements. Science **253:** 786–789.

98. VRONTAKIS, M.E., T. SANO, K. KOVACS & H.G. FRIESEN. 1990. Presence of galanin-like immunoreactivity in nontumorous corticotrophs and corticotroph adenomas of the human pituitary, J. Clin. Endocrinol. Metab. **70:** 747–751.

99. SANO, T., M.E. VRONTAKIS, K. KOVACS, S.L. ASA & H.G. FRIESEN. 1991. Galanin immunoreactivity in neuroendocrine tumors. Arch. Pathol. Lab. Med. **115:** 926–929.

100. HYDE, J.F., M.G. ENGLE & B.E. MALEY. 1991. Colocalization of galanin and prolactin within secretory granules of anterior pituitary cells in estrogen-treated Fischer 344 rats. Endocrinology **129:** 270–276.

101. MELANDER, T., T. HOKFELT & A. ROKAEUS. 1986. Distribution of galanin like immunoreactivity in the rat central nervous system. J. Comp. Neurol. **248:** 475–517.

102. SKOFITSCH, G. & D.M. JACOBOWITZ. 1986. Quantitative distribution of galanin-like immunoreactivity in the rat central nervous system. Peptides **7:** 609–613.

103. CH'NG, J.L., N.D. CHRISTOFIDES, P. ANAND, S.J. GIBSON, Y.S. ALLEN, H.C. SU, K. TATEMOTO, J.F. MORRISON, J.M. POLAK & S.R. BLOOM. 1985. Distribution of galanin immunoreactivity in the central nervous system and the responses of galanin-containing neuronal pathways to injury. Neuroscience **16:** 343–354.

104. LOPEZ, F.J., Z. LIPOSITS & I. MERCHENTHALER. 1992. Evidence for a negative ultrashort loop feedback regulating galanin release from the arcuate nucleus-median eminence functional unit. Endocrinology **130:** 1499–1507.

105. NIIMI, M., J. TAKAHARA, M. SATO & K. KAWANISHI. 1990. Immunohistochemical identification of galanin and growth hormone-releasing factor-containing neurons projecting to the median eminence of the rat. Neuroendocrinology **51:** 572–575.

106. LIPOSITS, Z., I. MERCHENTHALER, J.J. REID & A. NEGRO-VILAR. 1993. Galanin-immunoreactive axons innervate somatostatin-synthesizing neurons in the anterior periventricular nucleus of the rat. Endocrinology **132:** 917–923.

107. MAITER, D.M., S.C. HOOI, J.I. KOENIG & J.B. MARTIN. 1990. Galanin is a physiological regulator of spontaneous pulsatile secretion of growth hormone in the male rat. Endocrinology **126:** 1216–1222.

108. OTTLECZ, A., W.K. SAMSON & S.M. MCCANN. 1986. Galanin: Evidence for a hypothalamic site of action to release growth hormone. Peptides **7:** 51–53.

109. GIUSTINA, A., C. BONFANTI, M. LICINI, C. DE RANGO & G. MILANI. 1994. Inhibitory effect of galanin on growth hormone release from rat pituitary tumor cells (GH1) in culture. Life Sci. **55:** 1845–1851.

110. SATO, M., J. TAKAHARA, M. NIIMI, R. TAGAWA & S. IRINO. 1991. Characterization of the stimulatory effect of galanin on growth hormone release from the rat anterior pituitary. Life Sci. **48:** 1639–1644.

111. GABRIEL, S.M., C.M. MILBURY, J.A. NATHANSON & J.B. MARTIN. 1988. Galanin stimulates rat pituitary growth hormone secretion in vitro. Life Sci. **42:** 1981–1986.

112. BLOCH, G.J., S.M. KURTH, T.R. AKESSON & P.E. MICEVYCH. 1992. Estrogen-concentrating cells within cell groups of the medial preoptic area: Sex differences and co-localization with galanin-immunoreactive cells. Brain Res. **595:** 301–308.

113. GABRIEL, S.M., D.L. WASHTON & J.R. RONCANCIO. 1992. Modulation of hypothalamic galanin gene expression by estrogen in peripubertal rats. Peptides **13:** 801–806.

114. GABRIEL, S.M., L.M. KAPLAN, J.B. MARTIN & J.I. KOENIG. 1989. Tissue-specific sex differences in galanin-like immunoreactivity and galanin mRNA during development in the rat. Peptides **10:** 369–374.

115. MERCHENTHALER, I., F.J. LOPEZ, D.E. LENNARD & A. NEGRO-VILAR. 1991. Sexual differences in the distribution of neurons coexpressing galanin and luteinizing hormone-releasing hormone in the rat brain. Endocrinology **129:** 1977–1986.

116. MERCHENTHALER, I. 1991. The hypophysiotropic galanin system of the rat brain. Neuroscience **44:** 643–654.

117. MERCHENTHALER, I., F.J. LOPEZ & A. NEGRO-VILAR. 1990. Colocalization of galanin and luteinizing hormone-releasing hormone in a subset of preoptic hypothalamic neurons: Anatomical and functional correlates. Proc. Natl. Acad. Sci. USA **87:** 6326–6330.

118. LOPEZ, F.J., I. MERCHENTHALER, M. CHING, M.G. WISNIEWSKI & A. NEGRO-VILAR. 1991. Galanin: A hypothalamic-hypophysiotropic hormone modulating reproductive functions. Proc. Natl. Acad. Sci. USA **88:** 4508–4512.

119. LOPEZ, F.J., E.H. MEADE, JR. & A. NEGRO-VILAR. 1993. Endogenous galanin modulates the gonadotropin and prolactin proestrous surges in the rat. Endocrinology **132:** 795–800.

120. KOSHIYAMA, H., A. SHIMATSU, Y. KATO, H. ASSADIAN, N. HATTORI, Y. ISHIKAWA, T. TANOH, N. YANAIHARA & H. IMURA. 1990. Galanin-induced prolactin release in rats: Pharmacological evidence for the involvement of alpha-adrenergic and opioidergic mechanisms. Brain Res. **507:** 321–324.

121. OTTLECZ, A., G.D. SNYDER & S.M. MCCANN. 1988. Regulatory role of galanin in control of hypothalamic-anterior pituitary function. Proc. Natl. Acad. Sci. USA **85:** 9861–9865.

122. MELANDER, T., K. FUXE, A. HARFSTRAND, P. ENEROTH & T. HOKFELT. 1987. Effects of intraventricular injections of galanin on neuroendocrine functions in the male rat. Possible involvement of hypothalamic catecholamine neuronal systems. Acta Physiol. Scand. **131:** 25–32.

123 INVITTI, C., F. PECORI-GIRALDI, A. TAGLIAFERRI, M. SCACCHI, A. DUBINI & F. CAVAGNINI. 1993. Enhanced prolactin responsiveness to galanin in patients with Cushing's disease. Clin. Endocrinol. Oxf. **39:** 213–216.

124. TANOH, T., A. SHIMATSU, Y. ISHIKAWA, C. IHARA, N. YANAIHARA & H. IMURA. 1993. Galanin-induced growth hormone secretion in conscious rats: Evidence for a possible involvement of somatostatin J. Neuroendocrinol. **5:** 183–187.

125. TORSELLO, A., R. SELLAN, S.G. CELLA, V. LOCATELLI & E.E. MULLER. 1990. Age-dependent modulation by galanin of growth hormone release from rat pituitary cells in culture. Life Sci. **47:** 1861–1866.

126. BURDMAN, J.A., M.T. CALABRESE & R.M. MACLEOD. 1983. Hyperprolactinaemia and DNA synthesis in the pituitary gland of the rat. J. Endocrinol. **97:** 65–74.

127. JAHN, G.A., G.A. MACHIAVELLI, L.E. KALBERMANN, I. SZIJAN, G.E. ALONSO & J.A. BURDMAN. 1982. Relationships among release of prolactin, synthesis of DNA and growth of the anterior pituitary gland of the rat: Effects of oestrogen and sulpiride. J. Endocrinol. **94:** 1–10.

128. PEREZ, R.L., G.A. MACHIAVELLI, M.I. ROMANO & J.A. BURDMAN. 1986. Prolactin release, oestrogens and proliferation of prolactin-secreting cells in the anterior pituitary gland of adult male rats. J. Endocrinol. **108:** 399–403.

129. LLOYD, R.V. 1983. Estrogen-induced hyperplasia and neoplasia in the rat anterior pituitary gland. An immunohistochemical study. Am. J. Pathol. **113:** 198–206.

130. LLOYD, R.V., M. CANO & T.D. LANDEFELD. 1988. The effects of estrogens on tumor growth and on prolactin and growth hormone mRNA expression in rat pituitary tissues. Am. J. Pathol. **133:** 397–406.

131. LLOYD, R.V., L. JIN, K. FIELDS & E. KULIG. 1991. Effects of estrogens on pituitary cell and pituitary tumor growth. Pathol. Res. Pract. **187:** 584–586.

132. ASSCHEMAN, H., L.J. GOOREN, J. ASSIES, J.P. SMITS & R. DE-SLEGTE. 1988. Prolactin levels and pituitary enlargement in hormone-treated male-to-female transsexuals. Clin. Endocrinol. Oxf. **28:** 583–588.

133. GOOREN, L.J., J. ASSIES, H. ASSCHEMAN, R. DE-SLEGTE & H. VAN-KESSEL. 1988. Estrogen-induced prolactinoma in a man. J. Clin. Endocrinol. Metab. **66:** 444–446.

134. GOOREN, L.J., W. HARMSEN-LOUMAN & H. VAN-KESSEL. 1985. Follow-up of prolactin levels in long-term oestrogen-treated male-to-female. Clin. Endocrinol. Oxf. **22:** 201–207.

135. HEMMER, A. & J.F. HYDE. 1992. Regulation of galanin secretion from pituitary cells in vitro by estradiol and GHRH. Peptides **13:** 1201–1206.

136. GABRIEL, S.M., L.M. KAPLAN, J.B. MARTIN & J.I. KOENIG. 1989. Tissue-specific sex differences in galanin-like immunoreactivity and galanin mRNA during development in the rat. Peptides **10:** 369–374.

137. KAPLAN, L.M., S.M. GABRIEL, J.I. KOENIG, M.E. SUNDAY, E.R. SPINDEL, J.B. MARTIN & W.W. CHIN. 1988. Galanin is an estrogen-inducible, secretory product of the rat anterior pituitary. Proc. Natl. Acad. Sci. USA **85:** 7408–7412.

138. WYNICK, D., P.J. HAMMOND, K.O. AKINSANYA & S.R. BLOOM. 1993. Galanin regulates basal and oestrogen-stimulated lactotroph function. Nature **364:** 529–532.

139. HAMMOND, P.J., D.M. SMITH, K.O. AKINSANYA, W.A. MUFTI, D. WYNICK & S.R. BLOOM. 1996. Signalling pathways mediating secretory and mitogenic responses to galanin and pituitary adenylate cyclase-activating polypeptide in the 235-1 clonal rat lactotroph cell line. J. Neuroendocrinol. **8:** 457–464.

140. HSU, D.W., S.C. HOOI, E.T. HEDLEY WHYTE, R.M. STRAUSS & L.M. KAPLAN. 1991. Coexpression of galanin and adrenocorticotropic hormone in human pituitary and pituitary adenomas, Am. J. Pathol. **138:** 897–909.

141. XU, Z.Q., T.J. SHI & T. HOKFELT. 1996. Expression of galanin and a galanin receptor in several sensory systems and bone anlage of rat embryos. Proc. Natl. Acad. Sci. USA **93:** 14901–14905.

142. POLAK, J.M., S.J. GIBSON, S. GENTLEMAN, J.H. STEEL & S. VAN NOORDEN. 1991. *In* Galanin: Distribution, Ontogeny and Expression following Manipulation of the Endocrine and Nervous System.: 117–131.

143. SKOFITSCH, G. & D.M. JACOBOWITZ. 1985. Galanin-like immunoreactivity in capsaicin sensitive sensory neurons and ganglia. Brain Res. Bull. **15:** 191–195.

144. FARKAS SZALLASI, T., J.M. LUNDBERG, Z. WIESENFELD-HALLIN, T. HOKFELT & A. SZALLASI. 1995. Increased levels of GMAP, VIP and nitric oxide synthase, and their mRNAs, in lumbar dorsal root ganglia of the rat following systemic resiniferatoxin treatment. Neuroreport **6:** 2230–2234.

145. VILLAR, M.J., R. CORTES, E. THEODORSSON, Z. WIESENFELD-HALLIN, M. SCHALLING, J. FAHRENKRUG, P.C. EMSON & T. HOKFELT. 1989. Neuropeptide expression in rat dorsal root ganglion cells and spinal cord after peripheral nerve injury with special reference to galanin. Neuroscience **33:** 587–604.

146. ZHANG, X., A.P. NICHOLAS & T. HOKFELT. 1995. Ultrastructural studies on peptides in the dorsal horn of the rat spinal cord. 2. Co-existence of galanin with other peptides in local neurons. Neuroscience **6:** 875–891.

147. TUCHSCHERER, M.M. & V.S. SEYBOLD. 1989. A quantitative study of the coexistence of peptides in varicosities within the superficial laminae of the dorsal horn of the rat spinal cord. J. Neurosci. **9:** 195–205.

148. KAR, S. & R. QUIRION. 1994. Galanin receptor binding sites in adult rat spinal cord respond differentially to neonatal capsaicin, dorsal rhizotomy and peripheral axotomy. Eur. J. Neurosci. **6:** 1917–1921.

149. WIESENFELD-HALLIN, Z., X.J. XU, M.J. VILLAR & T. HOKFELT. 1989. The effect of intrathecal galanin on the flexor reflex in rat: Increased depression after sciatic nerve section. Neurosci. Lett. **105:** 149–154.

150. WIESENFELD-HALLIN, Z., M.J. VILLAR & T. HOKFELT. 1989. The effects of intrathecal galanin and C-fiber stimulation on the flexor reflex in the rat. Brain Res. **486:** 205–213.

151. KURAISHI, Y., M. KAWAMURA, T. YAMAGUCHI, T. HOUTANI, S. KAWABATA, S. FUTAKI, N. FUJII & M. SATOH. 1991. Intrathecal injections of galanin and its antiserum affect nociceptive response of rat to mechanical, but not thermal, stimuli. Pain **44:** 321–324.

152. CRIDLAND, R.A. & J.L. HENRY. 1988. Effects of intrathecal administration of neuropeptides on a spinal nociceptive reflex in the rat: VIP, galanin, CGRP, TRH, somatostatin and angiotensin II. Neuropeptides **11:** 23–32.

153. PINCUS, D.W., E.M. DICICCO BLOOM & I.B. BLACK. 1990. Vasoactive intestinal peptide regulates mitosis, differentiation and survival of cultured sympathetic neuroblasts. Nature **343:** 564–567.

154. WAKISAKA, S., K.C. KAJANDER & G.J. BENNETT. 1991. Increased neuropeptide Y (NPY)-like immunoreactivity in rat sensory neurons following peripheral axotomy. Neurosci. Lett. **124:** 200–203.

155. NUEZ, B., D. MICHALOVICH, A. BYGRAVE, R. PLOEMACHER & F. GROSVELD. 1995. Defective hae-matopoiesis in fetal liver resulting from inactivation of the EKLF gene. Nature **375:** 316–318.
156. O'HALLORAN, D.J., P.M. JONES, J.H. STEEL, G. GON, A. GIAID, M.A. GHATEI, J.M. POLAK & S.R. BLOOM. 1990. Effect of endocrine manipulation on anterior pituitary galanin in the rat. Endocrinology **127:** 467–475.
157. KNIGHT, C.H., D.T. CALVERT & D.J. FLINT. 1986. Inhibitory effects of bromocriptine on mam-mary development and function in lactating mice. J. Endocrinol. **110:** 263–270.
158. KANDAN, S., V. GOPALAKRISHNAN, P. GOVINDARAJULU, R. INDIRA & T. MALATHI. 1983. Role of pro-lactin in human milk composition and serum lipids studied during suppression of galactorrhea with bromocriptine. Horm. Res **17:** 93–102.
159. RAINS, C.P., H.M. BRYSON & A. FITTON. 1995. Cabergoline. A review of its pharmacological properties and therapeutic potential in the treatment of hyperprolactinaemia and inhibition of lactation. Drugs **49:** 255–279.
160. ORMANDY, C.J., A. CAMUS, J. BARRA, D. DAMOTTE, B. LUCAS, H. BUTEAU, M. EDERY, N. BROUSSE, C. BABINET, N. BINART & P.A. KELLY. 1997. Null mutation of the prolactin receptor gene pro-duces multiple reproductive defects in the mouse. Genes Dev. **11:** 167–178.
161. SHAW, B.C., S.J. PIRRUCELLO & J.D. SHULL. 1997. Expression of the prolactin gene in normal and neoplastic human breast tissues and human mammary cell lines: Promoter usage and alterna-tive mRNA splicing. Breast Cancer Res. Treat. **44:** 243–253.
162. KIM, J.Y., Y. MIZOGUCHI, H. YAMAGUCHI, J. ENAMI & S. SAKAI. 1997. Removal of milk by suck-ling acutely increases the prolactin receptor gene expression in the lactating mouse mammary gland. Mol. Cell Endocrinol. **131:** 31–38.
163. ERIKSSON, M., B. LINDH, K. UVNAS MOBERG & T. HOKFELT. 1996. Distribution and origin of pep-tide-containing nerve fibres in the rat and human mammary gland. Neuroscience **70:** 227–245.
164. ORMANDY, C.J., C.S. LEE, H.F. ORMANDY, V. FAND, J. SHINE, G. PETERS & R.L. SUTHERLAND. 1998. Cancer Res. In press.
165. HYDE, J.F., D.G. MORRISON, K.W. DRAKE, J.P. MOORE, JR. & B.E. MALEY. 1996. Vasoactive intes-tinal polypeptide mRNA and peptide levels are decreased in the anterior pituitary of the human growth hormone- releasing hormone transgenic mouse. J. Neuroendocrinol. **8:** 9–15.
166. SAIARDI, A., Y. BOZZI, J.H. BAIK & E. BORRELLI. 1997. Antiproliferative role of dopamine: Loss of D2 receptors causes hormonal dysfunction and pituitary hyperplasia. Neuron **19:** 115–126.
167. LIU, X., G.W. ROBINSON, K.U. WAGNER, L. GARRETT, B.A. WYNSHAW & L. HENNIGHAUSEN. 1997. Stat5a is mandatory for adult mammary gland development and lactogenesis. Genes Dev. **11:** 179–186.
168. LANDRY, M., D. ROCHE & A. CALAS. 1995. Short-term effects of centrally administered galanin on the hyperosmotically stimulated expression of vasopressin in the rat hypothalamus. An in situ hybridization and immunohistochemistry study. Neuroendocrinology **61:** 393-labeled.
169. SEUFFERLEIN, T. & E. ROZENGURT. 1996. Galanin, neurotensin, and phorbol esters rapidly stimu-late activation of mitogen-activated protein kinase in small cell lung cancer cells. Cancer Res. **56:** 5758–5764.

Galanin in Normal and Hyperplastic Anterior Pituitary Cells

From Pituitary Tumor Cell Lines to Transgenic Mice

JAMES F. HYDE,[a] JOSEPH P. MOORE, JR., AND AIHUA CAI

Department of Anatomy and Neurobiology, University of Kentucky Medical Center, Lexington, Kentucky 40536, USA

ABSTRACT: Studies on the regulation of galanin expression in the epithelial cells of the anterior pituitary gland have provided a wealth of insight into the cellular and molecular biology of this unique peptide. Galanin is localized within subpopulations of specific pituitary cell types, and hypothalamic as well as gonadal factors including dopamine, somatostatin, thyrotropin-releasing hormone, growth hormone-releasing hormone (GHRH), estrogen, and progesterone dynamically regulate its expression and release. Galanin gene expression and peptide secretion are markedly increased in estrogen-induced prolactinomas, wherein galanin serves as both an autocrine and paracrine hormone regulating prolactin secretion. Galanin mRNA and peptide levels are also dramatically elevated in somatotroph adenomas of human GHRH transgenic mice. Moreover, galanin secretion is increased from the hyperplastic somatotrophs of hGHRH transgenic mice. However, not all pituitary adenomas are associated with increased galanin gene expression; galanin synthesis is repressed in ^{131}I-induced thyrotroph adenomas. Thus, galanin acts locally to regulate pituitary hormone secretion and appears to act as a mitogenic factor to increase the proliferation of pituitary cells in a cell-type specific manner.

The anterior pituitary gland is one of only several non-neuronal tissues expressing the galanin gene in mammals. Soon after the discovery of the amino acid sequence of galanin, its cDNA sequence was reported and the remarkable sensitivity of pituitary galanin gene expression to estrogen was described.[1,2] During the last several years we studied the role and regulation of galanin in the anterior pituitary gland with particular emphasis on pituitary tumors. We employed a variety of animal models as well as cell culture systems in order to begin to elucidate the functions of galanin within the diverse cell populations comprising the anterior pituitary gland. Over the last two decades numerous peptides were localized to the pituitary gland. These small, biologically active peptides are much less abundant than the classic pituitary hormones, and their study has been difficult due to a lack of sensitive assay systems. Thus, many functions of these peptides in the anterior pituitary remain unknown. The dramatic induction of galanin gene expression in the rat anterior pituitary by estrogen made this 29 amino acid peptide a prime candidate for further study. Immunocytochemical studies showed that galanin is localized in somatotrophs and thyrotrophs of the male rat pituitary, whereas lactotrophs in female rats also express immunoreactive galanin.[3,4] Therefore, much of our work with galanin has focused on these pituitary cell types. Moreover, the coincidence of increased galanin gene expression with certain pituitary tumors has directed our experimental approaches.

[a]Address for correspondence: James F. Hyde, Ph.D., Department of Anatomy and Neurobiology, University of Kentucky Medical Center, 800 Rose Street (MN224), Lexington, KY 40536-0084. Phone, 606-323-6684; fax, 606-323-5946; e-mail, jfhyde00@pop.uky.edu

GALANIN SECRETION FROM PITUITARY CELLS *IN VITRO*

The ovariectomized, estrogen-treated Fischer 344 rat serves as an excellent model system to study estrogen-responsive genes due to its inherent hypersensitivity to estrogen.[5] We used this animal model to demonstrate that galanin peptide is, in fact, secreted from anterior pituitary cells through a regulated, rather than constitutive, secretory pathway.[6] We showed that dopamine and somatostatin directly inhibit galanin secretion from pituitary cells *in vitro* in a concentration-dependent manner and that thyrotropin-releasing hormone stimulates galanin release from estrogen-treated pituitary cells.[6] Pituitary cells from estrogen-treated female Fischer 344 rats secreted significantly greater amounts of galanin *in vitro* than did those cells obtained from estrogen-treated male Fischer 344 rats. This observation was directly correlated to the more dramatic pituitary hyperplasia observed in estrogen-treated female Fischer 344 rats than in males.[6] Moreover, we showed that estrogen increases galanin release by a direct effect on pituitary cells *in vitro* and that growth hormone-releasing hormone (GHRH) is capable of stimulating galanin release from pituitary cells when estrogen levels are low and galanin is principally localized in somatotrophs.[7] Using immunogold histochemistry at the level of the electron microscope, we demonstrated that galanin is stored in secretory granules.[8] In addition, dual-labeling experiments indicated that galanin and prolactin are localized in the same secretory granules. Interestingly, only a subpopulation of the hyperplastic lactotrophs contained immunoreactive galanin. These data provided direct morphologic evidence for the cosecretion of prolactin and galanin and provided a mechanism for the dual regulation of their secretion by either hypothalamic factors or autocrine/paracrine factors. Furthermore, these data suggested that colocalization of galanin in only a subset of lactotrophs might underlie the well-described heterogeneity of lactotrophs.

Recently we examined the role of galanin in regulating prolactin secretion in hyperplastic lactotrophs.[9] In estrogen-treated Fischer 344 rats, one third of the lactotrophs contained galanin mRNA, and more than 90% of the galanin mRNA-containing cells were lactotrophs. We quantified prolactin secretion at the level of the single cell by using the reverse hemolytic plaque assay and subsequently quantified galanin mRNA levels in the same individual lactotrophs. We found that prolactin secretion from galanin-positive lactotrophs was significantly greater than that from galanin-negative lactotrophs. Furthermore, treatment with galanin antiserum significantly decreased prolactin secretion from galanin-positive cells. Treatment with synthetic galanin significantly increased prolactin secretion from galanin-negative lactotrophs. These data provide direct evidence that galanin derived from the estrogen-treated rat pituitary stimulated prolactin secretion in both autocrine and paracrine manners.

GALANIN IN ESTROGEN-INDUCED PROLACTINOMAS: REGULATION OF PITUITARY GALANIN GENE EXPRESSION AND SECRETION BY HYPOTHALAMIC FACTORS *IN VIVO*

To further examine the possible role of galanin in the genesis of estrogen-induced prolactinomas, we used two pharmacologic treatments known to inhibit prolactin secretion. Estrogen-treated Fischer 344 rats were administered either the dopamine receptor agonist bromocriptine[10] or the somatostatin receptor agonist SMS 201-995 (octreotide)[11] for at least 2 weeks. Both drugs significantly reduced plasma levels of galanin and prolactin, reduced galanin mRNA levels in the pituitary, and profoundly inhibited the estrogen-induced pituitary tumor formation. These data further support the notion the galanin may serve a role in regulating the proliferation of lactotrophs and may mediate some of the actions of estrogen on altered pituitary function. Furthermore, these data support and extend our *in vitro* studies on the regulation of galanin gene expression and secretion to the whole animal and further implicate an important role for galanin in regulating prolactin secretion when estrogen levels are elevated.

GALANIN IN SOMATOTROPH ADENOMAS: HUMAN GHRH TRANSGENIC MICE AS AN ESTROGEN-INDEPENDENT ANIMAL MODEL OF PITUITARY TUMOR FORMATION

To evaluate the possible role of galanin in estrogen-independent pituitary adenomas we used the male human GHRH (hGHRH) transgenic mouse. These transgenic mice produce high plasma levels of hGHRH and mouse GH and develop a somatotroph hyperplasia that eventually progresses to become a mammosomatotroph adenoma.[12] When we initiated these studies, little was known about galanin in the mouse. Although the specific pituitary cell types expressing the galanin gene in the mouse had not been reported, we showed that the Ames dwarf mouse, which harbors a mutation in the *Pit-1* gene and lacks lactotrophs, somatotrophs, and thyrotrophs, fails to express the galanin gene in the anterior pituitary gland.[13] Using dual fluorescent immunocytochemistry we showed that lactotrophs, somatotrophs, and thyrotrophs contain galanin peptide in the normal and hGHRH transgenic mouse.[14] Galanin gene expression and peptide content were dramatically increased in the anterior pituitary gland of the male hGHRH transgenic mouse than in normal control mice.[15] Moreover, the development of somatotroph hyperplasia in hGHRH transgenic mice was directly correlated to the increase in galanin mRNA and peptide concentrations. We also showed that galanin secretion was increased at the level of the single pituitary cell in hGHRH transgenic mice,[16] further supporting the hypothesis that increased galanin secretion may result in pituitary cell hyperplasia.

To determine if the changes in pituitary galanin gene expression in the hGHRH transgenic mouse are specific for galanin or represent a more generalized phenomenon, we examined a variety of other pituitary peptides. Vasoactive intestinal polypeptide (VIP) has been implicated as an important regulator of prolactin release,[17] and like galanin, VIP has been proposed to act as a growth-promoting factor in a variety of systems.[18,19] In contrast to galanin, VIP peptide and mRNA concentrations in the anterior pituitary of hGHRH transgenic mice were significantly reduced 50%.[20] As determined by quantifying the number of VIP-containing pituitary cells, these changes were determined to be due to a decrease in the density of VIP-containing pituitary cells in the hyperplastic pituitary (i.e., a dilutional effect). Thus, the increase in galanin gene expression in the hGHRH transgenic is not a global pituitary peptide effect. As shown in TABLE 1, we have also examined calcitonin gene-related peptide (CGRP), neuropeptide Y (NPY), and substance P in the anterior pituitary gland of the male hGHRH transgenic mouse. Similar to VIP, CGRP, and NPY concentrations in the anterior pituitary gland were significantly decreased in hGHRH transgenic mice. By contrast, substance P concentrations were increased nearly sevenfold. In the rat, substance P was localized in gonadotrophs and lactotrophs,[21] and may play a role in regulating pituitary hormone secretion.[22,23] However, the precise cellular localization and role of substance P in mouse pituitary function remain to be determined.

GALANIN IN THYROTROPH ADENOMAS

The association of increased galanin gene expression with hyperplastic lactotrophs and somatotrophs led us to examine galanin gene expression in an animal model of thyrotroph hyperplasia/adenoma formation. We used ^{131}I-treated mice (radiothyroidectomy) as a model system to study the potential role of galanin in the development of thyrotroph adenomas.[24] After destruction of the thyroid gland, the anterior pituitary gland becomes hyperplastic and eventually develops a thyrotroph adenoma over the course of a 10-month period. In opposition to our results with somatotroph and lactotroph adenomas, we found that pituitary galanin mRNA and peptide levels were decreased more than 80% in the radiothyroidectomy-induced thyrotroph adenomas.[24] Treatment of ^{131}I-treated mice with T_3 increased pituitary galanin peptide levels fourfold, but did not fully restore galanin peptide expression. Estrogen increased pituitary galanin peptide levels 30-fold in radiothyroidectomized mice, but these levels of peptide were still below those attained in control mice. These data showed that thyroid hormones are important positive regulators of galanin gene expression in the mouse and that galanin does not have a critical stimulatory role in the proliferation of thyrotrophs.

GALANIN IN PITUITARY TUMOR CELL LINES

We examined a variety of established pituitary cell lines to begin to elucidate the cellular and molecular actions of galanin and the regulation of its expression. The transplantable MtTW-10 mammosomatotroph pituitary tumor expresses the galanin gene at very high levels and has retained its regulation by estrogen.[25] Unfortunately, the regulation of galanin secretion in these pituitary tumor cells is aberrant. Although somatostatin inhibited galanin, prolactin, and growth hormone release from MtTW-10 cells *in vitro*, only pharmacologic doses of dopamine inhibited hormone secretion and thyroid-releasing hormone (TRH) failed to alter hormone release. Some of the normal complement of cell sur-

TABLE 1. Anterior Pituitary Concentrations of Immunoreactive Peptides in Male hGHRH Transgenic Mice and Normal Siblings[a]

	Calcitonin Gene-Related Peptide	Neuropeptide Y	Substance P
hGHRH transgenic mice	22.4 ± 1.7^b	143.6 ± 20.5^b	218.6 ± 42.7^b
Normal sibling mice	33.6 ± 3.6	264.5 ± 41.6	30.3 ± 6.4

[a]Immunoreactive peptide concentrations in acetic acid extracts were determined by using specific radioimmunoassays (Peninsula Laboratories, Inc., Belmont, California). Each value ($n = 4$–6 mice per group) is expressed as picogram of peptide per milligram of total protein (mean ± SEM).

[b]Significantly different from normal sibling mice ($p < 0.05$).

face receptors apparently are either absent or nonfunctional. Nevertheless, MtTW-10 pituitary tumor cells are a useful tool for studying the transcriptional regulation of the galanin gene by estrogen.[26] Another lactotroph cell line, 235-1 cells, has also been shown to produce and secrete galanin.[27] Like MtTW-10 cells, 235-1 pituitary cells also retain their sensitivity to estrogen but do not respond normally to hypothalamic factors.[27] We recently described a pluripotential pituitary cell line, RC-4B/C, that robustly expresses the galanin gene, but unlike MtTW-10 and 235-1 cells, has lost its responsiveness to estrogen.[28] A comparison of galanin gene expression in MtTW-10, RC-4B/C, and 235-1 pituitary cells is shown in Figure 1. MtTW-10 and RC-4B/C cells show high levels of galanin mRNA expression, whereas galanin mRNA was undetectable in 235-1 and GH3 pituitary cells by Northern blot analysis. Immunoreactive galanin peptide is also undetectable in GH3 cells (J.F. Hyde, unpublished observation). Finally, α-TSH pituitary cells express low levels of galanin mRNA and do not appear sensitive to estradiol.[24] Despite their individual idiosyncrasies, some of these cell lines will undoubtedly be useful in the years to come as model cell culture systems in further exploring the function and regulation of galanin in pituitary cells.

OVEREXPRESSION OF GALANIN IN GH3 PITUITARY TUMOR CELLS

The recent cloning of a variety of galanin receptor subtypes showed that at least one of these receptors (GALR2) is expressed in the anterior pituitary gland.[29] GH3 pituitary tumor cells do not express the galanin gene (Figure 1), but do express GALR2 mRNA.[29] We exploited this property of GH3 pituitary cells and generated several GH3 cell lines stably expressing the mouse galanin gene. These new cell lines should be powerful tools to explore the regulation of GALR2 gene expression by chronic exposure to galanin peptide as well as to provide important information about the regulation of mammosomatotroph function by galanin. In particular, the effects on basal and stimulated prolactin and growth hormone gene expression and secretion will provide information about the potential consequences of chronic exposure to high levels of galanin, such as those associated with certain pituitary adenomas.

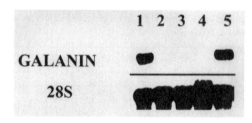

FIGURE 1. Northern blot analysis of galanin gene expression in pituitary tumor cell lines. *Lane 1,* 5μg RC-4B/C pituitary cell RNA; *Lane 2,* 5μg GH3 pituitary cell RNA; *Lane 3,* 5μg 235-1 pituitary cell RNA; *Lane 4,* 10μg 235-1 pituitary cell RNA; and *Lane 5,* 5μg MtTW-10 pituitary tumor RNA. The radiolabeled oligonucleotide probes (galanin and 28SrRNA) used for Northern blot analysis were previously described.[13]

TRANSGENIC MICE: DISRUPTION AND
OVEREXPRESSION OF THE GALANIN GENE

Recently, transgenic mice with a disrupted galanin gene have been generated.[30] Thus far, abnormalities in lactation, pituitary responsiveness to estrogen, and peripheral nerve injury have been described. These mice will undoubtedly uncover additional physiologic roles for galanin in the years to come. Overexpression of the galanin gene in the anterior pituitary of transgenic mice has been achieved by using either 310 bp of the rat growth hormone promoter[31] or 2.5 kb of the rat prolactin promoter (Cai and Hyde, manuscript in preparation). Because of the incidence of upregulated galanin gene expression in somatotroph and lactotroph adenomas, the use of transgenic mice to study the direct effects of pituitary cell-specific overexpression of galanin is particularly relevant to these pathophysiologic conditions. The development of pituitary adenomas and/or aberrant pituitary hormone gene expression and/or secretion in these animal models will provide direct evidence for a causal link between increased galanin secretion from pituitary cells and pituitary dysfunction.

SUMMARY

The prevailing data show that galanin plays a variety of important roles in anterior pituitary function. Accumulating evidence shows that galanin of pituitary origin can act as (1) a stimulatory autocrine factor to augment pituitary hormone secretion, (2) a stimulatory paracrine factor regulating hormone secretion from neighboring cells, (3) an endocrine hormone regulating peripheral functions, and (4) a mitogenic factor regulating the proliferation and possibly differentiation of anterior pituitary cells. FIGURE 2 depicts some of these interactions. Somatotrophs and lactotrophs currently appear to be the predominant pituitary cell types impacted directly by galanin. However, the role of pituitary galanin in regulating other pituitary cell types remains to be determined. One of the more confounding issues remaining with regard to elucidating the physiologic functions of galanin in the

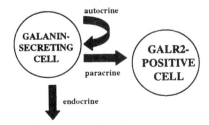

Peripheral Blood/Peripheral Galanin Receptors

FIGURE 2. Schematic diagram of galanin as an endocrine, paracrine, and autocrine pituitary peptide. Galanin-containing pituitary cells (notably lactotrophs, somatotrophs, and thyrotrophs in the rodent pituitary gland) secrete galanin that may then interact with (1) galanin receptors (i.e., GAL2) on the same cells; (2) galanin receptors on neighboring pituitary cells; or (3) peripheral galanin receptors (i.e., GALR1, GALR2, GALR3, etc).

anterior pituitary gland is to distinguish the exact roles for galanin from either hypothalamic or pituitary origin. Clearly in an environment with high levels of estrogen, the anterior pituitary gland synthesizes and secretes more galanin than does the hypothalamus. Thus, one must consider galanin of anterior pituitary origin to be of primary importance when estrogen levels are elevated. However, when estrogen levels are low, the impact of hypothalamic galanin on anterior pituitary function must be carefully weighed and considered because its impact will likely be considerable. Furthermore, the influence of hypothalamic galanin on neurotransmitter/neuropeptide release from nerve terminals in the median eminence requires further study, for this too may dramatically regulate pituitary hormone secretion, albeit in an indirect manner.

REFERENCES

1. KAPLAN, L.M., S.M. GABRIEL, J.I. KOENIG, M.E. SUNDAY, E.R. SPINDEL, J.B. MARTIN & W.W. CHIN. 1988. Galanin is an estrogen-inducible secretory product of the rat anterior pituitary. Proc. Natl. Acad. Sci. USA **85:** 7408–7412.
2. VRONTAKIS, M.E., L.M. PEDEN, M.L. DUCKWORTH & H.G. FRIESEN. 1987. Isolation and characterization of a complementary DNA (galanin) clone from estrogen-induced pituitary tumor messenger RNA. J. Biol. Chem. **262:** 16755–16758.
3. STEEL, J.H., G. GON, D.J. O'HALLORAN, P.M. JONES, N. YANAIHARA, H. ISHIKAWA, S.R. BLOOM & J.M. POLAK. 1989. Galanin and vasoactive intestinal polypeptide are colocalised with classical pituitary hormones and show plasticity of expression. Histochemistry **93:** 183–189.
4. HSU, D.W., M. EL-AZOUZI, P. McL. BLACK, W.W. CHIN, E.T. HEDLEY-WHITE & L.M. KAPLAN. 1990. Estrogen increases galanin immunoreactivity in hyperplastic prolactin-secreting cells in Fischer 344 rats. Endocrinology **126:** 3159–3167.
5. WIKLUND, J., N. WERTZ & J. GORSKI. 1981. A comparison of estrogen effects on uterine and pituitary growth and prolactin synthesis in F344 and Holtzman rats. Endocrinology **109:** 1700–1707.
6. HYDE, J.F. & B.K. KELLER. 1991. Galanin secretion from anterior pituitary cells in vitro is regulated by dopamine, somatostatin, and thyrotropin-releasing hormone. Endocrinology **128:** 917–922.
7. HEMMER, A. & J.F. HYDE. 1992. Regulation of galanin secretion from pituitary cells in vitro by estradiol and GHRH. Peptides **13:** 1201–1206.
8. HYDE, J.F., M.G. ENGLE & B.E. MALEY. 1991. Colocalization of galanin and prolactin within secretory granules of anterior pituitary cells in estrogen-treated Fischer 344 rats. Endocrinology **129:** 270–276.
9. CAI, A., R.C. BOWERS, J.P. MOORE, JR. & J.F. HYDE. 1998. Function of galanin in the anterior pituitary of estrogen-treated Fischer 344 rats: Autocrine and paracrine regulation of prolactin secretion. Endocrinology **139:** 2452–2458.
10. HYDE, J.F., B.K. KELLER & G. HOWARD. 1992. Dopaminergic regulation of galanin gene expression in the rat anterior pituitary gland. J. Neuroendocrinol. **4:** 449–454.
11. HYDE, J.F. & G. HOWARD. 1992. Regulation of galanin gene expression in the rat anterior pituitary gland by the somatostatin analog SMS 201–995. Endocrinology **131:** 2097–2102.
12. MAYO, K.E., R.E. HAMMER, L.W. SWANSON, R.L. BRINSTER, M.G. ROSENFELD & R.M. EVANS. 1988. Dramatic pituitary hyperplasia in transgenic mice expressing a human growth hormone-releasing factor gene. Mol. Endocrinol. **2:** 606–612.
13. HYDE, J.F., A. BARTKE & B.M. DAVIS. 1993. Galanin gene expression in the hypothalamic-pituitary axis of the Ames dwarf mouse. Mol. Cell. Neurosci. **4:** 298–303.
14. MOORE, J.P., JR., B.E. MALEY & J.F. HYDE. 1997. Evaluation of the distribution, secretion, and function of the peptide galanin in the anterior pituitary glands of human growth hormone-releasing hormone transgenic and normal mice. Soc. Neurosci. Abstr. **23:** 1250.
15. MOORE, J.P., JR., D.G. MORRISON & J.F. HYDE. 1994. Galanin gene expression is increased in the anterior pituitary gland of the human growth hormone-releasing hormone transgenic mouse. Endocrinology **134:** 2005–2010.

16. MOORE, J.P., JR. & J.F. HYDE. 1996. Effect of chronic growth hormone releasing hormone on individual mouse pituitary cell secretion of growth hormone, prolactin and galanin as measured by the cell immunoblot assay. 10th International Congress of Endocrinology, San Francisco, CA. (Abstr).

17. KATO, Y., Y. IWASAKI, J. IWASAKI, H. ABE, N. YANAIHARA & H. IMURA. 1978. Prolactin release by vasoactive intestinal polypeptide in rats. Endocrinology 103: 554–558.

18. GRESSENS, P., J.M. HILL, I. GOZES, M. FRIDKIN & D.E. BRENNEMAN. 1993. Growth factor function of vasoactive intestinal peptide in whole cultured mouse embryos. Nature 362: 155–158.

19. GOZES I. & D.E. BRENNEMAN. 1993. Neuropeptides as growth and differentiation factors in general and VIP in particular. J. Mol. Neurosci. 4: 1–9.

20. HYDE, J.F., D.G. MORRISON, K.W. DRAKE, J.P. MOORE, JR. & B.E. MALEY. 1996. Vasoactive intestinal polypeptide mRNA and peptide levels are decreased in the anterior pituitary of the human growth hormone-releasing hormone transgenic mouse. J. Neuroendocrinol. 8: 9–15.

21. MOREL, G., J.A. CHAYVIALLE, B. KERDELHUE & P.M. DUBOIS. 1982. Ultrastructural evidence for endogenous substance-P-like immunoreactivity in the rat pituitary gland. Neuroendocrinol. 35: 86–92.

22. KATO, Y., S. CHIHARA, S. OGHO, Y. IWASAKI, H. ABE & H. IMURA. 1976. Growth hormone and prolactin release by substance P in rats. Life Sci. 19: 441–446.

23. VIJAYAN E. & S.M. MCCANN. 1979. In vitro and in vivo effects of substance P and neurotensin on gonadotropin and prolactin release. Endocrinology 105: 64–68.

24. HYDE, J.F., J.P. MOORE, JR., K.W. DRAKE & D.G. MORRISON. 1996. Galanin gene expression in radiothyroidectomy-induced thyrotroph adenomas. Am. J. Physiol. 271: E24–E30.

25. HYDE, J.F., D.G. MORRISON, J.P. MOORE, JR. & G. HOWARD. 1993. MtTW-10 pituitary tumor cells: Galanin gene expression and peptide secretion. Endocrinology 133: 2588–2593.

26. HOWARD, G., L. PENG & J.F. HYDE. 1997. An estrogen receptor binding site within the human galanin gene. Endocrinology 138: 4649–4656.

27. WYNICK, D., P.J. HAMMOND, K.O. AKINSANYA & S.R. BLOOM. 1993. Galanin regulates basal and oestrogen-stimulated lactotroph function. Nature 364: 529–532.

28. HYDE, J.F., A. CAI & J.P. MOORE, JR. 1996. Characterization of a pituitary cell line producing the peptide galanin. Soc. Neurosci. Abstr. 22: 1591.

29. FATHI, Z., A.M. CUNNINGHAM, L.G. IBEN, P.B. BATTAGLINO, S.A. WARD, K.A. NICHOL, K.A. PINE, J. WANG, M.E. GOLDSTEIN, T.P. IISMAA & I.A. ZIMANYI. 1997. Cloning, pharmacological characterization and distribution of a novel galanin receptor. Mol. Brain Res. 51: 49–59.

30. WYNICK, D., C. SMALL, M. GHATEI, S.R. BLOOM & V. PACHNIS. 1996. Targeted disruption of the murine galanin gene lowers serum prolactin levels and abolishes lactation. 10th International Congress of Endocrinology, San Francisco, CA. (Abstr).

31. VRONTAKIS, M.E., P. PERUMAL & C. FARACI. 1996. Galanin gene expression in the pituitary of transgenic mice. 10th International Congress of Endocrinology, San Francisco, CA. (Abstr).

Structural Organization and Chromosomal Localization of Three Human Galanin Receptor Genes

TIINA P. IISMAA,[a,d] ZAHRA FATHI,[b] YVONNE J. HORT,[a]
LAWRENCE G. IBEN,[b] JULIE L. DUTTON,[a] ELIZABETH BAKER,[c]
GRANT R. SUTHERLAND,[c] AND JOHN SHINE[a]

[a]Neurobiology Program, The Garvan Institute of Medical Research, St. Vincent's Hospital,
384 Victoria Street, Sydney NSW 2010, Australia

[b]Neuroscience Drug Discovery, Bristol-Myers Squibb Pharmaceutical Research Institute,
5 Research Parkway, Wallingford, Connecticut 06492, USA

[c]Centre for Medical Genetics, Department of Cytogenetics and Molecular Genetics,
Women's and Children's Hospital, North Adelaide, South Australia 5006

ABSTRACT: Human galanin receptor subtypes GALR1, GALR2, and GALR3 are
encoded by separate genes that are located on human chromosomes 18q23, 17q25.3,
and 22q13.1, respectively. The exon:intron organization of the gene encoding GALR2
(*GALNR2*) and GALR3 (*GALNR3*) is conserved, with exon 1 encoding the NH_2-ter-
minus to the end of transmembrane domain 3 and exon 2 encoding the remainder of
the receptor, from the second intracellular loop to the COOH-terminus. This conser-
vation of structural organization is indicative of a common evolutionary origin for
GALNR2 and *GALNR3*. The exon:intron organization of the gene encoding GALR1
(*GALNR1*) is different from that of *GALNR2* and *GALNR3*, with exon 1 encoding the
NH_2-terminus to the end of transmembrane domain 5, exon 2 encoding the third
intracellular loop, and exon 3 encoding the remainder of the receptor, from transmembrane domain 6 to the COOH-terminus. The structural organization of
GALNR1 suggests convergent evolution for this gene and represents a structural
organization that is unique among genes encoding G-protein–coupled receptors.

The neuropeptide galanin occurs in the nervous system of vertebrate and invertebrate
species, and the sequence of the peptide has been reported for 15 species to date.
Human galanin is a 30 amino acid nonamidated peptide. In other species for which the
entire sequence is known, galanin comprises 29 amino acids and is COOH-terminally amidated. Amino acids 1-14 are conserved in all species, except for a single substitution of
Ala for Ser6 in tuna fish galanin.[1]

Consistent with widespread distribution throughout the central and peripheral nervous
system, galanin has a broad range of neuroendocrine and physiologic actions. These
include modulation of pituitary hormone secretion, inhibition of the release of neurotransmitters that may play a role in memory acquisition or contribute to anoxic damage in the
brain, modulation of appetite and sexual behavior, as well as effects on pain, gastrointestinal motility, heart rate, and blood pressure.[2,3] Galanin is also expressed in human breast

[d]Address for correspondence: Tiina Iismaa, Neurobiology Program, Garvan Institute of Medical
Research, 384 Victoria Street, Sydney NSW 2010, Australia. Phone, +61 2 9295 8293;
fax, +61 2 9295 8281; e-mail, t.iismaa@garvan.unsw.edu.au

cancer cells and has mitogenic effects in certain types of cancer.[4–6] The use of truncated forms and analogs of galanin, together with chimeric galanin peptides that behave as agonists or antagonists in different physiologic assays, initially provided pharmacologic evidence for the existence of galanin receptor subtypes, which may mediate specific effects of galanin in discrete tissues or organ systems. To date, three galanin receptor subtypes, designated GALR1, GALR2, and GALR3, have been cloned. They are members of the G-protein–coupled receptor superfamily and are each encoded by a different gene. In this report, we describe the structural organization of these genes and their chromosomal localization.

STRUCTURAL ORGANIZATION OF THE
GENE ENCODING GALR1 (*GALNR1*)

The isolation and characterization of genomic DNA clones containing the gene encoding GALR1 in human (*GALNR1*) and mouse (*Galnr1*) have revealed a structural organization that is conserved between the two species and is unique among genes encoding G-protein–coupled receptors.[7] The coding sequence of human and mouse GALR1, which gives rise to proteins of 349 and 348 amino acid residues, respectively, is contained on three exons. Exon 1 encodes the NH_2-terminal end and the first five transmembrane (TM) domains, exon 2 encodes the third intracellular loop, and exon 3 encodes the remainder of the receptor, from TM6 to the COOH-terminus. Coding of the third intracellular loop of GALR1 on a discrete exon is of interest, as this segment of many G-protein–coupled receptors is involved in interaction with G-proteins and, in some receptors, is the site of alternative splicing to generate functional diversity in receptor subtypes.[8,9] The structural organization of *GALNR1* raises the possibility of alternative splicing of exon 2 within the GALR1 transcript, but the isolation and characterization of several human and rat GALR1 cDNA clones have not yet provided evidence for this[7,10–14] (Ross [1995]: GenBank Accession U23854).

The sizes of the introns in *GALNR1* were determined by long-range polymerase chain reaction (PCR) amplification of human genomic DNA and Southern blotting of amplification products using oligonucleotide probes generated against intron sequence (FIG. 1). The sizes of introns 1 and 2 were determined to be ~5 and ~11 kb, respectively, consistent with restriction endonuclease mapping data of the cloned *GALNR1* locus.[7]

The transcription start site of the human GALR1 transcript has not been defined, but the sequence of both hypothalamic and human Bowes melanoma cDNA clones encoding GALR1[7,15] (GenBank Accession A46237) is contiguous with genomic sequence for approximately 720 nucleotides upstream of the translation inititation codon. This suggests that the start of transcription occurs at least this distance upstream of the translation initiation codon. The 5′ upstream region of *GALNR1* does not contain consensus TATA or CCAAT boxes or putative transcription factor recognition sites within approximately 1 kb of the translation initiation codon. In human Bowes melanoma cells, the 3′-untranslated region of the GALR1 transcript comprises 1234 nucleotides of 3′ untranslated sequence followed by a poly(A) tail of approximately 30 residues.[7]

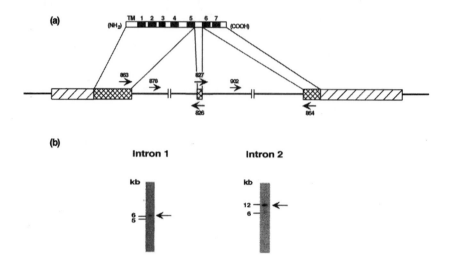

FIGURE 1. (a) Genomic organization of the gene encoding the human GALR1 galanin receptor (*GALNR1*). At the top is a schematic representation of the mature GALR1 galanin receptor protein. Putative transmembrane (TM) domains are shown as *black boxes* and are numbered 1-7, and other parts of the receptor protein are shown as *white boxes*. The *lower line* depicts the exon:intron organization of *GALNR1*. *Cross-hatched boxes* represent coding sequence. *Lightly hatched boxes* represent noncoding exon sequence. Segments of the mature GALR1 galanin receptor protein encoded by each of the exons are indicated. The positions of oligonucleotide primer pairs [863, 826] and [827, 864], which were used in long-range PCR amplification of fragments spanning introns 1 and 2, respectively, are shown, as are the positions of oligonucleotide probes 878 and 902, which were used for Southern hybridization detection of PCR amplification products. **(b)** Autoradiograph of long-range PCR amplification products spanning introns 1 and 2 of *GALNR1*. *Arrows* indicate hybridizing bands.

STRUCTURAL ORGANIZATION OF
THE GENE ENCODING GALR2 (*GALNR2*)

Both cDNA and genomic clones encoding human GALR2 were recently isolated.[16,17] Human GALR2 is a 387 residue protein that exhibits 40% identity with human GALR1 protein sequence (FIG. 2). The exon:intron organization of *GALNR2* is different from that of *GALNR1*, with the coding sequence of human GALR2 being encoded on two exons that are separated by an intron of approximately 1.4 kb.[17] Exon 1 encodes the NH_2-terminal end and the first three TM domains of GALR2, and exon 2 encodes the remainder of the receptor, from intracellular loop 2 to the COOH-terminus (FIG. 3). This structural organization is conserved in the rat, as indicated by the isolation and characterization of a partially processed hypothalamic cDNA transcript encoding rat GALR2.[18]

```
                    TM1
hGALR1   1   MELAVGNLSEGNASWPEPPAPEPGPLFGIGVENFVTLVVFGLIFALGVLGNSLVITVLARSKPG---K    65
hGALR2   1                    MNVSGCPGAGNASQAGGGGWHPEAVIVPLLFALIFLVGTVGNTLVLAVLLRGG----Q    55
hGALR3   1                      MADAQNISLDSPGSVGAVAVPVVFALIFLLGTVGNGLVLAVLLQPGPSAWQE         52

                   TM2                                    TM3
hGALR1  66   PRSTTNLFILNLSIADLAYLLFCIPFQATVYALPTWVLGAFICKFIHYFFTVSMLVSIFTLAAMSVDR   133
hGALR2  56   AVSTTNLFILNLGVADLCFILCCVPFQATIYTLDGWVFGSELCKAVHFLIFLTMHASSFTLAAVSLDR   123
hGALR3  53   PGSTTDLFILNLAVADLCFILSCVPFQATIYTLDAWLFGALVCKAVHLLIYLTMYASSFTLAAVSVDR   120

                                          TM4
hGALR1 134   YVAIVHSRRSSSLRVSRNATLGVGCIWALSIAMASPVAYHQGLFHPRASNQTFCWEQWPDPRHKKAYV   201
hGALR2 124   YLAIRYPLHSRELRTPRNALAAIGLIWGLSLLFSGPYSYYRQSQL--ANLTVCHPAWSAP-RRRAMD    198
hGALR3 121   YLAVRHPLRSRALRTPRNARAAVGLVWLLAALFSAPYLSYYGTVRY--GALELCVPAWEDA-RRRALD   185

                TM5                                      TM6
hGALR1 202   VCTFVFGYLLPLLLICFCYAKVLNHLHKKLKNMSKKSEASK----KKTAQTVLVVVVFGISWLPHHI    265
hGALR2 189   ICTFVFSYLLPVLVLGLTYARTLRYLWRAVDPVAAGSGARR--AKRKVTRMILIVAALFCLCWMPHHA   254
hGALR3 186   VATFAAGYLLPVAVVSLAYGRTLRFLWAAVGPAGAAEARRRATGRAGRAMLAVAALYALCWGPHHA    253

                  TM7
hGALR1 266   IHLWAEFGVFPLTPASFLFRITAHCLAYSNSSVNPIIYAFLSENFRKAYKQVFKC------HIRKDSH   327
hGALR2 255   LILCVWFGQFPLTRATYALRILSHLVSYANSCVNPIVYALVSKHFRKGFR--TICAGLLGRAPGRASG   320
hGALR3 254   LILCFWYGREAFSPATYACRLASHCLAYANSCLNPLVYALASRHFRARFRRLWPCGRRRHRARRALR    321

hGALR1 328   LSDTKEN---KSRIDTPPSTNCTHV                                             349
hGALR2 321   RVCAAARGTHSGSVLERESSDLLHMSEAAGALRPCPGASQPCILEPCPGPSWQGPKAGDSILTVDVA    387
hGALR3 322   RVRPASSGPPGCPGDARPSGRLLAGGGQGPEPREGPVHGGEAARGPE                       368
```

FIGURE 2. Alignment of human GALR1, GALR2, and GALR3 amino acid sequences. Identical residues are shaded and putative transmembrane (TM) domains are indicated by overlining.

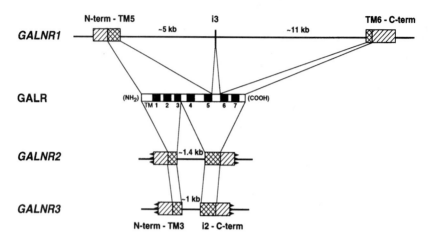

FIGURE 3. Genomic organization of *GALNR1, GALNR2,* and *GALNR3* galanin receptor genes. Within schematic representations of the exon:intron organization of the three genes encoding galanin receptors, *cross-hatched boxes* represent coding sequence and *lightly hatched boxes* represent noncoding exon sequence. The precise limits of noncoding exon sequence are not known for *GALNR2* and *GALNR3*. Below the representation of *GALNR1* is depicted a schematic of mature galanin receptor (GALR) protein. Putative transmembrane (TM) domains are shown as *black boxes* and are numbered 1-7, and other parts of the receptor protein are shown as *white boxes*. Segments of mature GALR protein encoded by each of the exons are indicated.

STRUCTURAL ORGANIZATION OF THE
GENE ENCODING GALR3 (*GALNR3*)

Putative exons identified in sequences isolated as part of the Human Genome Project (GenBank Accession Z82241, Z97630) exhibit homology on the order of 52% and 67% at the nucleic acid level with the coding region of human GALR1 and human GALR2, respectively. The deduced amino acid sequence of putative contiguous exons of this sequence predicts a protein of 368 residues, which is 92% identical to the sequence of rat GALR3,[19] and is 36% and 58% identical to human GALR1 and human GALR2, respectively (FIG. 2). Although functional activation of this putative human receptor protein in response to galanin has not yet been reported, the sequence data suggest it comprises a member of the galanin receptor family and is the human homolog of rat GALR3. Consequently, for the remainder of this discussion, the putative human receptor sequence will be referred to as human GALR3 and the gene encoding it will be identified as *GALNR3*. The structural organization of *GALNR3* is identical to that of *GALNR2* with respect to the position of the exon:intron boundaries (FIG. 3). The NH_2-terminal end and the first three TM domains of GALR3 are encoded on exon 1 (359 bp of coding sequence), and the remainder of the receptor is encoded on exon 2 (748 bp of coding sequence). The exons are separated by an intron of 954 bp.

Using a probe fragment corresponding to a segment of exon 2 of *GALNR3*, we isolated three independent P1 human genomic DNA clones encoding GALR3. Restriction endonuclease analysis and sequencing of the cloned DNAs identified a *Pst*I site within the intron which is polymorphic. Using oligonucleotide primers flanking the polymorphic *Pst*I site, *GALNR3* DNA was amplified by PCR from 21 human genomic DNA samples, and the amplified DNA was detected following incubation with *Pst*I restriction endonuclease using nested oligonucleotide probes in Southern hybridization. This preliminary analysis indicated that the allele containing the *Pst*I site within the intron of *GALNR3* occurred at a frequency of approximately 14%, with none of the DNA samples tested being homozygous for absence of the *Pst*I site. The significance of the *Pst*I polymorphism in the intron of *GALNR3* is currently unknown.

CHROMOSOMAL LOCALIZATION

A ~1-kb fragment corresponding to the coding region of human GALR1 was used to localize *GALNR1* to chromosome 18q23, in the vicinity of genes encoding cytochrome b5 (*CYB5*) and peptidase A (*PEPA*), and telomeric of the gene encoding myelin basic protein (*MBP*) at 18q22.1.[20] The gene encoding GALR1 in the mouse (*Galnr1*) occurs on mouse chromosome 18E4,[7,21] homologous with the human localization. Disease loci mapped to human chromosome 18q23 comprise a locus for bipolar disorder (manic-depressive illness) identified by analysis of two Costa Rican pedigrees[22] and a chromosomal deletion that gives rise to growth hormone insufficiency syndrome.[23]

A 1.6-kb fragment encompassing exon 2 of *GALNR2* was used in fluorescence *in situ* hybridization (FISH) to localize *GALNR2* to chromosome 17q25.3.[17] Disease loci for hereditary neuralgic amyotrophy (HNA) and Russell-Silver syndrome have been mapped

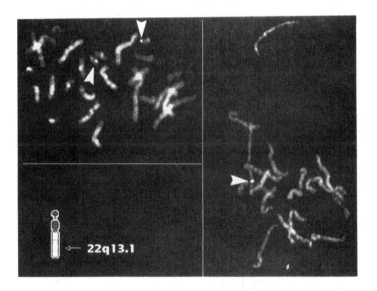

FIGURE 4. Chromosomal localization of *GALNR3*. *Arrows* indicate sites of hybridization at 22q13.1 on chromosomes counterstained with DAPI (4,6-diamino-2-phenylindole; for chromosome identification).

to 17q25.[24] (Genome Data Base - GDB™ Online Mendelian Inheritance in Man [NCBI]). HNA is a rare autosomal dominant disorder of the peripheral nervous system. It is a recurrent focal neuropathy characterized by painful episodes of brachial palsy and is often associated with short stature, hypotelomerism, and facial dysmorphic features. The main features of RSS are lateral asymmetry and low-birthweight dwarfism, and most patients with the disorder apparently have normal levels of growth hormone.[25,26]

An *Eco*RI 6-kb genomic DNA fragment containing human GALR3 coding sequences was used for FISH localization of the *GALNR3* locus, essentially as described previously[17,27] (FIG. 4). Of 20 metaphase spreads from one normal male that were examined for fluorescent signal, 19 showed signal on one or both chromatids of chromosome 22 in the region 22q12-q13.3; 71% of this signal was at 22q13.1. A total of eight non-specific background dots was observed in these 20 metaphases. A similar result was obtained from hybridization of the probe to 20 metaphase spreads from a second normal male. The gene encoding the G-protein–coupled receptor, somatostatin receptor 3 (*SSTR3*), was also localized to 22q13.1. No disease locus has yet been assigned to this location.

SUMMARY

Human galanin receptor subtypes GALR1, GALR2, and GALR3 are each encoded by separate genes, located on different human chromosomes. The structural organization of *GALNR2* and *GALNR3* suggests a common evolutionary origin, presumably involving gene duplication. Convergent evolution is indicated for *GALNR1*, which exhibits a structural organization that is unique among genes encoding members of the G-protein–coupled receptor superfamily. The *GALNR1* locus at 18q23 co-localizes with a locus reported for bipolar disorder and with a chromosomal deletion that gives rise to a growth hormone insufficiency syndrome. The *GALNR2* locus at 17q25 co-localizes with loci for Russell-Silver syndrome and hereditary neuralgic amyotrophy. Precise mapping studies using polymorphic microsatellite markers will allow assessment of the potential involvement of galanin and its receptors in these and other disorders.

REFERENCES

1. FATHI, Z., W.B. CHURCH & T.P. IISMAA. 1998. Galanin receptors: Recent developments and potential use as therapeutic targets. Ann. Reports Medicinal Chem. **33:** 41–50.
2. CAREY, D.G., T.P. IISMAA, K.Y. HO, I.A. RAJKOVIC, J. KELLY, E.W. KRAEGEN, J. FERGUSON, A.S. INGLIS, J. SHINE & D.J. CHISHOLM. 1993. Potent effects of human galanin in man: Growth hormone secretion and vagal blockade. J Clin. Endocrinol. Metab. **77:** 90–93.
3. CRAWLEY, J.N. 1995. Biological actions of galanin. Regul. Pept. **59:** 1–16.
4. WYNICK, D., P.J. HAMMOND, K.O. AKINSANYA & S.R. BLOOM. 1993. Galanin regulates basal and oestrogen-stimulated lactotroph function. Nature **364:** 529–532.
5. SUEFFERLEIN, T. & E. ROZENGURT. 1996. Galanin, neurotensin, and phorbol esters rapidly stimulate activation of mitogen-activated protein kinase in small cell lung cancer cells. Cancer Res. **56:** 5758–5764.
6. ORMANDY, C.J., C.S.L. LEE, H.F. ORMANDY, V. FANTL, J. SHINE, G. PETERS & R.L. SUTHERLAND. 1998. Amplification, expression, and steroid regulation of the preprogalanin gene in human breast cancer. Cancer Res. **58:** 1353–1357.
7. JACOBY, A.S., G.C. WEBB, M.L. LIU, B. KOFLER, Y.J. HORT, Z. FATHI, C.D.K. BOTTEMA, J. SHINE & T.P. IISMAA. 1997. Structural organization of the mouse and human GALR1 galanin receptor genes (*Galnr* and *GALNR*) and chromosomal localization of the mouse gene. Genomics **45:** 496–508.

8. HAYES, G., T.J. BIDEN, L.A. SELBIE & J. SHINE. 1992. Structural subtypes of the dopamine D2 receptor are functionally distinct: Expression of the cloned $D2_A$ and $D2_B$ subtypes in a heterologous cell line. Mol. Endocrinol. **6:** 920–926.

9. SPENGLER, D., C. WAEBER, C. PANTALONI, F. HOLSBOER, J. BOCKAERT, P.H. SEEBURG & L. JOURNOT. 1993. Differential signal transduction by five splice variants of the PACAP receptor. Nature **365:** 170–175.

10. HABERT-ORTOLI, E., B. AMIRANOFF, I. LOQUET, M. LABURTHE & J. MAYAUX. 1994. Molecular cloning of a functional galanin receptor. Proc. Natl Acad. Sci. USA **91:** 9780–9783.

11. LORIMER, D.D. & R.V. BENYA. 1996. Cloning and quantification of galanin-1 receptor expression by mucosal cells lining the human gastrointestinal tract. Biochem. Biophys. Res. Commun. **222:** 379–385.

12. SULLIVAN, K.A., L.-L. SHIAO & M.A. CASCIERI. 1997. Pharmacological characterization and tissue distribution of the human and rat GALR1 receptors. Biochem. Biophys. Res. Commun. **233:** 823–828.

13. PARKER, E.M., D.G. IZZARELLI, H.P. NOWAK, C.D. MAHLE, L.G. IBEN, J. WANG & M.E. GOLDSTEIN. 1995. Cloning and characterization of the rat GALR1 galanin receptor from Rin14B insulinoma cells. Mol. Brain Res. **34:** 179–189.

14. BURGEVIN, M.-C., I. LOQUET, D. QUARTERONET & E. HABERT-ORTOLI. 1995. Cloning, pharmacological characterization, and anatomical distribution of a rat cDNA encoding for a galanin receptor. J. Mol. Neurosci. **6:** 33–41.

15. AMIRANOFF, B., E. HABERT-ORTOLI & I. LOQUET, inventors; Rhone Poulenc Rohrer, assignee. 1995. Galanin receptor, nucleic acids, transformed cells and uses thereof. Patent WO 9522608-A 1. Date: August 24, 1995.

16. BLOOMQUIST, B.T., M.R. BEAUCHAMP, L. ZHELNIN, S.E. BROWN, A.R. GORE-WILLSE, P. GREGOR & L.J. CORNFIELD. 1998. Cloning and expression of the human galanin receptor GalR2. Biochem. Biophys. Res. Commun. **243:** 474–479.

17. FATHI, Z., P.M. BATTAGLINO, L.G. IBEN, H. LI, E. BAKER, D. ZHANG, R. MCGOVERN, C.D. MAHLE, G.R. SUTHERLAND, T.P. IISMAA, K.E.J. DICKINSON & I. ANTAL ZIMANYI. 1998. Molecular characterization, pharmacological properties and chromosomal localization of the human GALR2 galanin receptor. Mol. Brain Res. **58:** 156–169.

18. HOWARD, A.D., C. TAN, L.-L. SHIAO, O.C. PALYHA, K.K. MCKEE, D.H. WEINBERG, S.D. FEIGHNER, M.A. CASCIERI, R.G. SMITH, L.H.T. VAN DER PLOEG & K.A. SULLIVAN. 1997. Molecular cloning and characterization of a new receptor for galanin. FEBS Lett. **405:** 285–290.

19. WANG, S., C. HE, T. HASHEMI & M. BAYNE. 1997. Cloning and expressional characterization of a novel galanin receptor: Identification of different pharmacophores within galanin for the three galanin receptor subtypes. J. Biol. Chem. **272:** 31949–31952.

20. NICHOLL, J., B. KOFLER, G.R. SUTHERLAND, J. SHINE & T.P. IISMAA. 1995. Assignment of the gene encoding human galanin receptor (*GALNR*) to 18q23 by *in situ* hybridization. Genomics **30:** 629–630.

21. SIMONEAUX, D.K., R.J. LEACH & P. O'CONNELL. 1997. Galanin receptor 1 gene (*Galnr1*) is tightly linked to the myelin basic protein gene on Chromosome 18 in mouse. Mammalian Genome **8:** 875.

22. FREIMER, N.B., V.I. REUS, M.A. ESCAMILLA, L.A. MCINNES, M. SPESNY, P. LEON, S.K. SERVICE, L.B. SMITH, S. SILVA, E. ROJAS, A. GALLEGOS, L. MEZA, E. FOURNIER, S. BAHARLOO, K. BLANKENSHIP, D.J. TYLER, S. BATKI, S. VINOGRADOV, J. WEISSENBACH, S.H. BARONDES & L.A. SANDKUIJL. 1996. Genetic mapping using haplotype, association and linkage methods suggests a locus for severe bipolar disorder (BPI) at 18q22-q23. Nature Genet. **12:** 436–441.

23. CODY, J.D., D.E. HALE, Z. BRKANAC, C.I. KAYE & R.J. LEACH. 1997. Growth hormone insufficiency associated with haploinsufficiency at 18q23. Am. J. Med. Genet. **71:** 420–425.

24. PELLEGRINO, J.E., R.A.V. GEORGE, J. BIEGEL, M.R. FARLOW, K. GARDNER, J. CARESS, M.J. BROWN, T.R. REBBECK, T.D. BIRD & P.F. CHANCE. 1997. Hereditary neuralgic amyotrophy: Evidence for genetic heterogeneity and mapping to chromosome 17q25. Hum. Genet. **101:** 277–283.

25. TANNER, J.M. & T.J. HAM. 1969. Low birthweight dwarfism with asymmetry (Silver's syndrome): Treatment with human growth hormone. Arch. Dis. Childhood **44:** 231–243.

26. GALASSO, C., G. SCIRÈ & B. BOSCHERINI. 1995. Growth hormone and dysmorphic syndromes. Horm. Res. **44:** 42–48.

27. CALLEN D.F., E. BAKER, H.J. EYRE, J.E. CHERNOS, J.A. BELL & G.R. SUTHERLAND. 1990. Reassessment of two apparent deletions of chromosome 16p to an ins(11;16) and a t(1;16) by chromosome painting. Ann. Genet. **33:** 219–221.

Galanin Causes Cl⁻ Secretion in the Human Colon

Potential Significance of Inflammation-Associated NF-κB Activation on Galanin-1 Receptor Expression and Function

RICHARD V. BENYA,[a] KRISTINA A. MATKOWSKYJ, ALEXEY DANILKOVICH, AND GAIL HECHT

Department of Medicine, University of Illinois at Chicago, and Chicago Veterans Administration (West Side) Medical Center, Chicago, Illinois 60612, USA

ABSTRACT: Galanin is widely distributed in enteric nerves and nerve terminals throughout the gastrointestinal (GI) tract. Within the GI tract galanin is best known for its ability to alter smooth muscle contractility and regulate intestinal motility. However, recent studies also indicate that galanin can modulate epithelial ion transport. We previously showed that epithelial cells lining the human GI tract, including those of colonic origin, express Gal1 galanin receptors (Gal1-R). We herein demonstrate that epithelial cells lining the human colon only express Gal1-R receptors and do not express other galanin receptor subtypes. We previously showed that Gal1-R expression was transcriptionally regulated by the transcription factor NF-κB. Consistent with this transcription factor being activated in a number of inflammatory conditions, we show increased colonic Gal1-R expression in patients with colitis due to a variety of causes. To further evaluate the physiology of Gal1-R activation, we studied this receptor expressed by the human colon epithelial cell line T84. Gal1-R activation resulted in a dose-dependent increase in Cl⁻ secretion; whereas infection of T84 cells with pathogens known to activate NF-κB augmented Gal1-R expression and Cl⁻ secretion. Thus, galanin acts as a secretagogue in epithelial cells lining the human colon, with alterations in Gal1-R expression possibly playing an important role in the diarrhea associated with various inflammatory processes affecting the GI tract.

Galanin is a neuropeptide originally isolated from porcine small intestine[1] that is 30 amino acids long in humans[2] and 29 amino acids long in all other species (reviewed in ref. 3). Galanin is widely distributed along the length of the gastrointestinal (GI) tract, with immunoreactivity to this peptide restricted to enteric nerve bodies and fibers.[4] When secreted by enteric nerves, galanin binds to specific receptors expressed by smooth muscle cells, thereby causing either relaxation and/or contraction depending on the species and the exact location considered (reviewed in ref. 5). In addition to galanin's established role in altering intestinal smooth muscle motility and intestinal transit, recent investigations as will be described also suggest a role for this peptide hormone in regulating intestinal fluid homeostasis. We herein review the few studies describing galanin as a modulator of GI epithelial ion flux, and report our data showing that this peptide causes Cl⁻ secretion in

[a]Address for correspondence: Dr. Richard V. Benya, Division of Digestive and Liver Diseases, University of Illinois at Chicago, 840 South Wood Street (M/C 787), Chicago, IL 60612. Phone, 312/996-6651; fax, 312/455-5877; e-mail, rvbenya@uic.edu

epithelial cells lining the human colon. We also show that inflammatory disorders associated with NF-κB activation result in increased galanin-1 receptor (Gal1-R) expression. Thus, the Gal1-R may represent an important yet hitherto unappreciated modulator of intestinal secretion in inflammatory disorders.

GALANIN-1 RECEPTOR EXPRESSION AND FUNCTION IN EPITHELIAL CELLS LINING THE GASTROINTESTINAL TRACT

Relatively few investigators have studied galanin's effects on epithelial cells lining the GI tract. Furthermore, the four available reports provide conflicting information, as they demonstrate that galanin has different effects in different species as well as in different regions of the GI tract (TABLE 1). In all studies galanin's effects were evaluated by mounting intestine, as either an epithelial sheet or the entire organ containing all transmural layers, in an Ussing chamber and measuring alterations in short circuit current (Isc) (as originally described in ref. 6). Within the small intestine, galanin alone decreased Isc and thus net ion secretion in pig jejunum[7] and rabbit ileum.[8] In contrast, galanin had no effect on basal Isc in rat jejunum.[9] Whereas galanin had no effect on basal Isc in guinea pig colon,[10] this peptide caused a massive and prolonged increase in net electrogenic ion secretion in rat colon.[9]

Because galanin is ubiquitously present in nerves and nerve terminals throughout the GI tract,[4] application of electrical field stimulation (EFS) and tetrodotoxin (TTX) is commonly used to study the potential effects of neurally mediated stimuli. Within the small intestine, galanin attenuated EFS-induced increases in Isc in pig jejunum,[7] and potentiated TTX-induced decreases in net ion secretion observed in rabbit ileum (TABLE 1). In contrast, studies evaluating the colon reveal a mixed picture, as galanin attenuated EFS-induced increases in Isc in guinea pigs[10] but had no effect in rats.[9] Furthermore, galanin reversed the effects observed with TTX in rat colon and actually increased Isc after preincubating with this compound[9] (TABLE 1).

Only a single study has evaluated the pharmacology underlying galanin's ability to alter electrogenic ion flux in the GI tract. In the report studying rabbit ileum,[8] the investigators found that [^{125}I]galanin bound specifically and with high affinity (K_d = 0.4 ± 0.1 nM) to membrane vesicles prepared from isolated epithelial cells. Although relatively few binding sites were present (B_{MAX} = 28.0 ± 1.7 fmol/mg protein, or ~300 binding sites/cell using the conversion factor described in ref. 11), galanin rapidly altered rabbit ileum Isc with maximal decreases observed within 3 minutes and a return to baseline observed within 15 minutes.[8] Interestingly these investigators also showed that alterations in Isc were not diminished by repetitive stimulations with galanin, suggesting that *in vivo* endopeptidases may be critically involved in regulating this peptide's physiologic effects. In other studies, half-maximal effects for galanin were observed between 1 and 10 nM (TABLE 1), suggesting that this peptide is equally efficacious despite it having different effects on altering Isc.

Recent molecular studies indicate that galanin acts by binding to one of three different receptor subtypes now identified as the galanin-1 (Gal1-R), galanin-2 (Gal2-R), and galanin-3 (Gal3-R) receptors. The Gal1-R has been cloned and sequenced in humans,[12] rats,[13,14] and mice,[15] whereas the Gal2-R[16] and Gal3-R[17] have been cloned only in rats. We recently determined that mRNA for at least the Gal1-R is expressed by epithelial cells lin-

TABLE 1. Summary of Studies Evaluating Galanin's Effect in Modulating Cl⁻ Secretion from Epithelial Cells Lining the GI Tract[a]

Species	Location	Ref.	Ligand	Short Circuit Current (Isc)						
				Basal (Δ μA/cm²)	100 nM Gal (Δ μA/cm²)	EC_{50} (nM)	EFS (Δ μA/cm²)	Gal+EFS (% change)	TTX (Δ μA/cm²)	Gal+TTX (% change)
Pig	Jejunum	7	Porcine	9	↓8 ± 2	~10	↑31 ± 3	↓~60%	nd	nd
Rat	Jejunum	9	Rat	~35	NE	nd	↑~20	NE	nd	nd
Rabbit	Ileum	8	Porcine	2	↓18 ± 4	6 ± 1	nd	nd	↓~35	↓~33%
Human	Colon-T84	Current	Human	2-3	↑~20	~1	nd	nd	nd	nd
Guinea pig	Colon	10	Human	15	NE	nd	↑168 ± 21	↓~40%	nd	nd
Rat	Colon	9	Rat	~45	↑62 ± 3	~10	↑81 ± 11	NE	↓~25	↑~50%

[a]All data reported as means ± SEM, with values estimated from graphed results shown by (–). NE, no effect; nd, not determined or not determinable because of a small reported effect.

ing the human GI tract.[18] To confirm that mucosal epithelial cells lining the human GI tract express only Gal1-R, we performed RT-PCR on RNA isolated from colonic epithelia obtained from volunteers during elective endoscopy. Using primers for regions that appear to be conserved among the three subtypes, only mRNA for the Gal1-R could be detected in epithelial cells lining the human colon (FIG. 1). We also used RT-PCR to determine that Gal1-R mRNA is present in all human cell lines of colonic origin that we evaluated (FIG. 1, top panel). We performed quantitative PCR using a mimic to determine how this expression compared with that observed in nature. Overall, an eightfold range in Gal1-R mRNA amount was observed, with LoVo and DLD cells expressing the least amount of message and T84 cells expressing approximately the same amount of mRNA as detected in the epithelial cells from the distal human colon (FIG. 1, bottom panel). To determine the physio-

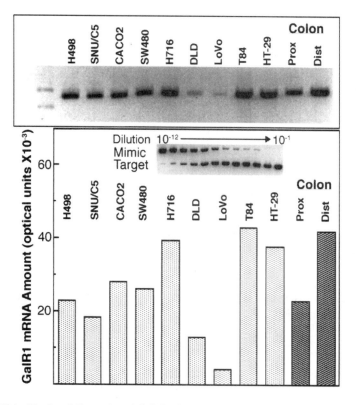

FIGURE 1. (*Top Panel*) Expression of Gal1-R mRNA in human colonic epithelial tissues as determined by RT-PCR. Pinch biopsies of mucosal epithelium lining the human colon were obtained during routinely scheduled endoscopy; while RNA was extracted from these tissues as well as the indicated human colon cell lines using Trizol (Gibco BRL, Gaithersburg, Maryland), RT-PCR was performed using gene-specific primers as described in ref. 18. (*Bottom Panel*) Quantitative PCR performed showing relative amount of Gal1-R mRNA expression. In all instances, 5 μg total RNA was subject to reverse transcription using gene-specific primers, and PCR was performed using a mimic (as shown in *inset*). The amount of PCR product at the appropriate dilution was then assessed by determining the optical density at 260 nm.

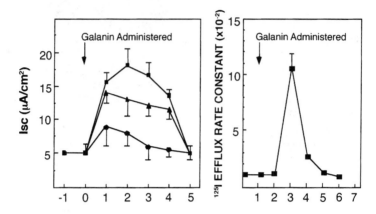

FIGURE 2. Cl⁻ secretion from T84 cells in response to stimulation with galanin. (*Left Panel*) Changes in short circuit current (Isc) over time in response to different concentrations of galanin. T84 cells were cultured to confluence on Transwells (Costar, Cambridge, Massachusetts) as previously described,[6] and Isc measured in response to 1 µM (■), 1 nM (▲), or 10 pM (●) galanin. (*Right Panel*) [¹²⁵I] efflux over time in response to stimulation with 1 µM galanin (■). T84 cells were loaded with [¹²⁵I], and efflux was recorded as a measure of chloride secretion as previously described.[22]

logic function of Gal1-R expressed by human colon epithelial cells, we focused our subsequent efforts on T84 cells.

Originally isolated from an adenocarcinoma of the colon, T84 cells are a well accepted model for studying the events that regulate apical Cl⁻ secretion.[19] Competitive binding experiments using [¹²⁵I]galanin revealed that T84 cells express low numbers (B_{MAX} = 330 ± 50 binding sites/cell) of high affinity (K_i = 1.6 ± 0.3 nM) receptors,[20] which by RT-PCR only express message for the Gal1-R (FIG. 1). To determine if galanin alters ion transport in the human colon as shown in guinea pigs and rats (TABLE 1), we studied confluent T84 cell monolayers in a modified Ussing chamber.[21] Porcine galanin increases Isc in a dose-dependent fashion (FIG. 2, left panel). Similar to what has been shown in rabbits but in contrast to that in rats,[9] galanin's peak action is rapid (within 2 minutes) and transient (return to baseline within 5–10 minutes) (FIG. 2, left panel). Both the magnitude and transient nature of the response are similar to those observed when T84 cells are stimulated with 100µM carbachol (as previously shown in ref. 21). To confirm that this increase in Isc is due to Cl⁻ secretion, we loaded T84 cells with ¹²⁵I as previously described[22] and demonstrated increased tracer efflux after stimulation with 1µM galanin (FIG. 2, right panel). Thus, in the human T84 colonocyte cell line, galanin binds to Gal1-R, causing Cl⁻ secretion.

CHARACTERIZATION AND REGULATION OF THE GAL1R GENE

Since the Gal1-R mediates multiple different physiologic functions, including modulating ion transport and regulating intestinal motility within the GI tract alone, we cloned the human GAL1R gene[23] to gain additional insight into this receptor's ability to alter cell behavior. The gene for GAL1R contains 2 introns, unusual insofar as both are located within the coding regions of the receptor's third intracellular loop. The third intracellular loop of many heptaspanning receptors is involved in coupling to heterotrimeric G-proteins.[24-28] Because alternative splicing may occur around intron-exon borders, we[23] and others[29] initially suggested that Gal1-R splice variants could exist. We determined the location of conserved intron-exon boundaries of all peptide hormone receptors for which the genomic sequence is known for at least two subtypes, or was derived from at least two different species (FIG. 3). Whereas intron-less receptors exist, the prevalent finding is for peptide receptors to possess one or more introns whose location is highly conserved despite poor sequence homology (i.e., <20% amino acid homology within the dopamine family of receptors). The number and location of these introns appear to be a distinguishing feature of peptide receptor genomic organization, with at least a single intron present in the third intracellular loop common to the receptor

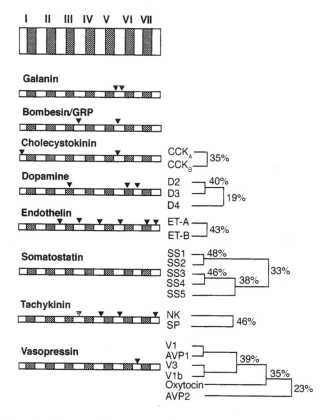

FIGURE 3. Location of conserved intron-exon splice sites for known heptaspanning receptor genes. The intron-exon splice sites that are conserved by genes for heptaspanning receptor subtypes are shown. The transmembrane-spanning regions (I to VII) of the receptor protein are indicated by the *dark boxes. Arrowheads* indicate the intron-exon splice sites. The percent nucleotide homology for the cDNAs of the indicated receptor subtypes is shown at the right.

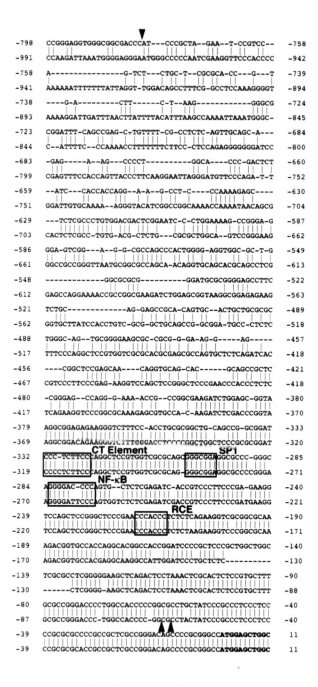

FIGURE 4. *See legend on facing page.*

FIGURE 4. Comparison of the ~1 Kb of 5′ flanking/UTR for the human GAL1-R gene cloned by Lorimer *et al.*[23] (*bottom sequence*) and Jacoby *et al.*[29] (*top sequence*). The *vertical lines* identify sequence identity. The sites of transcriptional initiation in colonic epithelia as shown by Lorimer *et al.*[23] are indicated by the *triangles* (▲), whereas the presumed site in the pituitary as described by Jacoby *et al.*[29] is indicated by the *arrowhead* (▼). Translated sequence is shown in *bold*, with all numbering relative to the translational initiation ATG. Potential regulatory sites conserved between the two sequences are *boxed*. NF-κB, nuclear factor kappa B; RCE, retinoblastoma control element.

◀──

families for bombesin, cholecytokinin, endothelin, the tachykinins, and perhaps galanin (FIG. 3). Interestingly, the frequent presence of introns in the third intracellular loop has no correlation with the existence of splice variants. Thus, the location of two introns in the GAL1R gene does not by itself indicate the existence of splice variants.

Jacoby *et al.*[29] simultaneously cloned the human GAL1R gene. However, differences exist between the study by Jacoby *et al.* and ours[23] (TABLE 2). Although Jacoby *et al.*[29] reported the existence of two introns in the same location, they differed in the analysis of their size. Whereas we found the two introns were 2.1 and 2.9 kb, respectively, Jacoby *et al.* reported them to be 5 and 11 kb in size. Furthermore, significant differences between the findings of the two groups are apparent in analyses of the 5′ untranslated region (UTR)/ flanking region of this gene (FIG. 4). Overall there is 65% homology for the two reported sequences in the ~1 kb region upstream of the site of translation initiation, with high homology observed downstream and increasing divergence observed as one progresses upstream (FIG. 4). Specifically, the 0.5 kb closest to the transitional initiation site is 82% homologous, whereas the next 0.5 kb is only 47% homologous. A possible explanation for these differences could be that we cloned the human GAL1R gene from a P1 clone, which may have undergone a recombination event ~0.5 kb upstream from the site of translation initiation. Indeed, we sequenced two independently identified P1 clones and generated the same 5′ upstream sequence for both, whereas our sequencing of the coding region itself was completely identical to that previously reported for the Gal1-R cDNA.[12] Although this finding suggests the existence of multiple GAL1R genes, no evidence currently exists to suggest

TABLE 2. Comparison of Pertinent Similarities and Differences between the Human GALR1 Gene Described by Jacoby *et al.*[29] and Lorimer *et al.*[23]

	Jacoby *et al.*	Lorimer *et al.*	Comment
Genomic organization	3 Exons	3 Exons	
Intron size	•*Intron 1* = 5 kb •*Intron 2* = 11 kb	•*Intron 1* = 2.1 kb •*Intron 2* = 2.9 kb	Error in long PCR vs evidence for multiple gene copies
5′ UTR	400–900 nt	61–63 nt	Likely reflects differences in transcription between pituitary and colon
5′ Flanking region similarities	•No TATA boxes •NF-κB at nt –274	•No TATA boxes •NF-κB at nt –259	Is NF-κB functional only in colonic transcription?

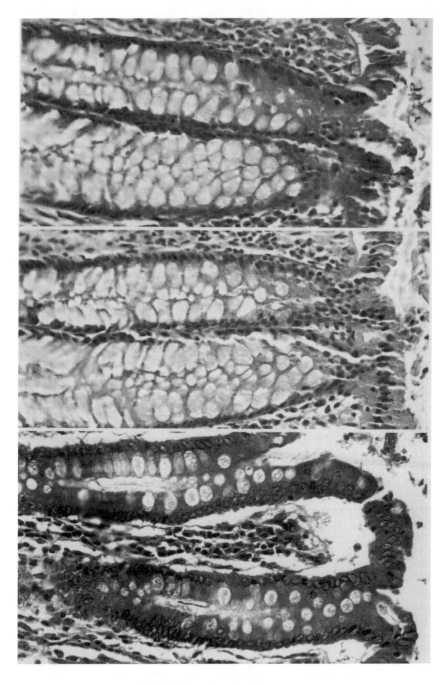

FIGURE 5. *See legend on facing page.*

FIGURE 5. Immunohistochemistry performed on human colonic epithelium using an antipeptide antibody unique for the Gal1-R. Normal human colon expresses relatively little Gal1-R, mostly in epithelial cells lining the lumen (*top panel*). In contrast, inflammatory conditions such as diverticulitis show markedly increased expression in cells lining the surface and crypts (*bottom panel*). Tissues representing negative controls (*middle panel*) were processed identically except for the absence of exposure to primary antibody. Photographs acquired at 400X using a MicroLumina digital scanning camera (Leaf, Fort Washington, Pennsylvania).

the presence of more than a single gene copy. Thus, differences between the two published reports regarding the GAL1R gene[23,29] cannot currently be satisfactorily resolved. Despite these differences, however, a number of important features are conserved between the two published sequences (TABLE 2). These include: (1) the absence of TATA boxes, features of housekeeping genes and associated with multiple sites of transcription initiation;[30] and (2) the conserved presence of recognition sites for the inflammation-associated transcription factor nuclear factor κB (NF-κB) (FIG. 4).

The absence of TATA boxes and the likelihood of multiple different sites of transcriptional initiation possibly account for the difference in the start of exon 1 reported by Jacoby *et al.*[29] and us. Whereas we used primer extension studies and circular PCR performed on RNA isolated from human colonic epithelial tissues to show that transcription started at -61 and -63 nt upstream from the initiation ATG,[23] Jacoby *et al.* compared their sequence with that of a human pituitary cDNA clone to argue that exon 1 started -772 nt

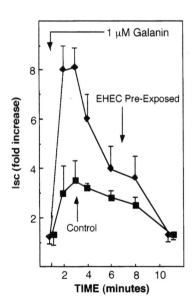

FIGURE 6. Change in short circuit current (Isc) over time in T84 cells with and without prior exposure to enterohemorrhagic *E. coli* (EHEC). Confluent T84 cells were exposed to log-growth EHEC for 1 hour, treated with gentamicin, and then studied in an Ussing chamber 23 hours later after treating with 1 μM galanin (◆). Control T84 cells not exposed to EHEC were otherwise processed similarly and in parallel (■).

upstream of the site of translation initiation. By contrast, Jacoby *et al.* estimate the 5′UTR in Bowes human melanoma cells to be ~0.4 to 0.9 kb and suggest that GAL1R gene transcription likely differs in different tissues. In both sequences, however, the location of potential NF-κB recognition sites is conserved (FIG. 4). We assessed the functional significance of these sites by evaluating various 5′ flanking region constructs linked to a gene for chloramphenicol acetyltransferase (CAT) in vector pCAT(An).[31] When studied in transiently transfected Bowes human melanoma cells, a cell line natively expressing the Gal1-R,[12] alterations in CAT activity were observed only in constructs eliminating NF-κB recognition sites.[23] The finding of functional NF-κB sites for the GAL1R gene is particularly interesting, because the human gene for the peptide galanin likewise contains a recognition site for this inflammation-associated transcription factor.[32] These data therefore raised the possibility that expression of both peptide and receptor could be increased in at least the colon subsequent to various inflammatory events.

FUNCTIONAL CONSEQUENCE OF ACTIVATED NF-κB ON GAL1-R EXPRESSION IN HUMAN COLONOCYTES

NF-κB is a transcription factor that, when activated, exists as a dimer containing several potential subunits including p50, p52, rel, p65 (Rel A), rel B, and c-rel (reviewed in refs. 33 and 34). The variability in NF-κB composition likely contributes to the specificity of gene regulation, as a particular nucleotide sequence may bind some NF-κB complexes but not others.[35–37] In unstimulated cells, NF-κB is cytoplasmic and associated with an inhibitor protein, IκB, that prevents its movement to the nucleus and acts as a transcription factor.[38] Appropriate stimulation results in IκB phosphorylation and degradation, allowing newly released NF-κB to translocate to the nucleus, where it binds to a variety of specific sequences located in the promoter region of target genes. NF-κB increases the transcription of many proteins in the colon involved in the host immune response including cytokines and chemokines (reviewed in ref. 38). Not surprisingly, NF-κB has been shown to be activated in response to colonic infection with enteric pathogens[39–41] and in inflammatory bowel disease, particularly ulcerative colitis.[42,43]

To determine if Gal1-R expression could be altered in humans with various inflammatory disorders of the colon, we performed immunohistochemistry on surgical and endoscopic tissues randomly selected from our tissue library from 1990 to the present. We used an antipeptide antibody that does not recognize the GalR2 or GalR3 and whose epitope is 100% conserved between rats, humans, and mice. Immunohistochemistry revealed minimal Gal1-R expression by epithelial cells lining the normal human colon, with the few cells expressing this receptor limited to the colonic surface and none observed in the crypts (FIG. 5, top panel). By contrast, grossly increased expression could be observed in the colon, including crypts, removed from a patient with diverticulitis (FIG. 5, bottom panel). Increased expression of Gal1-R was also observed in patients with active pseudomembranous colitis (*Clostridium difficile* infection), ulcerative colitis, and Crohn's disease. These findings demonstrate that whereas normal colonic epithelia express minimal amounts of Gal1-R, dramatically increased expression is observed in the colon of patients suffering with a variety of inflammatory diseases.

Regardless of the underlying cause, most if not all patients with colonic inflammation respond clinically with diarrhea. This is particularly true of patients with enteric pathogen infections of the colon. Although enteric pathogens cause increased fluid secretion by a variety of processes (reviewed in ref. 44), it is increasingly appreciated that all share the common feature of activating NF-κB.[39–41] We therefore returned to our T84 cell model to study the functional consequence of colonic epithelial cell exposure to enteric pathogens on Gal1-R expression and Cl⁻ secretion. We infected T84 cells with enterohemorrhagic *Escherichia coli* (EHEC) for 1 hour, an exposure time that does not alter T84 cell morphology, and then killed the bacteria by treating with gentamicin. We then studied these T84 cells 23 hours later to allow for Gal1-R synthesis and expression. As compared to control T84 cells (B_{MAX} = 330 ± 50 receptors/cell), infection with EHEC markedly increased Gal1-R expression (B_{MAX} = 4250 ± 760 receptors/cell). Whereas 1 μM galanin increased the Isc response 4.3 ± 0.9-fold, this same concentration of peptide increased Isc in EHEC-treated cells 8.5 ± 0.8-fold (FIG. 6).[20] We also evaluated enterotoxigenic and enteroinvasive *E. coli* under the same conditions. In all instances exposure to these enteric pathogens increased galanin-induced Isc between 10- and 20-fold as compared to control cells processed in parallel. Thus infection with pathogenic *E. coli* known to activate NF-κB allows for increased Gal1-R expression and ultimately increased Cl⁻ secretion when stimulated with ligand.

CONCLUSIONS

Galanin secreted by enteric nerves is known to act upon receptors expressed by smooth muscle cells lining the GI tract, thereby altering intestinal motility. We show that Gal1-R also are expressed by epithelial cells lining the GI tract, and when stimulated in the human colon cell line T84, they cause Cl⁻ secretion. Gal1-R expression is transcriptionally regulated by the inflammation-associated transcription factor NF-κB, with increased receptor expression observed in the colons of patients with inflammatory bowel disease and infectious diarrhea. These findings outline a hitherto unappreciated role for galanin and suggest that this peptide and receptor may be involved in a common pathway for the diarrhea associated with a variety of inflammatory disorders.

REFERENCES

1. TATEMOTO, K., A. ROKAEUS, H. JORNVALL, T.J. MCDONALD & V. MUTT. 1983. Galanin, a novel biologically active peptide from porcine intestine. FEBS Lett. **164:** 124–128.
2. BERSANI, M., A.H. JOHNSEN, P. HOJRUP, B.E. DUNNING, J.J. ANDREASEN & J.J. HOST. 1991. Human galanin: Primary structure and identification of 2 molecular forms. FEBS Lett. **283:** 189–194.
3. KASK, K., U. LANGEL & T. BARTFAI. 1995. Galanin, a neuropeptide with inhibitory actions. Cell Mol Neurobiol. **15:** 653–673.
4. WANG, Y.F., Y.K. MAO, T.J. MCDONALD & E.E. DANIEL. 1995. Distribution of galanin-immunoreactive nerves in the canine gastrointestinal tract. Peptides **16:** 237–247.
5. RATTAN, S. 1991. Role of galanin in the gut. Gastroenterology **100:** 1762–1768.
6. USSING, H.H. & K. ZERAHN. 1950. Active transport of sodium as the source of electric current in the short-circuited isolated frog skin. Acta Phys. Scandinav. **23:** 110–127.
7. BROWN, D.R., K.R. HILDEBRAND, A.M. PARSONS & G. SOLDANI. 1990. Effects of galanin on smooth muscle and mucosa of porcine jejunum. Peptides **11:** 497–500.
8. HOMAIDAN, F.R., S.H. TANG, M. DONOWITZ & G.W. SHARP. 1994. Effects on galanin on short circuit current and electrolyte transport in rabbit ileum. Peptides **15:** 1431–1436.
9. KIYOHARA, T., M. OKURA & H. ISHIKAWA. 1992. Galanin-induced alteration of electrolyte transport in the rat intestine. Am. J. Physiol. **263:** G502–G507.

10. McCulloch, C.R., A. Kuwahara, C.D. Condon & H.J. Cooke. 1987. Neuropeptide modification of chloride secretion in guinea pig distal colon. Regul. Pept. **19:** 35–43.
11. Ferris, H.A., R.E. Carroll, D.L. Lorimer & R.V. Benya. 1997. Location and characterization of the human GRP receptor expressed by gastrointestinal epithelial cells. Peptides **18:** 663–672.
12. Habert-Ortoli, E., B. Amiranoff, I. Loquet, M. Laburthe & J.-F. Mayaux. 1994. Molecular cloning of a functional human galanin receptor. Proc. Natl. Acad. Sci. USA **91:** 9780–9783.
13. Burgevin, M.C., I. Loquet, D. Quarteronet & E. Habert-Ortoli. 1995. Cloning, pharmacological characterization, and anatomical distribution of a rat cDNA encoding for a galanin receptor. J. Mol. Neurosci. **6:** 33–41.
14. Parker, E.M, D.G. Izzarelli, H.P. Nowak, C.D. Mahle, L.G. Iben, J. Wang & M.E. Goldstein. 1995. Cloning and characterization of the rat GAL1-R galanin receptor from Rin14B insulinoma cells. Mol. Brain Res. **34:** 179–189.
15. Wang, S., C. He, T. Maguire, A.L. Clemmons, R.E. Burrier, M.F. Guzzi, C.D. Strader, E.M. Parker & M.L. Bayne. 1997. Genomic organization and functional regulation of the mouse *Gal1-R* galanin receptor. FEBS Lett. **411:** 225–230.
16. Wang, S., T. Hashemi, C. He, C.D. Strader & M. Bayne. 1997. Molecular cloning and pharmacological characterization of a new galanin receptor subtype. Mol. Pharmacol. **52:** 337–343.
17. Howard, A.D., C. Tan, L.-L. Shiao, O.C. Palyha, K.K. McKee, D.H. Weiger, S.D. Feighner, M.A. Cascieri, R.G. Smith, L.H.T. Van Der Ploeg & K.A. Sullivan. 1997. Molecular cloning and characterization of a new receptor for galanin. FEBS Lett. **405:** 285–290.
18. Lorimer, D.D. & R.V. Benya. 1996. Cloning and quantification of human galanin-1 receptor expression by mucosal cells lining the gastrointestinal tract. Biochem. Biophys. Res. Commun. **222:** 379–385.
19. Dharmsathaphorn, K., J.A. McRoberts, K.G. Mandel, L.D. Tisdale & H. Masui. 1984. A human colonic tumor cell line that maintains vectorial electrolyte transport. Am. J. Physiol. **246:** G204–G208.
20. Marrero, J.A., A. Koutsouris, D.A. Ostrovskiy, S.D. Savkovic, G. Hecht & R.V. Benya. 1998. Galanin causes Cl⁻ secretion in T84 cells: Identification of a novel mechanism for infectious diarrhea. Gastroenterology **114:** A395.
21. Madara, J.L. and G. Hecht. 1991. Tight junctions in cultured epithelial cells. *In* Functional Epithelial Cells in Culture.:131–163. Alan Liss. New York.
22. Vlengarik, C.J., R.J. Bridges & R.A. Frizzell. 1990. A simple assay for agonist-regulated Cl and K conductances in salt-secreting epithelial cells. Am. J. Physiol. **259:** C358–C364.
23. Lorimer, D.D., K. Matkowskjy & R.V. Benya. 1997. Cloning, chromosomal localization, and transcriptional regulation of the human galanin-1 receptor gene (GALN1R). Biochem. Biophys. Res. Commun. **241:** 558–564.
24. Strader, C.D., I.S. Sigal & R.A. Dixon. 1989. Structural basis of β-adrenergic receptor function. FASEB J. **3:** 1825–1832.
25. Kjelsberg, M.A., S. Cotecchia, J. Ostrowski, M.G. Caron & R.J. Lefkowitz. 1992. Constitutive activation of the α_{1B}-adrenergic receptor by all amino acid substitutions at a single site. J. Biol. Chem. **267:** 1430–1433.
26. Samama, P., S. Cotecchia, T. Costa & R.J. Lefkowitz. 1993. A mutation-induced activated state of the beta 2-adrenergic receptor. Extending the ternary complex model. J. Biol. Chem. **268:** 4625–4636.
27. Probst, W.C., L.A. Snyder, D.I. Schuster, J. Brosius & S.C. Sealfon. 1992. Sequence alignment of the G-protein coupled receptor superfamily. DNA Cell Biol. **11:** 1–20.
28. Bluml, K., E. Mutschler & J. Wess. 1994. Insertion mutagenesis as a tool to predict the secondary structure of a muscarinic receptor domain determining specificity of G-protein-coupling. Proc. Natl. Acad. Sci. USA **91:** 7980–7984.
29. Jacoby, A.S., G.C. Webb, M.L. Liu, B. Kofler, Y.J. Hort, Z. Fathi, C.D.K. Bottema, J. Shine & T.P. Lismaa. 1997. Structural organization of the mouse and human GAL1-R galanin receptor genes (*Galnr* and *GALNR*) and chromosomal localization of the mouse gene. Genomics **45:** 496–508.
30. Dynan, W.S. & M.Z. Gilman. 1986. Transcriptional control and signal transduction: of soap operas and reductionism. Trends Genet. **2:** 196–197.

31. JACOBY, D.B., N.D. ZILZ & H.C. TOWLE. 1989. Sequence within the 5'-flanking region of the S$_{14}$ gene confer responsiveness to glucose in primary hepatocytes. J. Biol. Chem. **264:** 17623–17626.
32. KOFLER, B., H.F. EVANS, M.J. LIU, V. FALLS, T.P. IISMAA, J. SHINE & H. HERZOG. 1995. Characterization of the 5'-flanking region of the human preprogalanin gene. DNA Cell Biol. **14:** 321–329.
33. BARNES, P.J. & M. KARIN. 1997. Nuclear factor-κB, a pivotal transcription factor in chronic inflammatory diseases. N. Engl. J. Med. **336:** 1066–1071.
34. BAEUERLE, P.A. 1991. The inducible transcription activator NF-κB: Regulation by distinct protein subunits. Biochem. Biophys. Acta **1072:** 63–80.
35. KUNSCH, C., S.M. RUBEN & C.A. ROSEN. 1992. Selection of optional κB/Rel DNA-binding motifs: Interaction of both subunits of NF-κB with DNA is required for transcriptional activation. Mol. Cell Biochem. **12:** 4412–4442.
36. MUKAIDA, N., Y. MAHE & K. MATSUSHIMA. 1993. Cooperative interaction of nuclear factor-κB- and cis-regulatory enhancer binding protein-like factor binding elements in activating the interleukin-8 gene by proinflammatory cytokines. J. Biol. Chem. **21128:** 21133.
37. OETH, P.A., G.C.N. PARRY, C. KUNSCH, P. NANTERMET, C.A. ROSEN & N. MACKMAN. 1994. Lipopolysaccharide induction of tissue factor gene expression in monocytic cells is mediated by binding of c Rel/p65 heterodimers to a κB-like site. Mol. Cell Biochem. **14:** 3772–3781.
38. BAEUERLE, P.A. & D. BALTIMORE. 1996. NF-κB: Ten years after. Cell **87:** 13–20.
39. SAVAKOVIC, S.D., A. KOUTSOURIS & G. HECHT. 1997. Activation of NF-κB in intestinal epithelial cells by enteropathogenic *Escherichia coli*. Am. J. Physiol. **273:** C1160–C1167.
40. ZUNJIC, M., S.D. SAVAKOVIC, A. KOUTSOURIS & G. HECHT. 1997. Increased IL-8 expression induced by *Salmonella*, as compared to pathogenic *E. coli*, results from synergism between NF-κB and NF-IL6. Gastroenterology **112:** A1128.
41. DYER, R.B., C.R. COLLACO, D.W. NIESEL & N.K. HERZOG. 1993. *Shigella flexneri* invasion of HeLa cells induces NF-κB DNA binding activity. Infect. Immun. **61:** 4427–4433.
42. NEURATH, M.F., S. PETTERSSON, K.H. MEYER ZUM BUSCHENFELDE & W. STROBER. 1996. Local administration of antisense phosphorothioate oligonucleotides to the p65 subunit of NK-κB abrogates established experimental colitis in mice. Nat. Med. **2:** 998–1004.
43. JOURD'HEUIL, D., Z. MORISE, E.M. CONNER, I. KUROSE & M.B. GRISHAM. 1997. Oxidant-regulation of gene expression in the chronically inflamed intestine. Keio J. Med. **46:** 10–15.
44. SEARS, C.L. & J.B. KAPER. 1996. Enteric bacterial toxins: Mechanisms of action and linkage to intestinal function. Microbiol. Rev. **60:** 167–215.

Mutagenesis Study on Human Galanin Receptor GalR1 Reveals Domains Involved in Ligand Binding[a]

KALEV KASK,[c,g] MALIN BERTHOLD,[d] ULRIKA KAHL,[e] ANDERS JURÉUS, GUNNAR NORDVALL,[b] ÜLO LANGEL, AND TAMAS BARTFAI[f]

Department of Neurochemistry and Neurotoxicology, Stockholm University, S-106 91 Stockholm, Sweden

[b]Astra Arcus AB, S-151 85 Södertälje, Sweden

ABSTRACT: Many receptor mutants were generated and several NH_2-terminally modified galanin analogs synthesized to define the regions of hGalR1 involved in galanin binding. Ligand binding properties and functionality of mutant receptors were evaluated. The His264Ala and Phe282Ala receptor mutants, although deficient in binding in the concentration range of galanin used, remained functional albeit at least 20-fold less efficient than the wild-type receptor in the inhibition of stimulated cAMP production. Hence, His264 and Phe282 of hGalR1 are directly involved in galanin binding. NH_2-terminal carboxylic acid analogs of galanin (1-16) have a very low affinity for the wild-type receptor, but substantially increased affinity for the Glu271Lys-hGalR1, suggesting that the NH_2-terminus of galanin binds to the receptor near the transmembrane (TM) VI. Based on these findings and computer-aided molecular modeling, we propose a binding site model for the hGalR1 receptor (possibly also for other galanin receptor subtypes): galanin binds with its NH_2-terminus to the pocket between TM III and TM VI, Trp^2 of galanin interacts with His264 of the receptor, and Tyr^9 is involved in an aromatic-aromatic type of interaction with Phe282 of ECIII of GalR1.

Galanin's important involvement in pain signalling, acquisition, body weight control, and hormone release (for reviews, see refs. 1 and 2) is at the cellular level mediated by 7-transmembrane (7-TM)[1] spanning domain type of receptors coupled via inhibitory G-proteins (G_i/G_o) to effector systems such as adenylate cyclase, K^+ channels, and Ca^{2+} channels.[3]

[a]This work was supported by grants from the Swedish Medical Research Council, the Swedish Technical Board of Development, and The National Institute of Ageing Drug Discovery Programme.

[c]Present address: Max-Planck-Institute for Medical Research, 69120 Heidelberg, Germany.

[d]Present address: Department of Neuroscience, Karolinska Institute, 171 77 Stockholm, Sweden.

[e]Present address: Department of Neurological Sciences, Rush Presbyterian-St. Luke's Medical Center, Chicago, Illinois 60612, USA.

[f]Present address: CNS Department, Preclinical Research, Hoffmann-La Roche Ltd, CH-4070 Basle, Switzerland.

[g]Corresponding author. E-mail, kask@mpimf-heidelberg.mpg.de; fax, +49-6221-486110; phone, +49-6221-486118.

[1]TM - transmembrane; EC - extracellular; hGalR1 - human galanin receptor type 1; cAMP - 3′,5′-cyclic adenosine monophosphate.

Structure-activity relationship studies using galanin fragments and analogs show that amino acid residues responsible for the high affinity binding as well as agonist action reside in the evolutionarily conserved NH_2-terminal part of galanin. Studies on L-Ala substituted galanin analogs demonstrate that Trp^2 and Tyr^9 as well as the free NH_2-terminal amino group are the main pharmacophores.[4]

Recent cloning of galanin receptors (FIG. 1)[5–11] has made it possible to study which domains and/or single amino acid residues of the receptor form the binding pocket for galanin. In recent years, a picture has emerged on the mode of binding of monoamines and intermediately sized peptides such as substance P and angiotensin II to their receptors,[12–14] but it has remained largely unclear how a large peptide ligand such as galanin binds to its G-protein coupled receptor. Due to the bulkiness and hydrophilicity of galanin, one would assume that the receptor-ligand interactions take place near the top of membrane-spanning helices or at the extracellular domains of the receptor, as described for instance in substance P binding to NK-1 receptors[15–17] and angiotensin II binding to AT1 receptors.[18]

To identify the contact sites between galanin and the human galanin receptor hGalR1, we have undertook a mutational analysis of hGalR1 in combination with molecular modeling. Systematic deletions and mutations of amino acid residues in the NH_2-terminal extracellular domain and in extracellular loops II and III, transmembrane helices III, VI, and VII, and L-alanine-scanning of the majority of residues on the hydrophilic side of transmembrane domain V of the receptor have revealed the amino acid residues of hGalR1 which are important for the high affinity galanin binding. Furthermore, by mutually substituting functional groups in the NH_2-terminus of the peptide ligand and Glu271 near the top of TM VI of the receptor we created a new, nonendogenous interaction. This "gain-of-binding" indicates that the NH_2-terminal amino group of galanin binds to the receptor near the top of TM VI and thereby enables us to orient the ligand relative to the receptor. The combination of approaches used in this study has permitted us to delineate the galanin binding site of the human galanin receptor type 1.

RESULTS AND DISCUSSION

Addressing Some Methodologic Issues Related to This Study

The detailed description of methods used in this study was published elsewhere.[19,20] It is important, however, to mention here a couple of relevant methodologic issues. When studying galanin-galanin receptor interactions, one main concern is the lack of ligands to the galanin receptor, radiolabeled and nonlabeled, other than galanin itself or fragments thereof. Therefore, mutant receptors whose apparent affinity for ^{125}I-galanin was too low to show specific binding were assessed for their ability to mediate the inhibition by galanin of the isoproterenol-stimulated adenylate cyclase activity. Correct insertion of mutant receptors into the plasma membrane was demonstrated by immunostaining of cells expressing FLAG-tagged mutant receptors. Throughout binding studies, the cDNA constructs harboring wild-type or mutant galanin receptors were transiently expressed in either HEK 293 or COS-7 cells. Functionality of those mutant receptors that displayed an apparent loss-of-binding was evaluated, but only in COS cells, as these cells displayed more robust stimulation of cAMP production.

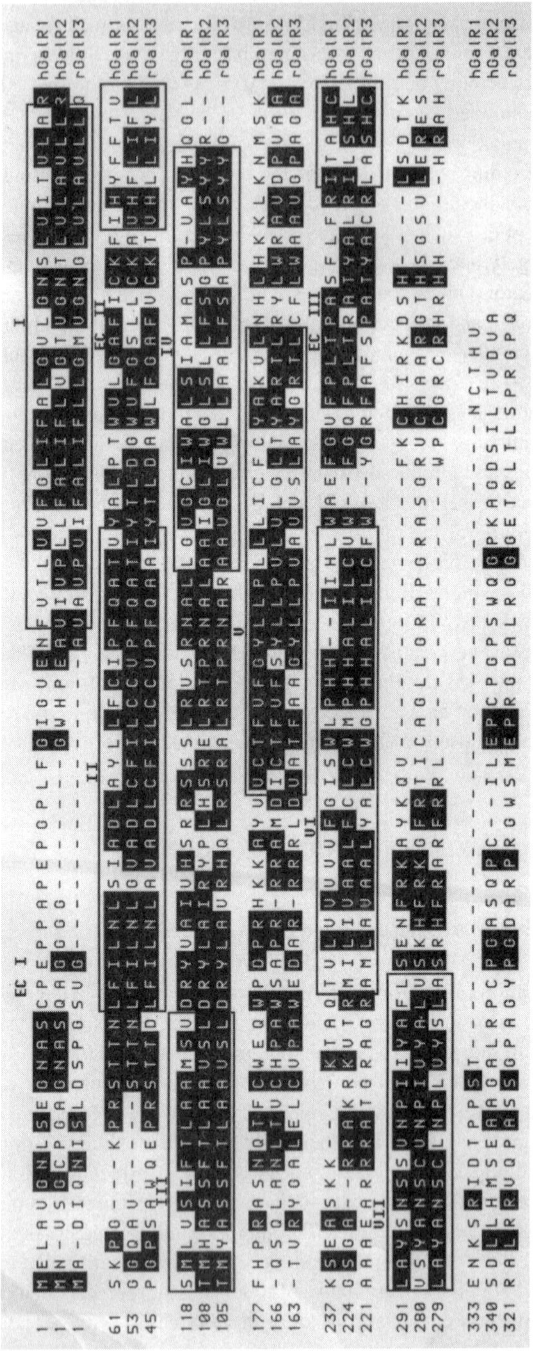

FIGURE 1. Comparison of amino acid sequences of the cloned galanin receptor subtypes. The putative transmembrane domains are *boxed*, and extracellular regions are *numbered*. Identical residues are in *black*.

Deletion of the NH₂-Terminal Extracellular Region of hGalR1 Has No Effect on Galanin Binding

Two NH_2-terminal deletion mutants of hGalR1 were generated; one in which amino acids 7-15 were replaced by three alanine residues, and a second mutant in which the residues 17-23 were deleted. Despite removal of both of its putative *N*-glycosylation sites Asn7 and Asn12 in the former mutant, neither deletion affects the ability of mutant receptors to bind galanin. Because the NH_2-terminal extracellular regions of other cloned galanin receptor subtypes have very little sequence homology to each other (Fig. 1), we conclude that these domains do not participate in ligand binding.

Substitutions of Residues Lining the Hydrophilic Sides of TMs III and V and in Extracellular Loop II

Residues of TMs III and V which reside close to the extracellular surface pointing towards the interior of the helical bundle were mutated by site-directed mutagenesis. None of the following substitutions, including His112Val in TM III, and Lys197Ala, Val201Ala, Phe205Ala, and Thr204Val in TM V, resulted in any significant change in galanin binding (Fig. 2 and Table 1). Similarly without impact on galanin binding are the mutations of two acidic and one aromatic residue (Glu189Ala, Asp193Ala, and Trp191Ala) in extracellular loop II (Fig. 2 and Table 1). Only the Phe115Ala mutation in TM III of hGalR1 led to a 10-fold drop in the binding affinity of galanin. As the hydrophobic nature of the amino acid residue in this position has been conserved in other galanin receptor subtypes (Fig. 1),

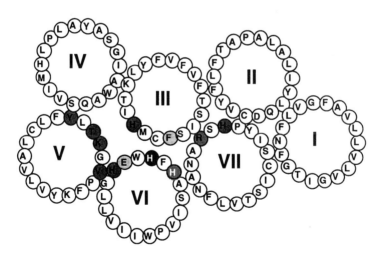

FIGURE 2. A helical wheel plot of hGalR1 as viewed from the extracellular side. The transmembrane helices are arranged according to the two-dimensional structure of bovine rhodopsin,[21] taking into account mutagenesis studies on mutual positioning of transmembrane domains of heptahelical receptors.[22] Amino acid residues mutated in this study, but without impact on galanin binding, are indicated in *dark grey*, His264 is in *black*, and other residues affecting galanin binding are in *light grey*. Phe282 of EC III is not indicated, as it remains above the plane of transmembrane domains.

TABLE 1. Relative Affinities of Galanin to Galanin Receptor Mutants as Compared to the Wild-Type Receptor (amino acids given in one-letter codes)

Region of hGalR1	GalR1 Wild-Type Mutation	K_D (nM) 3.1 ± 2.1 K_D mut / K_D wt
EC I	Δ7-15	0.8
	Δ17-23	0.5
TM III	H112V	1.4
	F115A	10.1
EC II	E189A	1.3
	W191A	0.4
	D193A	0.7
TM V	K197A	0.3
	V201A	2.0
	T204A	0.4
	F205V	0.7
TM VI	H263A	0.5
	H264A	≥ 20
	H267A	≥ 100
	E271S	12.5
	E271K	0.4
EC III	F282A	≥ 20
	F282Y	1.9
TM VII	R285A	0.4
	H289S	0.9

we propose that a hydrophobic interaction between galanin and its receptor in this position contributes to the high affinity binding.

Amino Acid Residues Critical for Galanin Binding Are at the Top of TM VI and in Extracellular Loop III

Several amino acid residues in the EC III and near the top of TMs VI and VII were mutated (Fig. 2 and Table 1). The following substitutions, including His264Ala and His267Ala of TM VI and Phe282Ala of ECIII, yielded apparent "loss-of-binding" hGalR1 mutants. These mutant receptors were correctly inserted into the cell membrane as shown by immunostaining of their FLAG-tagged analogs.[19] The extent of loss of the binding affinity towards galanin of these mutant hGalR1s was indirectly assessed in a functional assay. His264Ala and Phe282Ala mutant receptors, although about 20-fold less efficient than the wild-type hGalR1, can mediate the galaninergic inhibition of isoproterenol-stimulated cAMP production in COS-7 cells. Therefore, these two amino acid residues of hGalR1 very likely interact directly with galanin. Furthermore, because Phe282Tyr-hGalR1 and the wild-type hGalR1 bind galanin equally well (the tyrosine residue is present in this position in other galanin receptor subtypes [FIG. 1]), it is likely that this residue of the receptor mediates the aromatic-aromatic type of interactions with galanin. The His267Ala mutant receptor, however, is nonfunctional even at very high concentrations of galanin (>100μM), and as a histidine residue in this position is not conserved in other galanin receptor subtypes (FIG. 1), it is likely that the residue in this position plays an important role in maintaining the overall structure of the receptor. Replacement of Glu271 with serine leads to a 10-fold diminished binding affinity, but the Glu271Lys substitution does not affect galanin binding to hGalR1 (FIG. 2 and TABLE 1). As this amino acid residue is not conserved in other galanin receptor subtypes (FIG. 1), Glu271 may be close to the binding site, but is not directly involved in binding galanin. All other mutations in that region of hGalR1 have no impact on galanin binding.

Binding of NH_2-Terminally Modified Galanin Analogs to Wild-Type and Glu271Lys Mutant Receptors

Computer-aided modeling of the putative galanin binding site of hGalR1 predicts that the two important pharmacophores of galanin, Trp^2 and Tyr^9, may interact with His264 and Phe282 of hGalR1, but leaves open the orientation of galanin relative to the receptor surface. To test if the docking site for the NH_2-terminus of galanin is near the top of TM VI, we attempted a series of gain-of-binding interactions generated between NH_2-terminally negatively charged galanin analogs and Glu271Lys-hGalR1. Three galanin-(1-16) analogs in which the NH_2-terminal glycine was replaced by functional free carboxylic acids of increasing carbon chain length (malonic, succinic, and glutaric acids, respectively) were synthesized and tested for binding to the wild-type and Glu271Lys-hGalR1. The NH_2-terminally modified galanin (1-16) analogs show a drastic drop in affinity for wild-type receptors with an IC_{50} value of 2.5μM for malonyl-galanin(2-16), whereas both succinyl-galanin(2-16) and glutaryl-galanin (2-16) failed to displace ^{125}I-galanin even at the concentration of 10μM (TABLE 2). The binding of these NH_2-terminally substituted analogs to the Gly271Lys receptor mutant, however, shows a markedly improved affinity as compared to galanin (1-16) (cf. TABLE 2). The affinity of malonyl (2-16)-galanin to the Glu271Lys-hGalR1 is indeed comparable to the binding affinity of galanin-(1-16) to the wild-type receptor. This improvement in affinity can be contributed to the gain-of-binding owing to the new electrostatic interaction taking place between the positively charged Lys271 and the negatively charged NH_2-termini of synthetic galanin analogs. This finding indicates that galanin binds with its NH_2-terminus near the TM VI and enables us to orient galanin on the

TABLE 2. Relative Affinities (IC_{50}analog/IC_{50}wt) of Gly^1-Substituted Galanin-(1-16) Analogs Compared to Galanin (1-16) for the Wild-Type and Glu271Lys-Mutant hGalR1

Galanin Analog	Wild-Type-hGalR1	E271K-hGalR1
Malonyl-gal(2-16)	20	1
Succinyl-gal(2-16)	>50	6
Glutaryl-gal(2-16)	>200	5

receptor surface so that Trp^2, the most important pharmacophore of galanin, interacts with His264 and Tyr^9 of galanin binds to Phe282 of hGalR1 (in other galanin receptor subtypes, a tyrosine residue in the same position is likely to provide the same kind of interaction) (FIG. 2).

In conclusion, we propose that the main interactions between galanin and its receptor occur at the outermost parts of transmembrane domains VI, VII, and III as well as extracellular loop III. In our model, His264 and Phe282 are the amino acid residues of hGalR1 which by interacting with the main pharmacophores of galanin account for most of the free energy of binding. Other interactions should therefore be of a weaker nature, as scanning most of the residues lining the hydrophilic sides of the transmembrane helices did not reveal any additional significant contact points between galanin and its receptor.

REFERENCES

1. MERCHENTHALER, I. *et al.* 1993. Anatomy and physiology of central galanin-containing pathways. Prog. Neurobiol. **40:** 711–769.
2. BARTFAI, T. *et al.* 1993. Galanin: A neuroendocrine peptide. Crit. Rev. Neurobiol. **7:** 229–274.
3. KASK, K. *et al.* 1995. Galanin: A neuropeptide with inhibitory actions. Cell. Mol. Neurobiol. **15:** 653–673.
4. LAND, T. *et al.* 1991. Linear and cyclic NH$_2$-terminal galanin fragments and analogs as ligands at the hypothalamic galanin receptor. Int. J. Peptide Protein Res. **38:** 267–272.
5. HABERT-ORTOLI, E. *et al.* 1994. Molecular cloning of a functional human galanin receptor. Proc. Natl. Acad. Sci. USA **91:** 9780–9783.
6. HOWARD, A.D. *et al.* 1997. Molecular cloning and characterization of a new receptor for galanin. FEBS Lett. **405:** 285–290.
7. WANG, S. *et al.* 1997. Molecular cloning and pharmacological characterization of a new galanin receptor subtype. Mol. Pharmacol. **52:** 337–343.
8. SMITH, K.E. *et al.* 1997. Expression cloning of a rat hypothalamic galanin receptor coupled to phosphoinositide turnover. J. Biol. Chem. **272:** 24612–24616.
9. WANG, S. *et al.* 1997. Cloning and expressional characterization of a novel galanin receptor subtype. Identification of different pharmacophores within galanin for the three galanin receptor subtypes. J. Biol. Chem. **272:** 31949–31952.
10. FATHI, Z. *et al.* 1997. Pharmacological characterization and distribution of a novel galanin receptor. Brain Res. **51:** 49–59.
11. BLOOMQUIST, B.T. *et al.* 1998. Cloning and expression of the human galanin receptor GalR2. Biochem. Biophys. Res. Comm. **243:** 474–479.
12. STRADER, C.D. *et al.* 1994. Structure and function of G protein-coupled receptors. Annu. Rev. Biochem. **63:** 101–132.
13. SCHWARTZ, T.W. *et al.* 1995. Molecular mechanism of action of non-peptide ligands for peptide receptors. Curr. Pharmaceut. Design **1:** 325–342.
14. SCHWARTZ, T.W. *et al.* 1994. Locating ligand-binding sites in 7TM receptors by protein engineering. Curr. Opin. Biotechnol. **5:** 424–444.
15. FONG, T.M. *et al.* 1992. The extracellular domain of the neurokinin-1 receptor is required for high-affinity binding of peptides. Biochemistry **31:** 11806–11811.
16. YOKOTA, Y. *et al.* 1992. Delineation of structural domains involved in the subtype specificity of tachykinin receptors through chimeric formation of substance P/ substance K receptors. EMBO J. **11:** 3585–3591.
17. HUANG, R.-R.C. *et al.* 1994. Interaction of substance P with the second and seventh transmembrane domains of the neurokinin-1 receptor. Biochemistry **33:** 3007–3013.
18. HJORTH, S.A. *et al.* 1994. Identification of peptide binding residues in the extracellular domains of the AT1 receptor. J. Biol. Chem. **269:** 30953–30959.
19. KASK, K. *et al.* 1996. Delineation of the peptide binding site of the human galanin receptor. EMBO J. **15:** 236–244.

20. BERTHOLD, M. *et al.* 1997. Mutagenesis and ligand modification studies on galanin binding to its GTP-binding-protein-coupled receptor GalR1. Eur. J. Biochem. **249:** 601–606.
21. UNGER, V.M. & G.F.X. SCHERTLER. 1995. Low resolution structure of bovine rhodopsin determined by electron cryo-microscopy. Biophys. J. **68:** 1776–1786.
22. BALDWIN, J.M. 1993. The probable arrangements of the helices in G protein-coupled receptors. EMBO J. **12:** 1693–1703.

Chemistry and Molecular Biology of Galanin Receptor Ligands[a]

ÜLO LANGEL[b] AND TAMAS BARTFAI[c]

Department of Neurochemistry and Neurotoxicology, Stockholm University, S-106 91 Stockholm, Sweden

ENDOGENOUS LIGANDS

Galanin was discovered in porcine intestinal extracts as a 29 amino acid long COOH-terminally amidated peptide.[1] TABLE 1 lists the known amino acid sequences of galanin from several species. It is noteworthy that the NH$_2$-terminal 1-14 amino acids are fully conserved, and there are regions of homology within the 15–29 portion of galanin from different species. The human galanin is a 30 amino acid long peptide with a free COOH-terminus because of the replacement of the amide donor Gly in other species by Ser in the human galanin.

TABLE 1. Endogenous Galanin Sequences from 13 Species

Species	Sequence
Human	GWTLNSAGYLLGPH AVGNHRSFSDKNGLTS [32]
Porcine	GWTLNSAGYLLGPH AIDNHRSFHDKYGLA amide[1]
Bovine	GWTLNSAGYLLGPH ALDSHRSFQDKHGLA amide[33]
Canine	GWTLNSAGYLLGPH AIDNHRSFHEKPGLT amide[34]
Sheep	GWTLNSAGYLLGPH AIDNHRSFHDKHGLA amide[35]
Rat	GWTLNSAGYLLGPH AIDNHRSFSDKHGLT amide[36]
Mouse	GWTLNSAGYLLGPH AIDNHRSFSDKHGLT amide[37]
Chicken	GWTLNSAGYLLGPH AVDNHRSFSDKHGFT amide[38]
Quail	GWTLNSAGYLLGPH AVDNHRSFNDKHGFT amide[39]
Alligator	GWTLNSAGYLLGPH AIDNHRSFNEKHGIA amide[40]
Frog	GWTLNSAGYLLGPH AIDNHRSFNDKHGLA amide[41]
Trout	GWTLNSAGYLLGPH GIDGHRTLSDKHGLA amide[42]
Bowfin	GWTLNSAGYLLGPH AVDNHRSLNDKHGLA amide[43]

[a]This work was supported by grants from the Swedish Medical Research Council, the Swedish Board of Natural Sciences, and the EC Biomed 2 program BMH4 CT95 0172.

[b]Address for correspondence: Dr. Ülo Langel, Department of Neurochemistry and Neurotoxicology, Stockholm University, S-106 91 Stockholm, Sweden. Phone, +46-8-161 793; fax, +46-8-161 371; e-mail, ulo@neurochem.su.se

[c]Present address: CNS Department, Preclinical Research, Hoffmann-La Roche Ltd, CH-4070 Basel, Switzerland; on leave of absence from Stockholm University.

There are some NH_2-terminally extended forms of galanin found by immunologic methods in porcine adrenals[2,3] and isolated from porcine brain.[4] These peptides, similar to NH_2-terminally modified galanin(1–29), have lower affinity for spinal cord[5] galanin receptors. Also, truncated galanin fragments were recognized by antisera to porcine galanin.[4]

The secondary and tertiary structure of galanin in solution, in the presence or absence of SDS micelles[6] or phospholipid vesicles,[7,8] was investigated. ^{1}H-NMR studies[9] showed that the COOH-terminal portion of galanin may adopt an α-helical structure. Förster resonance energy transfer[10] between the endogenous fluorophore Trp^2 of galanin and the exogenous fluorescence quencher, dansyl group attached at the ϵ-amino group of Lys^{25} was analyzed to suggest that about 60–70% of the galanin molecule is bent around the Gly^{12}-Pro^{13} structure carrying the only Pro in the peptide. This tertiary structure confined upon galanin by the β-bend in the middle of the molecule places galanin in the small group of neuropeptides, such as neuropeptide Y (NPY) and peptide YY, that have a tertiary structure despite their short length. This structural feature may also be important for the recognition of galanin by the galanin receptor subtype present in the jejunum, because binding to this receptor requires both the NH_2- and COOH-termini of galanin.[11,12]

EXOGENOUS LIGANDS

Peptide Analogs and Fragments

The pharmacophores in galanin have been mapped by the L-Ala substitution of subsequent amino acids[13] in galanin(1-16), which is a high affinity short peptide agonist with an EC_{50} value of ≈ 10 nM. The free NH_2-terminus, Trp^2, Asn^5, and Tyr^9, respectively, was the most important pharmacophore in the 1-16 portion of galanin. Replacement of any of these amino acids one by one with L-Ala led to a 100-fold or more reduced affinity for the hippocampal or hypothalamic galanin receptors.

TABLE 2. The Affinity of Some Elongated and Truncated Forms of Galanin and Synthetic Fragments at Rat Hypothalamic[13] and Spinal Cord[5,a] Galanin Receptors

Peptide	K_D, nM
Galanin(1-29) amide	0.8
Galanin(1-16) amide	6.3
Galanin(1-15) amide	200
Galanin(1-13) amide	150
Galanin(1-12) amide	3,000
Galanin(1-9) amide	100,000
Galanin(-9-29) amide[a]	140
Galanin(-7-29) amide[a]	130
Galanin(17-29) amide	>10,000

The NH_2-terminal fragments 1-12, 1-15, and 1-16 are all relatively high affinity ligands and behave as agonists in *in vitro* and *in vivo* experiments[13,14] (TABLE 2). The peptide fragment experiments showed that for hippocampal galanin receptors the NH_2-terminal 1-12 amino acids are sufficient for recognition of the ligands.[15]

Chimeric Peptides and Substituted Peptides Carrying Galanin(1-13) As the NH₂-Terminus

A series of high affinity chimeric peptides, M15, M35, M40, M32, and C7, were synthesized (TABLE 3) that share the NH_2-terminal 1-13 amino acids of galanin and have different sequences covalently attached to Pro[13] through its carboxylic group. These peptides show distinction between several galanin receptor subtypes; their Hill coefficient in displacing ^{125}I-galanin has been lower than unity.

Most importantly, these high affinity ligands (IC_{50} is 0.1–10 nM) act as antagonists of exogenous galanin action in the ventral hippocampus, hypothalamus, and pancreas, respectively. More significantly, in the study of the spinal flexor reflex, M35 (intrathecally) blocked the effects of endogenous galanin in neuropathic pain models.[16] These ligands carry the full NH_2-terminus of galanin, that is, galanin(1-13), that is required for agonist activity, and *in vitro* models using transiently or stably transfected cell lines expressing 20,000–500,000 galanin receptors per cell (i.e., 5–500 times more receptors than those that endogenously occur) may act as partial agonists,[17] as reported during this conference. This is not surprising and it does not deduct anything from the value of these

TABLE 3. Chimeric and Substituted Galanin Receptor Ligands and Their Affinity for Hypothalamic Galanin Receptors

Peptide	K_D, nM
Galanin(1-29)[13]	0.8
Galanin(1-13)[13]	150
Galanin(1-12)[13]	3,000
M15[a], galanin(1-13)-substance P(5-11) amide[44]	0.1
M32[a], galanin(1-13)-neuropeptide Y(25-36) amide[20]	0.1
M35[a], galanin(1-13)-bradykinin(2-9) amide[20]	0.3
M40[a], galanin(1-13)-(Ala-Leu)₂-Ala amide[20]	10
C7[a], galanin(1-13)-spantide[44]	0.2
Galanin(1-13)-Lys[14](εNH-DOPA) amide[20]	0.4
Galanin(1-13)-Lys[14](εNH-AdoC) amide[20]	1.6
Galanin(1-13)-Lys[14](εNH-Tyr) amide[20]	2.3

[a]A significant amount of *in vivo* data exists on the effects of these ligands on memory, sexual function, and feeding behavior.

chimeric peptides *in vivo* where they helped us to establish the physiologic and pharmacologic roles of galanin (for review see refs. 18 and 19).

Substituted Galanin Receptor Ligands

Attachment of $Lys^{14}(\varepsilon NH-X)$ to galanin (1-13), where X is DOPA, Tyr, or AdoC, produced surprisingly high affinity for these peptide ligands with IC_{50} values in the nanomolar range.[20] These may serve as starting points for peptidomimetic ligand development together with the knowledge in line that Gly^1, Trp^2, Asn^5, and Tyr^9 are the major pharmacophores within these peptide derivatives.

NONPEPTIDE LIGANDS TO GALANIN RECEPTORS

With cells that express cloned galanin receptors (mostly human GalR1), several large scale, high throughput screening programs were carried out at pharmaceutical companies in search of low molecular weight (MW <600) galanin receptor ligands. So far only one patent application has been published (Derwant, patents in CNS, 1998) showing a nonpeptide ligand of moderate affinity ($IC_{50} \approx 1\,\mu M$). This compound is a starting point for synthesis of more improved nonpeptidic galanin receptor ligands.

USE OF ANTISENSE TECHNIQUE TO OBTAIN INFORMATION ON GALANIN ACTION AND ON GALANIN RECEPTOR SUBTYPE INVOLVEMENT

Galanin Antisense Has the Same Effects As Galanin Antagonists in the Spinal Cord

Because galanin expression is highly inducible and galanin turnover is high with galanin half-life being short,[21] the biosynthesis of galanin is ongoing. Under such circumstances, antisense oligonucleotides (AS-ON) antiparallel to galanin mRNA can substantially reduce galanin expression. We showed that galanin AS can be taken up by several axons and retrogradely transported into dorsal root ganglion cells and suppress galanin synthesis and subsequent release.[22] The effects of galanin AS on spinal flexor reflex are similar to those of galanin receptor antagonists, causing increased autotomy upon axotomy.[16] These experiments show that in the absence of good antagonists, AS-ON directed to the neuropeptide ligand may be used successfully.

Receptor Subtype Specificity Explored by Antisense Oligonucleotides to the Receptor Subtypes

Using cell-penetrating peptides with attached peptide nucleic acid type oligonucleotide antisense to GalR1 mRNA(18-38) and-(1-21), we suppressed the galanin effect by 70–80% in the spinal flexor reflex.[23] These experiments suggest that of the three galanin receptor subtypes described so far,[17,24–31] the GalR1 mediates most of the effects of galanin on the flexor reflex (FIG. 1).

Facilitation of flexor reflex, %

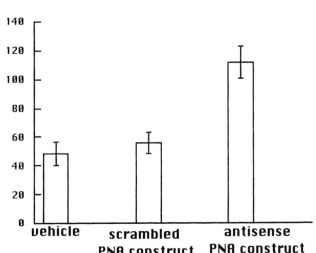

FIGURE 1. Antisense peptide nucleic acid (PNA), 21-mer construct with pAntp peptide, to GalR1 administered intrathecally blocks the effects of 2 ng of galanin on the spinal flexor reflex. 1.5 nmol of cell penetrating PNA antisense construct is administered 3 times in 12 hours. Data are presented as percentage of control facilitation following the conditioning stimulation without preceding galanin treatment. Modified from ref. 23; $n = 3$.

Until the receptor subtype specific/selective ligands for galanin receptor subtypes become available, this approach using receptor subtype-directed antisense oligonucleotides provides a fast and reliable qualitative answer to the involvement of a given subtype in a given function.

CONCLUSIONS

Several more galanin receptor subtypes will likely be discovered in the near future in addition to the three subtypes already known. Finding receptor subtype selective high affinity ligands for these receptors is a major challenge in exploiting the pharmacologic opportunities from occupying galanin receptors in different tissues in different pathophysiologic states with agonists or antagonists, respectively. TABLE 4 shows the expected therapeutic use of galanin receptor ligands.

TABLE 4. Therapeutic Potential of Galanin Receptor Ligands

Receptor Subtype	Ligand	Site of Action	Indication
GalR1/R2	Antagonist	Hippocampus	Alzheimer's disease
GalR2	Antagonist	Locus ceruleus, dorsal raphe nucleus	Depression
GalR2	Antagonist	Pituitary	Regulation of growth hormone secretion
GalR1/R2	Agonist	Spinal cord	Neuropathic pain

ACKNOWLEDGMENTS

We are fortunate to have been introduced to the field of galanin research by its discoverer, Professor Viktor Mutt, to whom we dedicate this manuscript. He helped us in innumerable ways when we found ourselves in a new country, in a new field, and with a new peptide.

We have had the privilege of collaborating with a host of excellent scientists in all areas of neurobiology. In particular we are grateful to Tomas Hökfelt, Zsuzsanna Wiesenfeld-Hallin, Silvana Consolo, Jacqueline Crawley, Astrid Gräslund, Rudolf Rigler, Y. Ben-Ari, and Bo Ahrén. Several doctoral dissertations were written in the course of the work on galanin receptor ligands by G. Fisone, T. Land, K. Bedecs, M. Berthold, K. Kask, S. Andell, M. Pooga, and A. Juréus. Their work is gratefully acknowledged.

REFERENCES

1. TATEMOTO, K., Å. RÖKAEUS, H. JÖRNVALL et al. 1983. Galanin: A novel biologically active peptide from porcine intestine. FEBS Lett. **164:** 124–128.

2. BAUER, F.E., T.E. ADRIAN, N. YANAIHARA et al. 1986. Chromatographic evidence for high-molecular-mass galanin immunoreactivity in pig and cat adrenal glands. FEBS Lett. **201:** 327–331.

3. BERSANI, M., L. THIM, T.N. RASMUSSEN et al. 1991. Galanin and galanin extended at the N-terminus with seven and nine amino acids are produced in and secreted from the porcine adrenal medulla in almost equal amounts. Endocrinology **129:** 2693–2698.

4. SILLARD, R., Å. RÖKAEUS, Y. XU et al. 1992. Variant forms of galanin isolated from porcine brain. Peptides **13:** 1055–1060.

5. BEDECS, K., Ü. LANGEL, X.-J. XU et al. 1994. Biological activities of two endogenously occurring N-terminally extended forms of galanin in the rat spinal cord. Eur. J. Pharmacol. **259:** 151–156.

6. WENNERBERG, A.B.A., M. JACKSON, A. ÖHMAN et al. 1994. The structure of the rodent and porcine neuropeptide galanin and antagonists as determined by FTIR and CD spectroscopy. Can. J. Chem. **72:** 1495–1499.

7. ÖHMAN, A., P.O. LYCKSELL, S. ANDELL et al. 1995. Solvent stabilized solution structures of galanin and galanin analogs, studied by circular dichroism spectroscopy. Biochim. Biophys. Acta **1236:** 259–265.

8. ÖHMAN, A., R. DAVYDOV, B.-M. BACKLUND et al. 1996. A study of melittin, motilin and galanin in reversed micellar environments, using circular dichroism spectroscopy. Biophys. Chem. **59:** 185–192.

9. WENNERBERG, A.B.A., R.M. COOKE, M. CARLQUIST et al. 1990. A ^{1}H NMR study of the solution conformation of the neuropeptide galanin. Biochem. Biophys. Res. Commun. **166:** 1102–1109.

10. KULINSKI, T., A.B. WENNERBERG, R. RIGLER et al. 1997. Conformational analysis of galanin using end to end distance distribution observed by Förster resonance energy transfer. Eur. Biophys. J. **26:** 145–154.

11. ROSSOWSKI, W.J., T.M. ROSSOWSKI, S. ZACHARIA et al. 1990. Galanin binding sites in rat gastric and jejunal smooth muscle membrane preparation. Peptides **11:** 333–338.

12. JURÉUS, A., Ü. LANGEL & T. BARTFAI. 1997. L-Ala-substituted rat galanin analogs distinguish between hypothalamic and jejunal galanin receptor subtypes. J. Pept. Res. **49:** 195–200.

13. LAND, T., Ü. LANGEL, M. LÖW et al. 1991. Linear and cyclic N-terminal galanin fragments and analogs as ligands at the hypothalamic galanin receptor. Int. J. Pept. Protein Res. **38:** 267–272.

14. FISONE, G., Ü. LANGEL, T. LAND et al. 1991. Galanin receptor ligands in the hippocampus: Galanin, N-terminal galanin fragments and analogues. In Galanin: A New Multifunctional Peptide in the Neuro-endocrine System. T. Hökfelt, T. Bartfai, D. Jacobowitz, & D. Ottoson, Eds.: 213–220. McMillan Press. London.

15. GIROTTI, P., R. BERTORELLI, G. FISONE et al. 1993. N-Terminal galanin fragments inhibit the hippocampal release of acetylcholine in vivo. Brain Res. **612:** 258–262.
16. WIESENFELD-HALLIN, Z., X.J. XU, Ü. LANGEL et al. 1992. Galanin-mediated control of pain: Enhanced role after nerve injury. Proc. Natl. Acad. Sci. USA **89:** 3334–3337.
17. SMITH, K.E., C. FORRAY, M.W. WALKER et al. 1997. Expression cloning of a rat hypothalamic galanin receptor coupled to phosphoinositide turnover. J. Biol. Chem. **272:** 24612–24616.
18. KASK, K., Ü. LANGEL & T. BARTFAI. 1995. Galanin: A neuropeptide with inhibitory actions. Cell. Mol. Neurobiol. **15:** 653–673.
19. JURÉUS, A. & Ü. LANGEL. 1996. Galanin and galanin antagonists. Acta Chim. Slovenica **43:** 51–60.
20. POOGA, M., A. JURÉUS, K. RAZAEI et al. 1998. Novel galanin receptor ligands. J. Pept. Res. **51:** 65–74.
21. LAND, T., Ü. LANGEL & T. BARTFAI. 1991. Hypothalamic degradation of galanin(1-29) and galanin(1-16): Identification and characterization of the peptidolytic products. Brain Res. **558:** 245–250.
22. JI, R.R., Q. ZHANG, K. BEDECS et al. 1994. Galanin antisense oligonucleotides reduce galanin levels in dorsal root ganglia and induce autotomy in rats after axotomy. Proc. Natl. Acad. Sci. USA **91:** 12540–12543.
23. POOGA, M., M. HÄLLBRINK, A. VALKNA et al. 1998. Cell penetrating PNA constructs down regulate galanin receptor expression and modify pain transmission in vivo. Nature Biotechnol. Submitted.
24. HABERT-ORTOLI, E., B. AMIRANOFF, I. LOQUET et al. 1994. Molecular cloning of a functional human galanin receptor. Proc. Natl. Acad. Sci. USA **91:** 9780–9783.
25. PARKER, E.M., D.G. IZZARELLI, H.P. NOWAK et al. 1995. Cloning and characterization of the rat GALR1 galanin receptor from Rin14B insulinoma cells. Mol. Brain Res. **34:** 179–189.
26. LORIMER, D.D. & R.V. BENYA. 1996. Cloning and quantification of galanin-1 receptor expression by mucosal cells lining the human gastrointestinal tract. Biochem. Biophys. Res. Commun. **222:** 379–385.
27. BURGEVIN, M.-C., I. LOQUET, D. QUARTERONET et al. 1995. Cloning, pharmacological characterization, and anatomic distribution of a rat cDNA encoding for a galanin receptor. J. Mol. Neurosci. **6:** 1–8.
28. WANG, S., C. HE, T. HASHEMI et al. 1997. Cloning and expressional characterisation of a novel galanin receptor. J. Biol. Chem. **272:** 31949–31952.
29. WANG, S., T. HASHEMI, C. HE et al. 1997. Molecular cloning and pharmacological characterisation of a new galanin receptor subtype. Mol. Pharmacol. **52:** 337–343.
30. HOWARD, A.D., C. TAN, L.L. SHIAO et al. 1997. Molecular cloning and characterization of a new receptor for galanin. FEBS Lett. **405:** 285–290.
31. BLOOMQUIST, B.T., M.R. BEAUCHAMP, L. ZHELNIN et al. 1998. Cloning and expression of the human galanin receptor GalR2. Biochem. Biophys. Res. Commun. **243:** 474–479.
32. SCHMIDT, W.E., H. KRATZIN, K. ECKART et al. 1991. Isolation and primary structure of pituitary human galanin, a 30-residue nonamidated neuropeptide. Proc. Natl. Acad. Sci. USA **88:** 11435–11439.
33. LINDSKOG, S., B. AHRÉN, I. LEIBIGER et al. 1992. The neuropeptide galanin occurs in two conformations. Neuropeptides **23:** 153–155.
34. BOYLE, M.R., C.B. VERCHERE, G. MCKNIGHT et al. 1994. Canine galanin: Sequence, expression and pancreatic effects. Regul. Pept. **50:** 1–11.
35. SILLARD, R., Ü. LANGEL & H. JÖRNVALL. 1991. Isolation and characterization of galanin from sheep brain. Peptides **12:** 855–859.
36. KAPLAN, L.M., E.R. SPINDEL, K.J. ISSELBACHER et al. 1988. Tissue-specific expression of the rat galanin gene. Proc. Natl. Acad. Sci. USA **85:** 1065–1069.
37. LUNDKVIST, J., T. LAND, U. KAHL et al. 1995. cDNA sequence, ligand binding, and regulation of galanin/GMAP in mouse brain. Neurosci. Lett. **200:** 121–124.
38. NORBERG, Å., R. SILLARD, M. CARLQUIST et al. 1991. Chemical detection of natural peptides by specific structures isolation of chicken galanin by monitoring for its N-terminal dipeptide and determination of the amino acid sequence. FEBS Lett. **288:** 151–153.
39. LI, D., K. TSUTSUI, Y. MUNEOKA et al. 1996. An oviposition-inducing peptide: Isolation, localization, and function of avian galanin in the quail oviduct. Endocrinology **137:** 1618–1626.

40. WANG, Y. & J. M. CONLON. 1994. Purification and primary structure of galanin from the alligator stomach. Peptides **15:** 603–606.

41. CHARTREL, N., Y.X. WANG, A. FOURNIER *et al.* 1995. Frog vasoactive intestinal polypeptide and galanin: Primary structures and effects on pituitary adenylate cyclase. Endocrinology **136:** 3079–3086.

42. ANGLADE, I., Y.X. WANG, J. JENSEN *et al.* 1994. Characterization of trout galanin and its distribution in trout brain and pituitary. J. Comp. Neurol. **350:** 63–74.

43. WANG, Y. & J. CONLON. 1994. Purification and characterization of galanin from the phylogenetically ancient fish, the bowfin (*Amia calva*) and dogfish (*Scyliorhinus canicula*). Peptides **15:** 981–986.

44. LANGEL, Ü., T. LAND & T. BARTFAI. 1992. Design of chimeric peptide ligands to galanin receptors and substance P receptors. Int. J. Pept. Protein Res. **39:** 516–522.

Molecular Biology and Pharmacology of Galanin Receptors

THERESA BRANCHEK,[a] KELLI E. SMITH, AND MARY W. WALKER

Synaptic Pharmaceutical Corporation, 215 College Road,
Paramus, New Jersey 07652, USA

ABSTRACT: Galanin was first isolated 15 years ago. Diversity of galanin receptors has been suspected from the study of native tissues and functional responses to galanin and galanin-like peptides *in vitro* and *in vivo*. The recent application of molecular biologic techniques to clone galanin receptors has extended this diversity. So far, three galanin receptor subtypes, GALR1, GALR2, and GALR3, have been cloned from both human and rat. Their molecular structure, pharmacologic profiles, tissue distribution, and signal transduction properties have been partially elucidated.

THE PEPTIDE TRANSMITTER

Galanin is a widely distributed peptide neurotransmitter that activates G-protein–coupled receptors to regulate a variety of physiologic processes, including feeding, insulin release, lactation, spinal reflex, gut contractility, growth, learning, memory, and depression.[1-4] All 14 species homologs studied to date contain 29 amino acids and a carboxy-terminal amide, with the exception of human galanin which contains 30 residues (ending in Ser^{30}) and a carboxyl-free acid. All except tuna fish galanin[5] share an absolutely conserved NH_2-terminal region associated with biologic activity (residues 1-14) and a variant COOH-terminal region.[2,6]

Peptide analogs commonly used to explore galanin receptor pharmacology include fragments, point mutants, and peptide chimera in which the biologically active NH_2-terminal region of galanin[1-13] is linked with a COOH-terminal domain from another neurotransmitter (e.g., substance P_{5-11} for M15, NPY_{25-36} for M32, and bradykinin$_{2-9}$ for M35) or a novel sequence (e.g., spantide for C7 and a hydrophobic stretch for M40).[2,7] Many novel point mutants, cyclic peptides, and chimerae (including corticotropin-releasing factor, leuenkephalin, and endothelin hybrids) were recently described, with receptor binding affinities ranging from subnanomolar to micromolar.[7]

GALANIN RECEPTORS IN NATIVE TISSUES

Galanin binding sites in native cells may be labeled with full-length ^{125}I-galanin or a truncated analog such as ^{125}I-galanin 1-15.[8-10] With this approach, galanin binding sites have been characterized in brain from numerous species. In human brain, a relatively high density of binding sites is reported to be present in cerebral cortex, amygdala, and hypothalamus; lower levels are found in thalamus, pons, and cerebellum.[10] In rat, a relatively

---

[a]Corresponding author. Phone, 201-261-1331 ext 118; fax, 201-261-0623; e-mail, tabranchek@synapticcorp.com

high density of binding sites is found in prefrontal cortex, olfactory bulb, amygdaloid complex, hippocampus, and stria terminalis, with lower levels in nucleus accumbens, hypothalamus, thalamus, and superior colliculus.[11,12] Galanin receptors outside the brain have also been described, with localization in anterior pituitary,[13] pituitary tumors,[14] astrocytes,[15] spinal cord,[16] and gastric and jejunal smooth muscle,[17,18] and in cell lines such as RIN m5F,[19] Rin 14b[20] and human Bowes melanoma.[21] Typical K_d values for ^{125}I-galanin are ~0.05 to 2 nM,[11,12,16,19–22] and reported B_{max} values are as high as 270 fmol/mg membrane protein for RIN14b.[20] Binding of ^{125}I-galanin to membrane-bound receptors may be reduced by GTP analogs,[14,22] indicating that native galanin receptors are coupled to heterotrimeric G-proteins.

Full-length ^{125}I-galanin is displaced from native receptors in human Bowes melanoma cells with a distinctive rank order: human galanin 1-30 > galanin 1-16 > D-Trp[2]-galanin >> galanin 3-30.[21] Galanin binding sites with ≤10-fold difference in affinity for galanin and galanin 1-16 have been documented in rat ventral hippocampus[23] and hypothalamus.[8] Evidence for an NH_2-terminal preferring receptor in the rat dorsal hippocampal formation, neocortex, and neostriatum comes from a binding study using rat ^{125}I-galanin 1-15.[9] A COOH-terminal peptide receptor has also been proposed with the profile: porcine galanin ~ galanin 3-29 > galanin 1-15 and M15.[13] Yet another profile has been identified using binding of ^{125}I-galanin to guinea pig gastric smooth muscle cells; binding was displaced with equal affinity by rat or porcine galanin 1-29, galanin 1-20, galanin 1-15, and galanin 1-10, and also by porcine galanin 2-29 and galanin 3-29.[17] The complex binding profiles for galanin in native tissues and cells have been used to propose the existence of distinct receptor subtypes.[2,9,13,17,24]

Native galanin receptors activate multiple second messenger pathways to affect cell physiology. Selected examples include the following: inhibition of cAMP;[20] activation of channels including ATP-sensitive K^+ channels[25–27] and inwardly rectifying K^+ channels[28,29] such as GIRK-1;[30] inhibition of L-type calcium channels;[31] inhibition of N-type calcium channels[32]; stimulation of inositol phospholipid turnover[33,34]; stimulation *and* inhibition of inositol phospholipid turnover[35]; stimulation of calcium mobilization[34,36]; stimulation *and* inhibition of calcium mobilization[37]; stimulation of phospholipase A_2[38]; activation of MAP kinase[39]; mitogenesis[34,40]; and stimulation of cAMP accumulation.[41] Galanin can either stimulate exocytosis of hormones, such as prolactin and growth hormone, or inhibit exocytosis of hormones and transmitters, such as insulin, glutamate, dopamine, and norepinephrine.[4]

The pharmacology derived from second messenger and physiologic responses reveals a complex profile. The rank order for reduction of forskolin-stimulated cAMP in human Bowes melanoma cells was: galanin 1-30 > galanin 1-16 > D-Trp[2]-galanin >> galanin 3-30.[21] Like galanin itself, the peptide chimerae were agonists: galanin 1-30 ~ M15, M32, M35 > C7, M40. Galanin reduced forskolin-stimulated cAMP with 250-fold greater potency in rat ventral hippocampus (IC_{50} = 1.1 nM) versus dorsal hippocampus (IC_{50} = 270 nM), suggesting either receptor diversity or differences in signal transduction pathways.[42] In dorsal hippocampus, galanin 1-15 but not galanin 1-29 was shown to modulate the binding of [3][H]8-OH-DPAT to $5HT_{1A}$ receptors.[43] A similar pattern (centrally infused galanin 1-15 > galanin 1-29) was found for reduction of baroceptor reflex sensitivity in the rat.[44] Galanin and galanin 15-29 produced dissimilar effects in the opposum internal anal sphincter, where resting tension was reduced by galanin but stimulated by galanin 15-29, and electric-field–stimulated reduction in resting tension was enhanced by galanin but unaffected by galanin 15-29.[45] A distinctive agonist profile was reported for stimulation of prolactin release from rat anterior pituitary: galanin ~ galanin 3-29 > galanin 5-29 > galanin 1-15, M15.[13] In gastric smooth muscle, cAMP was stimulated by galanin ~ galanin 3-29 > galanin 9-29 > galanin 21-29.[17] It is noteworthy that M40, described as a galanin receptor antagonist in brain,[4] ventral hippocampus,[46] hypothalamus,[47,48] amygdala,[48] and spinal cord (where potency was relatively weak versus brain),[4,46] was characterized as a weak agonist in functional studies of Bowes melanoma,[21] RIN m5f,[49] and pancreatic islets.[49] M15, also described as an antagonist in hypothalamus,[50] hippocampus,[27,51] locus ceruleus, spinal cord,[51] and pancreas,[52] was characterized as an agonist in functional studies of Bowes melanoma[21] and gastric smooth muscle,[53] a partial agonist in RIN m5f,[37] and an inactive peptide in the pituitary.[13] The complex functional profiles for these and other peptides such as M35, M32, and C7 with a spectrum of antagonist/agonist activity[21,43,48,54,55] are consistent with the existence of multiple receptor subtypes.

THE CLONED GALR1 RECEPTOR

The first galanin receptor cDNA was isolated by expression cloning from a human Bowes melanoma cDNA library using ^{125}I-porcine galanin[56] and later isolated from human small intestine[57] and human fibroblast.[58] The receptor cDNA for human GALR1 encodes a protein of 349 amino acids with significant homology to the rhodopsin family of G-protein–coupled receptors (GPCRs), including seven predicted hydrophobic membrane-spanning domains common to the GPCR family.[59] The most closely related sequences are those of somatostatin and opioid receptors, although the amino acid identity between hGALR1 and its nearest neighbors did not exceed 32%. The gene for human GALR1 is localized to chromosome 18q23.[58] The rat GALR1 homolog was cloned by expression from the rat RIN14b cell line[60,61] and by homology from rat brain.[62] The rat GALR1 receptor cDNA encodes a protein of 346 amino acids with 92% amino acid identity to human GALR1 (FIG. 1a). Rat and human GALR1 receptors share the same consensus sites for NH_2-linked glycosylation in predicted extracellular domains. Consensus sites for phosphorylation by protein kinases are also conserved between rat and human GALR1 with the exception that human GALR1 contains two additional sites in the COOH-terminal domain. Recently, a mouse GALR1 homolog was also reported[63,64] with 91% identity to human GALR1 and 94% identity to rat GALR1.

The mRNA encoding rat GALR1 was ~9.5 kb with a limited distribution in rat tissues as determined by Northern blot analysis.[60] GALR1 transcripts were readily detected by Northern blot in pancreas-derived RIN14b cells as well as brain and spinal cord, but not in other rat tissues.[60] Within the nervous system, the distribution of rat GALR1 mRNA determined by in situ hybridization was in good agreement with ^{125}I-galanin binding and galanin peptide expression; highest levels were observed in hypothalamus (supraoptic nucleus), amygdala, ventral hippocampus, thalamus, brain stem (medulla oblongata, locus ceruleus, and lateral parabrachial nucleus), and spinal cord (dorsal horn),[60–62]). Thus, the cloned GALR1 receptor distribution appears to overlap with most of the ^{125}I-galanin binding observed within the central nervous system.[65] GALR1 mRNA was not detectable in the rat anterior pituitary,[60,66] suggesting that galanin-dependent effects in this region may be due to another subtype in rat.

a **Comparison of Rat GALR1 and Human GALR1 Receptors**

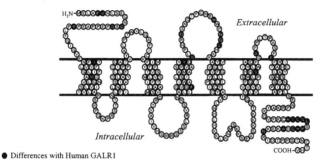

● Differences with Human GALR1

b **Comparison of Rat GALR2 and Human GALR2 Receptors**

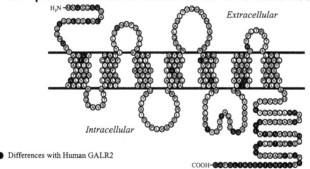

● Differences with Human GALR2

c **Comparison of Rat GALR3 and Human GALR3 Receptors**

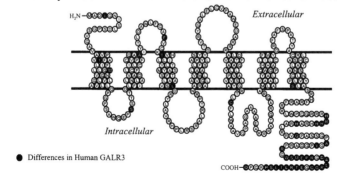

● Differences in Human GALR3

FIGURE 1. Amino acid sequence for rat GALR1, GALR2, and GALR3 receptors. Black residues are divergent from the human homolog. (**a**) Comparison of rat GALR1 and human GALR1 receptors. (**b**) Comparison of rat GALR2 and human GALR2 receptors. (**c**) Comparison of rat GALR3 and human GALR3 receptors.

Cloned GALR1 receptors expressed in COS cells bind porcine ^{125}I-galanin with high affinity, ~0.1–1 nM[56,60,62]; a second low affinity site was measured in one report.[60] Binding to rat GALR1 is displaced by galanin analogs with the following affinity rank order: porcine galanin > galanin 1-16, galanin 1-15 > galanin 3-29, D-Trp^2-galanin.[67] Rat GALR1 also binds the peptide chimerae: M15, M32, M35, C7, and M40.[60,67] The pharmacologic properties of GALR1 receptor binding are similar in rat and human, in parallel with the high level of amino acid identity.

Cloned GALR1 receptors expressed in transfected cells such as CHO and COS reduce forskolin-stimulated cAMP when stimulated with galanin peptide analogs, with a potency rank order matching the binding profile.[56,60,62] The peptide chimerae appear to be full agonists with the following rank order: M15, M32, M35 > C7, M40.[68] This agonist effect cannot be attributed to high receptor density as it persists even when receptor density is drastically reduced by clonal selection or alkylation. The GALR1-dependent reduction of cAMP is blocked by pertussis toxin,[60,67] supporting the involvement of Gi/Go-type G-proteins. A pertussis toxin-sensitive Gi/Go coupling pathway suggests a role for GALR1 in the modulation of native K^+ channels, Ca^{2+} channels, and exocytosis. Consistent with this proposal, GALR1 was shown to activate an inwardly rectifying K^+ current when cotransfected with GIRKs 1 and 4 into *Xenopus* oocytes.[69] The pharmacologic profile of the GALR1 receptor resembles that described for the human Bowes melanoma cell line[21] from which the human receptor was originally cloned.[56] The widespread distribution of GALR1 mRNA and GALR1-like pharmacology in brain and spinal cord[61,62] as well as gut[56,57] and pancreas-derived cells such as RIN14b[60] indicates that GALR1 may act broadly to inhibit neurotransmitter/hormone release, with potential effects on feeding, emotion, memory, nociception, insulin and glucose homeostasis, and gut secretion/motility. The relatively weak agonist activity of M40 in GALR1 cAMP assays resembles the weak agonist effect of M40 reported for the inhibition of glucose-stimulated insulin release from RIN m5f and pancreatic islets.[49] An autoinhibitory effect of GALR1 is suggested by the presence of GALR1 mRNA in galaninergic neurons of the rat basal forebrain.[70] The GALR1 gene is subject to transcriptional regulation by NF-kB, a transcription factor whose activity varies with inflammatory conditions.[58] Interestingly, GALR1 mRNA in dorsal root ganglia is decreased after inflammation or peripheral nerve injury.[71,72]

THE CLONED GALR2 RECEPTOR

Expression and homology-based strategies were used to clone a second galanin receptor subtype, termed GALR2, which displays a surprisingly low degree of amino acid identity with rat and human GALR1 of 38%.[67,73,74] The rat GALR2 cDNA encodes a protein of 372 amino acids with 7 predicted transmembrane domains (FIG. 1b), 3 consensus sites for NH$_2$-linked glycosylation in extracellular domains (1 shared with GALR1), and phosphorylation sites distinct from GALR1 in predicted intracellular regions. The mRNA for rat GALR2 is detected as ~1.8 kb transcript by Northern blot and contains an intron that may be incompletely spliced, as indicated by the cloning of the intron-containing GALR2 cDNAs from rat hypothalamic cDNA libraries.[67,73] By contrast with rat GALR1, the mRNA encoding rat GALR2 is more widely distributed; the GALR2 transcript was present in almost all rat tissues examined, including brain (with highest levels in hypothalamus, hippocampus, amygdala, and pyriform cortex[66]) and peripheral tissues such as vas deferens, prostate, uterus, ovary, stomach, large intestine, dorsal root ganglia, and pancreas-derived cells such as RIN m5f.[67,72–74] Notably, GALR2 mRNA was present in rat anterior pituitary by RNAse protection and RT-PCR, whereas GALR1 was not,[66] suggesting that GALR2 may mediate the effects of galanin on pituitary hormone secretion.

Cloning of the cDNA encoding the human GALR2 receptor has been reported.[75–77] Human GALR2 shares only 85% amino acid identity with rat GALR2 and is predicted to contain 387 amino acids, longer by 15 amino acids than the rat homolog in the carboxy terminus (FIG. 1b). Thus, the human and rat GALR2 receptors are less conserved than the human and rat GALR1 receptors.

Cloned GALR2 receptors expressed in COS cells bind porcine ^{125}I-galanin with high affinity, $K_d \sim 0.2$ nM.[66,67,73,74,78] Binding is displaced from rat GALR2 by galanin analogs with the following affinity rank order (porcine galanin > gal 1-16, galanin 1-15, D-Trp^2-galanin >> galanin 3-29[66,67,74]). Binding is also displaced by peptide chimerae (M32, M35, M40, M15, C7) within a relatively narrow affinity range.[67] Despite its sequence divergence from GALR1, the pharmacologic profile of rat GALR2 is similar to that of GALR1 in having high affinity for full-length and NH_2-terminal fragments of galanin ($\geq$ galanin 1-15) and also for the peptide chimerae, but no affinity for galanin 3-29 at concentrations up to 1 uM.[66,67,73,78] However, rat GALR2 may be distinguished from GALR1 by its ability to tolerate either D-Trp^2 [67] or the deletion of Gly^1, as in galanin 2-29.[78] NH_2-terminal extension of galanin to galanin -7 to 29 is more disruptive for GALR1 than for GALR2; this could indicate that GALR1 is more likely than GALR2 to mediate the reduced potency of galanin -7 to 29 versus galanin 1-29 in the spinal reflex assay.[79] The human GALR2 receptor displayed a similar pharmacologic profile in ^{125}I-galanin binding assays,[75] except that D-Trp^2-galanin bound with relatively reduced affinity.[75–77]

The consequences of GALR2 receptor activation include: pertussis toxin-resistant inositol phospholipid hydrolysis in CHO[67] and 293 cells[66]; calcium mobilization in CHO cells[67]; arachidonic acid efflux in CHO,[68] and activation of calcium-dependent Cl⁻ channels in *Xenopus* oocytes.[67] Rat GALR2 did not inhibit forskolin-stimulated cAMP in CHO cells under conditions supporting a pertussis toxin-sensitive reduction of cAMP by rat GALR1,[67] however, a small inhibitory effect of GALR2 on forskolin-stimulated cAMP accumulation was reported to occur in COS-1 cells.[74] The ability of rat GALR2 to produce a robust pertussis toxin-resistant stimulation of inositol phospholipid hydrolysis suggests a primary coupling to G-proteins of the Gq/G11 class activating phospholipase C. This coupling was surprising, because rarely do two rhodopsin-like receptor subtypes for a peptide neurotransmitter signal preferentially through different G-protein classes.

The pharmacology derived for rat GALR2-dependent stimulation of inositol phospholipid hydrolysis includes the following rank order: porcine galanin > D-Trp^2-galanin > galanin 1-15, galanin 1-16 >> galanin 3-29.[67] The peptide chimerae appear to be full agonists in inositol phosphate and arachidonic acid release assays.[67,68] The human GALR2 receptor also stimulates inositol phospholipid hydrolysis with a similar pharmacologic profile.[76,77] For both human and rat receptor homologs, the EC_{50}s for inositol phospholipid hydrolysis tend to be larger than the corresponding pK_i values derived from binding assays,[67] but the SAR is generally maintained.[67,68,77]

A structure-activity profile in support of a native GALR2-like pharmacology has not been documented previously; however native galanin receptors are linked to inositol phospholipid hydrolysis,[33–35] calcium mobilization,[34,36,37] and phospholipase A_2 activation,[38] all of which may underlie a stimulatory effect on exocytosis[13,36,40] and growth.[34,39,40]

Thus, GALR2 is a candidate receptor for the positive effects of galanin on calcium flux and related events in RIN m5f,[37] anterior pituitary,[13] GH3 cells,[36] mudpuppy neurons,[38] and small lung carcinoma cells.[34,39] Rat GALR2 mRNA is detected in brain, hypothalamus, pituitary, dorsal root ganglia, pancreas-derived cells, gut, spleen, lung, skeletal muscle, heart, kidney, liver, and reproductive organs.[66,67,72–74] The relative contribution of GALR2 to galanin signaling may be a function of development, nerve injury, and other factors. In Alzheimer's dementia, galanin-containing fibers hyperinnervate cholinergic neurons of the basal forebrain[80]; it would be interesting to know if GALR2 receptors are involved in this process. GALR2 may promote the survival of the dwindling population of cholinergic neurons. Outside the CNS, GALR2 mRNA is upregulated in dorsal root ganglia after inflammation, with a peak at 3 days[72]; again, GALR2 may promote survival in this paradigm. By contrast, GALR2 (like GALR1) mRNA is downregulated after axotomy, when galanin expression is dramatically upregulated,[72] suggesting a role for additional galanin receptor subtypes in the response to axotomy.

THE CLONED GALR3 RECEPTOR

A third rat galanin receptor subtype, GALR3, was recently described by two groups.[69,78] The receptor isolated by Wang and co-workers was derived from a homology-based screen of sequences deposited in GenBank using a GALR1 probe. A novel human gene fragment with similarity to GALR1 was identified; polymerase chain reaction primers were then used to isolate a partial coding sequence from rat liver cDNA. The full-length clone was subsequently isolated from rat hypothalamus. The receptor isolated by Smith and co-workers was obtained by a combination of homology and expression cloning techniques from a rat hypothalamic cDNA library.[69] The two reported sequences are divergent in four positions; the reason for the divergence remains to be determined. The rat GALR3 cDNA reported by Smith and co-workers encodes a protein of 370 amino acids sharing an amino acid identity of 35% with rat GALR1 and 52% with rat GALR2, the most closely related receptor. The sequence similarity to GALR2 is higher within TM domains II through IV, where amino acid identities range from 70% to over 90%. Although Wang and co-workers made no reference to an intron in the rat GALR3 sequence,[78] an intron contained in the human sequence from Genbank indicates conserved intron/exon boundaries for GALR3 and GALR2. The GALR3 receptor sequence contains a single consensus site for NH_2-linked glycosylation and several predicted intracellular sites for phosphorylation by protein kinases. Alignment of the three rat galanin receptors reveals a significant degree of sequence similarity: 83 residues are present in all three subtypes, representing ~23% shared amino acid identity. When compared with other GPCR sequences, galanin receptors show highest amino acid identity with the somatostatin sst_4 and sst_5 subtypes and with the orphanin FQ receptor (30–32%). Despite this degree of similarity, dendrogram analysis demonstrates that GALR1, GALR2, and GALR3 form a subfamily distinct from the somatostatin, opioid, and neurokinin subfamilies (FIG. 2). By Northern blot, Wang and co-workers detected GALR3 mRNA as a ~3-8 kb transcript (with molecular weight depending on the tissue) in heart, spleen, and testis but not in brain[78]; isolation of GALR3 from a rat hypothalamic cDNA library, however, indicates that it is present in rat CNS at low abundance. Using the more sensitive method of RPA, Smith and co-workers detected GALR3 transcripts in discrete regions of the rat CNS with

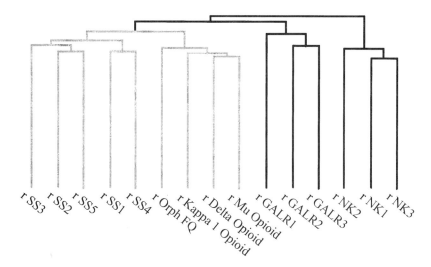

FIGURE 2. Dendrogram analysis of the galanin receptor subfamily and similar GPCR subfamilies in the rat.

highest levels in the hypothalamus, lower levels in the olfactory bulb, cerebral cortex, medulla oblongata, caudate putamen, cerebellum, and spinal cord, and no significant detection in hippocampus or substantia nigra. By the same method, GALR3 mRNA was detected in peripheral tissues with highest levels in pituitary, lower levels in liver, kidney, stomach, testicle, adrenal cortex, lung, adrenal medulla, spleen, and pancreas, and no significant detection in heart, uterus, vas deferens, choroid plexus, or dorsal root ganglia.[69]

The cloned GALR3 receptor bound porcine ^{125}I-galanin with an apparent K_d value of 0.6 nM when expressed transiently in COS-7[78] and 0.98 nM when expressed stably in 293 cells.[69] The apparent B_{max} measured in COS-7 by Wang and co-workers (27 fmol/mg membrane protein) was relatively low for a transiently expressed receptor.[78] By contrast, the apparent B_{max} measured in 293 cells by Smith and co-workers was over 10-fold higher, at 460 fmol/mg.[69] Binding was displaced by galanin analogs with the following affinity rank order: rat galanin > human galanin, galanin 1-16 >> galanin 3-29, D-Trp^2-galanin.[69] Binding was also displaced by peptide chimerae (C7, M32, M35, M40, and M15), with M40 displaying relatively weak activity.[69] Examination of peptides tested similarly in the separate GALR3 studies reveals general agreement in the structure-activity profiles;[69,78] slight differences in rank order may reflect differences in receptor expression and extent of G-protein–coupling in the host cell. Despite the clear evolutionary relatedness of GALR2 in amino acid identity (57%) and intron/exon structure, GALR3 pharmacology resembles GALR1 in many respects. Both GALR1 and GALR3 are relatively less tolerant of NH$_2$-terminal and COOH-terminal galanin deletion than are GALR2 receptors, and both GALR1 and GALR3 receptors display lower affinity for M40 than do other peptide chimerae.[69,78] All three cloned galanin receptor subtypes share a general preference for the conserved NH$_2$-terminal portion of galanin peptide (with no apparent affinity for galanin 3-29) and tolerance for galanin 2-29 as follows: GALR2 > GALR3 > GALR1. Diverse receptor subtype-selective ligands are needed to develop more definitive pharmacologic signatures (TABLE 1).

TABLE 1. Pharmacological Properties of Cloned Galanin Receptors

•GALR1	•GALR2	•GALR3
NH$_2$-terminus preferring	NH$_2$-terminus preferring	NH$_2$-terminus preferring
Coupled through Gα_i to inhibition of adenylylcyclase	Coupled through G$\alpha_{q/11}$ to PI turnover and calcium mobilization	Coupled through Gα_i/Gα_i
Chimeric antagonist peptides have agonist activity	Chimeric antagonist peptides have agonist activity	Chimeric antagonist peptides have agonist activity
Low affinity for [D-Trp^2] galanin and galanin 2-29	High affinity for [D-Trp^2] galanin and galanin 2-29	Moderate affinity for galanin 2-29
mRNA present in rat hypothalamus	mRNA present in rat hypothalamus	mRNA present in rat hypothalamus

The full-length human GALR3 receptor cDNA was isolated by homology approaches using the rat GALR3 sequence.[69] The human GALR3 receptor is predicted to contain 368 amino acids, with 90% identity to rat GALR3 (FIG. 1c). The human GALR3 shares an amino acid identity of 37% with human GALR1 and 57% with human GALR2. When compared with the human GALR3-like sequence deposited in Genbank, the human GALR3 receptor appears to differ in six amino acid positions. The human GALR3 receptor shares intron/exon boundaries with the GALR2 receptors, consistent with a relatively high homology between these two receptor subtypes. Human and rat GALR3 receptors both contain a single consensus site for NH$_2$-linked glycosylation in the NH$_2$-terminus and multiple intracellular consensus sites for phosphorylation. Human and rat GALR3 share a unique consensus phosphorylation site in the third intracellular loop which is absent in GALR1 and GALR2 and which could have implications for G-protein–coupling and receptor function. Human and rat GALR3 each contain a different consensus site for PKC phosphorylation in the COOH-terminal tail, suggesting the possibility of distinct regulatory mechanisms for human compared with rat GALR3 receptors. Human and rat GALR3 receptors share a similar pharmacologic profile in ^{125}I-galanin receptor binding assays.[69] Interestingly, both human and rat GALR3 receptors display lower affinity for human than for porcine and rat galanin.[69]

Human and rat GALR3 receptors expressed in *Xenopus* oocytes activate GIRKs in response to applied galanin.[69,81] Human GALR3 produced a more robust response than did rat GALR3, suggesting a difference in receptor expression or efficiency of G-protein activation. The human GALR3 response was completely blocked by pertussis toxin,[81] consistent with coupling to the Gi/Go-class of G proteins. The peptide ligand pharmacology is comparable to that derived in ^{125}I-galanin binding assays,[69,81] but the EC$_{50}$ values from the oocyte assays are larger than those of corresponding binding constants. This is similar to the pattern for GALR2, in which EC$_{50}$ values from inositol phosphate assays were larger than the corresponding binding constants. All chimeric peptides tested (C7, M32, M35, M15, and M40) were agonists in the GALR3 oocyte GIRK assay, with M40 displaying lowest potency.[81] Thus, both GALR1 and GALR3 share a common signal transduction pathway in the oocyte involving G proteins of the Gi/Go-class. Exactly which G proteins are involved for each receptor in native systems remains to be determined.

Discrete localization of GALR3 mRNA in such regions as hypothalamus, pituitary, spinal cord, pancreas, liver, kidney, stomach, and adrenal gland[69] suggests that GALR3 may be involved in feeding, digestion, pituitary hormone release, nociception, insulin, and glucose homeostasis. That GALR3 mRNA is detectable in spinal cord but not in dorsal root ganglia[69] is particularly intriguing, as a recent report documents the existence of a galanin-dependent inward current in dorsal root ganglia only after axotomy, at a time when galanin mRNA is dramatically upregulated but GALR1 and GALR2 mRNA are downregulated.[82] It would be of interest to determine whether GALR3 mRNA is upregulated in dorsal root ganglia in response to nerve injury.

OTHER RECEPTOR SUBTYPES

It is plausible that additional members of the galanin receptor family remain to be cloned. The cloned GALR1, GALR2, and GALR3 receptors do not readily account for all of the putative receptors proposed to exist based on structure-activity data (TABLE 1). Unexplained cases include the putative receptor for galanin 1-15 linked to $5HT_{1A}$ receptor modulation in dorsal hippocampus[43] and blood pressure modulation in locus ceruleus[44]; the receptor for galanin 15-29 linked to resting tension in the anal sphincter[45]; the receptor for galanin 3-29 linked to prolactin release in anterior pituitary[13]; and the receptor for galanin 3-29 linked to relaxation and cAMP accumulation in gastric smooth muscle.[17] Recently, galanin 3-29 was also reported to weakly inhibit synaptic transmission in the rat arcuate nucleus.[83] Furthermore, the cloned receptors do not explain why the peptide chimerae are reported to antagonize the effects of galanin in several systems, including hypothalamus, ventral hippocampus, dorsal hippocampus, amygdala, locus ceruleus, pituitary, spinal cord, pancreas, and RIN m5f cells.[4,43,46–48,50–52,54,55] In addition, it is difficult to align the cloned subtypes with published reports of galanin receptors studied *in vivo*. Essential for the clarification of these issues are the development of selective new agonists and antagonists, continued cloning efforts, and the construction of transgenic animals with targeted disruption of the galanin receptor genes.

ACKNOWLEDGMENT

We are grateful to George Moralishvili for his expert graphic design.

REFERENCES

1. BARTFAI, T., T. HOKFELT & U. LANGEL. 1993. Galanin: A neuroendocrine peptide. Crit. Rev. in Neurobiol. **7:** 229–274.
2. KASK, K., U. LANGEL & T. BARTFAI. 1995. Galanin: A neuropeptide with inhibitory actions. Cell. Mol. Neurobiol. **15:** 653–673.
3. BEDECS, K., M. BERTHOLD & T. BARTFAI. 1995. Galanin: 10 years with a neuroendocrine peptide. Int. J. Biochem. Bell. Biol. **27:** 337–349.
4. KASK, K., M. BERTHOLD & T. BARTFAI. 1997. Galanin receptors: Involvement in feeding, pain, depression and Alzheimer's disease. Life Sci. **60:** 1523–1533.
5. KAKUYAMA, H., A. KUWAHARA, T. MOCHIZUKI, M. HOSHINO & N. YANAIHARA. 1997. Role of N-terminal active sites of galanin in neurally evoked circular muscle contractions in the guinea-pig ileum. Eur. J. Pharmacol. **329:** 85–91.

6. LUNDKVIST, J., T. LAND, U. KAHL, K. BEDECS & T. BARTFAI. 1995. cDNA sequence, ligand binding, and regulation of galanin/GMAP in mouse brain. Neurosci. Lett. **200:** 121–124.
7. POOGA, M., A. JUREUS, K. REZAEI, H. HASANVAN, K. SAAR, K. KASK, P. KJELLEN, T. LAND, J. HALONEN, U. MAEORG, A. URI, S. SOLYOM, T. BARTFAI & U. LANGEL. 1998. Novel galanin receptor ligands. J. Pept. Res. **51:** 65–74.
8. LAND, T., U. LANGEL, G. FISONE, K. BEDECS & T. BARTFAI. 1991. Assay for galanin receptor. Methods Neurosci. **5:** 225–234.
9. HEDLUND, P.B., N. YANAIHARA & K. FUXE. 1992. Evidence for specific N-terminal galanin fragment binding sites in the rat brain. Eur. J. Pharmacol. **224:** 203–205.
10. JOHARD, H.A., C.T. LUNDQUIST, A. ROKAEUS & D.R. NASSEL. 1992. Autoradiographic localization of ^{125}I-galanin binding sites in the blowfly brain. Regul. Pept. **42:** 123–134.
11. SKOFITSCH, G., M.A. SILLS & D.M. JACOBOWITZ. 1986. Autoradiographic distribution of ^{125}I-galanin binding sites in the rat central nervous system. Peptides **7:** 1029–1042.
12. FISONE, G., U. LANGEL, M. CARLQUIST, T. BERGMAN, S. CONSOLO, T. HOKFELT, A. UNDEN, S. ANDELL & T. BARTFAI. 1989. Galanin receptor and its ligands in the rat hippocampus. Eur. J. Biochem. **181:** 269–276.
13. WYNICK, D., D.M. SMITH, M. GHATEI, K. AKINSANYA, R. BHOGAL, P. PURKISS, P. BYFIELD, N. YANAIHARA & S.R. BLOOM. 1993. Characterization of a high-affinity galanin receptor in the rat anterior pituitary: Absence of biological effect and reduced membrane binding of the antagonist M15 differentiate it from the brain/gut receptor. Proc. Natl. Acad. Sci. USA **90:** 4231–4235.
14. HULTING, A.L., T. LAND, M. BERTHOLD, U. LANGEL, T. HOKFELT & T. BARTFAI. 1993. Galanin receptors from human pituitary tumors assayed with human galanin as ligand. Brain Res. **625:** 173–176.
15. HOSLI, E., M. LEDERGERBER, A. KOFLER & L. HOSLI. 1997. Evidence for the existence of galanin receptors on cultured astrocytes of rat CNS: Colocalization with cholinergic receptors. J. Chem. Neuroanat. **13:** 95–103.
16. BEDECS, K., U. LANGEL, T. BARTFAI & Z. WIESENFELD-HALLIN. 1992. Galanin receptors and their second messengers in the lumbar dorsal spinal cord. Acta. Physiol. Scand. **144:** 213–220.
17. GU, Z.F., T.K. PRADHAN, D.H. COY & R.T. JENSEN. 1995. Interaction of galanin fragments with galanin receptors on isolated smooth muscle cells from guinea pig stomach: Identification of a novel galanin receptor subtype. J. Pharmacol. Exp. Ther. **272:** 371–378.
18. ROSSOWSKI, W.J., T.M. ROSSOWSKI, S. ZACHARIA, A. ERTAN & D.H. COY. 1990. Galanin binding sites in rat gastric and jejunal smooth muscle membrane preparations. Peptides **11:** 333–338.
19. LAGNY-POURMIR, I., B. AMIRANOFF, A.M. LORINET, K. TATEMOTO & M. LABURTHE. 1989. Characterization of galanin receptors in the insulin-secreting cell lineRin m 5F: Evidence for coupling with a pertussis toxin-sensitive guanosine triphosphate regulatory protein. Endocrinology **124:** 2635–2641.
20. AMIRANOFF, B., A.M. LORINET & M. LABURTHE. 1991. A clonal rat pancreatic delta cell line (Rin14B) expresses a high number of galanin receptors negatively coupled to a pertussis-toxin-sensitive cAMP-production pathway. Eur. J. Biochem. **195:** 459–463.
21. HEUILLET, E., Z. BOUAICHE, J. MENAGER, P. DUGAY, N. MUNOZ, H. DUBOIS, B. AMIRANOFF, A. CRESPO, J. LAVAYRE, J.C. BLANCHARD et al. 1994. The human galanin receptor: Ligand-binding and functional characteristics in the Bowes melanoma cell line. Eur. J. Pharmacol. **269:** 139–147.
22. WALLI, R., H. SCHAFER, C. MORYS-WORTMANN, G. PAETZOLD, R. NUSTEDE & W.E. SCHMIDT. 1994. Identification and biochemical characterization of the human brain galanin receptor. J. Mol. Endocrinol. **13:** 347–356.
23. FISONE, G., M. BERTHOLD, K. BEDECS, A. UNDEN, T. BARTFAI, R. BERTORELLI, S. CONSOLO, J. CRAWLEY, B. MARTIN, S. NILSSON et al. 1989. N-terminal galanin-(1-16) fragment is an agonist at the hippocampal galanin receptor. Proc. Natl. Acad. Sci. USA **86:** 9588–9591.
24. DEECHER, D.C., O.O. ODUSAN & E.J. MUFSON. 1995. Galanin receptors in human basal forebrain differ from receptors in the hypothalamus: Characterization using [^{125}I]galanin (porcine) and [^{125}I]galantide. J. Pharmacol. Exp. Ther. **275:** 720–727.
25. DUNNE, M.J., M.J. BULLETT, G.D. LI, C.B. WOLLHEIM & O.H. PETERSEN. 1989. Galanin activates nucleotide-dependent K+ channels in insulin-secreting cells via a pertussis toxin-sensitive G-protein. EMBO J. **8:** 413–420.
26. DE WEILLE, J., H. SCHMID-ANTOMARCHI, M. FOSSET & M. LAZDUNSKI. 1988. ATP-sensitive K+ channels that are blocked by hypoglycemia-inducing sulfonylureas in insulin-secreting cells

are activated by galanin, a hyperglycemia-inducing hormone. Proc. Natl. Acad. Sci. USA **85:** 1312–1316.

27. ZINI, S., M.P. ROISIN, U. LANGEL, T. BARTFAI & Y. BEN-ARI. 1993. Galanin reduces release of endogenous excitatory amino acids in the rat hippocampus. Eur. J. Pharmacol. **245:** 1–7.

28. PARSONS, R.L. & L.A. MERRIAM. 1993. Galanin activates an inwardly rectifying potassium conductance in mudpuppy atrial myocytes. Pflüger's Arch. **422:** 410–412.

29. DE WEILLE, J.R., M. FOSSET, H. SCHMID-ANTOMARCHI & M. LAZDUNSKI. 1989. Galanin inhibits dopamine secretion and activates a potassium channel in pheochromocytoma cells. Brain Res. **485:** 199–203.

30. PHILIPSON, L.H., A. KUZNETSOV, P.T. TOTH, J.F. MURPHY, G. SZABO, G.H. MA & R.J. MILLER. 1995. Functional expression of an epitope-tagged G protein-coupled K+ channel (GIRK1). J. Biol. Chem. **270:** 14604–14610.

31. KALKBRENNER, F., V.E. DEGTIAR, M. SCHENKER, S. BRENDEL, A. ZOBEL, J. HESCHLER, B. WITTIG & G. SCHULTZ. 1995. Subunit composition of G(o) proteins functionally coupling galanin receptors to voltage-gated calcium channels. EMBO J. **14:** 4728–4737.

32. PALAZZI, E., S. FELINSKA, M. ZAMBELLI, G. FISONE, T. BARTFAI & S. CONSOLO. 1991. Galanin reduces carbachol stimulation of phosphoinositide turnover in rat ventral hippocampus by lowering Ca2+ influx through voltage-sensitive Ca2+ channels. J. Neurochem. **56:** 739–747.

33. HARDWICK, J.C. & R.L. PARSONS. 1992. Galanin stimulates phosphatidylinositol turnover in cardiac tissue of the mudpuppy. J. Auton. Nerv. Syst. **40:** 87–90.

34. SETHI, T. & E. ROZENGURT. 1991. Galanin stimulates Ca2+ mobilization, inositol phosphate accumulation, and clonal growth in small cell lung cancer cells. Cancer Res. **51:** 1674–1679.

35. MALM, D., S. LINDSKOG, B. AHREN & J. FLORHOLMEN. 1997. Galanin exerts dual action on inositol-specific phospholipase C activity in isolated pancreatic islets. Endocrinol. J. **44:** 283–288.

36. DROUHAULT, R., N.C. GUERINEAU, P. MOLLARD, M.A. CADORET, J.B. CORCUFF, A.M. VACHER & N. VILAYLECK. 1994. Prolactin and growth hormone release and calcium influx are stimulated by galanin within a 'window' range of concentrations in pituitary GH3 B6 cells. Neuroendocrinology **60:** 179–184.

37. FRIDOLF, T. & B. AHREN. 1993. Dual action of the neuropeptide galanin on the cytoplasmic free calcium concentration in RIN m5F cells. Biochem. Biophys. Res. Commun. **191:** 1224–1229.

38. MULVANEY, J.M. & R.L. PARSONS. 1995. Arachidonic acid may mediate the galanin-induced hyperpolarization in parasympathetic neurons from *Necturus maculosus*. Neurosci. Lett. **187:** 95–98.

39. SEUFFERLEIN, T. & E. ROZENGURT. 1996. Galanin, neurotensin, and phorbol esters rapidly stimulate activation of mitogen-activated protein kinase in small cell lung cancer cells activation of mitogen-activated protein kinase in small cell lung cancer cells. Cancer Res. **56:** 5758–5764.

40. HAMMOND, P.J., D.M. SMITH, K.O. AKINSANYA, W.A. MUFTI, D. WYNICK & S.R. BLOOM. 1996. Signalling pathways mediating secretory and mitogenic responses to galanin and pituitary adenylate cyclase-activating polypeptide in the 235-1 clonal rat lactotroph cell line. J. Neuroendocrinol. **8:** 457–464.

41. GU, Z.F., T.K. PRADHAN, D.H. COY & R.T. JENSEN. 1994. Galanin-induced relaxation in gastric smooth muscle cells is mediated by cyclic AMP. Peptides **15:** 1425–1430.

42. VALKNA, A., A. JUREUS, E. KARELSON, M. ZILMER, T. BARTFAI & U. LANGEL. 1995. Differential regulation of adenylate cyclase activity in rat ventral and dorsal hippocampus by rat galanin. Neurosci. Lett. **187:** 75–78.

43. HEDLUND, P.B., U.B. FINNMAN, N. YANAIHARA & K. FUXE. 1994. Galanin-(1-15), but not galanin-(1-29), modulates 5-HT1A receptors in the dorsal hippocampus of the rat brain: Possible existence of galanin receptor subtypes. Brain Res. **634:** 163–167.

44. DIAZ, Z., J.A. NARVAEZ, P.B. HEDLUND, J.A. AGUIRRE, S. GONZALEZ-BARON & K. FUXE. 1996. Centrally infused galanin-(1-15) but not galanin-(1-29) reduces the baroreceptor reflex sensitivity in the rat. Brain Res. **741:** 32–37.

45. CHAKDER, S. & S. RATTAN. 1991. Effects of galanin on the opossum internal anal sphincter: Structure-activity relationship. Gastroenterology **100:** 711–718.

46. McDONALD, M.P. & J.N. CRAWLEY. 1996. Galanin receptor antagonist M40 blocks galanin-induced choice accuracy deficits on a delayed-nonmatching-to-position task. Behav. Neurosci. **110:** 1025–1032.

47. LEIBOWITZ, S.F. & T. KIM. 1992. Impact of a galanin antagonist on exogenous galanin and natural patterns of fat ingestion. Brain Res. **599:** 148–152.

48. CORWIN, R.L., J.K. ROBINSON & J.N. CRAWLEY. 1993. Galanin antagonists block galanin-induced feeding in the hypothalamus and amygdala of the rat. Eur. J. Neurosci. **5:** 1528–1533.

49. BARTFAI, T., U. LANGEL, K. BEDECS, S. ANDELL, T. LAND, S. GREGERSEN, B. AHREN, P. GIROTTI, S. CONSOLO & R. CORWIN. 1993. Galanin-receptor ligand M40 peptide distinguishes between putative galanin-receptor subtypes. Proc. Natl. Acad. Sci. USA **90:** 11287–11291.

50. SAHU, A., B. XU & S.P. KALRA. 1994. Role of galanin in stimulation of pituitary luteinizing hormone secretion as revealed by a specific receptor antagonist, galantide. Endocrinology **134:** 529–536.

51. BARTFAI, T., K. BEDECS, T. LAND, U. LANGEL, R. BERTORELLI, P. GIROTTI, S. CONSOLO, X.J. XU, Z. WIESENFELD-HALLIN & S. NILSSON. 1991. M-15: High-affinity chimeric peptide that blocks the neuronal actions of galanin in the hippocampus, locus coeruleus, and spinal cord. Proc. Natl. Acad. Sci. USA **88:** 10961–10965.

52. LINDSKOG, S., B. AHREN, T. LAND, U. LANGEL & T. BARTFAI. 1992. The novel high-affinity antagonist, galantide, blocks the galanin-mediated inhibition of glucose-induced insulin secretion. Eur. J. Pharmacol. **210:** 183–188.

53. GU, Z.F., W.J. ROSSOWSKI, D.H. COY, T.K. PRADHAN & R.T. JENSEN. 1993. Chimeric galanin analogs that function as antagonists in the CNS are full agonists in gastrointestinal smooth muscle. J. Pharmacol. Exp. Ther. **266:** 912–918.

54. KASK, K., M. BERTHOLD, J. BOURNE, S. ANDELL, U. LANGEL & T. BARTFAI. 1995. Binding and agonist/antagonist actions of M35, galanin(1-13)-bradykinin(2-9)amide chimeric peptide, in Rin m 5F insulinoma cells. Regul. Pept. **59:** 341–348.

55. XU, X.J., Z. WIESENFELD-HALLIN, U. LANGEL, K. BEDECS & T. BARTFAI. 1995. New high affinity peptide antagonists to the spinal galanin receptor. Br. J. Pharmacol. **116:** 2076–2080.

56. HABERT-ORTOLI, E., B. AMIRANOFF, I. LOQUET, M. LABURTHE & J.F. MAYAUX. 1994. Molecular cloning of a functional human galanin receptor. Proc. Natl. Acad. Sci. USA **91:** 9780–9783.

57. LORIMER, D.D. & R.V. BENYA. 1996. Cloning and quantification of galanin-1 receptor expression by mucosal cells lining the human gastrointestinal tract. Biochem. Biophys. Res. Commun. **222:** 379–385.

58. NICHOLL, J., B. KOFLER, G.R. SUTHERLAND, J. SHINE & T.P. IISMA. 1995. Assignment of the gene encoding human galanin receptor (GALNR) to 18q23 by in situ hybridization. Genomics **30:** 629–630.

59. PROBST, W.C., L.A. SNYDER, D.I. SCHUSTER, J. BROSIUS & S.C. SEALFON. 1992. Sequence alignment of the G-protein coupled receptor superfamily. DNA Cell Biol. **11:** 1–20.

60. PARKER, E.M., D.G. IZZARELLI, H.P. NOWAK, C.D. MAHLE, L.G. IBEN, J. WANG & M.E. GOLDSTEIN. 1995. Cloning and characterization of the rat GALR1 galanin receptor from Rin14B insulinoma cells. Brain Res. Mol. Brain Res. **34:** 179–189.

61. GUSTAFSON, E.L., K.E. SMITH, M.M. DURKIN, C. GERALD & T.A. BRANCHEK. 1996. Distribution of a rat galanin receptor mRNA in rat brain. NeuroReport **7:** 953–957.

62. BURGEVIN, M.C., I. LOQUET, D. QUARTERONET & E. HABERT-ORTOLI. 1995. Cloning, pharmacological characterization, and anatomical distribution of a rat cDNA encoding for a galanin receptor. J. Mol. Neurosci. **6:** 33–41.

63. WANG, S., C. HE, M.T. MAGUIRE, A.L. CLEMMONS, R.E. BURRIER, M.F. GUZZI, C.D. STRADER, E.M. PARKER & M.L. BAYNE. 1997. Genomic organization and functional characterization of the mouse GalR1 galanin receptor. FEBS Lett. **411:** 225–230.

64. JACOBY, A.S., G.C. WEBB, M.L. LIU, B. KOFLER, Y.J. HORT, Z. FATHI, C.D.K. BOTTEMA, J. SHINE & T.P. IISMAA. 1997. Structural organization of the mouse and human GALR1 galanin receptor genes (Galnr and GALNR) and chromosomal localization of the mouse gene. Genomics **45:** 496–508.

65. MELANDER, T., C. KOHLER, S. NILSSON, T. HOKFELT, E. BRODIN, E. THEODORSSON & T. BARTFAI. 1988. Autoradiographic quantitation and anatomical mapping of ^{125}I-galanin binding sites in the rat central nervous system. J. Chem. Neuroanat. **1:** 213–233.

66. FATHI, Z., A.M. CUNNINGHAM, L.G. IBEN, P.B. BATTAGLINO, S.A. WARD, K.A. NICHOL, K.A. PINE, J. WANG, M.E. GOLDSTEIN, T.P. IISMAA & I.A. ZIMANYI. 1997. Cloning, pharmacological characterization and distribution of a novel galanin receptor. Brain Res. Mol. Brain Res. **51:** 49–59.

67. SMITH, K.E., C. FORRAY, M.W. WALKER, K.A. JONES, J.A. TAMM, J. BARD, T.A. BRANCHEK, D.L. LINEMEYER & C. GERALD. 1997. Expression cloning of a rat hypothalamic galanin receptor coupled to phosphoinositide turnover. J. Biol. Chem. **272:** 24612–24616.

68. WALKER, M.W., K.E. SMITH, B. BOROWSKY, R. ZHOU, Z. SHAPOSHNIK, R. NAGORNY *et al.* 1997. Cloned galanin receptors: Pharmacology of GALR1 and GALR2 receptor subtypes. Soc. Neurosci. Abstr. **23:** 962.

69. SMITH, K.E., M.W. WALKER, K.A. JONES, R. ARTYMYSHYN, J. BARD, B. BOROWSKY, J.A. TAMM, W.-J. YAO, P.J.-J. VAYSSE, T.A. BRANCHEK, C. GERALD & K.A. JONES. 1998. Galanin GALR3 receptors: Cloning and functional expression of rat and human receptors. J. Biol. Chem. **273:** 23321–23326.

70. MILLER, M.A., P.E. KOLB & M.A. RASKIND. 1997. GALR1 galanin receptor mRNA is co-expressed by galanin neurons but not cholinergic neurons in the rat basal forebrain. Brain Res. Mol. Brain Res. **52:** 121–129.

71. XU, Z.Q., T.J. SHI, M. LANDRY & T. HOEKFELT. 1996. Evidence for galanin receptors in primary sensory neurones and effect of axotomy and inflammation. NeuroReport **8:** 237–242.

72. STEN SHI, T.J., X. ZHANG, K. HOLMBERG, Z.Q. XU & T. HOKFELT. 1997. Expression and regulation of galanin-R2 receptors in rat primary sensory neurons: effect of axotomy and inflammation. Neurosci. Lett. **237:** 57–60.

73. HOWARD, A.D., C. TAN, L.L. SHIAO, O.C. PALYHA, K.K. MCKEE, D.H. WEINBERG, S.D. FEIGHNER, M.A. CASCIERI, R.G. SMITH, L.H.T. VAN DER PLOEG & K.A. SULLIVAN. 1997. Molecular cloning and characterization of a new receptor for galanin. FEBS Lett. **405:** 285–290.

74. WANG, S., T. HASHEMI, C. HE, C. STRADER & M. BAYNE. 1997. Molecular cloning and pharmacological characterization of a new galanin receptor subtype. Mol. Pharmacol. **52:** 337–343.

75. BLOOMQUIST, B.T., M.R. BEAUCHAMP, L. ZHELNIN, S.E. BROWN, A.R. GORE-WILLSE, P. GREGOR & L.J. CORNFIELD. 1998. Cloning and expression of the human galanin receptor GalR2. Biochem. Biophys. Res. Commun. **243:** 474–479.

76. BOROWSKY, B., K.E. SMITH, J.A. BARD, M.W. WALKER, L.-Y. HUANG, T.A. BRANCHEK *et al.* 1997. Cloning and characterization of the human galanin GALR2 receptor. Soc. Neurosci. Abstr. **23:** 393

77. BOROWSKY, B., M. WALKER, L.-Y. HUANG, K.A. JONES, K.E. SMITH, J. BARD, T.A. BRANCHEK & C. GERALD. 1998. Cloning and characterization of the human galanin GALR2 receptor. Peptides. In press.

78. WANG, S., C. HE, T. HASHEMI & M. BAYNE. 1997. Cloning and expressional characterization of a novel galanin receptor. Identification of different pharmacophores within galanin for the three galanin receptor subtypes. J. Biol. Chem. **272:** 31949–31952.

79. BEDECS, K., U. LANGEL, X.J. XU, Z. WIESENFELD-HALLIN & T. BARTFAI. 1994. Biological activities of two endogenously occurring N-terminally extended forms of galanin in the rat spinal cord. Eur. J. Pharmacol. **259:** 151–156.

80. CHAN-PALAY, V. 1988. Galanin hyperinnervates surviving neurons of the human basal nucleus of Meynert in dementias of Alzheimer's and Parkinson's disease: A hypothesis for the role of galanin in accentuating cholinergic dysfunction in dementia. J. Comp. Neurol. **273:** 543–557.

81. YAO, W.-J., J.A. TAMM, K.E. SMITH, J. BARD, T. BRANCHEK, C. GERALD *et al.* 1998. GALR3 and GALR1 galanin receptors activate GIRK in *Xenopus* oocytes. Soc. Neurosci. Abstr. **24:** 1590.

82. XU, Z.Q., X. ZHANG, S. GRILLNER & T. HOKFELT. 1997. Electrophysiological studies on rat dorsal root ganglion neurons after peripheral axotomy: Changes in responses to neuropeptides. Proc. Natl. Acad. Sci. USA **94:** 13262–13266.

83. KINNEY, G.A., P.J. EMMERSON & R.J. MILLER. 1998. Galanin receptor-mediated inhibition of glutamate release in the arcuate nucleus of the hypothalamus. J. Neurosci. **18:** 3489–3500.

Cloning and Evaluation of the Role of Rat GALR-2, a Novel Subtype of Galanin Receptor, in the Control of Pain Perception

SULTAN AHMAD,[a] DAJAN O'DONNELL, KEM PAYZA, JULIE DUCHARME, DANIEL MÉNARD, WILLIAM BROWN, RALF SCHMIDT, CLAES WAHLESTEDT, S. H. SHEN,[b] AND PHILIPPE WALKER

Astra Research Centre Montreal and [b]Pharmaceutical Sector,
Biotechnology Research Institute, Montreal, Quebec, Canada

ABSTRACT: We have identified a novel subtype of galanin receptor (GALR-2) in rat dorsal root ganglia and spinal cord. The open reading frame of GALR-2 is 1116 nucleotides long, encoding a protein of 372 amino acids with a theoretical molecular mass of 40.7 kD. Membranes prepared from stable pools of 293 cells expressing GALR-2, but not wild-type 293 cells, demonstrated high affinity galanin binding sites. Rat galanin and galanin-related peptides M40, C7, M15, and galanin$_{1-16}$ effectively competed for binding; peptide C7 demonstrated a lower affinity for rGALR-2, and all these peptides were agonists at rGALR-2 when assessed on a microphysiometer. Studies on the expression of GALR-2 in various tissues by Northern and *in situ* hybridization analyses suggest a low abundance but wide distribution of GALR-2 mRNA, including several discrete areas in brain and spinal cord and a high abundance in the dorsal root ganglia.

Galanin is a 29 amino acid neuroendocrine peptide (30 amino acids in humans) that was initially isolated from pig intestine[1] and later shown to be widely distributed in the brain and spinal cord[2,3] and in several peripheral regions.[4,5]

Studies with exogenously applied galanin, galanin antagonists, galanin antibodies, and antisense to galanin suggest a wide array of central physiologic roles for galanin *in vivo*, such as modulation of cognitive, behavioral, and sensory functions (for a review see refs. 4 and 5).

Galanin-like immunoreactivity is present in the spinal cord[2,3,6–8] where it depresses the spinal nociceptive reflexes in rats.[9–11] This effect is enhanced after nerve section,[12] and galanin antagonizes the excitatory effect of vasoactive intestinal polypeptide.[13] Galanin is also present in a small number of dorsal root ganglion (DRG) neurons[2,3]; sciatic nerve section stimulates the levels of galanin-like immunoreactivity and galanin message in these neurons.[8,14,15] Galanin administered intrathecally is reported to cause analgesia[13] and potentiate the analgesic effect of morphine,[16] and the target application of galanin hyperpolarizes dorsal horn neurons.[17] Chronic administration of a galanin receptor antagonist, after axotomy, results in a marked increase in autotomy in rats.[4,18] Furthermore, galanin antisense also causes autotomy in rats after axotomy; this phenomenon is accompanied by suppression of axotomy-induced upregulation of galanin levels.[19] These observations strongly suggest that galanin, like morphine, has strong antinociceptive actions *in vivo*.

[a]Address for correspondence: Astra Research Centre Montreal, 7171 Frederick-Banting, Ville St Laurent, Quebec, H4S 1Z9. Phone, 514/832-3200 (ext 2100); fax, 514/832-3228.

One receptor for galanin (GALR-1) has been cloned.[20-22] Much of the pharmacologic data with the use of galanin fragments, galanin agonists, and galanin antagonists supports a multi-receptor system for galanin (for a review see refs. 4 and 5), because at many places the functional studies do not correlate well with the pharmacologic profile of GALR-1. The existence of galanin receptor subtypes was first suggested over a decade ago.[23] Since then, the concept of galanin receptor heterogeneity has been supported and extended by a large body of work.[4] Our interest in the area of analgesia and in the potential role of galanin in analgesia led us to investigate the pos

sible existence of a multi-receptor system for galanin.

We here describe cloning of a novel subtype of galanin receptor GALR-2 and evaluate the potential role of this novel receptor in the control of pain perception by performing a detailed analysis of the distribution of GALR-2 mRNA in tissues of the nociceptive pathways. While these studies were in progress, several other groups[24-28] also described the cloning of GALR-2 with essentially the same sequence as that described here.

MATERIALS AND METHODS

Cloning and Sequencing of Rat Galanin Receptor-2 (GALR-2)

Two degenerate oligonucleotides within the regions conserved among various G-protein–coupled receptors within putative transmembrane regions 2 and 7 (TM-2 and TM-7) with the following nucleotide sequence were designed: GG CCG TCG ACT TCA TCG TC[AT] [AC][TC]C TI[GT] CI[TC] TIG C[ACGT]G AC-3' (TM-2 primer) and 5'-[AG][CAT][AT] [AG]CA [AG]TA IAT IAT IGG [AG]TT-3' (TM-7 primer). Poly A+-messenger RNA from cultured fetal rat dorsal root ganglia neurons was subjected to first strand cDNA synthesis using the First Strand cDNA Synthesis Kit (Pharmacia Biotech) and then to amplification by polymerase chain reaction (PCR) under the following conditions using Ampli-Taq DNA polymerase (Perkin-Elmer Cetus): 3 minutes of denaturation at 94°C, then 40 cycles of 1 minute each at 94°C, 45°C, and 72°C. An amplification product at ~700 was subcloned into pGEM-T vector (Promega Corp.) which was used to transform competent DH5α bacteria. The recombinant clones were sequenced by the dideoxy chain termination reaction method using the T7-Sequencing Kit (Pharmacia Biotech).

One clone obtained by RT-PCR that had some degree of homology to the GALR-1 was used as a probe to screen the rat brain stem/spinal cord cDNA library (Stratagene), as described previously.[29] Positive and pure clones were excised *in vivo* according to the supplier's protocol. Several overlapping clones were obtained. One clone, 21RSC-4, of about 1,350 bp was sequenced in its entirety and appeared to contain the coding information for a seven-transmembrane G-protein–coupled receptor having the highest homology to the galanin receptor. This particular clone was complete at its 3'-end as far as the coding region was concerned; however, it was missing the initiation codon at the 5'-end, but it clearly had at least part of the sequence-coding first transmembrane region extending to the amino terminus extracellular region. A few reverse primers were designed in the 5'-region of this clone, and the missing 5'-region was amplified from another clone and pasted into a convenient Bsu36I site of 21RSC-4 to obtain a full-length composite sequence termed GALR-2.

Expression of GALR-2 in Mammalian Cells

GALR-2 was excised from pBluescript plasmid vector by *Hind*III/BstX-1 and was introduced directionally into *Hind*III/BstX-1 cut pcDNA3 mammalian expression vector (Invitrogen). The GALR-2/pcDNA3 construct was introduced into 293 cells by the calcium chloride/BES precipitation method. After overnight incubation in a reduced CO_2 (3%) atmosphere, cells were rinsed twice with the medium (DMEM containing 10% fetal bovine serum) and incubated overnight covered with the medium under regular atmosphere (5% CO_2). After overnight incubation, the selection (G418 at 600 µg/ml) was applied to obtain the stable pool. Cells were kept under selective medium for 18 days, with a medium change every 4 days, before harvesting them for the assays.

Membrane Preparation and Radioligand Binding Assays

The G418-resistant cells were washed on the plate once with cold phosphate-buffered saline, harvested, and centrifuged at $1,500 \times g$ at 4°C. The cell pellet was resuspended in membrane buffer (20 mM HEPES, pH 7.5, containing 10 µg/ml benzamidine, 5 µg/ml leupeptin, 5 µg/ml soybean trypsin inhibitor, and 0.1 mM phenyl methyl sulfonyl fluoride), and cells were disrupted with a polytron at a setting of ~20,000 rpm for 30 seconds. The disrupted cell suspension was centrifuged at $\sim 100,000 \times g$ for 60 minutes at 4°C in a fixed angle rotor in a Beckman ultracentrifuge. The pellet thus obtained was resuspended in the membrane buffer, aliquoted, and frozen at −80°C until used.

Radioligand binding experiments were performed by a modification of the method of Wynick *et al.*[30] in 100 µl reaction volume containing approximately 10-µg membranes, 0.1 nM ^{125}I-galanin (2,200 Ci/mmol, New England Nuclear), and 1 µM unlabeled galanin for determination of nonspecific binding which was ~5% of the total binding. Total binding was generally less than 10% of the total radiolabeled galanin present in the incubation medium. The binding buffer was made by adding 0.4% bovine serum albumin to the membrane buffer. Membranes, tracer, and unlabeled peptides were diluted in the binding buffer. Incubation at room temperature was carried out for 20 minutes in 96-well incubation plates, and the mixture was filtered through Unifilter™-96, GF/B filtration plates (Packard) using a Filtermate 196 filtration apparatus (Packard), washed 5 times with ice cold 20 mM HEPES, pH 7.5, and counted in a TopCount (Packard) scintillation counter. Pilot experiments had demonstrated that the equilibrium was attained at a 20-minute time point, remained stable up to 30 minutes, after which the specific binding decreased slowly (data not shown).

Functional Assay: Cytosensor Microphysiometer Analysis

Stable pools of transfected 293 cells were grown overnight, detached by tapping the flasks, pelleted by gentle centrifugation, and washed once with RPMI medium (Molecular Devices Corp.). The cells were then resuspended well in RPMI medium, agarose entrapment medium was then added to the cell suspension, and the cells were added to the cell capsule at 0.1 to 1 million cells per capsule. The cell capsule was loaded on the cytosensor sensor chamber and allowed to equilibrate for 1 hour; analysis was then performed in RPMI as the running medium. Cells were allowed to recover for at least 20 minutes between successive doses of the peptides. The experiment was performed in duplicate chambers, and nontransfected cells were used as controls for each peptide. Data were collected for at least three such separate experiments.

Northern Analysis

A rat multiple tissue Northern blot containing 2 μg of polyA RNA from various mouse tissues (Clonetech) was used to study the distribution of GALR-2 message. The blot was prehybridized for 3 hours and then hybridized overnight at 42°C in 50% (vol/vol) formamide/5X SSPE/10X Denhardt's solution/100 μg/ml denatured and sheared salmon sperm DNA/2% SDS (1X SSPE is 0.15 M NaCl, 0.01 M sodium phosphate, pH 7.4, 1 mM EDTA). The full-length GALR-2 cDNA was labeled with a Ready-to-Go DNA labeling kit (Pharmacia Biotech) to be used as a probe. After overnight hybridization, the blot was washed with several changes in 2X SSC (1X SSC: 0.15 M NaCl, 0.015 M Na-Citrate, pH 7.0), 0.05% SDS (sodium dodecyl sulfate) for 30 minutes. The blot was then washed with 0.1X SSC, 0.1% SDS at 50°C for 40 minutes with one change of the wash solution and exposed at −80°C to Kodak Biomax film for 14 days.

In Situ Hybridization

Animals and Tissue Preparation: Adult male Sprague-Dawley rats (~300 g; Charles River, St. Constant, Quebec) were sacrificed by decapitation. Frozen tissue was sectioned and thaw-mounted onto slides.

Riboprobe Synthesis: Sense and antisense GALR-2 and GALR-1 riboprobes were transcribed *in vitro* using either T7 or SP6 RNA polymerases in the presence of [35S]UTP (~800 Ci/mmol; Amersham) using linearized pCDNA3/GalR2/GalR1 as a template. Following transcription, the DNA template was digested with DNAse I (Pharmacia). Riboprobes were subsequently purified by phenol/chloroform/isoamyl alcohol extraction and precipitated in 70% ethanol.

In Situ Hybridization: Sections were postfixed in 4% paraformaldehyde in 0.1 M phosphate buffer (pH 7.4) for 10 minutes at room temperature and rinsed in three changes of 2X standard sodium citrate buffer (SSC; 0.15 M NaCl 0.015 M sodium citrate, pH 7.0). Sections were equilibrated in 0.1 M triethanolamine, treated with 0.25% acetic anhydride in triethanolamine, rinsed in 2X SSC, and dehydrated in an ethanol series (50–100%). Hybridization was performed in a buffer containing 75% formamide (Sigma, St. Louis, Missouri), 600 mM NaCl, 10 mM Tris (pH 7.5), 1 mM EDTA, 1X Denhardt's solution (Sigma), 50 mg/ml denatured salmon sperm DNA (Sigma), 50 mg/ml yeast tRNA (Sigma), 10% dextran sulfate (Sigma), 20 mM dithiothreitol and [35S]UTP-labeled cRNA probes (10×10^6 cpm/ml) at 55°C for 18 hours in humidified chambers. Following hybridization, slides were rinsed in 2X SSC at room temperature, treated with 20 mg/ml RNase IA in RNase buffer (10 mM Tris, 500 mM NaCl, 1 mM EDTA, pH 7.5) for 45 minutes at room temperature, and washed to a final stringency of 0.1X SSC at 65°C. Sections were then dehydrated and exposed to Kodak Biomax MR film for 17–21 days and/or dipped in Kodak NTB2 emulsion diluted 1:1 with distilled water and exposed for 6–8 weeks at 4°C before development and counterstaining with cresyl violet acetate (Sigma).

RESULTS AND DISCUSSION

Cloning of rGALR-2

Using degenerate primers in the conserved domains of the TM-2 and TM-7 regions, in the current studies we identified partial cDNA for some known and a few potentially novel receptors including the one that showed some homology to the GALR-1. We used this 700-bp product to probe a rat brain stem/spinal cord cDNA library (Stratagene) to obtain several overlapping clones. One of these clones, 21RSC-4, when aligned to galanin receptor and several other G-protein-coupled receptors, appeared to contain most of the coding region of the receptor; however, the initiation codon and perhaps a few more bases were missing from the 5′-end of this clone. Another clone (21RSC-21) contained this 5′-region; however, this particular clone also contained an intron of approximately 1,000 bp within the coding region right after the putative transmembrane 3 region (within the signature domain DRY). Therefore, a fragment of about 360 bases was amplified from the later clone and pasted into the Bsu36I site near the 5′-end of the former clone to obtain a full-length GALR-2 receptor. We confirmed, by polymerase chain reaction, the existence of this 5′-region of the clone using RNA samples from rat brain, dorsal root ganglia, and spinal cord as well as from several peripheral tissues (data not shown).

The full-length cDNA sequence and the translated amino acid sequence of GALR-2 are depicted in FIGURE 1A. The codon beginning at nucleotide number 36 appears to be the genuine initiation codon based on (1) consensus with Kozak's sequence, (2) upstream in-frame stop codons, and (3) the length of the protein and its comparison with hGALR-1 and rGALR-1 which are 349 and 346 amino acid long proteins, respectively.[20–22] Therefore, we putatively termed the codon starting at 36 as the initiation codon; an in-frame stop codon lies at nucleotide number 1151, which would translate into a protein of 372 amino acids with a predicted molecular mass of 40.70 kD and estimated pI of 10.80. The predicted amino acid sequences of rat and human GALR-1 and that of GALR-2 are aligned in FIGURE 1B. GALR-2 has an overall identity of about 53% at the nucleotide level and 35.5% identity at the amino acid level with rat GALR-1 and 34.8% with human GALR-1. Certain regions, such as the second and third transmembrane domains, are more conserved between GALR-1 and GALR-2 than between other regions. The homology at both termini is less significant. During the preparation of this manuscript, several other laboratories[24–28] published the cloning of GALR-2 from rat hypothalamus. The sequence of rat hypothalamic GALR-2 is identical to the sequence presented here with only one amino acid difference (S17 in the present sequence versus G17 in hypothalamic receptor) resulting from a single nucleotide change. This difference may reflect the genetic polymorphism that was also detected by Howard *et al.*,[26] albeit at a different site.

Characterization of rGALR-2

When transfected into HEK293 cells, pCDNA3/GALR-2 generated the expression of specific ^{125}I-galanin binding sites. No specific ^{125}I-galanin binding sites were generated by the transfection of the vector itself or a control pCDNA3 expression construct encoding a delta-opioid receptor. To pharmacologically characterize the GALR-2 receptor, we gener-

TABLE 1. Pharmacologic Profile of GALR-2 in Radioligand Binding Assays (Log IC_{50}) and in Microphysiometer Assays (Log EC_{50})

	Log IC_{50}	Log EC_{50}
Galanin	-8.6 ± 0.03	-7.6 ± 0.22
Galanin$_{1-16}$	-7.7 ± 0.04	-8.0 ± 0.13
M15	-7.5 ± 0.10	-6.5 ± 0.44
M40	-8.1 ± 0.09	-7.6 ± 0.27
C7	-6.8 ± 0.13	-6.1 ± 0.42

ated a pool of stable HEK293 cells expressing the GALR-2 receptor by selecting pCDNA3/GALR-2 transfected cells using G418. Binding experiments were performed on membranes prepared from the pools of G418-resistant pool. A single class of saturable ^{125}I-galanin binding sites was detected displaying an estimated K_d for ^{125}I-galanin of 1.68 ± 0.43 nM and a B_{max} of 1–2 pmol/mg of crude protein. Various galanin-related peptides were used in competition experiments. These experiments using ^{125}I-galanin as a tracer enabled us to evaluate the affinities of various galanin-related peptides for GALR-2. The Log IC_{50} values of tested peptides are summarized in TABLE 1. Overall, the affinities of the peptides at GALR-2 appear to be generally lower than those at GALR-1.[20–22] This fact is more apparent for peptide C7 which is equipotent to galanin at GALR-1 but is several-fold less potent at GALR-2.

A cytosensor microphysiometer was used to assess the functionality of rGALR-2 and to determine the agonistic/antagonistic profiles of galanin-related peptides at this receptor. All peptides used in this assay were agonists at GALR-2, whereas none of these peptides demonstrated stimulation of control HEK-293 cell acidification in the same assay. These results agree with those of Smith *et al.*[27] who also observed full agonist activity for these peptides in phosphoinositide turnover assay. The relative potency of peptides in the functional assay was similar to that in the radioligand binding assay; in the functional assay, however, the peptides were generally less potent than those in radioligand binding assays (TABLE 1).

Northern Analysis

Northern analysis of GALR-2 message reveals a sharp band at around 2.6 kb in skeletal muscle and a diffuse signal at ~1.8 kb in other tissues (FIG. 2, upper panel). The diffuse bands at ~1.8 kb do not appear to arise from degraded RNA in these samples, because hybridization with the actin probe yields sharp bands in all samples (FIG. 2, lower panel). The pattern of hybridization signal seen at around 1.8 kb is essentially similar to that observed by Smith *et al.*[27] We also see a signal in skeletal muscle at ~2.6 kb that was not observed by Smith *et al.*[27] The reason for this discrepancy is unclear. The presence of the message in the skeletal muscle, however, is not surprising, because it is becoming increasingly evident that skeletal muscle and neuronal cells demonstrate an overlapping program of gene expression; for example, in the developing neural tube, myogenic cells have been identified. Tajbakhsh *et al.*[31] and Edmundson *et al.*[32] identified the myogenic gene Mef-2

```
acagctgcggga gcggcgtccact ttggtgatacc ATG AAT GGC TCC GGC AGC CAG GGC GCG GAG AAC ACG AGC CAG GAA
                                       M   N   G   S   G   S   Q   G   A   E   N   T   S   Q   E
              90                                   120                                        150
               *                                    *                                          *
GGC AGT AGC GGC GGC TGG CAG CCT GAG GCG GTC CTT GTA CCC CTA TTT TTC GCG CTC ATC TTC CTC GTG GGC
 G   S   S   G   G   W   Q   P   E   A   V   L   V   P   L   F   F   A   L   I   F   L   V   G
                           180                                        210
                            *                                          *
ACC GTG GGC AAC GCG CTG GTG CTG GCG GTG CTG CTG CGC GGC GGC CAG GCG GTC AGC ACC ACC AAC CTG TTC
 T   V   G   N   A   L   V   L   A   V   L   L   R   G   G   Q   A   V   S   T   T   N   L   F
                   240                                       270
                    *                                         *
ATC CTC AAC CTG GGC GTG GCC GAC CTG TGT TTC ATC CTG TGC TGC GTG CCT TTC CAG GCC ACC ATC TAC ACC
 I   L   N   L   G   V   A   D   L   C   F   I   L   C   C   V   P   F   Q   A   T   I   Y   T
    300                                       330                                         360
     *                                         *                                           *
CTG GAC GAC TGG GTG TTC GGC TCG CTG CTC TGC AAG GCT GTT CAT TTC CTC ATC TTT CTC ACT ATG CAC GCC
 L   D   D   W   V   F   G   S   L   L   C   K   A   V   H   F   L   I   F   L   T   M   H   A
                       390                                       420
                        *                                         *
AGC AGC TTC ACG CTG GCC GCC GTC TCC CTG GAC AGG TAT CTG GCC ATC CGC TAC CCG CTG CAC TCC CGA GAG
 S   S   F   T   L   A   A   V   S   L   D   R   Y   L   A   I   R   Y   P   L   H   S   R   E
        450                                       480                                         510
         *                                         *                                           *
TTG CGC ACA CCT CGA AAC GCG CTG GCC GCC ATC GGG CTC ATC TGG GGG CTA GCA CTG CTC TTC TCC GGG CCC
 L   R   T   P   R   N   A   L   A   A   I   G   L   I   W   G   L   A   L   L   F   S   G   P
                           540                                       570
                            *                                         *
TAC CTG AGC TAC TAC CGT CAG TCG CAG CTG GCC AAC CTG ACA GTA TGC CAC CCA GCA TGG AGC GCA CCT CGA
 Y   L   S   Y   Y   R   Q   S   Q   L   A   N   L   T   V   C   H   P   A   W   S   A   P   R
               600                                       630
                *                                         *
CGT CGA GCC ATG GAC CTC TGC ACC TTC GTC TTT AGC TAC CTG CTG CCA GTG CTA GTC CTC AGT CTG ACC TAT
 R   R   A   M   D   L   C   T   F   V   F   S   Y   L   L   P   V   L   V   L   S   L   T   Y
    660                                       690                                         720
     *                                         *                                           *
GCG CGT ACC CTG CGC TAC CTC TGG CGC ACA GTC GAC CCG GTG ACT GCA GGC TCA GGT TCC CAG CGC GCC AAA
 A   R   T   L   R   Y   L   W   R   T   V   D   P   V   T   A   G   S   G   S   Q   R   A   K
                   750                                       780
                    *                                         *
CGC AAG GTG ACA CGG ATG ATC ATC ATC GTG GCG GTG CTT TTC TGC CTC TGT TGG ATG CCC CAC CAC GCG CTT
 R   K   V   T   R   M   I   I   I   V   A   V   L   F   C   L   C   W   M   P   H   H   A   L
        810                                       840                                         870
         *                                         *                                           *
ATC CTC TGC GTG TGG TTT GGT CGC TTC CCG CTC ACG CGT GCC ACT TAC GCG TTG CGC ATC CTT TCA CAC CTA
 I   L   C   V   W   F   G   R   F   P   L   T   R   A   T   Y   A   L   R   I   L   S   H   L
                           900                                       930
                            *                                         *
GTT TCC TAT GCC AAC TCC TGT GTC AAC CCC ATC GTT TAC GCT CTG GTC TCC AAG CAT TTC CGT AAA GGT TTC
 V   S   Y   A   N   S   C   V   N   P   I   V   Y   A   L   V   S   K   H   F   R   K   G   F
               960                                       990
                *                                         *
CGC AAA ATC TGC GCG GGC CTG CTG CGC CCT GCC CCG AGG CGA GCT TCG GGC CGA GTG AGC ATC CTG GCG CCT
 R   K   I   C   A   G   L   L   R   P   A   P   R   R   A   S   G   R   V   S   I   L   A   P
    1020                                      1050                                        1080
     *                                         *                                           *
GGG AAC CAT AGT GGC AGC ATG CTG GAA CAG GAA TCC ACA GAC CTG ACA CAG GTG AGC GAG GCA GCC GGG CCC
 G   N   H   S   G   S   M   L   E   Q   E   S   T   D   L   T   Q   V   S   E   A   A   G   P
                       1110                                      1140
                        *                                         *
CTT GTC CCA CCA CCC GCA CTT CCC AAC TGC ACA GCC TCG AGT AGA ACC CTG GAT CCG GCT TGT TAA aggacca
 L   V   P   P   P   A   L   P   N   C   T   A   S   S   R   T   L   D   P   A   C   *
        1170                                      1200                                        1230
         *                                         *                                           *
aaggcatctaacag cttctagacagt gtggcccgagga tccctgggggtt atgcttgaacgt tacagggttgag gctaaagactga
                1260
                 *
ggattgattgta gggaacctccag
```

FIGURE 1A. *See legend on facing page.*

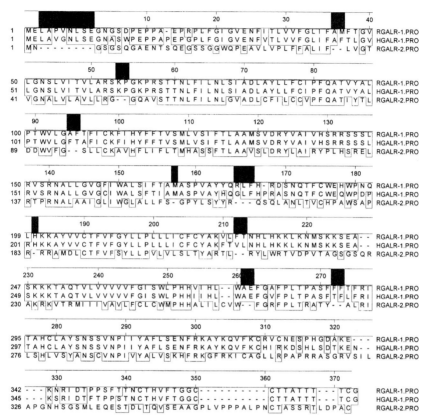

Decoration 'Decoration #1': Shade (with bright yellow at 50% fill) residues that match the Consensus exactly.

Decoration 'Decoration #2': Box residues that match the Consensus exactly.

FIGURE 1. (**A**) Nucleotide sequence and corresponding translated amino acid sequence (bold, in single letter code) of rat GALR-2. The predicted transmembrane regions (TM-1 to TM-7) are shaded and underlined. (**B**) Alignment of rat GALR-2 (RGALR-2.PR), rat GALR-1 (RGALR.PR), and human GALR-1 (HGALR.PR) amino acid sequence. Residues identical to rat GALR-2 are boxed. To optimize alignment, gaps were created at several places in GALR-2; these gaps are indicated by *black boxes*.

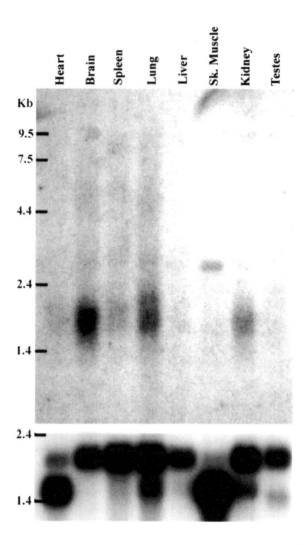

FIGURE 2. Northern blot of GALR-2 and β-actin. Multiple tissue northern blot from Clonetech was used. The blot contained 2 μg of polyA⁺RNA from various tissues. The blot was hybridized with the full-length clone for GALR-2 (*upper panel*) and a control β-actin probe (*lower panel*). The blot was exposed at −80°C for 14 days for the GALR-2 message and for 1 hour for the β-actin message.

in neural crest cells. The GALR-2 gene in skeletal muscle, however, may utilize a skeletal muscle-specific regulatory element distinct from the one used by neuronal cells. Furthermore, the diffuse band at ~1.8 kb may suggest the presence of either more than one alternatively spliced form of GALR-2 or more than one GALR-2–related gene. Studies are under way in our laboratory to clarify these issues.

In situ Hybridization

To gain insight into the potential contribution of GALR-2 and GALR-1 to the control of pain perception, we examined the regional distribution of GALR-2 and GALR-1 mRNA in neuroaxis of the rat using *in situ* hybridization. Adjacent rat brain and spinal cord sections with dorsal root ganglia attached were hybridized with ^{35}S-labeled GALR-2 and GALR-1 riboprobes.

In brain (FIG. 3A), the highest levels of GALR-2 mRNA are present in the mammillary nuclei of the hypothalamus, dentate gyrus, and cerebellar cortex. Moderate to weak GALR-2 labeling is observed in the olfactory bulb, in superficial layers of the neocortex, as well as in certain hypothalamic and brainstem nuclei. The thalamus and basal ganglia are generally devoid of GALR-2 hybridization signal. In spinal cord, GALR-2 labeling is low and distributed throughout gray matter of the dorsal and ventral horns (FIG. 3B). Interestingly, dorsal root ganglia (DRG) express by far the highest levels of GALR-2 mRNA observed in rat CNS as evidenced by dense patches of labeling seen on film autoradiograms (FIG. 3C). Emulsion autoradiography revealed that the hybridization signal is mainly concentrated over small and intermediate primary sensory neurons, although a few large neurons are also weakly labeled (data not shown).

By contrast, the pattern of GALR-1 mRNA expression in rat CNS is markedly different from that of GALR-2. In brain, high levels of GALR-1 mRNA are seen in the olfactory bulb, in several hypothalamic nuclei, as well as in certain thalamic and brainstem nuclei. Moderate GALR-1 labeling is observed in the diagonal band of Broca, septum, and periaqueductal gray. Neocortex and cerebellum are devoid of GALR-1 mRNA expression. In spinal cord, intense GALR-1 labeling is detected in the dorsal horn of the spinal cord, particularly over laminae I and II (FIG. 3D). GALR-1 mRNA is also highly expressed in the DRGs (FIG. 3D); however, labeling is associated predominantly with large sensory neurons (data not shown).

The pattern of GALR-2 distribution within rat CNS and DRG differs considerably from that of GALR-1, suggesting these receptors mediate different central actions of galanin. Given galanin's putative antinociceptive properties,[13–34] the differential distribution of these receptors in nociceptive pathways is of particular interest. On the one hand, GALR-2 mRNA is preferentially expressed in primary afferents, namely small and medium DRG neurons, and is thus a likely target for modulating primary input of pain and temperature. On the other hand, GALR-1 is highly expressed in most laminae I and II dorsal horn neurons, presumably some of which are second-order nociceptive neurons, as well as in supraspinal sites associated with pain perception such as the thalamus and periaqueductal gray. At this time, the individual contribution of GALR-2 and GALR-1 in altering pain perception is unclear; however, both receptors are ideally located to modulate ascending nociceptive input. Moreover, GALR-1's presence in supraspinal sites suggests that it is also poised to modulate descending pain pathways.

Preliminary experiments in our laboratory suggest that GALR-2 activation may be involved in the control of pain perception, because intrathecal injections of a GALR-2–selective agonist (to be disclosed later) reverse the allodynic response generated by Freund's complete adjuvant injection. Clearly, elucidation of the relative contribution of galanin receptor subtypes to the control of pain perception awaits the development of metabolically stable agonists selective for each of the galanin receptor subtypes.

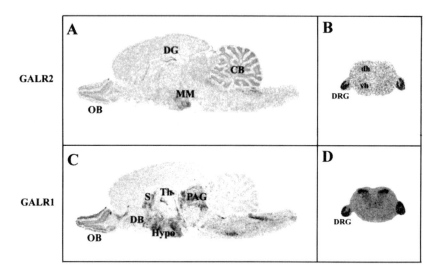

FIGURE 3. *In situ* hybridization film autoradiograms showing localization of GALR-2 and GALR-1 mRNA expression in CNS and dorsal root ganglia (DRG) of the rat. Series of adjacent sagittal brain (**A, C**) and spinal cord with DRGs still attached (**B, D**). Sections were hybridized in parallel with ^{35}S-labeled riboprobes directed to GALR-2 (**A, B**) and GALR-1 (**C, D**) and exposed to film for 17 days to obtain autoradiograms shown. The CNS expression pattern of novel GALR-2 differs markedly from that of GALR-1. No specific hybridization signal was observed with control ^{35}S-labeled sense probe (not shown). Abbreviations are as follows: CB, cerebellum; DB, diagonal band of Broca; DG, dentate gyrus; dh, dorsal horn; Hypo, hypothalamus; MM, mammillary nuclei; OB, olfactory bulb; PAG, periaqueductal gray; S, septum; Th, thalamus; vh, ventral horn.

REFERENCES

1. TATEMOTO, K. *et al.* 1983. Galanin: A novel biologically active peptide from porcine intestine. FEBS Lett. **164:** 124–128.
2. CH'NG, J.L.C. *et al.* 1985. Distribution of galanin immunoreactivity in the central nervous system and the responses of galanin-containing pathways to injury. Neuroscience **16:** 343–354.
3. SKOFITSCH, G. & G. JACOBOWITZ. 1985. Immunohistochemical mapping of galanin-like neurons in the rat central nervous system. Peptides **6:** 509–546.
4. BARTFAI, T. *et al.* 1992. Galanin and galanin antagonists: Molecular and biochemical perspectives. Trends Pharmacol. Sci. **13:** 312–316.
5. BEDECS, K. *et al.* 1995. Galanin: 10 years with a neuroendocrine peptide. Int. J. Biochem. Cell Biol. **4:** 337–349.
6. JOHNSON, H. *et al.* 1992. Galanin and CGRP-like immunoreactivity co-exist in rat spinal motoneurons. NeuroReport **3:** 303–306.
7. MELANDER, T. *et al.* 1986. Distribution of galanin-like immunoreactivity in rat central nervous system. J. Comp. Neurol. **248:** 475–517.
8. VILLAR, M.J. *et al.* 1989. Neuropeptide expression in rat dorsal root ganglion cells and spinal cord after peripheral nerve injury. Neuroscience **33:** 587–604.
9. WIESENFELD-HALLIN, Z. *et al.* 1989. The effects of intrathecal galanin on the flexor reflex in the rat. Brain Res. **486:** 205–213.

10. YANAGISAWA, M. *et al.* 1986. Inhibitory effects of galanin on the isolated spinal cord of the new born. Neurosci. Lett. **70:** 278–282.

11. XU, X.-J. *et al.* 1995. New high affinity peptide antagonists to the spinal galanin receptors. Br. J. Pharmacol. **116:** 2076–2080.

12. XU, X.-J. *et al.* 1990. On the role of galanin, substance P and other neuropeptides in primary sensory neurons of the rat: Studies on spinal reflex excitability and peripheral axotomy. Eur. J. Neurosci. **2:** 733–743.

13. WIESENFELD-HALLIN, Z. *et al.* 1989. The effect of intrathecal galanin on flexor reflex in rat: Increased depression after sciatic nerve section. Neurosci. Lett. **105:** 149–154.

14. HÖKFELT, T. *et al.* 1987. Increase of galanin-like immunoreactivity in rat dorsal root ganglion cells after peripheral axotomy. Neurosci. Lett. **83:** 217–220.

15. HÖKFELT, T. *et al.* 1994. Messenger plasticity in primary sensory neurons following axotomy and its functional implications. Trends. Neurosci. **17:** 22–30.

16. POST, C. *et al.* 1988. Intrathecal galanin increases the latency in the tail flick and hot plate test in mouse. Acta Physiol. Scand. **132:** 583–584.

17. RANDIC, M. *et al.* 1986. Inhibitory actions of galanin and somatostatin 28 on rat spinal dorsal horn neurons. Soc. Neurosci. Abstr. **13:** 1308.

18. VERGE, V.M.K. *et al.* 1993. Evidence for endogenous inhibition of autotomy by galanin in rat after sciatic nerve section demonstrated by chronic intrathecal infusion of a high affinity galanin receptor antagonist. Neurosci. Lett. **149:** 193–197.

19. JI, R. *et al.* 1994. Galanin antisense oligonucleotides reduce galanin levels in dorsal root ganglia and induce autotomy in rats after axotomy. Proc. Natl. Acad. Sci. USA **91:** 12540–12543.

20. HABERT-ORTOLI, E. *et al.* 1994. Molecular cloning of a functional human galanin receptor. Proc. Natl. Acad. Sci. USA **91:** 9780–9783.

21. BURGEVIN, M.-C. *et al.* 1995. Cloning, pharmacological characterization, and anatomical distribution of a rat cDNA encoding for a galanin receptor. J. Mol. Neurosci. **6:** 33–41.

22. PARKER, E.M. *et al.* 1995. Delineation of the peptide binding site of the human galanin receptor. Mol. Brain Res. **34:** 179–189.

23. EKBLAD, E. *et al.* 1985. Galanin: Neuromodulatory and direct contractile effects on smooth muscle preparations. Br. J. Pharmacol. **86:** 241–246.

24. BLOOMQUIST, B.T. *et al.* 1998. Cloning and expression of the human galanin receptor GALR-2. Biochem. Biophys. Res. Commun. **243:** 474–479.

25. FATHI, Z. *et al.* 1997. Cloning, pharmacological characterization and distribution of a novel galanin receptor. Brain Res. **51:** 49–59.

26. HOWARD, A.D. *et al.* 1997. Molecular cloning and characterization of a new receptor for galanin. FEBS Lett. **405:** 285–290.

27. SMITH, K.E. *et al.* 1997. Expression cloning of a rat hypothalamic galanin receptor coupled to phosphoinositide turnover. J. Biol. Chem. **272:** 24612–24616.

28. WANG, S. *et al.* 1997. Molecular cloning and pharmacological characterization of a new galanin receptor subtype. Mol. Pharmacol. **52:** 337–343.

29. AHMAD, S. *et al.* 1993. A widely expressed human protein tyrosine phosphatase containing src homology 2 domains. Proc. Natl. Acad. Sci. USA **90:** 2197–2201.

30. WYNICK, D. *et al.* 1993. Characterization of a high affinity galanin receptor in the rat anterior pituitary: Absence of biological effects and reduced membrane binding of the antagonist M15 differentiate it from the brain/gut receptor. Proc. Natl. Acad. Sci. USA **90:** 4231–4235.

31. TAJBAKHSH, S. *et al.* 1994. A population of myogenic cells derived from the mouse neural tube. Neuron **13:** 813–821.

32. EDMUNDSON, D.G. *et al.* 1994. Mef 2 gene expression marks the cardiac and skeletal muscle lineages during mouse embryogenesis. Development **120:** 1251–1263.

Distribution and Characterization of the Cell Types Expressing GALR2 mRNA in Brain and Pituitary Gland

B. DEPCZYNSKI, K. NICHOL, Z. FATHI,[a] T. IISMAA, J. SHINE, AND A. CUNNINGHAM[b]

Neurobiology Program, Garvan Institute of Medical Research, St. Vincent's Hospital, 384 Victoria Street, Darlinghurst, 2010, NSW, Australia

[a]*Neuroscience Drug Discovery, Bristol-Myers Squibb Pharmaceutical Research Institute, 5 Research Parkway, Wallingford, Connecticut 06492, USA*

ABSTRACT: The neuropeptide galanin mediates its activities through G-protein–coupled receptors, and three receptor subtypes have been described with distinctly different patterns of regional tissue expression. GALR1 is predominantly expressed in basal forebrain, hypothalamus, as well as spinal cord. GALR2 has a wider distribution in brain and is also present in the pituitary gland and peripheral tissues. GALR3 has been found to be widely distributed at low abundance. We examined the distribution of GALR2 in rat brain and pituitary by *in situ* hybridization histochemistry and found it abundant in regions of hippocampus, piriform and entorhinal cortex, basal nucleus of the accessory olfactory tract, amygdala, hypothalamic nuclei, Purkinje cells, and discrete brainstem nuclei. It is also highly expressed in the intermediate and anterior lobes of the pituitary. Using combined *in situ* hybridization immunohistochemistry we characterized the neurotransmitter and hormonal phenotype of cells expressing GALR2 mRNA in the hypothalamus and pituitary gland. Our findings suggest GALR2 is a receptor mediating important functions of galanin in the hypothalamic-pituitary axis and may also play a role in hippocampal and cerebellar function.

G alanin (GAL) modulates a diverse range of biologic processes and interacts with distinct receptor subtypes of the seven transmembrane, G-protein–coupled superfamily. Physiologic processes modulated by GAL include feeding, pituitary hormone secretion, nociception, cognition, and memory.[1–3] Support for the mediation of GAL's actions via multiple receptor subtypes arose initially from the differing pharmacologic effects of synthetic agonists and antagonists.[4–6]

With the cloning of the first GAL receptor, GALR1,[7] several studies reported its mRNA localization by *in situ* hybridization histochemistry (ISH).[8–10] GALR1 mRNA was found at high levels in ventral hippocampus, thalamic nuclei, amygdala, brainstem nuclei, hypothalamus, and posterior horns of the spinal cord, with some minor differences found between reports. More recently, GALR1 has been mapped in detail throughout the major regions of the rat hypothalamus and shown to be expressed in anterior hypothalamic nuclei as well as mediobasal and periventricular regions.[11]

[b]Address for correspondence: Dr. A. Cunningham, Head, Sensory Neurobiology Group, Neurobiology Program, The Garvan Institute of Medical Research, 384 Victoria St, Darlinghurst, NSW 2010, Australia. Phone, 61-2-9295-8282; fax, 61-2-9295-8281; e-mail, a.cunningham@garvan.unsw.edu.au

A second galanin receptor subtype, GALR2, was described by four groups, including ours, in 1997.[12–15] GALR2 shares less than 40% overall sequence identity with GALR1 and is distinguished by its high affinity for the ligand galanin-(2-29).[14] Additionally, GALR2 appears to have a broader distribution than does GALR1 outside the central nervous system.[14] We recently reported the first ISH analysis of GALR2 mRNA distribution in the CNS showing moderately high levels of expression in many areas of brain, including major hypothalamic nuclei, hippocampus, entorhinal and piriform cortex, amygdala and pituitary gland.[12] More recently, using radioactive ISH, Xu *et al.*[16] also reported GALR2 mRNA expression in the dentate gyrus of the hippocampus.

The finding of GALR2 in pituitary gland is important, as GAL modulates the release of prolactin and growth hormone (GH),[2] but the anatomic site at which GAL mediates its influence on anterior pituitary function has not been clearly delineated. Various *in vitro* studies have demonstrated direct effects of galanin on prolactin and GH secretion from rat pituitary cells,[17,18] and a paracrine role for GAL in anterior pituitary function has also been proposed.[19]

The report of GALR3, a third receptor subtype, which was amplified by polymerase chain reaction from a rat cDNA hypothalamic library, showed no significant signal detectable by Northern analysis in brain but significant levels in heart, spleen, and testes.[20]

We have mapped the expression of GALR2 mRNA at high resolution in the adult male rat brain and pituitary gland and used a double labeling technique to commence phenotyping the classes of neurons and other cells expressing GALR2. The aim of our studies is to define the neuroanatomic framework with which to understand how GAL functions through its receptors, and to further define GAL's mode of action on the pituitary.

MATERIALS AND METHODS

The details of the ISH method have been published.[12] Briefly, a 455-bp fragment, corresponding to the segment extending from transmembrane domain 6 to the COOH-terminus of the rat GALR2 receptor, was amplified over 30 cycles from the cloned receptor cDNA using the gene-specific sense/antisense primer pair (5′-GTGACTGCAGGCTCAGGTTCC-3′ and 5′-ACAAGCCGGATCCAGGGTTCT-3′) and AmpliTaq DNA polymerase. The fragment was cloned into pGEM-T (Promega, USA) and used as a template to synthesize digoxigenin-labeled sense and antisense riboprobes (DIG RNA labeling kit (SP6/T7), Boehringer Mannheim, Germany).

Adult male Wistar rats (200–250 g) were maintained on a 12-hour light:dark cycle with access to food and water ad libitum. Animals were anesthetized with barbiturate and transcardially perfused with phosphate-buffered saline solution followed by 4% paraformaldehyde. Paraffin sections (5 μm) were collected on gelatin and chromium potassium sulfate-coated slides. Sections were dewaxed, washed, and pretreated with proteinase K (Boehringer Mannheim, Germany). Sense and antisense digoxigenin-labeled riboprobes in hybridization buffer (2X SSPE, 50% formamide, 5% dextran sulfate, 1X Denhardt's reagent, 100 μg/ml tRNA type X-SA) were added to the sections and hybridized at moderate stringency for 16 hours using a Hybaid PCR Thermal Cycler (Hybaid, USA). After hybridization, sections were washed and processed for immunologic detection according to the manufacturer's instructions using an alkaline phosphatase conjugated anti-digoxigenin antiserum (Boehringer Mannheim, Germany). The labeled probes were visualized using nitroblue tetrazolium and bromochloro-indoyl phosphate (with 1 mM levamisole) as substrates for 16 hours in the dark. Sections were mounted and photographed using a Zeiss Axiophot photomicroscope with Nomarski optics.

The distribution of GALR2 mRNA was mapped throughout the brain by examination of sequential coronal sections from rostral to caudal regions. Brain regions and nuclei were identified by reference to Paxinos and Watson,[21] and hybridization was scored as negative, low, moderate, or high.

For combined *in situ* hybridization immunohistochemistry we used anti-digoxigenin alkaline phosphatase antibody for mRNA detection and fluorescent secondary antibodies for protein detection. Following *in situ* hybridization and color development, sections were washed, preincubated with 10% serum for 30 minutes at room temperature, and incubated for 2 hours with the various primary antibodies at room temperature. The primary antibodies used were: anti-tyrosine hydroxylase (Chemicon, USA); anti-thyroid stimulating hormone (TSH) (lot no AFP-1274789) and anti-prolactin (lot no AFP425-10-91); these antisera were obtained from NIDDK; anti-GH antibody (a kind gift from Dr. M. Brandon, University of Melbourne, Australia); anti-ACTH and anti-melanocyte-stimulating hormone (MSH) antibodies (Peninsula Laboratories, USA); and anti-luteinizing hormone (LH) antibody (BioGenex, USA). After washing, sections were incubated with fluorescein-conjugated anti-mouse or anti-rabbit immunoglobulin (Silenus, Australia). Sections were examined with a Zeiss Axiophot or a Leica TCS NT confocal microscope to simultaneously view the fluorescent and transmission mode channels. Controls for the double labeling technique consisted of sense riboprobes with substitution of normal serum from the same species as the primary antibody for the immunohistochemical step.

RESULTS AND DISCUSSION

The nonradioactive digoxigenin method of *in situ* hybridization is particularly suitable for this type of receptor mapping in CNS, as it offers excellent morphologic tissue preservation, allowing the identification of brain regions and nuclei at the single cell level of resolution. The sensitivity of the digoxigenin method has been addressed by studies such as those by Pohle *et al.*[22] who directly compared the digoxigenin and radioactive detection methods for individual probes and showed them to be equally sensitive. In addition, nonradioactive ISH is particularly amenable to the addition of double and triple labels using colorimetric and fluorescent probes.

GALR2 in Brain

The regional distribution of GALR2 mRNA was examined. The antisense riboprobe produced hybridization in a restricted and very distinctive pattern, whereas the sense probe was negative for hybridization in all regions examined. Generally, cortical regions did not show significant hybridization, but the piriform, entorhinal, and cingulate cortex showed a high hybridization signal. The amygdaloid nuclei and basal nucleus of the accessory olfactory tract were highly labeled. Brainstem nuclei which labeled moderately to highly included the pontine, trigeminal and deep cerebellar nuclei, the vagal complex, and the locus ceruleus. In cerebellum, there was significant expression in Purkinje cells, which complements the report of preprogalanin mRNA in these cells,[23] and some cells in the granule cell layer also hybridized.

Recently, Xu *et al.*[16] have shown the detailed innervation of the hippocampus by GALinergic fibers as well as the presence of GALR2 mRNA in the dentate gyrus by ISH using ^{35}S-labeled oligonucleotide probes. Using nonradioactive labeling we found a wide distribution of GALR2 in the hippocampus with definite gradients in expression. Expression in CA3 and the dentate, including the polymorphic region, was generally higher than that in other regions. In ventral areas, significant expression was noted in the pyramidal cells of CA1 which waned dorsally.

GALR2 in Hypothalamus

All major hypothalamic nuclei were moderately labeled for GALR2 mRNA with the most intense hybridization found in the lateral mammillary bodies, the magnocellular neurons of the supraoptic nucleus, the tuberomammillary nucleus, and somewhat less in the paraventricular nucleus (PVN) and arcuate.

In the PVN, the highest hybridization was found in the lateral magnocellular region (FIG. 1). Some heterogeneity of expression of mRNA was noted with the most strongly hybridizing magnocellular neurons intermingled with less labeled neurons. This is likely to be of functional importance, because these neurons are known to be heterogeneous in expression of hormones and neurotransmitters. Significant hybridization was also seen in the medial parvocellular subdivision and the periventricular region of PVN.

GALR2 in Pituitary Gland

In the pituitary gland, GALR2 mRNA was expressed at high levels by essentially all cells of the intermediate lobe. In the anterior lobe a subset of cells was positive for GALR2 mRNA, individual cells expressing at moderate to high levels. There was a tendency for GALR2 positive cells to be located more peripherally in the lobe with sparser distribution centrally. The posterior pituitary was negative for hybridization.

Phenotyping of the GALR2-Positive Cells

Determining the neurotransmitter, peptide, or hormonal phenotype of cells expressing GALR2 is of crucial importance to understanding its specialized function. To address this, we used a technique for simultaneously detecting mRNA hybridization and protein immunoreactivity. Hypothalamic sections taken from the region of the zona incerta were examined for GALR2 mRNA and tyrosine hydroxylase immunoreactivity. FIGURE 2A illustrates the alkaline phosphatase method of colorimetric detection for GALR2 mRNA, and FIGURE 2B, the simultaneous view showing fluorescent (FITC) labeling for tyrosine hydroxylase immunoreactivity. Two prominent large neurons are indicated which show coexpression of GALR2 and tyrosine hydroxylase.

Using this technique we examined GALR2 coexpression with a panel of anterior pituitary hormones in the pituitary gland. Data were analyzed on a confocal microscope which

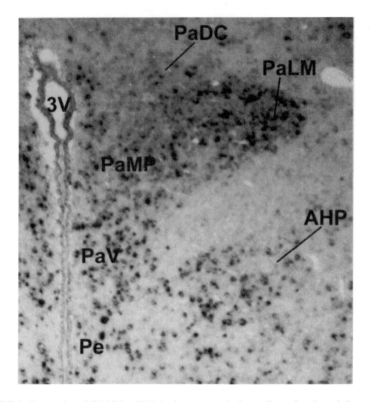

FIGURE 1. Expression of GALR2 mRNA in the paraventricular nucleus of rat hypothalamus by *in situ* hybridization histochemistry. Positive hybridization is seen as a dark reaction product in the body of cells of the PVN, adjacent to the third ventricle (3V). Dense hybridization is present in neurons of the lateral magnocellular division (PaLM) with moderate levels in the parvocellular regions dorsally (PaDC), medially (PaMP), and ventrally (PaV). Prominently hybridizing cells are also seen in the periventricular region of this nucleus (Pe). Less signal is seen in the anterior hypothalamic area (AHP). (150× original magnification.)

allowed us to simultaneously view the two detection channels and facilitate the scoring of positive or negative colocalization. We found that the intermediate lobe of the pituitary was highly immunoreactive for MSH and essentially all these cells expressed GALR2 mRNA. By contrast, in the anterior lobe, only a subset of prolactin, GH, TSH, and LH immunoreactive cells coexpressed GALR2. The frequency of colocalization was high for GH and prolactin and lower for TSH and LH. No colocalization was found with ACTH. Hence, cells in the anterior pituitary in the baseline state in a normal male were heterogeneous in their expression of GALR2 mRNA, but it was expressed by a percentage of lactotrophs, somatotrophs, thyrotrophs, and gonadotrophs. GAL in rodent anterior pituitary is present in lactotrophs, somatotrophs, and thyrotrophs.[24]

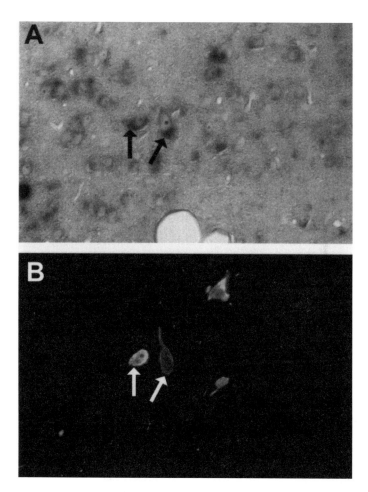

FIGURE 2. Localization of GALR2 mRNA and tyrosine hydroxylase immunoreactivity in rat zona incerta by simultaneous *in situ* hybridization immunohistochemistry. (**A**) GALR2 mRNA in large neurons is detected as a dark cytosolic reaction product. (**B**) Tyrosine hydroxylase immunoreactivity detected by immunofluorescence on the same field. Two large neurons are indicated (*arrows*) that coexpress GALR2 and tyrosine hydroxylase. Bar represents 25 μm. (400× original magnification.)

SUMMARY

Our studies show that GALR2 mRNA has a unique pattern of CNS distribution, distinguishing it from GALR1, but there are regions such as the hypothalamus, amygdala, and brainstem where their expression overlaps. GALR2 is highly expressed in the hippocampus, amygdala, piriform and entorhinal cortex, all regions of brain involved in learning, memory, and cognition. Recently, high binding of human GALR2 was demonstrated in entorhinal cortex, a region of brain affected early in Alzheimer's disease.[25]

The actions of GAL in modulating acetylcholine release[26] and, more recently, the demonstration that the neuropeptide Y (NPY) knockout mouse has a propensity for seizures[27] have focused new interest on the role of neuropeptides in cognition, memory, and learning as well as seizure pathogenesis. The detailed innervation of the hippocampus by GALinergic fibers was recently reported.[16] In view of our results showing significant GALR2 hybridization in pyramidal cells of CA regions of the hippocampus and the granule cell layer of the dentate, we might postulate that GAL-positive fibers may be targeting a postsynaptic receptor at these sites. It is notable that the pattern of GALR1 expression in hippocampus is different from that of GALR2, being high in the subiculum ventrally, moderate in ventral CA1, and negative in other regions.[8]

The expression of GALR2 mRNA in the soma of Purkinje cells in the cerebellum is fascinating, as we do not understand the role neuropeptides play in this brain region. It is notable, however, that in recent years our understanding of the role of the cerebellum has expanded from simply a motor integrator into the field of cognition. In fact, it has been shown that in cerebellar disorders there are defects in visuospatial attention.[28] It may be that the neuropeptide galanin modulates or facilitates aspects of this higher cognitive ability.

Expression of GALR2 mRNA in the hypothalamus and amygdala is of particular interest in view of the effects of galanin on feeding behavior. Direct injection of galanin into the paraventricular nucleus of the hypothalamus or amygdala has been reported to increase food intake, particularly fat consumption, in satiated rats.[1,29] Both GALR1 and GALR2 mRNA are expressed in the hypothalamus and amygdala; therefore, either or both receptors could mediate the effects of galanin on feeding. Comparison of the hypothalamic distribution of GALR2 mRNA with that of GALR1[11] showed a similar pattern of expression in the PVN and arcuate. By contrast, GALR2's high expression in the lateral mammillary body and the tuberomammillary body is quite distinctive from that reported for GALR1.

GALR1 mRNA has not been detected in the anterior pituitary even though galanin binding has been shown at that site.[4] Our finding of GALR2 in the anterior pituitary partially resolves this discrepancy, but it is likely that other pituitary galanin receptors will be described. GALR2 expression in lactotrophs, somatotrophs, gonadotrophs, and thyrotrophs in the baseline state suggests that this receptor plays a major functional role in hypothalamic-pituitary secretion. Our results also raise the possibility that overexpression of GALR2 may be involved in disorders of the pituitary, such as adenomas. The application of the double labeling technique to simultaneously view mRNA and protein immunoreactivity in individual cells has provided us with a powerful tool with which to further delineate the action of GAL in central neuroendocrine pathways.

ACKNOWLEDGMENTS

We wish to thank F. Pemper for expert technical assistance. We would also like to thank Dr. P. Smith and Dr. M. Brandon for the donation of antibodies. B.D. is the recipient of an NH&MRC Medical Postgraduate Research Scholarship and A.C. of a Garnett Passe and Rodney Williams Memorial Foundation Senior Research Fellowship.

Note added in proof: Smith *et al.* (1998. J. Biol. Chem. **273:** 23321–23326) recently reported rat GALR3 to be widely distributed, at low abundance, with the highest levels in hypothalamus and pituitary gland by RNase protection assays.

REFERENCES

1. TEMPEL, D.L., K.J. LEIBOWITZ & S.F. LEIBOWITZ. 1988. Effects of PVN galanin on macronutrient selection. Peptides **9:** 309–314.

2. OTTLECZ, A., G.D. SNYDER & S.M. McCANN. 1988. Regulatory role of galanin in control of hypothalamic-anterior pituitary function. Proc. Natl. Acad. Sci. USA **85:** 9861–9865.

3. CRAWLEY, J. 1995. Biological actions of galanin. Regul. Pept. **59:** 1–16.

4. WYNICK, D., D.M. SMITH, M. GHATEI, K. AKINSANYA, R. BHOGAL, P. PURKISS, P. BYFIELD, N. YANAIHARA & S.R. BLOOM. 1993. Characterization of a high-affinity galanin receptor in the rat anterior pituitary: Absence of biological effect and reduced membrane binding of the antagonist M15 differentiate it from the brain/gut receptor. Proc. Natl. Acad. Sci. USA **90:** 4231–4235.

5. BARTFAI, T., Ü. LANGEL, K. BEDECS, S. ANDELL, T. LAND, S. GREGERSEN, B. AHRÉN, P. GIROTTI, S. CONSOLO, R. CORWIN, J. CRAWLEY, X. XU & Z. WIESENFELD-HALLIN. 1993. Galanin-receptor ligand M40 peptide distinguishes between putative galanin-receptor subtypes. Proc. Natl. Acad. Sci. USA **90:** 11287–11291.

6. BARTFAI, T., T. HÖKFELT & Ü. LANGEL. 1993. Galanin: A neuroendocrine peptide. Crit. Rev. Neurobiol. **7:** 229–274.

7. HABERT-ORTOLI, E., B. AMIRANOFF, I. LOQUET, M. LABURTHE & J.F. MAYAUX. 1994. Molecular cloning of a functional human galanin receptor. Proc. Natl. Acad. Sci. USA **91:** 9780–9783.

8. PARKER, E.M., D.G. IZZARELLI, H.P. NOWAK, C.D. MAHLE, L.G. IBEN, J. WANG & M.E. GOLDSTEIN. 1995. Cloning and characterization of the rat GALR1 galanin receptor from Rin14B insulinoma cells. Mol. Brain Res. **34:** 179–189.

9. BURGEVIN, M.C., I. LOQUET, D. QUARTERONET & E. HABERT-ORTOLI. 1995. Cloning, pharmacological characterization, and anatomical distribution of a rat cDNA encoding for a galanin receptor. J. Mol. Neurosci. **6:** 33–41.

10. GUSTAFSON, E.L., K.E. SMITH, M.M. DURKIN, C. GERALD & T.A. BRANCHEK. 1996. Distribution of a rat galanin receptor mRNA in rat brain. Neuroreport **7:** 953–957.

11. MITCHELL, V., E. HABERT-ORTOLI, J. EPELBAUM, J.P. AUBERT & J.C. BEAUVILLAIN. 1997. Semi-quantitative distribution of galanin-receptor (GAL-R1) mRNA-containing cells in the male rat hypothalamus. Neuroendocrinology **66:** 160–172.

12. FATHI, Z., A.M. CUNNINGHAM, L.G. IBEN, P.B. BATTAGLINO, S.A. WARD, K.A. NICHOL, K.A. PINE, J. WANG, M.E. GOLDSTEIN, T.P. IISMAA & I. ZIMANYI. 1997. Cloning, pharmacological characterization and distribution of a novel galanin receptor. Mol. Brain Res. **51:** 49–59.

13. HOWARD, A.D., C. TAN, L.L. SHIAO, O.C. PALYHA, K.K. McKEE, D.H. WEINBERG, S.D. FEIGHNER, M.A. CASCIERI, R.G. SMITH, L.H. VAN DER PLOEG & K.A. SULLIVAN. 1997. Molecular cloning and characterization of a new receptor for galanin. FEBS Lett. **405:** 285–290.

14. WANG, S., T. HASHEMI, C. HE, C. STRADER & M. BAYNE. 1997. Molecular cloning and pharmacological characterization of a new galanin receptor subtype. Mol. Pharmacol. **52:** 337–343.

15. SMITH, K.E., C. FORRAY, M.W. WALKER, K.A. JONES, J.A. TAMM, J. BARD, T.A. BRANCHEK, D.L. LINEMEYER & C. GERALD. 1997. Expression cloning of a rat hypothalamic galanin receptor coupled to phosphoinositide turnover. J. Biol. Chem. **272:** 24612–24616.

16. XU, Z.Q.D., T.J.S. SHI & T. HÖKFELT. 1998. Galanin/GMAP- and NPY-like immunoreactivities in locus coeruleus and noradrenergic nerve terminals in the hippocampal formation and cortex with notes on the galanin-R1 and -R2 receptors. J. Comp. Neurol. **392:** 227–251.

17. WYNICK, D., P.J. HAMMOND, K.O. AKINSANYA & S.R. BLOOM. 1993. Galanin regulates basal and oestrogen-stimulated lactotroph function. Nature **364:** 529–532.

18. LINDSTRÖM, P. & L. SÄVENDAHL. 1993. Effects of galanin on growth hormone release in isolated cultured rat somatotrophs. Acta Endocrinol. **129:** 268–272.

19. O'HALLORAN, D.J., P.M. JONES & S.R. BLOOM. 1991. Neuropeptides synthesised in the anterior pituitary: Possible paracrine role. Mol. Cell. Endocrinol. **75:** C7–C12.

20. WANG, S., C. HE, T. HASHEMI & M. BAYNE. 1997. Cloning and expressional characterization of a novel galanin receptor. Identification of different pharmacophores within galanin for the three galanin receptor subtypes. J. Biol. Chem. **272:** 31949–31952.
21. PAXINOS, G. & C. WATSON. 1997. The Rat Brain in Stereotaxic Coordinates. Academic Press. San Diego.
22. POHLE, T., M. SHAHIN, A. GILLESSEN, D. SCHUPPAN, H. HERBST & W. DOMSCHKE. 1996. Expression of type I and IV collagen mRNAs in healing gastric ulcers: A comparative analysis using isotopic and non-radioactive in situ hybridization. Histochem. Cell Biol. **106:** 413–418.
23. RYAN, M.C. & A.L. GUNDLACH. 1996. Localization of preprogalanin messenger RNA in rat brain: Identification of transcripts in a subpopulation of cerebellar Purkinje cells. Neuroscience **70:** 709–728.
24. STEEL, J.H., G. GON, D.J. O'HALLORAN, P.M. JONES, N. YANAIHARA, H. ISHIKAWA & S.R. BLOOM. 1989. Galanin and vasoactive intestinal polypeptide are colocalised with classical pituitary hormones and show plasticity of expression. Histochemistry **93:** 183–189.
25. DEECHER, D.C., D.C. MASH, J.K. STALEY & E.J. MUFSON. 1998. Characterization and localization of galanin receptors in human entorhinal cortex. Regul. Pept. **73:** 149–159.
26. FISONE, G., C.F. WU, S. CONSOLO, Ö. NORDSTRÖM, N. BRYNNE, T. BARTFAI, T. MELANDER & T. HÖKFELT. 1987. Galanin inhibits acetylcholine release in the ventral hippocampus of the rat: Histochemical, autoradiographic, in vivo and in vitro studies. Proc. Natl. Acad. Sci. USA **84:** 7339–7343.
27. ERICKSON, J.C., K.E. CLEGG & R.D. PALMITER. 1996. Sensitivity to leptin and susceptibility to seizures of mice lacking neuropeptide Y. Nature **381:** 415–418.
28. YAMAGUCHI, S., H. TSUCHIYA & S. KOBAYASHI. 1998. Visuospatial attention shift and motor responses in cerebellar disorders. J. Cogn. Neurosci. **10:** 95–107.
29. SMITH, B.K., D.A. YORK & G. BRAY. 1996. Effects of dietary preference and galanin administration in the paraventricular or amygdaloid nucleus on diet self-selection. Brain Res. Bull. **39:** 149–154.

Endocrine and Gastrointestinal Action of Galanin

NOBORU YANAIHARA,[a,e] TOHRU MOCHIZUK,[b] ATSUKAZU KUWAHARA,[b]
MINORU HOSHINO,[b] HIROYOSHI KAKUYAMA,[b] KAZUOKI IGUCHI,[b]
TOSHIHIKO IWANAGA,[c] LI JUN,[a] YOKO FUTAI,[a] TOMIO KANNO,[a]
KAORU YAMABE,[d] AND CHIZUKO YANAIHARA[d]

[a]Yanaihara Institute Inc., Fujinomiya-shi, 418-0011, Japan

[b]Department of Pharmaceutical Sciences, University of Shizuoka, 422-8002, Japan

[c]Department of Biomedical Sciences, Graduate School of Veterinary Medicine,
Hokkaido University Sapporo, 060-0818, Japan

[d]Department of Pharmacy, Hyogo Medical University, Nishinomiya-shi, 663-8131, Japan

Rapid advances in the field of peptide chemistry and gene technology have resulted in a burst of determinations about the molecular structures not only of regulatory peptides such as galanins (Gal) of various species but also of their precursors and receptors. Based on information about mature peptides and precursor structures, Gal-related peptides and other peptides with related amino acid sequences were synthesized. Certain specifically designed synthetic peptides have enabled the investigation of such questions as the molecular basis of receptor binding and the active role of peptides.[1] Synthetic replicates of Gal of various species and its precursor-related peptides provide us with important immunogens for producing region-specific antibodies. Specific antibodies against Gal or its precursor-related peptides demonstrate well the posttranslational biosynthetic processing in cells and identify steps in the metabolite pathway of the regulatory peptide in tissues and tissue fluids.[2,3]

Exogenous administration of Gal has been shown to contract smooth muscle preparations[3–6] and to inhibit neurally induced smooth muscle contractility. Gal stimulates the release of growth hormone (GH),[7,8] prolactin,[9] and luteinizing hormone either from dispersed pituitary cells or at the hypothalamic level modulating dopamine, vasoactive intestinal polypeptide, (VIP), somatostatin, opioid, and GnRH release into the portal circulation[10–13] and inhibits insulin release.[14–23]

In this review, we describe structure-function studies of the endocrine and gastrointestinal action of Gal.

PEPTIDES AND ANTISERA

Peptides. All peptides used in the study were synthesized by solid phase methodology with BOC- or Fmoc- strategy using an automated peptide synthesizer (model 430A, Applied Biosystems, or model 9050, Perseptive, USA). The crude peptide was purified by reverse-phase HPLC on a column of YMC-Pack D-ODS-5 (2.0 × 25.0 cm) using 0.01 N HCl/CH₃CN. Purity of the peptides was assessed by analytic HPLC on a column of YMC

[e]Address for correspondence: Dr. Noboru Yanaihara, Yanaihara Institute Inc., Awakura 2480-1, Fujinomiya-shi, Shizuoka 418-0011, Japan. Phone, +81-544-22-2771; fax, +81-544-22-2770.

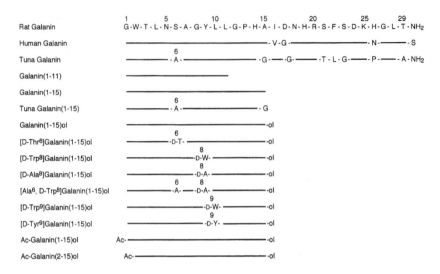

FIGURE 1. Synthetic galanin and galanin(1-15)ol analogs. *Bars* indicate the same amino acid residues as those of rat galanin. Only substituted or modified residues are presented. Ac, N^{α}-acetylated. D at positions 6 through 9 means D-form.

pack R-ODS-5 (0.46 × 25.0 cm), amino acid analysis of the acid hydrolysates using a Beckman system 7300 (Beckman, USA) (FIG. 1).

Antisera. Synthetic peptide (3 mg) was stirred with 50% (v/v) polyvinylpyrrolidone (MW 25,000, Merck, Darmstadt, Germany) in saline solution (1.5 ml) for 2 hours at 25°C. The mixture was emulsified with Freund's complete adjuvant (15 ml, Calbiochem Behring, La Jolla, California, USA) for 10 minutes in an ice bath. The emulsion was injected intradermally into multiple sites of two Japanese white male rabbits (about 2.0 kg). Each rabbit received approximately 1 mg of peptide for the primary immunization. Immunizations were performed at 2-week intervals using a half dose of the immunogen used for the primary immunization. Rabbits were bled from the marginal ear vein at 10 days after each immunization. Anti-Gal(1-15) serum, anti-rat Gal(1-29) serum, and anti-rat Gal(20-29) serum, and anti-preproGal(89-124) thus obtained were used in the study.

IMMUNOREACTIVE GAL

Especially in the COOH-terminal region, Gal is structurally similar to other neuropeptides, such as substance P and neurokinnis, which were found widely in the central and peripheral nervous systems. However, these posttranslational molecular variations must not be overlooked in immunochemical and immunohistochemical studies on immunoreactive Gal. We previously produced Gal monoclonal antibodies that can discriminate immunoreactive Gal from other structurally related peptides.[2]

In the study we used four kinds of new antisera against Gal(1-15), rat Gal(1-29), rat Gal(20-29), and preproGal(89-124) with the COOH-terminal 89-124 sequence of rat Gal mRNA-associated peptide, respectively. These antisera were extremely valuable for detection of Gal-containing nerve fibers (FIG. 2).

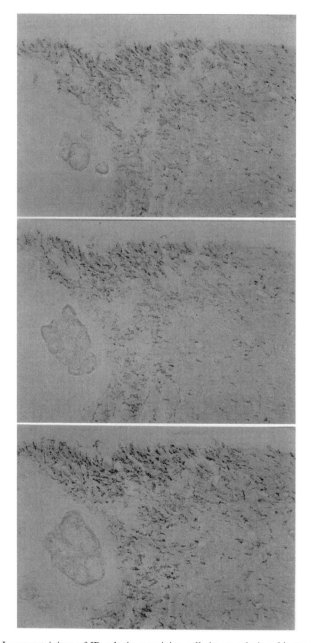

FIGURE 2. Immunostainings of IR-galanin containing cells in rat pyloric sphincter on serial sections using anti-rat preprogalanin(89-124) serum RY193(1:14,000 dilution) (*top*), anti-rat galanin serum Y182 (1:8,000 dilution) (*middle*), and anti-rat galanin(15-29) serum Y183 (*bottom*).

EFFECTS OF GAL AND ITS FRAGMENTS ON INSULIN RELEASE

Immunohistochemical studies in canine pancreas revealed Gal-immunoreactivity (IR) in a dense neural network surrounding the islets of Langerhans.[14,15] These data strongly support the finding Gal participates in pancreatic endocrine function.

Functional studies showed that intravenous infusion of Gal results in that mild but statistically significant sustained hyperglycemia in conscious dogs. Gal produces a transient decrease in the basal insulin level and significant blunt insulin responses to glucose or arginine challenge in dogs.[16–18] Gal also inhibits basal and stimulated insulin secretion in the mouse[19,20] and rat.[21–23]

We investigated the correlation between the structure of Gal and its activity on insulin release by the use of various synthetic Gal fragments. Gal(2-29) lacking Gly[1] did not inhibit insulin (IRI) release from the isolated perfused rat pancreas. By contrast, Gal(3-29) lacking Gly[1] and Trp[2] had a potentiating effect on IRI release.[24] This stimulatory effect of Gal on insulin release was maximum with Gal(15-29). Porcine gastrin-releasing peptide (GRP) and bombesin, which resemble the COOH-terminal region of Gal, can also increase IRI release in conscious dogs.[25]

Lagny-Puormir et al.[26] reported earlier that the NH_2-terminal portion of Gal was essential for interaction with central or peripheral Gal receptors, whereas the COOH-terminal fragment of Gal(10-29) was not essential for Gal binding. Fox et al.[27] also reported similar findings on canine intestinal motility. Consideration of our data along with previous findings suggests that the structural requirements of the Gal receptor for its ligand may be heterogeneous and vary according to the target site. Although speculative, Gal COOH-terminal fragments that show a stimulatory action may act at a different target site from that of Gal(1-29). In contrast to COOH-terminal fragments of Gal, Gal NH_2-terminal fragments, Gal(1-15) and Gal(1-19), had little influence on 13.9 mM glucose-induced IRI release.

In most cases, physiologically active peptides become less potent and inactive as residues regarded essential for biologic activity are deleted. By contrast, the inhibitory activity of porcine Gal(1-29) changed to a stimulatory one. Deletion of NH_2-terminal residues resulted in an augmentation of IRI release. This is the first report in which the biologic activity of Gal is reversed in a potent fashion. Boublic et al.[28] reported that a fragment of neuropeptide Y (NPY) has a potent hypotensive action in contrast to the hypertensive effect of intact NPY.

More importantly, we found that Gly and Trp in positions 1 and 2, respectively, were essential for the inhibitory effect of porcine Gal on IRI secretion. Trp is characterized by its aromatic ring and hydrophobicity and is considered important for maintenance of receptor binding. [D-Trp[2]]-Gal, [Phe[2]]-Gal, and [Ile[2]]-Gal had an inhibitory effect equal to that of Gal. [Tyr[2]]-Gal had no effect on insulin release. According to the secondary structures of the synthetic porcine Gal analogs, as predicted by the Chou-Fasman method,[29,30] the NH_2-terminal region of Gal has a high incidence of β-sheet structure. Such structure holds on [Phe[2]]-Gal, [Ile[2]]-Gal, and [Tyr[2]]-Gal. By contrast, [Ala[2]]-Gal has an insulinotropic effect and is predicted to have little β-sheet structure. It has a random coil structure, similar to that of Gal (3-29) in the NH_2-terminal region. Evidently, a subtle variation in molecular structure can modify the recognition of the peptide by its receptor, because the structural distinction between [Tyr[2]]-Gal and [Phe[2]]-Gal is only one phenolic hydroxyl introduced to the benzene ring. Alternatively, the structure of [Tyr[2]]-Gal in the perfusate may differ from that of Gal so that [Tyr^2]-Gal is easily degraded by vascular or tissue peptidases, resulting in a short biologic half-life.

With the goal of developing a specific antagonist of Gal(1-29), we synthesized Ac-Gal(2-29), Ac-Gal(1-29), and Ac-[Tyr^2]-Gal and examined their effects on glucose-induced insulin release. Acetylated Gal derivatives were thought to be resistant to aminopeptidases and more stable than Gal(1-29). Ac-Gal(2-29), desamino Gal, lacking NH$_2$ of Gly,[1] showed the same inhibitory effect as did Gal(1-29). These results may indicate that it is possible to design antagonists of Gal on the basis of Ac-Gal(2-29; acetyl in the NH$_2$-terminal of Gal) showed no effect on insulin secretion. Their potential was also revealed by the introduction of acetyl which converts the structure of Gal in the NH$_2$-terminal position and reduces its affinity for receptors. Ac-Gal(2-29) may not be degraded quickly or it may bind to the Gal receptor similar to that of Gal(1-29), based on the fact that Ac-Gal(2-29) showed an inhibitory effect on insulin release equal to that of Gal(1-29). Ac-[Tyr^2]-Gal(2-29) showed a marginal but not a significant inhibitory effect on insulin release, supporting the idea that it is easily degraded.

Since the NH$_2$-terminal 1-15 sequence of Gal does not vary among species (porcine, rat, bovine, and human), this portion of Gal is considered essential for Gal activity. Therefore, we designed and synthesized Gal(1-15)-ol. This analog has the COOH-terminal carboxyl replaced with an alcoholic hydroxyl, which was expected to resist carboxypeptidase with the same intention as the introduction of acetyl to NH$_2$-terminal of Gal. However, Gal(1-15)(COOH-terminal carboxyl) had no effect on insulin release, because it might have a short half-life. Gal(1-15)-ol (10^{-5} M) also had no effect on glucose-induced insulin release as did Gal(1-15) and Gal(1-19).

Previous reports indicate that the NH$_2$-terminal fragment of Gal(1-16) is recognized by its high-affinity receptor site in the ventral hippocampus of the rat.[31] Gal(1-15) retains high affinity for receptors present in rat brain.[26] Gal(1-15) had a significant inhibitory effect on neurally evoked circular muscle contraction to Gal,[32] and the NH$_2$-terminal Gal(1-16) fragment can depress the facilitation of the flexor reflex in rat.[33] The effects of Gal(1-15) closely parallel those of Gal(1-29).[34] Gal(1-15)-ol evoked a significant inhibitory effect on neurally evoked circular muscle contraction almost equal to the activity of Gal(1-29).[35] These data suggest that the NH$_2$-terminal region 1-15 of Gal is critical for the interaction with receptors of the central and peripheral nervous systems. Furthermore, differences in the recognition of Gal(1-29) and Gal derivatives or differences in the structure of Gal receptors may exist in the neural and endocrine systems.

Gal receptors have been characterized in the insulin-secreting β-cell line Rin m5F.[36,37] Gal(1-15) had a high affinity for receptors in this pancreatic cell line similar to Gal, and Gal(1-15) as well as Gal had inhibitory effects on insulin release from this cell line.[38] These findings suggest again that the Gal NH$_2$-terminal portion, 1-15, is crucial for its activity in the pancreatic endocrine system and that Gal fragments and analogs used in our study may stimulate other pancreatic insulinotropic hormones which act in a paracrine fashion. In addition, the Rin m5F cell line is a product of tumor and may have developed responsiveness to the NH$_2$-terminal of Gal.

Gal seems to inhibit the glucose-induced insulin release probably via sympathetic nerve terminals that innervate pancreatic islets.[39] The primary structure of the Gal receptor was recently deduced to be a member of the G-protein–coupled seven-transmembrane domain receptor superfamily.[40,41] On the other hand, autoradiographic study revealed that specific binding sites for radioiodinated Gal(1-15) existed in the rat brain.[42]

Recently, we found that [D-Trp[8]]Gal(1-15)-ol at position 8 showed a higher binding affinity than did Gal on plasma membranes in human small cell lung carcinoma cell line, SBC-3A, and rat hippocampus.[43] Interestingly, tuna Gal,[44] which substituted two amino acids at positions 6 and 15, showed lower binding affinity on rat hippocampal membranes than did mammalian Gal, and the tuna Gal at 10^{-8} M did not inhibit glucose-induced insulin release from the isolated perfused rat pancreas,[24] suggesting that the substitution at position 6 may result in the remarkable reduction in agonistic action. Based on these demonstrations, we synthesized several Gal(1-15)-ol analogs that were substituted with D-isomer amino acid residue at position 8 and/or at position 6.[45] Their activity was examined in terms of glucose-induced insulin release from the isolated perfused rat pancreas and binding affinity to the plasma membranes in rat insulinoma cell line Rin m5F. It has been reported that Gal inhibited forskolin-stimulated insulin release through inhibition of adenylate cyclase in Rin m5F cell[46] and that inhibition of adenylate cyclase activity by Gal was mediated by the G-protein G_{i3}. Thus, [Ala[6],D-Trp[8]]Gal(1-15)-ol significantly suppressed the inhibitory action of rat Gal on forskolin-stimulated insulin release from Rin m5F cells in a dose-dependent manner.[45] However, [Ala[6],D-Trp[8]]Gal(1-15)-ol alone did not suppress forskolin-stimulated insulin release even at a concentration of 10^{-6} M. These findings indicate clearly that [Ala[6],D-Trp[8]]Gal(1-15)-ol is a specific and potent Gal antagonist on insulin release.

Previously, several chimeric Gal analogs were reported to function as Gal receptor antagonists.[47–51] The chimeric antagonist M15, Gal(1-13)-substance P(5-11), and galantide[49] were shown to antagonize the action of Gal in the central nervous system and also the inhibitory effect of Gal on glucose-induced insulin release from mice pancreatic islets. By contrast, it acts as a full agonist in gastrointestinal motility in the rat.[51] There is a disadvantage of using the chimeric peptides such as M15 and galantide as Gal antagonists, because the COOH-terminal portion consisting of a partial sequence of substance P might interact with receptors of other regulatory peptides. In fact, M15 has been reported to recognize the substance P receptor.[52] Moreover, Gal is widely distributed and colocalized with other neuropeptides and hormones in various tissues. Accordingly, Gal antagonists should be developed to retain specificity to the Gal receptor alone. [Ala[6],D-Trp[8]]Gal(1-15)-ol developed in our laboratory was designed as a small-sized peptide consisting of the 1-15 sequence of active site with proteolysis-resistant substitution. In fact, [Ala[6],D-Trp[8]]Gal(1-15)-ol was found to be the most potent Gal antagonist among analogs synthesized in the study on glucose-induced insulin release from isolated perfused rat pancreas and the rat insulinoma cell line. These analogs will be useful for investigating the physiologic function of Gal.

EFFECT OF GALANIN ON GASTROINTESTINAL FUNCTION

Immunohistochemical studies have shown that Gal-IR is widely distributed in the mammalian peripheral and central nervous systems.[53] Gal has a wide variety of species-specific motor actions of the gastrointestinal tract.[54,55] Kuwahara et al.[32] reported that Gal inhibits neurally evoked circular muscle contractions via myentric neurons in the guinea pig ileum. This is in contrast to the rat jejunum and canine small intestine, where Gal probably acts directly on the smooth muscle to affect muscle activities. We further examined the structure-function relationship of Gal using synthetic Gal fragments and analogs to investigate their effects on neurally evoked muscle contractions of the guinea pig ileum *in vitro*.[35] The results showed clearly that the whole Gal molecule was required to exhibit the full potency and effectiveness of the peptide using the guinea pig ileum as a target for neuronal Gal receptors. This agrees with other studies of Gal using different organs such as rat pancreas, guinea pig taenia coli, and canine small intestine.[54,55] However, Gal(2-29) and Gal(1-15) showed a significant suppressing effect on neurally evoked circular muscle contractions, although both fragments were less potent than Gal(1-29). On the other hand, the COOH-terminal Gal fragments such as Gal(10-29) and Gal(21-29) did not affect the neurally evoked circular muscle in this system. This demonstrates that the active site of Gal resides in the NH_2-terminal half of the molecule in this system. These results are further supported by the observation that Gal(1-20) still possessed biologic activity in dog small intestine, but Gal(1-10) lost its activity in the guinea pig taenia coli.[27] With respect to Trp in position 2, substitution by other aromatic residues, as in [Tyr^2]Gal, [Phe^2], or [D-Trp^2]Gal, dramatically diminished the efficacy of the peptide.

As has been reported, the inhibitory action of Gal occurs at neural level,[56] because Gal does not affect acetylcholine (ACh)-induced muscle contractions in the presence of tetrodotoxin, suggesting that Gal receptors of guinea pig ileum may be located on enteric neurons. This is in contrast to the canine small intestine, where Gal acts directly on the smooth muscle.[54] Our study showed that Gal(3-29), Gal(10-29), and Gal(21-29) did not significantly affect neurally evoked muscle contractions. On the contrary, Fox *et al.*[55] showed that COOH-terminal fragments Gal(21-29) and Gal(15-29) produce inhibition of neurally evoked ileal muscle contraction in dogs,[55] suggesting that the COOH-terminal fragment of porcine Gal may be recognized by canine small intestine. It is noteworthy that Gal(3-29), lacking Gly^1 and Trp^2) had a potentiating effect on IR insulin release from the isolated perfused rat pancreas. It should be emphasized again that porcine Gal with 29 amino acid residues is structurally similar at the COOH-terminal residues to the tachykinins, physaelamin, substance P, and neurokinin A.[1]

EFFECT OF NH_2-TERMINAL GAL(1-15) AND ITS ANALOGS ON NEURALLY EVOKED CIRCULAR MUSCLE CONTRACTION IN GUINEA PIG ILEUM

Gal(1-15) and Gal(1-16) exert a wide range of biologic actions.[31,35,57] Recently, we found that [D-Trp^8]Gal(1-15)-ol showed an affinity higher than that of Gal on human small cell carcinoma cell membranes, suggesting the importance of D-Trp^8 for binding to the receptor.[43] On the basis of these observation, we examined nine Gal(1-l5)-ol analogs including six D-amino acid residue analogs to explore the structure-function relationships on Gal(1-15) as they affect neurally evoked muscle contractions in guinea pig ileum in detail. We focused on the importance of the amino acid residue at positions 6, 8, and 9, and NH_2-terminal Gly.[58]

[D-Thr^6]Gal(1-15)-ol, in which L-Ser was replaced by D-Thr, resulted in a remarkable reduction in activity. In contrast, the inhibitory activity of tuna Gal was equipotent to that of mammalian Gal on neurally evoked guinea pig ileal contraction, although the amino acid sequence of tuna Gal at positions 6 and 15 differs from the 1–15 sequence of mammalian Gal. The two peptides in which Ser^6 was replaced by Ala^6, such as tuna Gal(1-15) and [Ala^6, D-Trp^8]Gal(1-15)-ol, still retain significant inhibitory activity, although these peptides were less potent than mammalian form peptides such as mammalian Gal(1-15) and

[D-Trp^8]Gal(1-15)-ol on neurally evoked circular muscle contractions. These results confirmed that the replacement of L-Ser^6 by L-Ala^6 retained the inhibitory activity of Gal. Together, the results make it reasonable to speculate that the L configuration of position 6 is important in the inhibitory activity of Gal.

We previously reported that [D-Trp^8]Gal(1-15)-ol, in which Gly at position 8 was replaced by D-Trp, showed higher affinity than rat and human Gal in both rat hippocampal and human small cell lung carcinoma cell (SBC-3A) membranes, suggesting the importance of D-Trp at position 8 for receptor binding.[43] The inhibitory effect of [D-Trp^8]Gal(1-15)-ol was shown to be equipotent to that of Gal(1-15)-ol.

Neither [D-Tyr^9]Gal(1-15)-ol nor [D-Trp^9]Gal(1-15)-ol had any effect on neurally evoked circular muscle contractions in guinea pig ileum, showing results similar to the loss of binding in rat hippocampus and hypothalamus that resulted from replacement of L-Ala at position 9. Thus, Tyr at position 9 seems to be essential for the biologic activity of Gal. Moreover, [D-Thr^6]Gal(1-15)-ol, [D-Tyr^9]Gal(1-15)-ol, and [D-Trp^9]Gal(1-15)-ol, which were inactive in the system, did not show any antagonistic activity against the inhibitory action of Gal, although [Ala^6,D-Trp^8]Gal(1-15)-ol[46] or [D-Thr^6,D-Trp^{8,9}]Gal(1-15)-ol[59] have shown antagonistic activity against the inhibitory activity of Gal on insulin release.

Comparison of the inhibitory activity of rat, human, and tuna Gal revealed that these three Gal showed nearly identical potencies in the system using guinea pig ileum.[58] However, tuna Gal caused no significant effects on glucose-induced insulin release from the isolated perfused rat pancreas[24] and on basal gastrin release from the isolated perfused rat

TABLE 1. Comparison of the Potencies of Galanin and Related Peptides^a

Galanin-Related Peptides	Suppression of Insulin Release^b	Effects on the Neurally Evoked Guinea Pig Circular Muscle Contraction^c
Rat galanin	+++	+++
Human galanin	+++	+++
Tuna galanin		+++
Rat galanin(1-11)	–	–
Rat galanin(1-15)	–	+
Tuna galanin(1-15)	–	+
Acetylated galanin(2-15)	–	++
Rat galanin(1-15)ol	–	++
[D-Trp^8]Galanin(1-15)ol	+	++
[D-Ala^8]Galanin(1-15)ol	–	+
[Ala^6, D-Trp^8]Galanin(1-15)ol	–	+
[D-Thr^6]Galanin(1-15)ol	–	–
[D-Trp^9]Galanin(1-15)ol	–	–
[D-Tyr^9]Galanin(1-15)ol	–	–
[Trp^8]Galanin(2-15)ol	–	–

^{a}Values are mean ±SEM (n = 6): +++, very strong; ++, moderate; +, weak; –, not detectable in the experimental condition used.

^{b}13.9 mM glucose-induced insulin release from the isolated perfused rat pancreas (see ref. 45).

^{c}Percent contraction in the presence of 1-μM peptides (see ref. 58).

stomach.[60] These findings may have resulted from the different recognition sensitivity of these peptides among the neural and endocrine systems and/or different species (TABLE 1).

EFFECT OF GAL ON THE MESENTERIC MICROCIRCULATION, ARTERIAL SMOOTH MUSCLE, AND ELECTROLYTE TRANSPORT IN THE RAT INTESTINE

Gal(0.03–300 pmol) given intraarterially into the mesenteric arteriole caused intermittent interruption of blood flow within 40 seconds and finally stopped blood flow within a few minutes. The diameter of the arterioles was not changed or was slightly widened. Gal also relaxed the preconstricted small mesenteric artery in an endothelium-independent manner. Furthermore, the relaxing action of Gal was not antagonized by glibenclamide, indicating that activation of ATP-sensitive K^+ channels was not involved. These results suggest that Gal plays a modulatory role in the mesenteric circulation.[61] In addition, a recent study showed that Gal significantly decreased sodium and chloride net absorption and suggested that Gal acts as a secretory modulator in the rat via noncholinergic neural transmission.[62]

ENDOCRINE FUNCTION IN THE GUT

Gal inhibits the release of somatostatin and gastrin from the stomach, suggesting that Gal might be involved in the control of gastric endocrine secretions,[35,56,60,63] in addition to its effect on motility and blood flow. Gal may exert its action directly on the G cells and D Gal cells, because Gal-containing nerve fibers have been demonstrated in the lamina propria and musclaris mucosal area of the stomach. In addition, the inhibitory effect of Gal on gastrin release was observed during infusion of neuromeduline C or gastrin-releasing peptide (GRP) which stimulates gastrin release.[56] This inhibitory effect of Gal was also observed during infusion of tetrodotoxin, suggesting that the inhibitory effect is not mediated via neuronal pathways.[63]

An inhibitory effect of Gal on methacholine- or porcine GRP(14-27)-stimulated gastrin release was observed.[35,60] The inhibitory effect of Gal on gastrin release is not attributed to the action of somatostatin because Gal produces a decrease in somatostatin release rather than an increase. This suggests that the inhibitory effect of Gal is a direct action on the gastric G cell.

Recently, Herrmann-Rinke *et al.*[64] described that stimulation of GLP-1 secretion by methacholine was abolished by the addition of atropine and partly reduced by Gal. Gal dose-dependently antagonized the stimulatory effect of GIP on GLP-1 release. Double immunohistochemical labeling techniques revealed that Gal-containing nerves were detected in the vicinity of GLP-1–immunostained cells in the lower intestine.

These results suggest that inhibition of GLP-1 release by Gal may be mediated by peptidergic interneurons.

EFFECT OF GAL AND ITS RELATED PEPTIDES ON GASTRIN AND SOMATOSTATIN RELEASE

Rossowsky and Coy[65] demonstrated that the NH_2-terminal 1-14 sequence of Gal is important for exerting the inhibitory effect of Gal based on studies that examine the effects of Gal and two Gal fragments, Gal(9-25) and Gal(15-19), on gastric acid secretion in anesthetized rats. In our study using the isolated perfused rat stomach,[60] Gal(2-29) and Gal(3-29) at 10^{-8} M showed no significant effect on gastrin and somatostatin release, although Gal(1-29) at the same concentration significantly suppressed basal gastrin and somatostatin release, suggesting that the NH_2-terminal Gly is crucial for exerting the inhibitory effect on gastrin and somatostatin release. Furthermore, [Phe^2]Gal and des-α-amino-Gal(AcGal(2-29)) showed significant inhibitory effect, whereas [Ala^2]Gal, [Tyr^2]Gal, and [Ile^2]Gal at 10^{-8} M had no effect on methacholine- and GRP(14-27)-stimulated gastrin and somatostatin release. It is noteworthy that N^α-Ac-Gal(2-29) exhibited a significant and stronger inhibitory effect on GRP(14-27)-stimulated somatostatin release when compared with that of Gal(1-29). These demonstrations suggest that the aromatic ring in the second residue of Gal may be important in inhibiting gastrin release, and the potency of Gal-related peptides is different in the two cell populations (gastrin [G] and SRIF [D]).

ROLE OF GALANIN ON RELEASE OF ANTERIOR PITUITARY HORMONES

Gal is widely distributed in rat brain. In the central nervous system (CNS), the hypothalamus is rich in fibers and cell bodies containing Gal. Specific binding sites for the peptide were found in the hypothalamus, including the median eminence of the rat. These observations suggest that Gal is involved in regulating anterior pituitary function as a neuromodulator or a neurotransmitter in the CNS.

Gal affects the basal and stimulated release of the anterior pituitary hormones prolactin, growth hormone, and luteinizing hormone either from dispersed pituitary cells or at the hypothalamic level modulating dopamine, ACh, opioid, VIP, somatostatin, GRH, and GnRH release into the portal circulation.[10–13]

In human subjects, Gal plays a stimulating role in GH secretion,[7,66–70] whereas there are conflicting reports on prolactin release by Gal. Bauer et al.[7] reported a stimulatory effect of Gal on prolactin release in normal subjects, whereas Murakami et al.[70] failed to demonstrate elevation of the plasma prolactin level by intravenous injection of synthetic human Gal (33 pmol/kg body weight). However, a higher dose of human Gal elicited a slight but significant increase in plasma prolactin.

Recently, Murakami et al.[71] examined the effect of human Gal on GH and prolactin release in patients with nonfunctioning pituitary adenoma, acromegaly, and prolactinoma. Continuous intravenous infusion of synthetic human Gal (33.2 pmol/kg body weight · min for 60 min) resulted in elevation of plasma GH levels in patients with nonfunctioning adenoma and prolactinoma. By contrast, GH level was not changed by human Gal in acromegalic patients except one, in whom plasma GH levels were lowered. On the other hand, intravenous infusion of human Gal resulted in elevation of plasma prolactin levels in three of four patients with nonfunctioning adenoma and in two of four patients with acromegaly, whereas plasma prolactin levels were not affected by human Gal in patients with prolactinoma. These findings provide additional evidence that Gal stimulates GH secretion in humans but also stimulates prolactin secretion in patients with nonfunctional pituitary adenoma and acromegaly.

Gal plays a stimulating role in prolactin secretion in rats,[9] whereas human Gal at doses used in most clinical studies (33 pmol/kg body weight · min) does not apparently increase plasma prolactin levels in normal subjects, but elevates plasma prolactin levels in some populations of patients with pituitary adenoma. By contrast, human Gal had little effect on plasma prolactin levels in patients with prolactinoma, suggesting that prolactin-secreting adenoma cells lack responsiveness to the peptide.

By contrast to Gal-R$_1$, the first two NH$_2$-terminal amino acid residues were reported not to be important for interacting to pituitary Gal-R$_2$, because Gal(3-29) retains full biologic activity. Wynick *et al.*[72] showed that receptor binding and release of prolactin decreased with increasingly shorter COOH-terminal fragments. In fact, Gal(10-29) and (20-29) have no significant activity.

It is noteworthy that binding of NH$_2$-terminal labeled ^{125}I-BH porcine Gal in tissues that have been known to express Gal receptor was displaced with Gal and not with Gal(3-29), supporting the endocrine and gastrointestinal actions of Gal and its related peptides.

REFERENCES

1. YANAIHARA, N., C. YANAIHARA, M. HOSHINO, T. MOCHIZUKI & K. IGUCHI. 1988. Immunochemical and biochemical properties of purposely designed synthetic peptides. Ann. N.Y. Acad. Sci. **527:** 29–43.
2. YANAIHARA, N., C. YANAIHARA, T. MOCHIZUKI, M. HOSHINO & K. IGUCHI. 1987. Biochemical and immunological aspects of gastrointestinal hormones. Exp. Brain Res. Series **16:** 19–22.
3. EKBLAD, E.R., F. HÅKANSON, F. SUNDLER & C. WAHLESTEDT. 1985. Galanin: Neuromodulatory and direct contractile effects on smooth muscle preparations. Br. J. Pharmacol. **86:** 241–246.
4. TATEMOTO, K., A RÖKAEUS, H. JÖRNVALL, T.J. MCDONALD & V. MUTT. 1983. Galanin, a novel biologically active peptide from porcine intestine. FEBS Lett. **164:** 124–128.
5. FOX, J.E.T., T.J. MCDONALD, F. KOSTOLANSKA & K. TATEMOTO. 1986. Galanin: An inhibitory neural peptide of the canine small intestine. Life Sci. **39:** 103–110.
6. MURAMATSU, I. & N. YANAIHARA. 1988. Contribution of galanin to non-cholinergic non-adrenergic transmission in the rat ileum. Br. J. Pharmacol. **94:** 1241–1249.
7. BAUER, F.E., L. GINSBERG, M. VENETIKOU, D.J. MACKAY, J.M. BURRIN & S.R. BLOOM. 1986. Growth hormone release in man induced by galanin, a new hypothalamic peptide. Lancet **II:** 192–195.
8. OTTLECZ, A., W.K. SAMSON & S.M. MCCANN. 1986. Galanin: Evidence for a hypothalamic site of action to release growth hormone. Peptides **7:** 51–53.
9. KOSHIYAMA, H., Y. KATO, T. INOUE, Y. MURAKAMI, Y. ISHIKAWA, N. YANAIHARA & H. IMURA. 1987. Central galanin stimulates pituitary prolactin in rats: Possible involvement of hypothalamic vasoactive intestinal polypeptide. Neurosci. Lett. **75:** 49–54.
10. SHIMATSU, A., T. TANOH, H. KOSHIYAMA, Y. MURAKAMI, Y. KATO, N. YANAIHARA & H. IMURA. 1991. Role of galanin in prolactin and growth hormones secretion in rats. *In* Galanin. T. Hökfelt, T. Bartfai, D. Jacobowitz & D. Ottosen, Eds.: 321–327. Macmillan Education. London.
11. MCCANN, S.M., A.G. REZNIKOV, M.C. AQUILA, U. MARUBAYASHI, J. GUTKNOWSKA & V. RETTORI. 1991. Role of galanin in control of hypothalamic pituitary function. *In* Galanin. *Ibid.*: 307–319.
12. KOENIG, J.I., S.C. HOOI, D.M. MAITER, J.B. MARTIN, S.M. GABRIEL, R.M. STRAUSS & L.M. KAPLAN. 1991. On the interactions of galanin within the hypothalamic-pituitary axis of the rat. *In* Galanin. *Ibid* : 331–341.
13. SAHU, A., W.R. CROWLEY, K. TATEMOTO & S.P. BALASUBRAMANIAM-KALRA. 1987. Effects of neuropeptide Y, NPY analog (Norleucin⁴-NPY), galanin and neuropeptide K on LH release in ovariectomized (ovx) and ovx estrogen, progesterone-treated rats. Peptides **8:** 921–926.
14. DUNNING, B.E., B. AHREN, R.C. VEITH, G. BÖTTCHER, F. SUNDLER & G.J. TABORSKY. 1986. Galanin: A novel pancreatic neuropeptide. Am. J. Physiol. **251:** E127–E133.
15. DUNNING, B.E. & G.J. TADORSKY. 1988. Galanin-sympathetic neurotransmitter in endocrine pancreas? Diabetes **37:** 1157–1162.
16. MCDONALD, T.J., J. DUPRE, G.R. GREENBERG, F. TEPPERMAN, B. BROOKS, K. TATEMOTO & V. MUTT. 1986. The effect of galanin on canine plasma glucose and gastroenteropancreatic hormone responses to oral nutrients and intravenous arginine. Endocrinology **119:** 2340–2345.

17. McDonald, T.J., J. Dupre, K. Tatemoto, G.R. Greenberg, J. Radziuk & V. Mutt. 1985. Galanin inhibits insulin secretion and induces hyperglycemia in dogs. Diabetes **34:** 192–196.
18. Ahrén, B., P. Arkhammar, P.-O. Berggren & T. Nilsson. 1986. Galanin inhibits glucose-stimulated insulin release by a mechanism involving hyperpolarization and lowering of cytoplasmic free Ca^{2+} concentration. Biochem. Biophys. Res. Commun. **140:** 1059–1063.
19. Lindskog, S. & B. Ahrén. 1987. Galanin: Effects on basal and stimulated insulin and glucagon secretion in the mouse. Acta Physiol. Scand. **129:** 305–309.
20. Lindskog, S. & B. Ahrén. 1988. Galanin and pancreastatin inhibit stimulated insulin secretion in the mouse comparison of effects. Hormone Res. **29:** 237–240.
21. Dunning, B.E. & G.J. Taborsky. 1990. The effect of rat galanin in rats. Diabetologia **33:** 125–126.
22. Schnuerer, E.M., T.J. McDonald & J. Dupre. 1987. Inhibition of insulin release by galanin and gastrin-releasing peptide in the anesthetized rat. Regul. Peptides **18:** 307–320.
23. Takeda, Y., C. Yanaihara, Y. Hashimoto, Y. Yamamoto, R. Takeda, K. Tatemoto, V. Mutt & N. Yanaihara. 1987. Galanin: Suppressing effect on glucose-induced insulin and C-peptide release. Biomed. Res. **8** (Suppl.): 117–125.
24. Mochizuki, T., J. Ishikawa, K. Ohshima, G.H. Greeley, Jr. & N. Yanaihara. 1992. Effects of galanin fragments on insulin release from the isolated perfused rat pancreas. Biomed. Res. **13:** 203–213.
25. McDonald, T.J., M.A. Ghatei, S.R. Bloom, T.E. Adrian, T. Mochizuki, C. Yanaihara & N. Yanaihara. 1983. Dose-response comparisons of canine plasma gastroenteropancreatic hormone responses to bombesin and the porcine gastrin-releasing peptide (GRP). Regul. Peptides **5:** 125–137.
26. Lagny-Puormir, I., A.M. Lorinet, N. Yanaihara & M. Laburthe. 1989. Structural requirements for galanin interaction with receptors from pancreatic beta cells and from brain tissue of the rat. Peptides **10:** 757–761.
27. Fox, J.E.T., B. Brooks, T.J. McDonald, W. Barnett, F. Kostolanska, C. Yanaihara, N. Yanaihara & Å. Rökaeus. 1988. Actions of galanin fragments on rat, guinea-pig, and canine intestinal motility. Peptides **9:** 1183–1189.
28. Boublik, J.H., N.A. Scott, M.R. Brown & J.E. Rivier. 1989. Synthesis and hypertensive activity of neuropeptide Y fragments and analogues with modified N- or C-terminal or D-substitutions. J. Med. Chem. **32:** 597–601.
29. Chou, P.Y. & G.D. Fasman. 1974. Conformational parameters for amino acids in helical, β-sheet, and random coil regions calculated from proteins. Biochemistry **13:** 211–221.
30. Chou, P.Y. & G.D. Fasman. 1974. Prediction of protein conformation. Biochemistry **13:** 222–245.
31. Fisone, G., M. Berthold, K. Bedecs, A. Unden, T. Bartfai, R. Bertorelli, S. Consolo, J. Crawley, B. Martin, S. Nilsson & T. Hökfelt. 1989. N-terminal galanin(1-16) fragment is an agonist at the hippocampal galanin receptor. Proc. Natl. Acad. Sci. USA **86:** 9588–9591.
32. Kuwahara, A., T. Ozaki & N. Yanaihara. 1990. Structural requirements for galanin action in the guinea-pig ileum. Regul. Pept. **29:** 23–29.
33. Xu, X.-J., Z. Wiesenfeld-Hallin, G. Fisone, T. Bartfai & T. Hökfelt. 1990. The N-terminal 1-16, but not C-terminal 17-29, galanin fragment affects the flexor reflex in rats Eur. J. Pharmacol. **182:** 137–141.
34. Yanaihara, N., M. Kadowaki, N. Yagi, T. Inoue, M. Sakabe, J. Ishikawa, Y. Hashimoto, T. Mochizuki & C. Yanaihara. 1988. Galanin: A unique feature in structure-function relationship. *In* Peptide Chemistry 1987. T. Shiba & S. Sakakibara, Eds.: 487–490. Protein Research Foundation, Osaka.
35. Yanaihara, N., T. Mochizuki, K. Iguchi, M. Hoshino, N. Nagashima, N. Takatsuka, J. Ishikawa, G.H. Greeley, C. Yanaihara & A. Kuwahara. 1991. Structure-function relationships of galanin. *In* Galanin. T. Hökfelt, T. Bartfai, D. Jacobowitz & D. Ottosen, Eds.: 185–196. Macmillan Education. London.
36. Lagny-Pourmir, I., B. Amiranoff, A.M. Lorinet, K. Tatemoto & M. Laburthe. 1989. Characterization of galanin receptors in the insulin-secreting cell line Rin m 5F: Evidence for coupling with a pertussis toxin-sensitive guanosine triphosphate regulatory protein. Endocrinology **124:** 2635–2641.

37. AMIRANOFF, B., A.-M. LORINET & M. LABURTHE. 1989. Galanin receptor in the rat pancreatic β cell line Rin m 5F. J. Biol. Chem. **264:** 20714–20717.
38. AMIRANOFF, B., A.-M. LORINET, N. YANAIHARA & M. LABURTHE. 1989. Structural requirement for galanin action in the pancreatic β cell line Rin m 5F. Eur. J. Pharmacol. **163:** 205–207.
39. SHIMOSEGAWA, T. & T. TOYOTA. 1993. Galanin in pancreas. Biomed. Res. **14** (Suppl. 3): 97–106.
40. HABERT-ORTOLI, E., B. AMIRANOFF, I. LOQUET, M. LABURTHE & J.F. MAYAUX. 1994. Molecular cloning of a functional human galanin receptor. Proc. Natl. Acad. Sci. USA **91:** 9780–9783.
41. PARKER, E.M., D.G. IZZARELLI, H.P. NOWAK, C.D. MAHLE, L.G. IBEN, J. WANG & M.E. GOLDSTEIN. 1995. Cloning and characterization of the rat GALR1 galanin receptor from Rin 14B insulinoma cells. Mol. Brain Res. **34:** 179–189.
42. HEDLUND, P.B., N. YANAIHARA & K. FUXE. 1992. Evidence for specific N-terminal galanin fragment binding sites in the rat brain. Eur. J. Pharmacol. **224:** 203–205.
43. KAKUYAMA, H., M. SUZUKI, M. IIZUKA, T. MOSHIZUKI, K. IGUCHI, M. HOSHINO & N. YANAIHARA. 1995. Structural requirements of galanin for occupancy of galanin receptor and cell growth in human small cell lung carcinoma cell line SBC-3A. *In* Peptide Chemistry. M. Ohno, Ed.: 61–64. Protein Research Foundation. Osaka.
44. HABU, A., T. OHISHI, S. MIHARA, R. OHKUBO, Y.-M. HONG, T. MOCHIZUKI & N. YANAIHARA. 1994. Isolation and sequence determination of galanin from pituitary of yellow fin tuna. Biomed. Res. **15:** 357–362.
45. KAKUYAMA, H., T. MOCHIZUKI, K. IGUCHI, K. YAMABE, H. HOSOE, M. HOSHINO & N. YANAIHARA. 1997. [Ala⁶, D-Trp⁸]-Galanin(1-15)ol is a potent galanin antagonist on insulin release. Biomed. Res. **18:** 49–56.
46. AMIRANOFF, B., A.M. LORINET, I. LAGNY-POURMIR & M. LABURTHE. 1988. Mechanism of galanin-inhibited insulin release. Occurrence of a pertussis-toxin-sensitive inhibition of adenylate cyclase. Eur. J. Biochem. **177:** 147–152.
47. BARTFAI, T., K. BEDECS, T. LAND, U. LANGEL, R. BERTORELLI, P. GIROTTI, S. CONSOLO, X. XU, Z. WIESENFELD-HALLIN, S. NILSSON, V.A. PIERIBONE & T. HÖKFELT. 1991. M-15: High-affinity chimeric peptide that blocks the neuronal actions of galanin in the hippocampus, locus coeruleus, and spinal cord. Proc. Natl. Acad. Sci. USA **88:** 10961–10965.
48. GREGERSEN, S., S. LINDSKOG, T. LAND, Ü. LANGEL, T. BARTFAI & B. ANRÉN. 1993. Blockade of galanin-induced inhibition of insulin secretion from isolated mouse islets by the non-methionine containing antagonist M35. Eur. J. Pharmacol. **232:** 35–39.
49. LINDSKOG, S., B. AHRÉN, T. LAND, U. LANGEL & T. BARTFAI. 1992. The novel high-affinity antagonist, galantide, blocks the galanin-mediated inhibition of glucose-induced insulin secretion. Eur. J. Pharmacol. **210:** 183–188.
50. XU, X.-J., Z. WIESENFELD-HALLIN, Ü. LANGEL, K. BEDECS & T. BARTFAI. 1995. New high affinity peptide antagonists to the spinal galanin receptor. Brit. J. Pharmacol. **116:** 2076–2080.
51. GU, Z.-F.A., W.J. ROSSOWSKI, D.H. COY, T.K. PRADHAN & R.T. JENSEN. 1993. Chimeric galanin analogs that function as antagonists in the CNS are full agonists in gastrointestinal smooth muscle. J. Pharmacol. Exp. Ther. **266:** 912–918.
52. BARTFAI, T., T. HÖKFELT & U. LANGEL. 1993. Galanin—A neuroendocrine peptide. Crit. Rev. Neurobiol. **7:** 229–274.
53. MELANDER, T., T. HÖKFELT, Å. RÖKAEUS, J. FAHRENKRUG, K. TATEMOTO & V. MUTT. 1985. Distribution of galanin-like immunoreactivity in the gastro-intestinal tract of several mammalian species. Cell Tissue. Res. **239:** 253–270.
54. FOX-THRELKELD, J.-A.E.T. 1991. Galanin and gastrointestinal function. *In* Galanin. T. Hökfelt, T. Bartfai, D. Jacobowitz & D. Ottosen, Eds.: 275–286. Macmillan Education. London.
55. FOX, J.E.T., B. BROOKS, T.J. MCDONALD, W. BARNETT, F. KOSTOLANSKA, C. YANAIHARA, N. YANAIHARA & A. ROKAEUS. 1988. Actions of galanin fragments on rats, guinea-pig, and canine intestinal motility. Peptide **9:** 1183–1189.
56. KWOK, Y.W., C.B. VERCHERE, C.H.S. MCINTOSH & J.C. BROWN. 1988. Effect of galanin on endocrine secretions from the isolated perfused rat stomach and pancreas. Eur. J. Pharmacol. **145:** 49–54.
57. NARVAEZ, J.A., Z. DIAZ, J.A. AGUIRRE, S.G. BARÓN, N. YANAIHARA, K. FUXE & P.B. HEDLUND. 1994. Intracisternally injected galanin-(1-15) modulates the cardiovascular responses of galanin-(1-29) and the 5-HT$_{1A}$ receptor agonist 8-OH-DPAT. Eur. J. Pharmacol. **257:** 257.

58. KAKUYAMA, H., A. KUWAHARA, T. MOCHIZUKI, M. HOSHINO & N. YANAIHARA. 1997. Role of N-terminal active sites of galanin in neurally evoked circular muscle contractions in the guinea-pig ileum. Eur. J. Pharmacol. **329:** 85–91.

59. YANAIHARA, N., T. MOCHIZUKI, N. TAKATSUKA, K. IGUCHI, K. SATO, H. KAKUYAMA, M. LI & C. YANAIHARA. 1993. Galanin analogues: Agonist and antagonist. Regul. Pept. **46:** 93–101.

60. NAGASHIMA, T., N. TAKATSUKA, T. MOCHIZUKI, M. HOSHINO, C. YANAIHARA, G.H. GREELEY, JR. & N. YANAIHARA. 1992. Effects of galanin-related peptides on gastrin and somatostatin (SRIF) release from the isolated perfused rat stomach. Biomed. Res. **13** (Suppl. 2): 329–336.

61. NAKAYAMA, K., N. WATANABE, T. YAMAZAWA, N. TAKESHITA, Y. TANAKA & N. YANAIHARA. 1991. Effects of porcine galanin on the mesentoric microcirculation and arterial smooth muscle in the rat. Eur. J. Pharmacol. **193:** 75–80.

62. KIYOHARA, T., M. OKUNO, H. ISHIKAWA, T. NAKANISHI, Y. SHINOMURA, C. YANAIHARA & Y. MATSUZAWA. 1992. Galanin-induced alteration of electrolyte transport in the rat intestine. Am. J. Physiol. **263** (Gastrointest, Liver Physiol. **26**): G502–G507.

63. MADAUS, S., V. SCHUSDZIARRA, TH. SEUFFERLEIN & M. CLASSEN. 1988. Effect of galanin on gastrin and somatostatin release from the rat stomach. Life Sci. **42:** 2381–2387.

64. HERRMANN-RINKE, C., D. HÖRSCH, G.P. MCGREGOR & B. GÖKE. 1996. Galanin is a potent inhibitor of glucagon-like peptide-1 secretion from rat ileum. Peptides **17:** 571–576.

65. ROSSOWSKI, W.J. & D.H. COY. 1989. Inhibitory action of galanin on gastric acid secretion in pentobarbital-anesthetized rats. Life Sci. **44:** 1807–1813.

66. CAREY, D.G., T.P. IISMAA, K.Y. HO, I.A. RAIKOVIC, J. KELLY, E.W. KRAEGEN, J. FERGUSON, A.S. INGLIS, J. SHINE & D.J. CHISHOLM. 1993. Potent effects of human galanin in man: Growth hormone secretion and vagal blockade. J. Clin. Endocrinol. Metab. **77:** 90–93.

67. DAVIS, T.M.E., J.M. BURRIN & S.R. BLOOM. 1987. Growth hormone (GH) release in response to GH-releasing hormone in man is 3-fold enhanced by galanin. J. Clin. Endocrinol. Metab. **65:** 1248–1252.

68. GIUSTINA, A., M. LICINI, A.R. BUSSI, A. GIRELLI, G. PIZZOCOLO, M. SCHETTINO & A. NEGRO-VILAR. 1993. Effects of sex and age on the growth hormone response to galanin in healthy human subjects. J. Clin. Endocrinol. Metab. **76:** 1369–1372.

69. GIUSTINA, A., M. LICINI, M. SCHETTINO, M. DOGA, G. PIZZOCOLO & A. NEGRO-VILAR. 1994. Physiological role of galanin in the regulation of anterior pituitary function in humans. Amer. J. Physiol. **266:** E57–E61.

70. MURAKAMI, Y., K. OHSHIMA, T. MOCHIZUKI & N. YANAIHARA. 1993. Effect of human galanin on growth hormone prolactin, and antidiuretic hormone secretion in normal men. J. Clin. Endocrinol. Metab. **77:** 1436–1438.

71. MURAKAMI, Y., M. NISHIKI, J. TANAKA, K. KOSHIMURA, H. ISHIDA, N. YANAIHARA & Y. KATO. 1996. Effect of human galanin on growth hormone and prolactin secretion in patients with pituitary adenoma. Biomed. Res. **17:** 101–104.

72. WYNICK, D., D.M. SMITH, M. GHATEI, K. AKINSANYA, R. BHOGAL, P. PURKISS, P. BYFIELD, N. YANAIHARA & S.R. BLOOM. 1993. Characterization of a high-affinity galanin receptor in the rat anterior pituitary: Absence of biological effect and reduced membrane binding of the antagonist M15 differentiate it from the brain/gut receptor. Proc. Natl. Acad. Sci. USA **90:** 4231–4235.

Role of Galanin in the Gastrointestinal Sphincters[a]

SATISH RATTAN[b] AND WATARU TAMURA

Department of Medicine, Division of Gastroenterology and Hepatology,
Jefferson Medical College, Thomas Jefferson University,
Philadelphia, Pennsylvania 19107, USA

ABSTRACT: Galanin was present and exerted potent effects in all the gastrointestinal sphincters examined. Galanin-immunoreactive nerve fibers and neurons are present in both the myenteric and submucosal plexuses of sphincters. The neuropeptide exerts diverse effects in different sphincteric smooth muscles that may be species specific. For example, in the lower esophageal sphincter, it may cause an increase in basal tone and suppression of nonadrenergic noncholinergic (NANC) nerve-mediated relaxation. On the contrary, in the internal anal sphincter (IAS), the predominant effect of galanin is to cause smooth muscle relaxation and augmentation of NANC nerve-mediated relaxation. In other sphincters, galanin may either have no effect or cause either an increase or a decrease in basal tone. Most of the actions of galanin on basal smooth muscle sphincteric tone are due to its actions directly on smooth muscle cells. However, some of the relaxant actions of the peptide may also be due to activation of NANC inhibitory neurons. The basic mechanism/s responsible for sphincteric smooth muscle contraction or relaxation in response to galanin have not been investigated. The suppressive as well as the augmentatory effects of galanin on NANC nerve-mediated sphincteric smooth muscle relaxation may be due to inhibition or facilitation, respectively, of the release of NANC inhibitory neurotransmitters such as nitric oxide and vasoactive intestinal polypeptide. Diverse effects in different gastrointestinal sphincters suggest a neuromodulatory rather than a neurotransmitter role of galanin and a significant role of the neuropeptide and putative antagonists in the pathophysiology and potential therapy of gastrointestinal motility disorders especially those affecting sphincteric function.

Gastrointestinal sphincters are groups of distinct skeletal and smooth muscles located in specific areas throughout the gastrointestinal tract. In the basal state, the sphincters remain in a state of tonic contraction and closure to serve as one-way valves to regulate and coordinate the caudad flow of gastrointestinal contents. The skeletal muscle sphincters, upper esophageal sphincter (UES), and external anal sphincter (EAS) are under voluntary control. The smooth muscle sphincters are the lower esophageal sphincter (LES), pyloric sphincter, sphincter of Oddi (SO), ileocecal sphincter (ICS), and internal anal sphincter (IAS). These smooth muscle sphincters are autonomic organs and are controlled by complex interactions between extrinsic nerves from the CNS and intrinsic control by the enteric nervous system (ENS) and the myogenic properties of specialized smooth muscle cells. The regulation of the sphincters is species as well as site specific.

[a]This work was supported by US Public Health Service Grant DK-35385 from the National Institutes of Health and an institutional grant from Thomas Jefferson University.

[b]Address for correspondence: Dr. Satish Rattan, Professor of Medicine and Physiology, 901 College, Department of Medicine, Division of Gastroenterology & Hepatology, 1025 Walnut Street, Philadelphia, PA 19107. Phone, 215/955-6944; fax, 215/923-7697.

Sphincteric relaxation in response to an appropriate reflex is mediated by intramural nonadrenergic noncholinergic (NANC) neurons and is responsible for the caudad movements of gastrointestinal contents. The basal tone of the sphincters, on the other hand, is under variable control of myogenic activity, adrenergic, cholinergic, and NANC innervation. The primary NANC inhibitory neurotransmitters are postulated to be vasoactive intestinal polypeptide (VIP) and nitric oxide (NO). Immunohistochemical studies have also shown the presence of galanin-immunoreactive (IR) neurons in the ENS. In addition, galanin immunoreactivity colocalizes with nitric oxide synthase (NOS) and VIP-IR neurons. This suggests a dynamic role of galanin in the regulation and modulation of sphincteric function.

Since the initial report of Galanin in 1983 by Tatemoto et al.,[1] various functions of this neuropeptide have been studied. However, the exact role and significance in gastrointestinal physiology, especially in the sphincters, are not known. The neuropeptide is widely distributed in the central and peripheral nervous systems[2,3] including those of the gastrointestinal tract. It is distributed in all levels of the gastrointestinal tract[4] and is present in neurons of the myenteric, submucous, and mucous plexuses of the gut.[5] In the gastrointestinal tract, galanin modifies gastrointestinal motility by both increasing and decreasing the release of neurohumoral substances (neuromodulator role of galanin).[6] Certain actions of galanin may be mediated by the direct activation of the receptor/s located at the smooth muscle cells (neurotransmitter role of galanin).[7]

Examination of the effects and the mechanism of action of galanin in gastrointestinal smooth muscle sphincters offers a unique opportunity to explore its role in the pathophysiology and possibly in the therapy of gastrointestinal sphincteric motility disorders.

As compared to the COOH-terminal, the NH_2-terminal of galanin (residue 1-15) seems to be highly conserved among different species studied. It is possible therefore that the COOH-terminal portions are responsible for the species-specific actions of galanin.

This review focuses on the role of galanin as a NANC mediator and a modulator of basal tone and neurally mediated relaxation of smooth muscle sphincters in the gastrointestinal tract. The LES and IAS have been examined in most detail in our laboratory and serve as prototypes for the actions of galanin in gastrointestinal sphincters.

EFFECTS AND MECHANISMS OF ACTIONS OF GALANIN IN SPECIFIC SPHINCTERS

Lower Esophageal Sphincter

General.   The human LES is a 2–4 cm long high pressure zone of specialized smooth muscle that straddles the diaphragm and is considered to be the major component of the antireflux barrier. At the onset of swallowing, the LES relaxes promptly and stays relaxed until the esophageal peristaltic wave initiated at the upper part reaches the end of the esophagus. The LES is innervated primarily by the vagus nerve with its preganglionic nerve endings in the myenteric plexus. Basal LES tone is thought to be primarily due to the intrinsic myogenic activity that may partly be regulated by postganglionic cholinergic and adrenergic neurons and other NANC excitatory neurons. LES relaxation, on the other hand, is mediated by postganglionic NANC myenteric inhibitory neurons via the inhibitory neurotransmitters NO and VIP.[8-10]

Common Conditions Affecting the LES.   Achalasia is characterized by hypertensive LES, inadequate LES relaxation, and aperistalsis in the smooth muscle portion of the esophagus. The disorder may be due to a dramatic decrease in the number of postganglionic NANC inhibitory neurons in the myenteric plexus associated with a marked decrease in VIP and NOS immunoreactive neurons. The pathogenesis of spastic motility disorders such as diffuse esophageal spasm (DES) and nutcracker esophagus, although poorly understood, may involve CNS and myenteric neural dysfunction. In the pathogenesis of gastroesophageal reflux disease, transient LES relaxations (TLESRs) unassociated with swallowing are thought to play a major role. Interestingly, these reflux episodes are not seen in patients with achalasia and may be mediated by the NANC inhibitory neurons.

Effects and Mechanisms of Actions of Galanin.   The effect of galanin on the LES has been studied in the opossum,[11] pig,[12] and cat.[13] In the opossum and pig, galanin was very potent in causing contractions of the LES due to its direct action on smooth muscle, because this effect was not modified by different neurohumoral antagonists (atropine, phentolamine, methysergide, pyrilamine, and indomethacin) and the neurotoxin tetrodotoxin. In the opossum LES, another important effect of galanin in causing suppression of the neurally (vagal stimulation, esophageal distention, or intramural nerve stimulation) mediated LES relaxation was recognized.[11] In general, the *in vitro* actions of galanin were similar to those *in vivo*,[14] where galanin caused an increase in basal LES tone and suppression of LES relaxation in response to NANC nerve stimulation by electrical field stimulation. The suppressant action of galanin on the LES relaxation is speculated to be due to inactivation of the NANC inhibitory neuron and a decrease in the release of inhibitory neurotransmitters such as NO and VIP. Additionally, galanin caused a significant decrease in both the amplitude and the latency of onset of contractions of the lower esophagus by suppressing the cholinergic and noncholinergic components of peristalsis.[15,16] This may resemble the picture of the combination of DES and achalasia. Galanin in the esophagus and LES thus appears to have primarily a neuromodulatory role. Whether these modulatory actions of galanin are exerted by its interaction with neurons that contain NOS, VIP, substance P, and ACh remains to be determined.

In contrast to the pig and opossum, in the feline LES,[13] intraarterial injection of galanin caused no significant effect on basal tone, but it inhibited the contractions by the agonists that act directly on the LES smooth muscle (substance P and bethanechol) or indirectly by neural stimulation (bombesin). The precise mechanisms of the inhibitory effect of galanin on the agonist-induced contractions and the lack of its effect on basal LES tone in the cat are not known. Furthermore, in contrast to the opossum,[11] in the feline LES, galanin failed to modify LES relaxation induced by neural stimulation or VIP. In these experiments, however, the only mode of neural stimulation tested was esophageal balloon distention. The lack of observed effect of galanin on LES relaxation may be due to involvement of multiple sites of esophageal distention-induced LES relaxation. Interestingly, in opossum studies also, LES relaxation in response to higher volumes of esophageal distention was not significantly affected.[11]

The species-specific effects of galanin on the LES are not surprising, because the anatomy of the LES and physiologic regulation of basal LES tone are different in different species. Because of the complex regulation of the basal tone of the feline LES[17-19] and multiple neuromodulatory actions of galanin, it is therefore possible that the net effect of galanin after modulation of the complex network is nil.

Pyloric Sphincter

General.   The pyloric sphincter plays an important role in the regulation of gastric emptying of solids and liquids into the duodenum. Relaxation of the pyloric sphincter is also under the control of NANC inhibitory innervation via the release of NO, VIP, and ATP.[20–27] The exact mechanisms controlling pyloric sphincter tone in humans is not understood, but it is considered to be myogenic and under the modulation of adrenergic and cholinergic pathways. The gastric contents, once in the duodenum, stimulate receptors that respond to low pH, high osmolality, fatty acids, and caloric density. These receptors, in turn, trigger enterogastric reflexes which slow gastric emptying by the feedback regulation of the pyloric sphincter.

Common Conditions Affecting the Pyloric Sphincter.   Infantile hypertrophic pyloric stenosis is caused by gastric outlet obstruction manifested as regurgitation and projectile vomiting at 3–4 weeks after birth. The etiology is unknown, but the lack of NOS in the pylorus may be responsible.[28] Medical treatment is usually unsuccessful, but pyloromyotomy offers excellent results and prognosis. Diabetic gastroparesis characterized by a delay in emptying of solid meal is generally believed to result from impaired phasic motor activity in the antrum and an increase in the outflow resistance from either the pyloric sphincter or small intestine. The pathogenesis of this abnormal motility is also not well understood, but it seems to be due to a combination of neural and myogenic factors.

Effects and Mechanisms of Actions of Galanin.   Interestingly, as reported by Allescher *et al.,*[27] galanin generally causes no significant effect on basal pyloric sphincter activity. Galanin, on the other hand, did cause significant inhibition of the pyloric activity that was stimulated by nerve stimulation by electrical field stimulation or intraduodenal infusion of 0.1 N HCl. In this regard, VIP and peptide histidine isoleucine (PHI) were several-fold more potent than galanin. The data suggest that galanin in the pylorus works primarily by inhibiting the neural excitatory pathway. The inhibitory effects of galanin were observed *in vivo* and not in *in vitro* pyloric circular smooth muscle rings. The inhibitory effects of galanin are perhaps due to inhibition of cholinergic activation. Thus, in the pylorus, galanin rather than being the inhibitory neurotransmitter may serve as the NANC inhibitory modulator by its action at the excitatory nicotinic synapse.

Sphincter of Oddi

General.   In humans, the length of the SO varies from 4–10 mm. The sphincter regulates the flow of bile and pancreatic exocrine juice to prevent reflux of duodenal contents into the bile duct. The sphincter is under both hormonal and neural control. The anatomy of the SO is variable in different species. In humans, monkeys, and cats, the common bile duct is often joined by the main pancreatic duct to form the ampulla of Vater and is embedded in the wall of the duodenum.[29] In the opossum, the sphincter is longer (>1 cm) and lies outside the duodenum. This accessibility and its location make the opossum SO a favorite model for basic studies. Innervation of the common bile duct and SO is more dense than that of the proximal regions of the biliary tree and is variable among species.

The sphincter of Oddi is innervated with the cholinergic, adrenergic, and NANC nerves. The NANC nerves contain VIP, neuropeptide Y, somatostatin, substance P, calcitonin gene-related polypeptide (CGRP), and bombesin.[30–34] In the sphincter of Oddi, both VIP and NO may serve as NANC inhibitory neurotransmitters.[35–43]

Common Conditions Affecting the Sphincter of Oddi.   Sphincter of Oddi dysfunction (SOD) is a benign noncalculous obstructive disorder that causes pancreatobiliary pain. Other terms used to define the condition are papillary stenosis, biliary dyskinesia, and postcholecystectomy syndrome. The etiology of the syndrome is poorly understood.

Effects and Mechanisms of Actions of Galanin.   Baker *et al.*[44] examined the effects of galanin on the Australian brush-tailed opossum SO both *in vivo* and *in vitro*. *In vitro*, galanin caused an increased in the spontaneous contractions of the longitudinal but not the circular smooth muscle of the SO. The effect of galanin on the longitudinal smooth muscle was specific and direct, because it was blocked by galantide and was resistant to tetrodotoxin. *In vivo*, galanin produced a small decrease in transsphincteric flow, possibly related to the increase in activity in the longitudinal smooth muscle of the SO. Galanin produced interesting actions on the opossum SO rings (circular smooth activity) *in vitro*.[45] In the SO rings, galanin had no significant effect on the amplitude of contractions but it had a direct (myogenic) stimulatory effect on the frequency of contractions.

Interestingly, the extraduodenal segment was the most sensitive to the effect of galanin. These data suggest the specific role of SO circular and longitudinal smooth muscle towards the decrease in the transsphincteric flow. However, participation of the duodenum may be difficult to rule out completely, because it may cause either contraction or relaxation of the upper part of the small intestine.[46–48] The effects of galanin in the porcine SO were different from those in the opossum, where it produced a decrease in the frequency of phasic activity.[49] Interestingly, galanin had no effect on the gallbladder.

Ileocecal Sphincter

There are no published reports on the effects of galanin on the ICS. The effects of galanin in the ICS were recently examined in our laboratory. Preliminary studies showed that galanin caused a small but concentration-dependent rise in the basal tone of the opossum ICS that was blocked by the neurotoxin tetrodotoxin. Furthermore, ICS relaxation by NANC nerve stimulation was not significantly modified by galanin (Rattan *et al.*, unpublished observations).

Internal Anal Sphincter

General.   The IAS is a specialized smooth muscle with elevated basal tone as compared to the rectum and it plays a significant role in rectoanal continence. Rectoanal continence is maintained by the joint efforts of tonic contraction of the IAS and the continuous activity of the somatically innervated skeletal muscles puborectalis, levator ani, and external anal sphincter. Rectal distention by gas, stool, or experimentally by balloon distention elicits reflex relaxation of the IAS (defecation reflex or rectoanal inhibitory reflex). For successful completion of the reflex, the skeletal muscles undergo relaxation by the voluntary inhibition or cessation of pudendal nerve firing followed by relaxation of IAS smooth muscle.

The high pressures in the anal canal are primarily due to the myogenic properties of the IAS smooth muscle.[50] The IAS resting tone, however, may be modulated by adrenergic, cholinergic, and NANC excitatory and inhibitory neurons. The IAS relaxation in response to the rectal inhibitory reflex is mediated by the NANC inhibitory neurons which can be mimicked *in vitro* in the IAS smooth muscle strips by selecting the appropriate parameters of EFS. The major inhibitory neurotransmitters in the IAS are NO and VIP.[51–53]

Common Conditions Affecting the IAS. Hirschsprung's disease is characterized by the absence of appropriate IAS relaxation in response to the rectal inhibitory reflex that may lead to dilatation of the proximal part of the gut and severe constipation. There is either an absence or a dramatic decrease in the number of both VIP and NOS-immunoreactive myenteric neurons in the IAS. The usual treatment is surgical correction with myectomy, although recently botulinum toxin has also been successfully tried.[54,55] Fecal incontinence may be caused by hypotensive IAS, sphincteric trauma through injury or surgery, and pelvic floor neuropathies with associated weakness of the puborectalis. Patients with normal rectal sensation and compliance can be trained by biofeedback techniques to prevent incontinence. In the absence of any specific IAS dysfunction, the usual treatment is the use of antidiarrheals. Constipation and dyskinesia may result from paradoxic contraction of the striated musculature during attempts at defecation. Many such patients respond very well to biofeedback, because their rectal sensation, compliance, and rectoanal inhibitory reflex are normal.

Effects and Mechanisms of Actions of Galanin. The effects of galanin in the opossum IAS have been studied *in vitro* by Chakder and Rattan.[14] In contrast to that of the LES, galanin caused a dose-dependent decrease in the resting tension of the IAS. Additionally, galanin caused dose-dependent augmentation of the neurally mediated IAS relaxation. The relaxant responses of galanin in basal IAS tone were partly due to its neural (neuromodulatory) action and partly its actions directly at the smooth muscle. Both of these relaxant responses were due to the NH_2-terminal portion of the neuropeptide, because galanin (1–29) and galanin (1–10) produced similar effects and was not observed with COOH-terminal portion galanin (15–29). Interestingly, galanin (15–29) caused an increase in resting IAS tension by direct action at the smooth muscle, and it had no significant effect on neurally mediated IAS relaxation. The middle portion of galanin (7–16) had no significant effect on the IAS. It was interesting that although the relaxant actions of galanin reside in the NH_2-terminal, a whole molecule of galanin is required for the full effect, suggesting indirectly the importance of the COOH-terminal in the relaxation response. This action was similar to that in the guinea pig ileum circular muscle, where galanin and NH_2-terminal caused relaxation of the muscle by suppression of the release of ACh and substance P.[56] In the ileum also, the NH_2-terminal was less potent than the whole molecule of galanin. It is speculated that in the IAS, the contractile effect of the whole molecule of galanin (observed with galanin 15–29) must have been masked by the predominant inhibitory effect of galanin.

Interestingly, in a different laboratory, the effects of galanin in humans were similar to those in the opossum.[14,57] Galanin caused relaxation of the IAS smooth muscle and it failed to modify the fall in basal IAS tension caused by VIP. Other details of the actions of galanin in the human IAS were not examined. There are no *in vivo* studies to examine the actions of galanin in the IAS.

Two major possibilities responsible for the neurally mediated fall in resting IAS tension as well as the augmentatory effect of galanin on EFS-induced IAS relaxation are: (a) the facilitatory modulation of the release of an inhibitory neurotransmitter (NO and VIP) by galanin, and (b) the augmentation of the inhibitory effect of the released inhibitory neu-rotransmitter as in isolated smooth muscle cells of the guinea pig small intestine where galanin caused significant augmentation of the inhibitory effects of VIP, isoproterenol, and cAMP.[58] The possible potentiation of the inhibitory effect of the released inhibitory neu-rotransmitter in the IAS seems unlikely, because a VIP-induced fall in basal IAS tension was not modified by galanin. Interestingly, in canine ileum, galanin caused a decrease in the tonic release of VIP.[59]

PRESENCE AND DISTRIBUTION OF GALANIN IN DIFFERENT SPHINCTERS

Galanin is present in porcine,[12] human,[60] canine,[22] feline,[13] rat,[5] mouse,[5] and opossum[61] esophagus and LES. Galanin-like immunoreactivity has been observed in nerve cell bodies of the myenteric plexus and in nerve fibers along the smooth muscle bundles. The density of galanin innervation was considerably higher in the LES than in nonsphinc-teric regions of the esophageal body and stomach.[61] Contrary to previous reports, recent reports by Kuramoto et al.[62,63] have shown the presence of galanin-like immunoreactive motor end plates in the esophageal striated muscle of mice, guinea pigs, and rats. The studies showed dual innervation of GAL- and calcitonin gene-related peptide/acetylcho-line-containing nerve terminals,[64] suggesting a possible role of galanin as a neurotransmit-ter/neuromodulator in the cholinergic neurons of esophageal striated muscle.

Immunohistochemical studies show high densities of galanin as well as VIP immunore-active fibers in the pyloric sphincter and other sphincters of the canine gastrointestinal tract.[22,24] Galanin-like immunoreactive nerves have been demonstrated in the biliary tract including the SO smooth muscle of the dog,[22] pig,[49,65] American opossum,[45] Australian brush-tailed opossum,[44] and man.[66] In all cases, both galanin-immunoreactive cell bodies and nerve fibers were localized mostly in the muscle layers of the SO and the rest of the biliary tract.

The presence of galanin in the IAS was demonstrated in humans.[57,67] Galanin was shown to be present in the nerve fibers especially around the outside of and between the smooth muscle bundles in addition to its presence in the cell bodies seen either singly or in ganglia in both the myenteric and submucosal plexi. Interestingly, no significant differ-ences in the density of innervation were noted between the controls and the individuals affected with neurogenic fecal incontinence[57] and Hirschsprung's disease.[68] However, a trend towards a decrease in the density of galanin innervation was noted in the fecal incon-tinent patients.

It is well known that nNOS and VIP are highly colocalized in different parts of the ali-mentary tract including the IAS.[69,70] The colocalization of galanin with nNOS and VIP has been shown in different regions of the gastrointestinal tract including the sphincteric regions that have been examined.

SIGNIFICANCE AND POTENTIAL ROLE OF GALANIN, ITS ANALOGS, AND ITS ANTAGONISTS IN THE PATHOPHYSIOLOGY AND MANAGEMENT OF SPHINCTER DISORDERS

There is a paucity of information on the effect of galanin in human gastrointestinal sphincters. In some cases, the actions of galanin in human in vitro smooth muscle strips were described as just discussed[57] and were similar to those in the opossum.[14]

The exact role of galanin in basal LES tone and NANC relaxation awaits the determination of the effects of galanin and galanin antagonists. Animal data on the effects of galanin in the LES suggest that the neuropeptide is an important neuromodulator of basal tone, the NANC relaxation, in esophageal peristalsis and in the pathophysiology of achalasia and DES.[11,15,16] The potent effects of galanin in causing an increase in basal tone of the LES suggest the potential therapeutic role of galanin and analogs in LES disorders characterized by the weak LES tone such as gastrointestinal reflux disease or reflux esophagitis. Interestingly, in the esophageal body, the effects of galantide were opposite those of galanin. The galanin antagonist enhanced the amplitude of esophageal peristaltic contraction elicited by vagal stimulation,[16] suggesting the potential role of endogenous galanin and galanin antagonists in the pathophysiology and perhaps in the management of esophageal motility disorders.

Based on findings in the canine pyloric sphincter,[27] galanin seems to act as an inhibitory modulator of duodenopyloric activation. Galanin inhibits the slow synaptic transmission of myenteric neurons in the small intestine.[71,72] The actions of galanin in the pylorus may be due to its actions on the excitatory nicotinic synapses rather than directly on the smooth muscle.[73] The extrapolation of animal data in the pylorus may predict a corrective role of galanin in gastric emptying disorders such as diabetic gastroparesis (functional gastric outlet obstruction resulting from pylorospasm due to dysfunction in the NANC innervation). However, human studies showed that galanin causes an actual delay in gastric emptying.[74]

In the absence of detailed and systematic actions of galanin in the SO and the complexity of the SO apparatus combined with its anatomic variability, the clinical implications of galanin in the pathophysiology, pathogenesis, and potential therapy in SOD are difficult to speculate.

The augmentatory effect of galanin on the NANC nerve-mediated IAS relaxation as well as its own relaxant effect in basal IAS tone in *in vitro* smooth muscle strips from the opossum IAS suggests a potential role of galanin in IAS dysfunction involving incomplete IAS relaxation such as Hirschsprung's disease. The inhibitory effect of galanin in the IAS, whether a direct or an indirect effect, suggests a potential role of galanin in hypertensive IAS as in patients with hemorrhoids and fissures.

The actions of galanin in the gastrointestinal sphincters as just discussed are both species and tissue specific. Therefore, caution should be exercised when extrapolating data for galanin and antagonists, from one sphincter to the other for their physiologic, pathophysiologic, and therapeutic actions. For example, galanin exerts opposite effects in the LES and IAS. For the drug design, to avoid the blunders of beneficial effects in one sphincter at the cost of ill effects in the other, it is important that the galanin analogs and antagonists are receptor, tissue, and species specific.

The differences in the actions of galanin may be related to the COOH-terminal portion of the peptide, because the NH_2-terminal is highly conserved. The role of galanin in sphincteric function is primarily that of a neuromodulator. From the IAS studies,[14] it is evident that although some of the actions are dependent on the NH_2-terminal and the other actions on the COOH-terminal portion, the whole molecule is necessary for the full spectrum of actions of galanin.

The overall action of galanin is to cause significant slowing of gastrointestinal transport by decreasing gastric emptying and mouth to colon transit time.[74] However, galanin caused an increase in human intestinal contractions. The inhibitory actions of galanin on gastrointestinal motility may be either direct on the smooth muscle or indirect via inhibition of vagally mediated esophageal peristalsis and LES relaxation in the case of esophageal studies[11,61] or by inhibition of the excitatory neurotransmitter release, such as decreased contraction of guinea pig tenia coli via inhibition of acetylcholine and substance P.[7] On the other hand, galanin also exerts direct stimulatory actions on gastrointestinal motility. Such examples are the contractions of the fundus of the rat stomach *in vitro*.[1,75] By contrast, galanin suppressed antral and pyloric activity in anesthetized dogs[22,27] and increased LES pressure in the pig[12,76] and opossum,[11,61] contraction of rat jejunal/ileal longitudinal muscle,[1] and contraction of human small intestine longitudinal muscle,[77] increasing the amplitude of spontaneous contractions in porcine jejunal longitudinal muscle[78] and potentiating stimulated contractions of porcine ileal longitudinal muscle.[79] Another example of indirect

TABLE 1. Summary of Actions and Site(s) of Action of Galanin on Gastrointestinal Sphincters

Organ	Species	Action	Site of Action
LES	Opossum	↑Basal tone	Smooth muscle
		↓NANC relaxation	NANC neurons
	Pig	↓Basal tone	Smooth muscle
		↓NANC relaxation	?
	Cat	No effect on basal tone or NANC relaxation	
		↓In contraction by direct acting agonists (sub P, bethanechol)	Smooth muscle
		↓In contraction by neural stimulation with bombesin	Neural
Pylorus	Dog	No effect on basal tone	
		↓In contraction by NANC stimulation with high-threshold EFS and intraduodenal acid	Vagal fibers
SO	American opossum	No effect on amplitude of the SOC	
		↑Frequency of SOC contractions	Smooth muscle
		↓Transsphincteric flow	?
	Australian brush-tailed opossum	No effect on spontaneous SOC activity	
		↓Contractile activity of SOL	NANC neurons
		↓Transsphincteric flow	Smooth muscle
	Pig	↓Frequency and amplitude of contractions	?
		? Transsphincteric flow	
ICS	Opossum	↑Basal tone	Neural
IAS	Opossum	↓Basal tone	Neural + smooth muscle
		↑NANC relaxation	Neural
	Human	↓Basal tone	Smooth muscle?
		No effect on NANC relaxation	

↓, inhibits or decreases; ↑, contracts or increases, stimulates or facilitates; ?, not known; LES, lower esophageal sphincter; SO, sphincter of Oddi; SOC, circular muscle of the sphincter of Oddi; SOL, longitudinal muscle of the sphincter of Oddi; ICS, ileocecal sphincter; IAS, internal anal sphincter; sub P, substance P; EFS, electrical field stimulation; NANC, nonadrenergic, noncholinergic.

inhibitory actions of galanin is the potentiating VIP-induced relaxation by opening membrane K^+ channels in the circular muscle of guinea pig small intestine[80] and inhibiting neurally evoked acetylcholine release from myenteric longitudinal muscle strips of the guinea pig small intestine.[81] In the latter example, galanin also inhibited acetylcholine release induced by VIP and substance P,[82] but not basal release, suggesting the role of galanin as an important neuromodulator in the enteric nervous system.

Specific studies to characterize the nature of galanin receptor/s and the intracellular mechanism/s responsible for the gastrointestinal sphincteric smooth muscle contraction or relaxation in response to galanin have not been carried out.

Actions of galanin in different gastrointestinal sphincters are summarized in TABLE 1.

REFERENCES

1. TATEMOTO, K., A. ROKAEUS, H. JORNVALL, T.J. MCDONALD & V. MUTT. 1983. Galanin: A novel biologically active peptide from porcine intestine. FEBS Lett. 164: 124–128.
2. ROKAEUS, A., T. MELANDER, T. HOKFELT, J.M. LUNDBERG, K. TATEMOTO, M. CARLQUIST & V. MUTT. 1984. A galanin-like peptide in the central nervous system and intestine of the rat. Neurosci. Lett. 47: 161–166.
3. GOYAL, R.K. & I. HIRANO. 1996. The enteric nervous system. N. Engl. J. Med. 334: 1106–1115.
4. ROKAEUS, A. 1987. Galanin-a newly isolated biologically active neuropeptide. Trends Neurosci. 10: 158–164.
5. MELANDER, T., T. HOKFELT, A. ROKAEUS, J. FAHRENKRUG, K. TATEMOTO & V. MUTT. 1985. Distribution of galanin-like immunoreactivity in the gastro-intestinal tract of several mammalian species. Cell Tissue Res. 239: 253–270.
6. RATTAN, S. 1991. Role of galanin in the gut. Gastroenterology 100: 1762–1768.
7. EKBLAD, E., R. HAKANSON, F. SUNDLER & C. WAHLESTEDT. 1985. Galanin: Neuromodulatory and direct contractile effects on smooth muscle preparations. Br. J. Pharmacol. 86: 241–246.
8. GOYAL, R.K., S. RATTAN & S.I. SAID. 1980. VIP as a possible neurotransmitter of non-cholinergic non-adrenergic inhibitory neurones. Nature 288: 378–380.
9. BIANCANI, P., J.H. WALSH & J. BEHAR. 1984. Vasoactive intestinal polypeptide: A neurotransmitter for lower esophageal sphincter relaxation. J. Clin. Invest. 73: 963–967.
10. TOTTRUP, A., D. SVANE & A. FORMAN. 1991. Nitric oxide mediating NANC inhibition in opossum lower esophageal sphincter. Am. J. Physiol. 260: G385–G389.
11. RATTAN, S. & R.K. GOYAL. 1987. Effect of galanin on the opossum lower esophageal sphincter. Life Sci. 41: 2783–2790.
12. HARLING, H., T. MESSELL, S.L. JENSEN, J.J. HOLST & S.S. POULSEN. 1989. Occurrence, distribution and motor effects of galanin in the porcine lower esophageal sphincter. Digestion 42: 151–157.
13. LICHTENSTEIN, G.R., J.C. REYNOLDS, C.P. OGOREK & H.P. PARKMAN. 1994. Localization and inhibitory actions of galanin at the feline lower esophageal sphincter. Regul. Pept. 50: 213–222.
14. CHAKDER, S. & S. RATTAN. 1991. Effects of galanin on the opossum internal anal sphincter: Structure-activity relationship. Gastroenterology 100: 711–718.
15. KACZMAREK, J., S. RATTAN & R.K. GOYAL. 1987. Galanin selectively inhibits noncholinergic component of peristalsis in smooth muscle of opossum esophagus (abstr) Gastroenterology 92: 1802.
16. YAMATO, S., I. HIRANO & R.K. GOYAL. 1996. Role of galanin in esophageal peristalsis in opossum in vivo (abstr) Gastroenterology 110: A785.
17. PARKMAN, H.P., J.C. REYNOLDS, C.P. OGOREK & M.S. KREIDER. 1993. Thyrotropin releasing hormone: An inhibitory regulatory peptide of the feline lower esophageal sphincter. Am. J. Physiol. Gastrointest. Liver Physiol. 264: G522–G527.
18. REYNOLDS, J.C., M. DUKEHART, A. OUYANG & S. COHEN. 1986. Interactions of bombesin and substance P at the lower esophageal sphincter. J. Clin. Invest. 77: 436–440.

19. REYNOLDS, J.C., A. OUYANG & S. COHEN. 1984. A lower esophageal sphincter reflex involving substance P. Am. J. Physiol. Gastrointest. Liver Physiol. **256:** G345–G354.

20. HE, X.D. & R.K. GOYAL. 1995. Inhibitory junction potential in the mouse pyloric sphincter: Roles of ATP, VIP and NO. Gastroenterology **108:** A975.

21. ALLESCHER, H.-D. & E.E. DANIEL. 1994. Role of NO in pyloric, antral, and duodenal motility and its interaction with other inhibitory mediators. Dig. Dis. Sci. **39** (Suppl): 73S–75S.

22. GONDA, T., E.E. DANIEL, T.J. MCDONALD, J.E.T. FOX, B.D. BROOKS & M. OKI. 1989. Distribution and function of enteric GAL-IR nerves in dogs: Comparison with VIP. Am. J. Physiol. **256:** G884–G896.

23. DENT, J. & B. CHIR. 1976. A new technique for continuous sphincter pressure measurement. Gastroenterology **71:** 263–267.

24. ALUMETS, J., O. SCHAFFALITZKY DE MUCKADELL, J. FAHRENKRUG, F. SUNDLER, R. HAKANSON & R. UDDMAN. 1979. A rich VIP nerve supply is characteristic of sphincters. Nature **280:** 155–156.

25. TANGE, A. 1983. Distribution of peptide-containing endocrine cells and neurons in the gastrointestinal tract of the dog: Immunocytochemical studies using antisera to somatostatin, substance P, vasoactive intestinal polypeptide, metenkephalin and neurotensin. Biomed. Res. **4:** 9–14.

26. ALLESCHER, H.D., J. DENT, E.E. DANIEL, J.E.T. FOX & F. KOSTALANSKA. 1989. Extrinsic and intrinsic neural control of pyloric sphincter in the dog. J. Physiol. (Lond.) **401:** 17–38.

27. ALLESCHER, H.D., E.E. DANIEL, J. DENT & J.E.T. FOX. 1989. Inhibitory function of VIP-PHI and galanin in canine pylorus. Am. J. Physiol. **256:** G789–G797.

28. VANDERWINDEN, J.-M., P. MAILLEUX, S.N. SCHIFFMANN, J.-J. VANDERHAEGHEN & M.-H. DE LAET. 1992. Nitric oxide synthase activity in infantile hypertrophic pyloric stenosis. N. Engl. J. Med. **327:** 511–515.

29. TOOULI, J. & R.A. BAKER. 1991. Innervation of the sphincter of Oddi: Physiology and considerations of pharmacological intervention in biliary dyskinesia. Pharmacol. Ther. **49:** 269–281.

30. MELANDER, T., E. MILLBOURN & M. GOLDSTEIN. 1991. Distribution of opioidergic, sympathetic and neuropeptide Y-positive nerves in the sphincter of Oddi and biliary tree of the monkey, *Macaca fascicularis.* Cell Tissue Res. **266:** 597–604.

31. GOEHLER, L.E., C. STERNINI & N.C. BRECHA. 1988. Calcitonin gene-related peptide immunoreactivity in the biliary pathway and liver of the guinea-pig: Distribution and colocalization with substance P. Cell Tissue Res. **253:** 145–150.

32. KEAST, J.R., J.B. FURNESS & M. COSTA. 1985. Distribution of certain peptide containing nerve fibers and endocrine cells in the gastrointestinal mucosa in five mammalian species. J. Comp. Neurol. **236:** 403–422.

33. LUNDGREN, O., J. SVANVIK & L. JIVEGARD. 1989. Enteric nervous system. II. Physiology and pathophysiology of the gallbladder. Dig. Dis. Sci. **34:** 284–288.

34. RYAN, J.P. 1987. Motility of the gallbladder and biliary tree. *In* Physiology of the Gastrointestinal Tract. L.R. Johnson, Ed.:695. Raven Press. New York.

35. BAUER, A.J., V.L.W. GO, T.R. KOCH & J.H. SZURSZEWSKI. 1987. Non-adrenergic, non-cholinergic (NANC) inhibitory innervation of the canine and opossum sphincter of Oddi (SO) (abstr). Gastroenterology **92:** 1311A.

36. DAHLSTRAND, C., A. DAHSTROM & H. AHLMAN. 1989. Adrenergic and VIP-ergic relaxatory mechanisms of the feline extrahepatic biliary tree. J. Auton. Nerv. Syst. **26:** 97–106.

37. SAND, J., P. ARVOLA, V. JÄNTTI, S. OJA, C. SINGARAM, G. BAER, P.J. PASRICHA & I. NORDBACK. 1997. The inhibitory role of nitric oxide in the control of porcine and human sphincter of Oddi activity. Gut **41:** 375–380.

38. ALLESCHER, H.D., S. LU, E.E. DANIEL & M. CLASSEN. 1993. Nitric oxide as putative nonadrenergic noncholinergic inhibitory transmitter in the opossum sphincter of Oddi. Can. J. Physiol. Pharmacol. **71:** 525–530.

39. SLIVKA, A., R. CHUTTANI, D.L. CARR-LOCKE, L. KOBZIK, D.S. BREDT, J. LOSCALZO & J.S. STAMLER. 1994. Inhibition of sphincter of Oddi function by the nitric oxide carrier *S*-nitroso-*N*-acetylcysteine in rabbits and humans. J. Clin. Invest. **94:** 1792–1798.

40. THUNE, A., D.S. DELBRO, B. NILSSON, S. FRIMAN & J. SVANVIK. 1995. Role of nitric oxide in motility and secretion of the feline hepatobiliary tract. Scand. J. Gastroenterol. **30:** 715–720.

41. CULLEN, J.J., B.M. HERRMANN, R.M. THOMAS, S.Y. FANG, J.A. MURRAY, A. LEDLOW, J. CHRISTENSEN & J.L. CONKLIN. 1997. The role of antioxidant enzymes in the control of opossum sphincter of Oddi motility. Am. J. Physiol. Gastrointest. Liver Physiol. **272:** G1050–G1056.

42. WILEY, J.W., T.M. O'DORISIO & C. OWYANG. 1988. Vasoactive intestinal polypeptide mediates cholecystokinin-induced relaxation of the sphincter of Oddi. J. Clin. Invest. **81:** 1920–1924.

43. BAKER, R.A., G.T.P. SACCONE, S.J.H. BROOKES & J. TOOULI. 1993. Nitric oxide mediates nonadrenergic, noncholinergic neural relaxation in the Australian possum. Gastroenterology **105:** 1746–1753.

44. BAKER, R.A., T.G. WILSON, R.T.A. PADBURY, J. TOOULI & G.T.P. SACCONE. 1996. Galanin modulates sphincter of Oddi function in the Australian brush-tailed possum. Peptides **17:** 933–941.

45. PARODI, J.E., S.A. WYORAL, R.E. GLEASON, R. DIGEORGIO, C. STERNINI & J.M. BECKER. 1992. Immunohistochemical mapping and functional effects of galanin on the opossum sphincter of Oddi (abstr). Gastroenterology **102:** A328.

46. GREGERSEN, H., F.H. DALL, C.S. JORGENSEN, S.L. JENSEN & B. AHRÉN. 1992. Effects of noradrenaline and galanin on duodenal motility in the isolated perfused porcine pancreatico-duodenal block. Regul. Pept. **39:** 157–167.

47. CHEN, C.K., T.J. MCDONALD & E.E. DANIEL. 1994. Galanin receptor in plasma membrane of canine small intestinal circular muscle. Am. J. Physiol. **266:** G113–G117.

48. BOTELLA, A., M. DELVAUX, J. FIORAMONTI, J. FREXINOS & L. BUENO. 1995. Galanin contracts and relaxes guinea pig and canine intestinal smooth muscle cells through distinct receptors. Gastroenterology **108:** 3–11.

49. HARLING, H., T. MESSELL, S.L. JENSEN & S.S. POULSEN. 1991. Distribution and effect of galanin on gallbladder and sphincter of Oddi motility in the pig. HPB Surgery **3:** 279–288.

50. CULVER, P.J. & S. RATTAN. 1986. Genesis of anal canal pressures in the opossum. Am. J. Physiol. Gastrointest. Liver Physiol. **251:** G765–G771.

51. NURKO, S. & S. RATTAN. 1988. Role of vasoactive intestinal polypeptide in the internal anal sphincter relaxation of the opossum. J. Clin. Invest. **81:** 1146–1153.

52. RATTAN, S. & S. CHAKDER. 1992. Role of nitric oxide as a mediator of internal anal sphincter relaxation. Am. J. Physiol. Gastrointest. Liver Physiol. **262:** G107–G112.

53. CHAKDER, S. & S. RATTAN. 1996. Evidence for VIP-induced increase in NO production in myenteric neurons of opossum internal anal sphincter. Am. J. Physiol. Gastrointest. Liver Physiol. **270:** G492–G497.

54. LANGER, J.C. & E. BIRNBAUM. 1997. Preliminary experience with intrasphincteric botulinum toxin for persistent constipation after pull-through for Hirschsprung's disease. J. Pediatr. Surg. **32:** 1059–1062.

55. MARIA, G., E. CASSETTA, D. GUI, G. BRISINDA, A.R. BENTIVOGLIO & A. ALBANESE. 1998. A comparison of botulinum toxin and saline for the treatment of chronic anal fissure. N. Engl. J. Med. **338:** 217–220.

56. KUWAHARA, A., T. OZAKI & N. YANAIHARA. 1990. Structural requirements for galanin action in the guinea-pig ileum. Regul. Pept. **29:** 23–29.

57. SPEAKMAN, C.T.M., C.H.V. HOYLE, M.A. KAMM, M.M. HENRY, R.J. NICHOLLS & G. BURNSTOCK. 1993. Neuropeptides in the internal anal sphincter in neurogenic faecal incontinence. Int. J. Colorect. Dis. **8:** 201–205.

58. GRIDER, J.R., K.S. MURTHY, J.-G. JIN & G.M. MAKHLOUF. 1992. Stimulation of nitric oxide from muscle cells by VIP: Prejunctional enhancement of VIP release. Am. J. Physiol. Gastrointest. Liver Physiol. **262:** G774–G778.

59. FOX-THRELKELD, J.-A.E.T., T.J. MCDONALD, S. CIPRIS, Z. WOSKOWSKA & E.E. DANIEL. 1991. Galanin inhibition of vasoactive intestinal polypeptide release and circular muscle motility in the isolated perfused canine ileum. Gastroenterology **101:** 1471–1476.

60. SINGARAM, C., A. SENGUPTA, D.J. SUGARBAKER & R.K. GOYAL. 1991. Peptidergic innervation of the human esophageal smooth muscle. Gastroenterology **101:** 1256–1263.

61. SENGUPTA, A. & R.K. GOYAL. 1988. Localization of galanin immunoreactivity in the opossum esophagus. J. Auton. Nerv. Syst. **22:** 49–56.

62. KURAMOTO, H. & Y. ENDO. 1995. Galanin-immunoreactive nerve terminals innervating the striated muscle fibers of the rat esophagus. Neurosci. Lett. **188:** 171–174.

63. KURAMOTO, H., Y. KATO, H. SAKAMOTO & Y. ENDO. 1996. Galanin-containing nerve terminals that are involved in a dual innervation of the striated muscles of the rat esophagus. Brain Res. **734:** 186–192.

64. NEUHUBER, W.L., J. WÖRL, H.-R. BERTHOUD & B. CONTE. 1994. NADPH-diaphorase-positive nerve fibers associated with motor endplates in the rat esophagus: A new evidence for co-innervation of striated muscle by enteric neurons. Cell Tissue Res. **276:** 23–30.

65. SAND, J., H. TAINIO & I. NORDBACK. 1993. Neuropeptides in pig sphincter of Oddi, bile duct, gall-bladder, and duodenum. Dig. Dis. Sci. **38:** 694–700.

66. SAND, J., H. TAINIO & I. NORDBACK. 1994. Peptidergic innervation of human sphincter of Oddi. Dig. Dis. Sci. **39:** 293–300.

67. CHRISTIANSEN, J., M. LORENTZEN & J. HOLST. 1990. Influence of peptides on anorectal function. Ann. Med. **22:** 413–418.

68. LARSSON, L.T., G. MALMFORS & F. SUNDLER. 1988. Neuropeptide Y, calcitonin gene-related peptide, and galanin in Hirschsprung's disease: An immunoctytochemical study. J. Pediatr. Surg. **23:** 342–345.

69. LYNN, R.B., S.L. SANKEY, S. CHAKDER & S. RATTAN. 1995. Colocalization of NADPH-diaphorase staining and VIP immunoreactivity in neurons in opossum internal anal sphincter. Dig. Dis. Sci. **40:** 781–791.

70. GUO, R., O. NADA, S. SUITA, T. TAGUCHI & K. MASUMOTO. 1997. The distribution and co-localization of nitric oxide synthase and vasoactive intestinal polypeptide in nerves of the colons with Hirschsprung's disease. Virchows Arch. Int. J. Pathol. **430:** 53–61.

71. PALMER, J.M., M. SCHEMANN, K. TAMURA & J.D. WOOD. 1986. Galanin mimics slow synaptic inhibition in myenteric neurons. Eur. J. Pharmacol. **124:** 379–380.

72. TAMURA, K., J.M. PALMER & J.D. WOOD. 1987. Galanin suppresses nicotinic synaptic transmission in the myenteric plexus of guinea-pig small intestine. Eur. J. Pharmacol. **136:** 445–446.

73. FOX, J.E.T., T.J. MCDONALD, F. KOSTOLANSKA & K. TATEMOTO. 1986. Galanin: An inhibitory neural peptide of the canine small intestine. Life Sci. **39:** 103–110.

74. BAUER, F.E., A. ZINTEL, M.J. KENNY, D. CALDER, M.A. GHATEI & S.R. BLOOM. 1989. Inhibitory effects of galanin on postprandial gastrointestinal motility and gut hormone release in humans. Gastroenterology **97:** 260–264.

75. KATSOULIS, S., W.E. SCHMIDT, H. SCHWORER & W. CREUTZFELDT. 1990. Effects of galanin, its analogues and fragments on rat isolated fundus strips. Br. J. Pharmacol. **101:** 297–300.

76. HARLING, H. 1993. Galanin: A candidate neurotransmitter in the porcine gastrointestinal tract. Danish Med. Bull. **40:** 511–518.

77. MAGGI, C.A., R. PATACCHINI, P. SANTICIOLI, S. GIULIANI, D. TURINI, G. BARBANTI, P. BENEFORTI, D. MISURI & A. MELI. 1989. Human isolated small intestine: Motor responses of the longitudinal muscle to field stimulation and exogenous neuropeptides. Naunyn Schmiedeberg's Arch. Pharmacol. **339:** 415–423.

78. BROWN, D.R., K.R. HILDEBRAND, A.M. PARSONS & G. SOLDANI. 1990. Effects of galanin on smooth muscle and mucosa of porcine jejunum. Peptides **11:** 497–500.

79. HARLING, H. & A. TOTTRUP. 1991. Motility regulating effects of galanin on smooth muscle of porcine ileum. Regul. Pept. **34:** 251–260.

80. GRIDER, J.R. & G.M. MAKHLOUF. 1988. The modulatory action of galanin: Potentiation of VIP-induced relaxation in isolated smooth muscle cells (Abstr) Gastroenterology **94:** A157.

81. KUWAHARA, A., T. OZAKI & N. YANAIHARA. 1989. Galanin suppresses neurally evoked contractions of circular muscle in the guinea-pig ileum. Eur. J. Pharmacol. **164:** 175–178.

82. YAU, W.M., J.A. DORSETT & M.L. YOUTHER. 1986. Evidence for galanin as an inhibitory neuropeptide on myenteric cholinergic neurons in the guinea pig small intestine. Neurosci. Lett. **72:** 305–308.

Galanin Activates an Inwardly Rectifying Potassium Conductance and Inhibits a Voltage-Dependent Calcium Conductance in Mudpuppy Parasympathetic Neurons[a]

RODNEY L. PARSONS,[b,d] JENNIFER M. MULVANEY,[c]
AND LAURA A. MERRIAM[b]

[b]Department of Anatomy and Neurobiology,
University of Vermont College of Medicine,
Burlington, Vermont, 05405, USA

[c]Department of Physiology, Veterinary Medicine,
Cornell University, Ithaca, New York, USA

ABSTRACT: Galanin-induced activation of an inwardly rectifying membrane potassium (K^+) current and inhibition of barium current (I_{Ba}) were studied using whole cell voltage clamp recording techniques in parasympathetic neurons dissociated from the mudpuppy cardiac ganglion. Both activation of the K^+ current and inhibition of I_{Ba} were concentration-dependent with an EC_{50} (or IC_{50}) of ~35 nM and ~0.4 nM, respectively. Both actions of galanin were eliminated by pretreatment with pertussis toxin, which suggested involvement of G_i/G_o protein activation. Galantide antagonized the galanin-induced activation of K^+ current with an IC_{50} equal to 4 nM. By contrast, galantide, by itself, inhibited I_{Ba} with an EC_{50} equal to 16 nM. Another galanin analog, M40, primarily antagonized the galanin-induced activation of K^+ current, but in some cells, M40 also acted as a weak agonist. M40, like galantide, inhibited I_{Ba}. The NH_2-terminal fragment galanin-(1-16) activated the K^+ current and inhibited I_{Ba}, indicating that the first 16 amino acids of the galanin peptide were sufficient for both actions. In summary, it is postulated that the effects of galanin on mudpuppy parasympathetic neurons might be mediated by activation of two different subtypes of galanin receptor, one that regulates membrane K^+ conductance and a second that modulates calcium conductance.

The 29 amino acid neuropeptide galanin, which was initially identified in porcine gut,[1] is known to be widely distributed in peripheral and central neurons across species.[2-4] Galanin stimulation of various cell types elicits diverse physiologic responses in many tissues.[3,5-7] The actions of galanin are believed to be mediated through multiple receptor subtypes that may be coupled to different intracellular pathways.[3-5]

In 1989 we reported that a neuropeptide antigenically very similar to mammalian galanin was present in neurons and fibers within mudpuppy cardiac tissues.[8] Later studies demonstrated that the distribution of this galanin-like neuropeptide in different tissues of the mudpuppy was similar to that reported for other species.[9] We have developed the mud-

[a]This work was supported by National Institutes of Health Grant NS-23978.

[d]Corresponding author: Rodney L. Parsons, PhD, Department of Anatomy and Neurobiology, College of Medicine, University of Vermont, Burlington, Vermont 05405. Phone, 802/656-2230; fax, 802/656-8704; e-mail, rparsons@zoo.uvm.edu

puppy cardiac ganglion as a model system for examining the different effects of galanin on membrane conductance in a single neuronal cell type.

Within the mudpuppy parasympathetic cardiac ganglia, virtually all of the parasympathetic postganglionic neurons and ~40% of the small intensely fluorescent (SIF) cells exhibited galanin-immunoreactivity (FIG. 1A), whereas neither the afferent nor the sympathetic postganglionic fibers were galanin positive.[10] Thus, galanin-like neuropeptide innervation of the mudpuppy myocardium (FIG. 1B) is derived from parasympathetic postganglionic fibers. Our initial studies demonstrated that galanin inhibited contraction of mudpuppy cardiac muscle.[8] Galanin hyperpolarized cardiac myocytes by activating a voltage-dependent, inwardly rectifying potassium conductance.[11,12] The galanin-induced increase in potassium conductance required activation of a G-protein.[12] Galanin also inhibited voltage-dependent calcium currents in mudpuppy atrial myocytes, an action that most likely contributed to the galanin-induced decrease in tension development (Merriam and Parsons, unpublished observations). Based on these initial observations, Parsons *et al.*[8] proposed that an amphibian galanin-like neuropeptide was the previously unidentified, noncholinergic, inhibitory transmitter released by vagal stimulation from postganglionic fibers innervating the mudpuppy heart.[13]

Many postganglionic neurons in the mudpuppy cardiac ganglion appear to receive innervation from galanin-immunoreactive SIF cells (FIG. 1A) as well as by collateral fiber processes from nearby postganglionic neurons, which also contain a galanin-like peptide.[10] Thus, it was not surprising that most mudpuppy parasympathetic neurons responded to exogenously applied galanin. Konopka *et al.*[14] showed that approximately 70% of the postganglionic neurons in the mudpuppy cardiac ganglia responded to galanin application. Roughly 90% of the responsive neurons were hyperpolarized by galanin, whereas the remaining cells either were depolarized or exhibited a biphasic response consisting of early depolarization followed by hyperpolarization.[8,14–16] The depolarization initiated by galanin was suggested to result from activation of a nonselective cationic conductance, because the depolarization appeared to have a reversal potential close to 0 mV.[15] However, the depolarizing response initiated by galanin occurred very infrequently and was not studied in any detail. Therefore, because the predominant effect of galanin on the membrane potential of mudpuppy cardiac neurons was hyperpolarization, many of our subsequent studies focused on elucidation of the ionic conductance underlying the galanin-induced hyperpolarization. Studies completed on cardiac neurons in intact ganglia suggested that the galanin-induced hyperpolarization is due to activation of a potassium conductance.[14] Support for this conclusion was drawn from the observations that the hyperpolarization recorded in current-clamped cells and outward currents recorded with single electrode voltage clamp recording techniques reversed near the expected equilibrium potential for potassium. In addition, the reversal potential for the galanin-induced hyperpolarization was shifted appropriately by an increase in extracellular potassium.[14] The galanin-induced hyperpolarization was eliminated during exposure to 1–10 µM *N*-ethylmaleimide (NEM),[17] a sulphydryl-alkylating agent that is proposed to alkylate the α subunit of pertussis-sensitive G-proteins.[18,19] Oxotremorine M-induced hyperpolarizations of the mud-puppy parasympathetic neurons were also inhibited in the presence of NEM, an observation consistent with activation of a pertussis-sensitive G-protein required for the increase in potassium conductance by both galanin and muscarinic agonists.[17] In a brief report, Parsons and Merriam[20] provided evidence that the galanin-induced hyperpolarization, like that initiated by muscarinic agonists, was produced by activation of a time- and

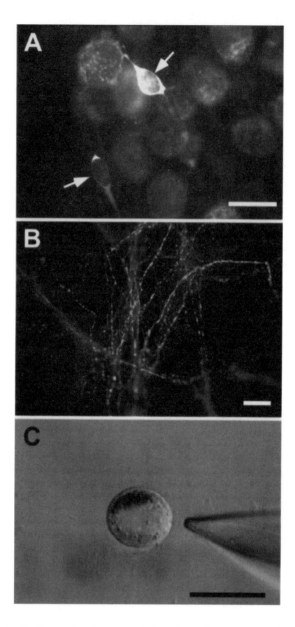

FIGURE 1. Photomicrographs of neurons and fibers in whole mount preparations (**A, B**) or of a dissociated neuron (**C**). (**A**) Two galanin-immunopositive SIF cells (*arrows*) within a cluster of mudpuppy parasympathetic neurons, many of which also exhibited galanin immunoreactivity.[8,10] (**B**) Galanin-immunopositive nerve fibers covering muscle strands in the mudpuppy cardiac septum. (**C**) A patch pipette approaching a dissociated mudpuppy parasympathetic neuron. Scale bar in all three panels equals 50 μM.

voltage-dependent inwardly rectifying potassium conductance. This conclusion was based on results obtained from whole cell recordings from enzymatically dissociated mudpuppy cardiac neurons.

In addition to initiating membrane hyperpolarization, galanin depressed excitability of the mudpuppy parasympathetic neurons.[14,21] The galanin-induced decrease in excitability remained even when the hyperpolarization was negated electrotonically or in those neurons that exhibited very little hyperpolarization.[14,21] Thus, even though membrane hyperpolarization must contribute to the galanin-induced depression of action potential generation, effects of galanin on other conductances underlying spike initiation may be involved. In fact, the decrease in excitability appeared to result from a shift in the threshold for spike generation to more positive values of membrane potential and occurred whether the major inward current carrier was sodium or calcium.[11,21] Galanin also decreased the rate of rise of sodium spikes and decreased the amplitude and duration of calcium spikes, which suggested that galanin may modulate voltage-gated sodium or calcium conductances.[14,21]

In most systems in which galanin actions were studied at the cellular level, it acts primarily as an inhibitory neurotransmitter/neuromodulator substance.[2,5,7] The predominant inhibitory action of galanin on parasympathetic neurons within the mudpuppy cardiac ganglia is similar to the major actions of galanin on mammalian peripheral and central neurons.[22–24] Thus, we have continued to use mudpuppy parasympathetic postganglionic neurons as a model neuronal system to elucidate galanin-induced modulation of membrane ionic conductances. Our recent work, summarized in the following sections, has focused on an analysis of the galanin-activated potassium conductance and galanin-induced inhibition of voltage-dependent calcium conductances. It remains to be determined whether the modulation of these two membrane conductance systems results from the action of galanin on a common receptor or occurs through the action of galanin on subtypes of galanin receptors expressed by the mudpuppy parasympathetic neurons. In addition, the contribution of putative galanin-stimulated signaling molecules to modulation of membrane conductances is of interest.

GALANIN-ACTIVATED POTASSIUM CONDUCTANCE

Galanin-activated potassium currents have been studied in parasympathetic neurons dissociated from the mudpuppy cardiac ganglia (FIG. 1C).[20,25] Perforated patch recordings of membrane currents were made at room temperature 21–22°C with the neurons kept in a HEPES-buffered sodium-deficient bath solution containing in mM: 100 n-methyl-d-glucamine-Cl (NMG), 2.5–12.5 KCl, 3.6 $CaCl_2$, 2 $MgCl_2$, and 3×10^{-4} tetrodotoxin; pH = 7.3. The sodium-deficient, NMG-substituted solution was used to eliminate any potential contribution of the galanin-induced activation of a nonselective cationic conductance to the measured currents. Most of the recordings were made with the bath K^+ concentration kept at 12.5 mM in order to facilitate measurement of inwardly rectifying K^+ currents.[20] The pipette solution contained in mM: 90 K-aspartate, 20 KCl, 10 HEPES, 8 $MgCl_2$; pH = 7.15. The pipettes were backfilled with an identical solution, which also contained 0.33 mg/ml nystatin. The cells were continuously perfused with fresh bath solution (~3 ml/min into a 0.5 ml bath), and galanin was applied by bath superfusion.

Experiments were done initially to characterize more fully the membrane current activated by galanin in dissociated neurons kept in the 12.5 K$^+$/NMG solution. The cells were voltage-clamped to -50 mV and stepped for 300 ms to different test potentials (-30 to -120 mV in 10-mV increments) before and after the addition of 10^{-7} M galanin. The agonist-induced current was determined by subtracting the control current from the

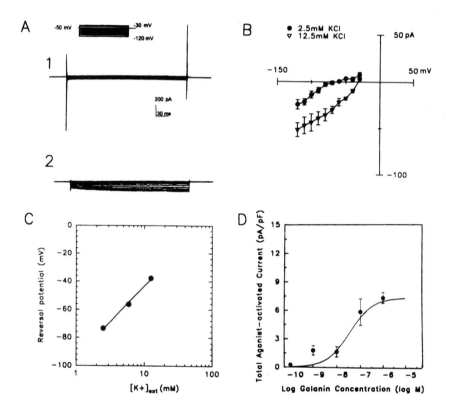

FIGURE 2. Galanin activates an inwardly rectifying potassium current. (**A**) Galanin-induced currents evoked by 300-ms voltage steps from a holding potential of -50 mV to potentials between -30 and -120 mV. The cell was bathed in the NMG-substituted, 12.5 mM K$^+$ solution. The protocol is shown above trace 1, which shows control membrane currents recorded prior to galanin application. Trace 2 shows 10^{-7} M galanin-activated currents determined after subtraction of control currents from total current recorded in the presence of galanin. (**B**) The averaged current-voltage (I-V) relationship for galanin-induced currents (10^{-7} M) recorded in 2.5 mM K$^+$ (9 cells) and 12.5 mM K$^+$ (8 cells). (**C**) The potassium dependence of the reversible potential for galanin-activated currents (10^{-7} M or 10^{-6} M). Each point represents results from at least 4 cells with the standard error bars obscured by the symbols. The reversal potentials were determined using voltage protocols similar to those in FIGURE 2A. (**D**) Concentration dependence of the galanin-induced activation of K$^+$ current. The current values are normalized to cell capacitance (pA/pF) and the vertical bars give SEM values for mean currents from 3, 11, 6, 6, and 14 neurons at 10^{-10} to 10^{-6} M galanin, respectively. The estimated EC$_{50}$ was 35 nM.

total current recorded in the presence of galanin. With galanin there was very little additional outward current with steps to voltages more positive than the holding potential (FIG. 2A). In contrast, during galanin exposure, a marked increase in current was noted with voltage steps to potentials more negative than the holding potential (FIG. 2A). This observation confirmed the previous conclusion that galanin activated an inwardly rectifying membrane current in the mudpuppy cardiac neurons.[20] To ensure that the current activated by galanin under these recording conditions was due to activation of K^+ conductance, we tested whether the reversal potential for this current was shifted by changes in extracellular K^+ concentration. FIGURE 2B shows the ~40 mV shift in reversal potential for the galanin-induced current that occurred when the external K^+ concentration was reduced from 12.5 to 2.5 mM. The reversal potential for the galanin-induced current at different external K^+ concentrations is shown in FIGURE 2C. The slope of the relationship between the reversal potential of the galanin-induced current and bath K^+ concentration was ~53, a value close to that expected (58 mV) if the galanin-induced current was primarily potassium selective.

Experiments were also done to determine the concentration dependence of the galanin-induced increase in K^+ current. As the parasympathetic neurons range in size from 30–50 μM, the galanin-induced currents were normalized to cell capacitance (pA/pF) to minimize variability of maximum current amplitude due to cell size. For these experiments, the neurons were maintained in the 12.5 mM K^+/NMG solution, held at −40 mV, and stepped every 5 seconds to −100 mV for 300 ms prior to and during exposure to different concentrations of galanin (10^{-10} to 10^{-6} M). As evident from FIGURE 2D, the galanin-induced increase in K^+ current was concentration dependent with an EC_{50} equal to ~35 nM.

We also tested if the galanin-induced activation of the K^+ current was maintained during prolonged exposure to agonist. With continued exposure to galanin, the current reached a peak value and then declined gradually (FIG. 3A). This progressive decline from the peak value occurred at both high and low concentrations of galanin. However, although not quantitated, the rate and extent of the decline of the galanin-induced current from the peak value appeared to be greater with the higher concentrations.

Previously, Konopka *et al.*[17] reported that the galanin-induced hyperpolarization was eliminated in the presence of NEM, suggesting that activation of a pertussis toxin (PTX)-sensitive G-protein was involved in the generation of the galanin-induced hyperpolarization. Because NEM actions are diverse, we tested directly whether PTX treatment, which selectively inhibits G_i/G_o proteins, also inhibited the galanin-induced activation of the K^+ conductance. Pretreatment with PTX (10–20 μg/ml) for 20–30 hours essentially eliminated the galanin-activated currents (FIG. 3B).

Previously, Hardwick and Parsons[26] reported that galanin stimulated phosphoinositide (PI) turnover in mudpuppy myocardium. Agonist-induced PI turnover has often been correlated with the activation of protein kinase C (PKC) through the diacyglycerol (DAG) pathway. Given that PKC has been shown to modulate the function of numerous ion channels, we tested whether inhibition of PKC by a 15–30 minute pretreatment with 0.5 μM staurosporine interfered with the generation of the galanin-induced current. At this concentration, staurosporine also should effectively inhibit a number of protein kinases in addition to PKC. As shown in FIGURE 3C, treatment with staurosporine had no effect on the amplitude of the galanin-induced K^+ current. Also, staurosporine treatment did not produce any noticeable effect on the time course of the galanin-activated K^+ conductance.

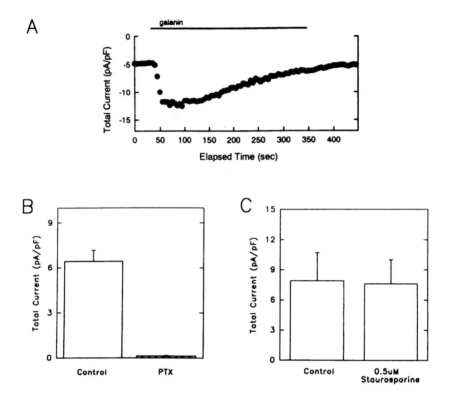

FIGURE 3. Pretreatment with pertussis toxin (PTX) but not staurosporine inhibits galanin-induced currents. (**A**) The increase in K^+ current fades during a prolonged exposure to 10^{-6} M galanin. Currents were produced by 300-ms voltage steps (delivered at 5-second intervals) from a holding potential of -40 mV to -110 mV before, during, and after removal of galanin. The *solid horizontal line* indicates the duration of galanin application. (**B**) Comparison of galanin-induced current in 4 control and 4 PTX-pretreated cells. Treatment with PTX (10 µg/ml) for 24–36 hours at room temperature essentially eliminated the 10^{-6} M galanin-induced currents. (**C**) Pretreatment with 0.5 µM staurosporine did not affect the magnitude of the galanin-induced current. In all three panels the galanin-induced K^+ current is normalized to cell capacitance.

Galantide (10^{-6} M), a chimeric peptide that is reported to act as a galanin receptor antagonist in some systems,[27] blocked the galanin-induced increase in K^+ current and did not by itself activate the K^+ current (FIG. 4B).[25] The antagonism by galantide of the 10^{-6} M galanin-induced activation of the K^+ current was concentration-dependent with an IC_{50} of 4 nM (FIG. 4D).[25] Similar experiments were completed using M40, another putative galanin receptor antagonist.[28] M40 (10^{-6} M) consistently blocked the 10^{-6} M galanin-induced activation of the K^+ current. However, unlike galantide, M40 also acted like a weak agonist so that in some cells at high concentrations, it activated a small K^+ current. In the example result shown in FIGURE 4C, M40 did not activate any noticeable K^+ current, but it did effectively inhibit the galanin-induced current. Additional studies demonstrated that

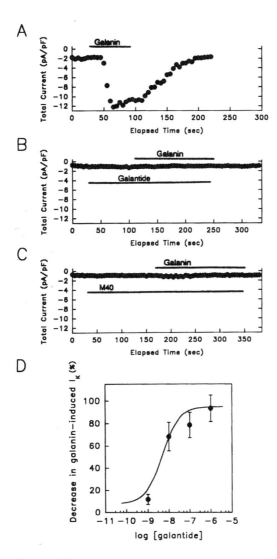

FIGURE 4. Galantide and M40 antagonize the galanin-induced activation of K⁺ current. Results from three different cells. In each, membrane currents produced by 300-ms voltage steps (delivered every 5 seconds) from a holding potential of -40 to -110 mV were recorded before, during, and after drug application. *Solid lines* indicate the duration of exposure to the different drugs. (**A**) An example of the galanin-induced K⁺ current in the absence of galantide or M40. (**B**) Galantide (10^{-6} M) did not activate a membrane current but inhibited the K⁺ current activation by 10^{-6} M galanin. (**C**) M40 (10^{-6} M) did not activate a membrane current in this cell, but it did inhibit the 10^{-6} M galanin-induced activation of a K⁺ current. (**D**) The concentration dependence of the galantide inhibition of the 10^{-6} M galanin activation of K⁺ current. *Vertical bars* give the SEM of the mean current recorded from at least three cells. The estimated IC$_{50}$ for galantide was 4 nM. Panels **A**, **B**, and **D** are reprinted with permission from Mulvaney *et al.*[25]

the NH_2-terminal fragment, galanin-(1-16), also effectively activated the inwardly rectifying K^+ current.[25] Thus, the first 16 amino acids of the galanin peptide are sufficient to activate the K^+ conductance in mudpuppy cardiac neurons.

GALANIN-INDUCED INHIBITION OF VOLTAGE-DEPENDENT CALCIUM CONDUCTANCE

In mudpuppy cardiac neurons, both sodium influx and calcium influx can contribute to the inward current underlying the depolarizing phase of action potentials.[14] We have shown that galanin can affect the rising phase of both sodium-dependent and calcium-dependent spikes.[14,21] The effect of galanin on the amplitude and duration of calcium-dependent action potentials was very striking, indicating that galanin had a marked inhibitory action on voltage-dependent calcium conductances in these neurons. Previously, galanin was reported to inhibit voltage-dependent calcium currents in endocrine cells.[29] Consequently, we tested whether galanin inhibited voltage-dependent calcium conductance in the mudpuppy cardiac neurons. All experiments were completed on dissociated neurons voltage-clamped with either the standard whole cell or nystatin perforated patch whole cell recording technique.[30] The composition of the external bath solutions and pipette solutions was designed to ensure that calcium currents were isolated from other voltage-gated currents, and in most experiments barium was used as the charge carrier (I_{Ba}) through calcium channels.[30]

When cells were voltage-clamped to -80 mV and stepped to more positive potentials, I_{Ba} was first evident with depolarizing steps to -30 or -20 mV, reached a peak at approximately $+10$ mV, and decreased with steps to more positive voltages.[30] Galanin produced a concentration-dependent inhibition of I_{Ba}, with the concentration that produced half-maximal (IC_{50}) inhibition being 0.42 nM (FIG. 5B). The maximum inhibition, which occurred with galanin concentrations $>10^{-8}$ M, was approximately 50%. Example records, which illustrate the galanin-induced decrease in I_{Ba} at different voltage steps, are shown in FIGURE 5A. When standard whole cell recordings were used, inhibition of I_{Ba} by galanin reached a maximum value and then tended to slowly reverse even though the galanin application continued. In contrast, when the perforated patch recording mode was used, the galanin-induced inhibition of I_{Ba} appeared to be sustained throughout galanin exposure.[30] Thus, most analysis of the galanin-induced inhibition of I_{Ba} was done using the perforated patch whole cell recording technique.

The galanin-induced inhibition of I_{Ba} was eliminated by a 24–30 hour pretreatment with PTX (10–15 µg/ml) (FIG. 5C). Thus, the galanin-induced inhibition of I_{Ba} required activation of a G_i/G_o protein.

Galanin did not alter the onset or extent of inactivation with long depolarizing voltage steps. In addition, the inhibition of I_{Ba} was not due to an alteration in inactivation kinetics or due to an affect on steady-state levels of inactivation. Furthermore, the inhibition of I_{Ba} by galanin in mudpuppy neurons appeared to involve both voltage-dependent and voltage-independent mechanisms.[30] Mudpuppy neurons contain at least two pharmacologically distinguishable calcium channel types, channels inhibited by dihydropyridines such as nifedipine and channels blocked by ω-conotoxin-GVIA. The ω-conotoxin-GVIA-sensitive calcium channels appeared to be preferentially inhibited by galanin.[30]

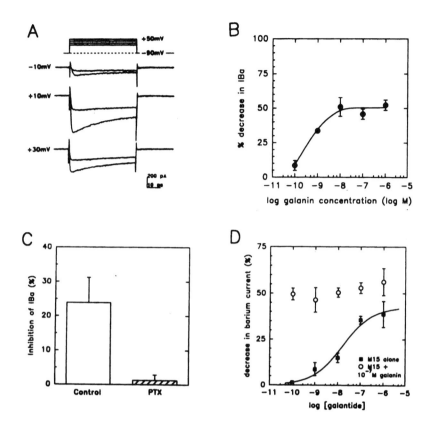

FIGURE 5. Galanin inhibits I_{Ba} flowing through voltage-dependent calcium channels. (A) The 10^{-7} M galanin-induced decrease of I_{Ba} elicited by steps from a holding potential of -90 mV to more positive voltages. In each example, the current recorded in the presence of galanin is the *upper trace*; the control current is the *lower trace*. (B) The concentration dependence of the galanin-induced inhibition of I_{Ba}. The decrease of I_{Ba} by galanin was determined from peak current measured during steps to $+10$ mV from holding potential of -80 or -90 mV. *Vertical bars* give mean ± SEM obtained from at least three cells. (C) Pretreatment with 10–15 μg/ml pertussis toxin (PTX) for ~24 hours eliminated the galanin-induced inhibition of I_{Ba}. (D) The concentration dependence of the inhibition of I_{Ba} by galantide (M15) compared with various concentrations of galantide plus 10^{-7} M galanin. The IC_{50} for inhibition of I_{Ba} by galantide was 16 nM. Peak current was recorded at $+10$ mV from a holding potential of -80 mV. *Symbols* and *error bars* represent mean ± SEM from at least four cells. Panels **A** and **B** are reprinted with permission from Merriam and Parsons.[30] Panel **D** is reprinted with permission from Mulvaney *et al.*[25]

We also tested whether activation of a staurosporine-sensitive protein kinase was required for inhibition of I_{Ba} by galanin. Pretreatment with 0.5 μM staurosporine had no effect on the inhibition of I_{Ba} produced by 10^{-7} M galanin (Merriam and Parsons, unpublished observations). Thus, we concluded that activation of protein kinases, in particular PKC, was not involved in the galanin-induced inhibition of I_{Ba}.

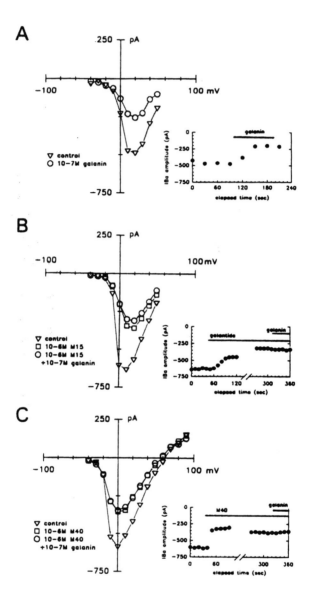

FIGURE 6. Galanin, galantide (M15), and M40 inhibit I_{Ba}. **(A-C)** I-V relationship of I_{Ba} recorded in three different cells. **(A)** I_{Ba} in control solution and in the presence of 10^{-6} M galanin. **(B)** I_{Ba} in control solution, in the presence of 10^{-6} M galantide, and in the presence of 10^{-6} M galantide and 10^{-7} M galanin. **(C)** I_{Ba} in control solution, in the presence of 10^{-6} M M40, and in the presence of 10^{-6} M M40 and 10^{-7} M galanin. The *inset* in each panel shows the time of exposure to galanin, galantide, or M40 and effect on I_{Ba}. Panel **B** was reproduced with permission from Mulvaney *et al.*[25]

Experiments also have been done to test whether galanin analogs antagonized the ability of galanin to inhibit I_{Ba} (FIG. 6A and B). Galantide did not act as an antagonist. Instead, galantide, in the absence of galanin, produced a concentration-dependent inhibition of I_{Ba} with an IC_{50} equal to 16 nM (FIG. 5D).[25] The maximum inhibition of I_{Ba} by galantide, which occurred at a concentration of galantide of 10^{-6} M, was ~40%. This extent of inhibition was slightly less than the maximum inhibition (50%) produced by galanin. However, the maximum inhibition of I_{Ba} by galantide and 10^{-7} M galanin together was the same as that produced by galanin alone (FIG. 5D). Thus, we concluded that galantide and galanin were acting through the same receptors.[25]

Additional experiments were completed to test whether M40 inhibited I_{Ba} or reduced the galanin-induced inhibition of I_{Ba}. M40 also inhibited I_{Ba} in the mudpuppy cardiac neurons. As shown in FIGURE 6C, with a concentration of 10^{-6} M, M40 inhibited I_{Ba} by ~45% and the addition of 10^{-7} M galanin did not produce a further inhibition of I_{Ba}. Thus, the galanin- and M40-induced inhibition of I_{Ba} appeared to be mediated by the same receptor. The NH_2-terminal fragment, galanin-(1-16), also effectively inhibited I_{Ba}.[25]

CONCLUSIONS

The results of these recent studies demonstrated that galanin has concentration-dependent effects on two distinct ionic conductances in mudpuppy parasympathetic neurons. Both actions of galanin on mudpuppy parasympathetic neurons require activation of a PTX-sensitive G-protein and are mimicked by galanin-(1-16) as in mammalian CNS neurons.[25, 31] The latter result indicated that the NH_2-terminal portion of the galanin molecule responsible for the galanin-induced activation of K^+ current and inhibition of I_{Ba}. The chimeric peptides, galantide and M40, had different effects on these two actions of galanin. Galantide only acted as an antagonist on the galanin-induced activation of the K^+ current, whereas it effectively replaced galanin as an inhibitor of I_{Ba}. M40 predominantly antagonized the galanin-induced activation of K^+ currents, although it also activated the K^+ current to a small extent in some cells. M40 and galantide effectively inhibited I_{Ba} and at 10^{-6} M occluded any further inhibition of I_{Ba} by galanin.

It is possible that the actions of galanin in the mudpuppy cardiac neurons are mediated by a single receptor that is coupled to different G-proteins and/or different intracellular transduction mechanisms. However, we postulate that the effects of galanin on mudpuppy neurons are mediated by activation of two different subtypes of galanin receptor, one that regulates K^+ conductance and a second that mediates the inhibition of I_{Ba}. The presence of at least two different subtypes of galanin receptor is now well established.[32-34] We demonstrated that the mudpuppy neurons provide a convenient model system to analyze the basic mechanisms of galanin-induced modulation of membrane conductances in a cell endogenously expressing more than one galanin receptor subtype.

ACKNOWLEDGMENT

The authors thank the *European Journal of Pharmacology* and the *Journal of Neurophysiology* for permission to reproduce portions of figures published previously.

REFERENCES

1. TATEMOTO, K., Å. ROKAEUS, H. JÖRNVALL, T.J. McDONALD & V. MUTT. 1983. Galanin: A novel biologically active peptide from porcine intestine. FEBS. Lett. **164:** 124–128.
2. BARTFAI, T., G. FISONE & Ü. LANGEL. 1992. Galanin and galanin antagonists: Molecular and biochemical perspectives. TiPS **13:** 312–317.
3. BARTFAI, T., T. HÖKFELT & Ü. LANGEL. 1993. Galanin: A neuroendocrine peptide. Crit. Rev. Neurobiol. **7:** 229–274.
4. BEDECS, K., M. BERTHOLD & T. BARTFAI. 1995. Galanin: 10 years with a neuroendocrine peptide. Int. J. Biochem. Cell Biol. **27:** 337–349.
5. CRAWLEY, J.N. 1995. Biological actions of galanin. Regul. Pept. **59:** 1–16.
6. KASK, K., M. BERTHOLD & T. BARTFAI. 1997. Galanin receptors: Involvement in feeding, pain, depression and Alzheimer's disease. Life Sci. **60:** 1523–1533.
7. KASH, K., Ü. LANGEL & T. BARTFAI. 1995. Galanin: A neuropeptide with inhibitory actions. Cell. Mol. Neurobiol. **15:** 653–673.
8. PARSONS, R.L., D.S. NEEL, L.M. KONOPKA & T.W. McKEON. 1989. The presence and possible role of a galanin-like peptide in the mudpuppy heart. Neuroscience **29:** 749–759.
9. McKEON, T.W., R.E. CARRAWAY, L.M. KONOPKA & R.L. PARSONS. 1990. Distribution of galanin-like peptide in various tissues of Necturus maculosus. Cell Tiss. Res. **262:** 461–466.
10. McKEON, T.W. & R.L. PARSONS. 1990. Galanin immunoreactivity in the mudpuppy cardiac ganglion. J. Auton. Nerv. Syst. **31:** 135–140.
11. KONOPKA, L.M., T.W. McKEON, L.A. MERRIAM, J.C. HARDWICK & R.L. PARSONS. 1991. Galanin in a parasympathetic ganglion. *In* Galanin: A new multifunctional peptide in the neuroendocrine system. T. Hökfeld & T. Bartfai, Eds. :261–274, Macmillan Press, New York.
12. PARSONS, R.L. & L.A. MERRIAM. 1993. Galanin activates an inwardly rectifying potassium conductance in mudpuppy atrial muscles. Pflügers Arch. **422:** 410–412.
13. AXELSSON, M. & S. NILSSON. 1985. Control of the heart in the mudpuppy, *Necturus maculosus.* Exp. Biol. **44:** 229–239.
14. KONOPKA, L.M., T.W. McKEON & R.L. PARSONS. 1989. Galanin-induced hyperpolarization and decreased membrane excitability of neurones in mudpuppy cardiac ganglia. J. Physiol. **410:** 107–122.
15. KONOPKA, L.M. & R.L. PARSONS. 1989. Characteristics of the galanin-induced depolarization of mudpuppy parasympathetic postganglionic neurons. Neurosci. Lett. **99:** 142–146.
16. PARSONS, R.L. & L.M. KONOPKA. 1990. Galanin-induced hyperpolarization of mudpuppy neurons is calcium dependent. Neurosci. Lett. **115:** 207–212.
17. KONOPKA, L.M., L.A. MERRIAM, J.C. HARDWICK & R.L. PARSONS. 1992. Aminergic and peptidergic elements in a cardiac parasympathetic ganglion. Can. J. Physiol. Pharmacol. **70:** S32–S43.
18. NAKAJIMA, T., H. INISAWA & W. GILES. 1990. *N*-ethlmaleimide uncouples muscarinic receptors from acetylcholine-sensitive potassium channels in bullfrog atrium. J. Gen. Physiol. **96:** 887–903.
19. SHAPIRO, M.S., L. P. WOLLMUTH & B. HILLE. 1994. Modulation of Ca^{++} channels by PTX-sensitive G-proteins is blocked by *N*-ethylmaleimide in rat sympathetic neurons. J. Neurosci. **14:** 7109–7116.
20. PARSONS, R.L. & L.A. MERRIAM. 1992. Galanin and bethanechol appear to activate the same inwardly rectifying potassium current in mudpuppy parasympathetic neurons. Neurosci. Lett. **140:** 33–36.
21. PARSONS, R.L. & L.M. KONOPKA. 1991. Analysis of the galanin-induced decrease in membrane excitability in mudpuppy parasympathetic neurons. Neuroscience **43:** 647–660.
22. PAPAS, S. & C.W. BOURQUE. 1997. Galanin inhibits continuous and phasic firing in rat hypothalamic magnocellular neurosecretory cells. J. Neurosci. **17:** 6048–6056.
23. PIERIBONE, V.A., Z.-Q. XU, X. ZHANG, S. GRILLNER, T. BARTFAI & T. HÖKFELT. 1995. Galanin induces a hyperpolarization of norepinephrine-containing locus coeruleus neurons in the brainstem slice. Neuroscience **64:** 861–874.

24. TAMURA, K., J.M. PALMER, C.K. WINKELMANN & J.D. WOOD. 1988. Mechanism of action of galanin on myenteric neurons. J. Neurophysiol. **60:** 966–979.
25. MULVANEY, J.M., L.A. MERRIAM & R.L. PARSONS. 1995. Galantide distinguishes putative subtypes of galanin receptors in mudpuppy parasympathetic neurons. Eur. J. Pharmacol. **287:** 97–100.
26. HARDWICK, J.C. & R.L. PARSONS. 1992. Galanin stimulates phosphatidylinositol turnover in cardiac tissue of the mudpuppy. J. Auton. Nerv. Syst. **40:** 87–90.
27. BARTFAI, T., K. BEDECS, T. LAND, Ü. LANGEL, R. BERTORELLI, P. GRIOTTI, S. CONSOLO, X. XU, Z. WEISENFELD-HALLIN, S. NILSSON, V.A. PIERBONE, & T. HÖKFELT. 1991. M-15: High-affinity chimeric peptide that blocks the neruonal actions of galanin in the hippocampus, locus coeruleus, and spinal cord. Proc. Natl. Acad. Sci. USA **88:** 10961–10965
28. BARTFAI, T., Ü. LANGEL, K. BEDECS, S. ANDELL, T. LAND, S. GREGERSEN, B. AHRÉN, P. GIROTTI, S. CONSOLO, R. CORWIN, J. CRAWLEY, X. XU, Z. WEISENFELD-HALLIN & T. HÖKFELT. 1993. Galanin-receptor ligand M40 peptide distinguishes between putative galanin-receptor subtypes. Proc. Natl. Acad. Sci. USA **90:** 11287–11291.
29. HOMAIDAN, F.R., G.W.G. SHARP & L.M. NOWAK. 1991. Galanin inhibits a dihydropyridine-sensitive Ca^{2+} current in the RINm5f cell line. Proc. Natl. Acad. Sci. USA **88:** 8744–8748.
30. MERRIAM, L.A. & R.L. PARSONS. 1995. Neuropeptide galanin inhibits (ω-conotoxin GVIA-sensitive calcium channels in parasympathetic neurons. J. Neurophysiol. **73:** 1374–1382.
31. FISONE, G., M. BERTHOLD, K. BEDECS, A. UNDÉN, T. BARTFAI, R. BERTORELLI, S. CONSOLO, J. CRAWLEY, B. MARTIN, S. NILSSON & T. HÖKFELT. 1989. N-terminal galanin-(1-16) fragment is an agonist at the hippocampal galanin receptor. Proc. Natl. Acad. Sci. USA **86:** 9588–9591.
32. HABERT-ORTOLI, E., B. AMIRANOFF, I. LOQUET, M. LABURTHE & J.–F. MAYAUX. 1994. Molecular cloning of a functional human galanin receptor. Proc. Natl. Acad. Sci. USA. **91:** 9780–9783.
33. HOWARD, A.D., C. TAN, L.-L. SHIAO, O.C. PALYHA, K. KULJU MCKEE, D.H. WEINBERG, S.D. FEIGHNER, M.A. CASCIERI, R.G. SMITH, L.H. T. VAN DER PLOEG & K.A. SULLIVAN. 1997. Molecular cloning and characterization of a new receptor for galanin. FEBS Lett. **405:** 285–290.
34. WANG, S., T. HASHEMI, C. HE, C. STRADER & M. BAYNE. 1997. Molecular cloning and pharmacological characterization of a new galanin receptor subtype. Mol. Pharmacol. 1997 **52:** 337–343.

Cardiovascular Actions of Galanin[a]

ERICA POTTER[b]

*Prince of Wales Medical Research Institute, Prince of Wales Hospital,
High Street, Randwick, 2031 Australia*

In the dog, attenuation of the slowing of the heart evoked by vagal stimulation following stimulation of the cardiac sympathetic nerve has been attributed to inhibition of acetylcholine release by neuropeptide Y (NPY) released from sympathetic nerves.[1,2] NPY was identified as a sympathetic cotransmitter in 1982[3] and seemed an obvious candidate for this effect which has a long duration of action, lasting many minutes beyond the effects of noradrenaline. The attenuation of cardiac vagal action also survives α- and β-adrenoceptor blockade, suggesting a neurotransmitter other than noradrenaline. However, since 1982, other neuropeptides have been identified in sympathetic nerves, and their role as modulators of autonomic neurotransmission has been systematically investigated. One of these, galanin (GAL), a 29 amino acid peptide (30 in humans), has been identified in sympathetic nerves in the cat[4] and dog.[5] In the Australian marsupial *Trichosurus vulpecula*, the thoracic sympathetic ganglia contain GAL but not NPY colocalized with noradrenaline.[6] We have examined a possible role for GAL as a modulator of autonomic neurotransmission in several species, including the cat, dog, and Australian possum, *Trichosurus vulpecula*.

All animals were anesthetized with pentobarbitone sodium (Nembutal; Abbott Laboratories, Sydney; 30 mg/kg). Anesthesia was induced in possums by intramuscular injection of ketamine (Ketavet; Delta Veterinary Laboratories, Australia; 70 mg/kg) and xylazine (Rompun; Bayer; 10 mg/kg). All experiments were approved by the Institutional Animal Care and Ethics Committee and with the appropriate licences. All animals were artificially ventilated and held at constant temperature. Blood pressure and beat by beat pulse interval (PI, time between each heart beat) were measured. Both vagus nerves were cut and the right vagus stimulated supramaximally (1 ms, ≈ 4 Hz). The frequency of stimulation was chosen to increase pulse interval 100–300 ms, a submaximal effect for vagal slowing. The stellate ganglion was identified after dissection which allowed forward reflection of the foreleg and removal of the second rib. The cardiac sympathetic nerve was identified by acceleration of the heart when stimulated electrically. The sympathetic nerve was stimulated supramaximally at high frequency (16–20 Hz) for 2–3 minutes.

In the cat, as in the dog, stimulation of the cardiac sympathetic nerve evokes a prolonged attenuation of cardiac vagal action in the presence of effective β-adrenoceptor blockade. FIGURE 1 is a polygraph record taken from an experiment on one anesthetized cat in which prolonged attenuation of cardiac vagal action is clearly seen following sympathetic stimulation.

In a group of cats the magnitude of the attenuation of cardiac vagal action following sympathetic stimulation was 41 ± 5%, and the time to half recovery of this effect was 8 ± 1.5 min[7] ($n = 6$). As in the dog, guanethidine abolished the inhibitory effect following

[a]This work was supported by the National Health and Medical Research Council of Australia and the National Heart Foundation of Australia.

[b]Phone, 61 2 9382 2683; fax, 61 2 93822722; e-mail, e.potter@unsw.edu.au

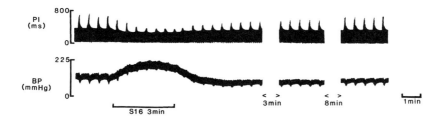

FIGURE 1. Record of pulse interval (PI) and blood pressure (BP) from an anesthetized cat, showing the effects of stimulation of the cardiac sympathetic nerve. An increase in PI was evoked every 30 seconds by stimulating the peripheral cut end of the right vagus. Sympathetic stimulation caused long-lasting inhibition of vagal effects on PI.

sympathetic stimulation, suggesting that the effect was mediated by a sympathetic cotransmitter.

Intravenous injection of GAL (1.6–3.1 nmol/kg) mimics the effect of sympathetic stimulation and an example from one cat is shown in FIGURE 2.

In the group of cats the maximum percentage of inhibition of cardiac vagal action following injection of GAL was 41 ± 8% with a time to half recovery of 14 ± 3 minutes ($n = 9$). Intravenous injection of GAL evoked a decrease in BP of 10 ± 2 mm Hg, and this depressor effect returned to control levels in 8 minutes.[7] The sequence of cat GAL is not known, but GAL from several species has similar depressor effects. In a second study in cats, porcine GAL showed a significantly greater depressor effect than did rat or human GAL; 24 ± 3, 17 ± 3.5, and 12 ± 2 mm Hg, respectively. Recovery time was 3 ± 1, 6 ± 1, and 4 ± 0.5 minutes, respectively.[8] In the cat, NPY does not cause attenuation of cardiac vagal action as it does in the dog, but it does increase blood pressure. In the dog, GAL does not attenuate cardiac vagal action, but it does have a transient depressor response of 9 ± 4 mm Hg for 2 minutes for porcine GAL.

In the possum, the magnitude of the attenuation of cardiac vagal activity following stimulation of the cardiac sympathetic nerve is 31 ± 10% with a time to half recovery of 5 ± 1 minute ($n = 8$). Following exogenous GAL the magnitude of the response was

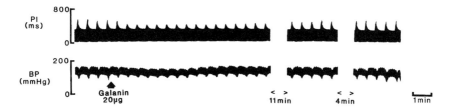

FIGURE 2. Record of pulse interval (PI) and blood pressure (BP) from an anesthetized cat. An increase in PI was evoked every 30 seconds by stimulating the peripheral cut end of the right vagus. Intravenous injection of galanin evoked long-lasting inhibition of cardiac vagal action. Galanin also had a slight depressor action.

$41 \pm 4\%$ with a time to half recovery of 13 minutes. GAL evoked a pressor response of 57 ± 5 mm Hg. NPY had no effect on cardiac vagal action.[9]

Both the cat and the dog have NPY, GAL, and noradrenaline colocalized in sympathetic nerves. In the cat, GAL not NPY mimics the attenuation of cardiac vagal action following sympathetic stimulation, whereas in the dog it is NPY not GAL that mimics the effect of sympathetic stimulation. In the possum, the sympathetic nerves contain GAL but not NPY, and consistent with this it is GAL, not NPY, that mimics the effect of sympathetic stimulation.

Many GAL antagonists are now available. These are chimeric molecules of GAL and can help define a physiological role for GAL.[10,11] We have used three of these chimeric GAL antagonists to look at the role of GAL in the cardiovascular system. We and others have shown that the N-terminal of GAL is important for recognition of its receptor and subsequent biological action.[12,13] The chimeric antagonists have the N-terminal of GAL (usually GAL 1-13) linked to the C-terminal of other molecules. Galantide or M15 con-

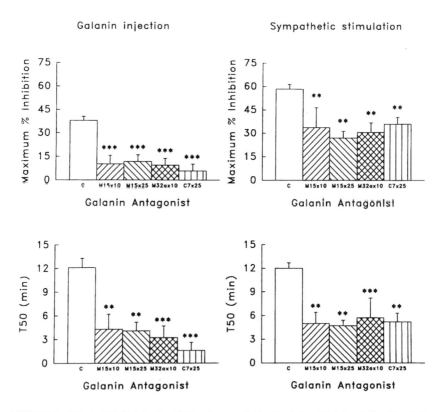

FIGURE 3. Effects of GAL injection (*left*) and sympathetic stimulation (*right*) and after the administration of the GAL antagonists M15, M32a, and C7 in ×10 or ×25 the molar dose of GAL. *Top graphs* show maximum % inhibition of cardiac vagal action and the *bottom graphs* show the time to half recovery (** $p < 0.01$, *** $p < 0.001$).

sists of GAL 1–13 + substance P 5–11; C7 consists of GAL 1–13 + spantide (the substance P antagonist); M32a consists of GAL 1–13 + NPY 24–36. Pretreatment with each of these chimeric peptides has shown that the attenuation of cardiac vagal action following sympathetic stimulation or exogenous GAL is significantly reduced in both magnitude and duration. These effects are summarized in FIGURE 3.

Interestingly, none of the chimeric antagonists had any effect on the decrease in blood pressure evoked by intravenous injection of GAL.[14] The chimeric antagonist M15 did not modify the cardiac vagal inhibitory effects following sympathetic stimulation in the dog.[15]

GAL appears to have powerful modulating actions on the cardiovascular system which are species specific. In the cat and possum it is proposed that GAL released from sympathetic nerves inhibits subsequent cardiac vagal action. In a study on human subjects, intravenous injection of human GAL decreased sinus arrhythmia, an effect consistent with inhibition of vagal activity.[16] The doses used in this study did not affect blood pressure. In the cat, however, GAL significantly decreased blood pressure. The vagus nerves and right sympathetic nerve were cut in the animal studies, thus removing the major baroreceptor pathways, possibly unmasking a depressor effect on blood pressure which would have been buffered in the human study.

Three GAL receptors have now been cloned. One of these, GalR3, shows significant peripheral expression particularly in the heart.[13] This receptor may mediate the inhibitory effects of GAL on cardiac vagal action following sympathetic stimulation. However, our studies suggest that there should be a second peripheral GAL receptor, on blood vessels, which mediates the depressor effects of GAL. In the studies using the chimeric antagonists the depressor action of galanin was not modified by any of the antagonists, even when large doses were used.

The studies described here demonstrate that GAL has powerful actions in the cardiovascular system. It is suggested that GAL released from sympathetic nerves in the cat, possum, and possibly human subjects inhibits acetylcholine release and subsequent slowing of the heart mediated by the GalR3 receptor. We also suggest that GAL has a direct vasodilator action mediated by a possible GalR4 receptor.

ACKNOWLEDGMENTS

The help of my colleagues, Maureen Revington, Lesley Ulman, Gillian Courtice, and Ian McCloskey, is acknowledged.

REFERENCES

1. POTTER, E.K. 1985. Prolonged non-adrenergic inhibition of cardiac vagal action following sympathetic stimulation. Neurosci. Lett. **54:** 117–121.
2. POTTER, E.K. 1987. Presynaptic inhibition of cardiac vagal postganglionic nerves by neuropeptide Y. Neurosci. Lett. **83:** 101–106.
3. TATEMOTO, K. 1982. Neuropeptide Y: The complete amino acid sequence of the brain peptide. Proc. Natl. Acad.Sci. USA **79:** 5485–5489.
4. KUMMER, W. 1987. Galanin- and neuropeptide Y-like immunoreactivities coexist in paravertebral sympathetic neurones of the cat. Neurosci. Lett. **78:** 127–131.
5. MORIARTY, M., I.L. GIBBINS, E.K. POTTER & D.I. MCCLOSKEY. 1992. Comparison of the inhibitory roles of neuropeptide Y and galanin on cardiac vagal action in the dog. Neurosci. Lett. **136:** 275–279.

6. MORRIS,J.L., I.L. GIBBINS & R. MURPHY. 1986. Neuropeptide Y-like immunoreactivity is absent from most perivascular noradrenergic axons in a marsupial, the brush-tailed possum. Neurosci. Lett. **71:** 264–270.

7. REVINGTON, M.L., E.K. POTTER & D.I. MCCLOSKEY. 1990. Prolonged inhibition of cardiac vagal action following sympathetic stimulation and galanin in anaesthetised cats. J. Physiol. **431:** 495–503.

8. ULMAN. L.G., H.F. EVANS, T.P. IISMAA, E.K. POTTER, D.I. MCCLOSKEY & J. SHINE. 1992. Effects of human, rat and porcine galanins on cardiac vagal action and blood pressure in the anaesthetised cat. Neurosci. Lett. **136:** 105–108.

9. COURTICE, G.P., E.K. POTTER & D.I. MCCLOSKEY. 1993. Inhibition of cardiac vagal action by galanin but not neuropeptide Y in the brush tailed possum *Trichosurus vulpecula*. J. Physiol. **461:** 379–386.

10. LINDSKOG, S., B. AHRÉN, T. LAND, U. LANGEL & T. BARTFAI. 1992. The novel high affinity antagonist galantide blocks the galanin mediated inhibition of glucose-induced insulin secretion. Eur. J. Pharmacol. **210:** 183–188.

11. CRAWLEY, J.N., J.K. ROBINSON, U. LANGEL & T. BARTFAI. 1993. Galanin receptor antagonists M40 and C7 block galanin induced feeding. Brain Res. **600:** 268–272.

12. ULMAN, L.G., E.K. POTTER & D.I. MCCLOSKEY. 1993. The effects of galanin and galanin fragments on cardiac vagal action and blood pressure in the anaesthetised cat. Reg. Pept. **44:** 85–92.

13. WANG, S., C. HE, T. HASHEMI & M. BAYNE. 1997. Cloning and expressional characterisation of a novel galanin receptor. Identification of different pharmacophores within galanin for the three galanin receptor subtypes. J. Biol. Chem. **272:** 31949–31952.

14. ULMAN, L.G., E.K. POTTER & D.I. MCCLOSKEY. 1994. Functional effects of a family of galanin antagonists on the cardiovascular system in anaesthetised cats. Reg. Pept. **51:** 17–23.

15. ULMAN, L.G., M. MORIARTY, E.K. POTTER & D.I. MCCLOSKEY. 1993. Galanin antagonist effects on cardiac vagal inhibitory actions of sympathetic stimulation in anaesthetised cats and dogs. J. Physiol. **464:** 491–499.

16. CAREY, D.G., T.P. IISMAA, K.Y. HO, I.A. RAJKOVIC, J. KELLY, E.W. KRAEGEN, J. FERGUSON, A.S. INGLIS, J. SHINE & D.J. CHISHOLM. 1993. Potent effects of human galanin in man: Growth hormone secretion and vagal blockade. J. Clin. Endocrinol. Metab. **77:** 90–93.

LHRH and Sexual Dimorphism

ISTVAN MERCHENTHALER[a]

Women's Health Research Institute, Wyeth-Ayerst Research, Radnor, Pennsylvania 19087, USA

ABSTRACT: An increasing amount of evidences suggests that galanin plays an important role in the regulation of reproduction in the rat. Galanin is colocalized with luteinizing hormone–releasing hormone (LHRH) in a subset of LHRH neurons, and the pattern of coexpression is sexually dimorphic, with a higher incidence of colocalization and level of galanin mRNA and peptide expression in females than in males. Therefore, the role of galanin may be unique to females, as are the LH surge and ovulation. The colocalization of LHRH and galanin is neonatally determined by an epigenetic mechanism involving the testis, whereas the expression of galanin in adult LHRH neurons is upregulated by estrogen and modulated by progesterone. The action of these sex steroids requires intact neurotransmission towards LHRH neurons, indicating that their action is mediated by interneurons.

Sex differences in the control of gonadotropin secretion and reproductive functions are a distinct characteristic in all mammalian species. Ovulation and cyclicity are among the most distinct neuroendocrine markers of female brain differentiation, along with sex behavioral traits that are also evident in different species. The luteinizing hormone–releasing hormone (LHRH), also called gonadotropin-releasing hormone (GnRH), neuronal system is the primary regulator of neuroendocrine events leading to ovulation and hormonal changes during the menstrual cycle in primates and the estrous cycle in rodents. Therefore, the LHRH neuronal system is the potential site where many of these sex differences are expressed or integrated.

Until 1989, LHRH was considered a unique peptide in that it did not colocalize with any other neuropeptides or neurotransmitters. In 1989, Charnay *et al.*[1] reported that delta sleep-inducing peptide (DSIP), a peptide isolated from rabbit plasma during sleep, was colocalized with LHRH in the rat brain. A year later, our group[2] and Coen *et al.*[3] reported that galanin (GAL) is also colocalized with LHRH in a subset of LHRH neurons. The brain area in which the LHRH/GAL neurons are present is restricted to a small region around the organum vasculosum of the lamina terminalis (OVLT), which includes portions of the diagonal band of Broca and the medial preoptic area. Neurons that are immunoreactive only for GAL, not for LHRH, occupy a similar area; however, they are larger, multipolar neurons compared to the smaller, fusiform LHRH/GAL immunoreactive (IR) cells (Figs. 1–3). The colocalization of LHRH and GAL was later confirmed at the mRNA level with double label *in situ* hybridization histochemical studies.[4,5–7,8–10] This paper summarizes data on the colocalization of GAL and LHRH in rats, describes the effect of sex steroids on the incidence of colocalization of these two peptides, and summarizes the potential role of GAL colocalization with LHRH.

[a]Address for correspondence: Istvan Merchenthaler, MD, DSc, Women's Health Research Institute, Wyeth-Ayerst Research, 145 King of Prussia Road, Radnor, PA 19087. Phone, 610/341-2791; fax, 610/989-4832; e-mail, merchei@war.wyeth.com

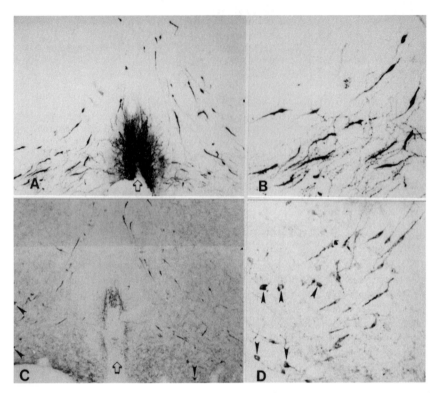

FIGURE 1. LHRH-IR **(A,B)** and galanin-IR **(C,D)** perikarya in the vertical limb of the diagonal band of Broca, around the organum vasculosum of the lamina terminalis (*open arrows*) with lower **(A,C)** and higher **(B,D)** magnifications. The LHRH IR neurons are fusiform **(B)** and arranged in a tent-like manner **(A)**. In the brain of a female rat, the majority of galanin-IR neurons are also fusiform (LHRH-like); however, some of them are larger and located more laterally and closer to the basal surface of the brain (*arrowheads*). The LHRH-like shape of galanin-IR perikarya suggests that the two peptides are colocalized in these neurons.

REGULATION OF GALANIN EXPRESSION WITHIN LHRH NEURONS DURING THE ESTROUS CYCLE: LIGHT MICROSCOPIC IMMUNOCYTOCHEMICAL AND *IN SITU* HYBRIDIZATION HISTOCHEMICAL OBSERVATIONS

Estrogen has a profound effect on GAL gene expression in the pituitary and, to a lesser extent, the hypothalamus.[11,12] The studies aimed at verifying the effect of estrogen on the colocalization of GAL and LHRH utilized (1) cycling female rats, sacrificed on different days of the estrous cycle and (2) ovariectomized animals treated with vehicle or estrogen. The data were compared to results obtained from male rats. During the estrous cycle, the highest number of cells colocalizing GAL and LHRH can be seen in estrus, when approximately 85% of LHRH neurons contain GAL.[13] The number of LHRH/GAL-IR cells is about five times higher in estrous female than in male animals. The incidence of colocal-

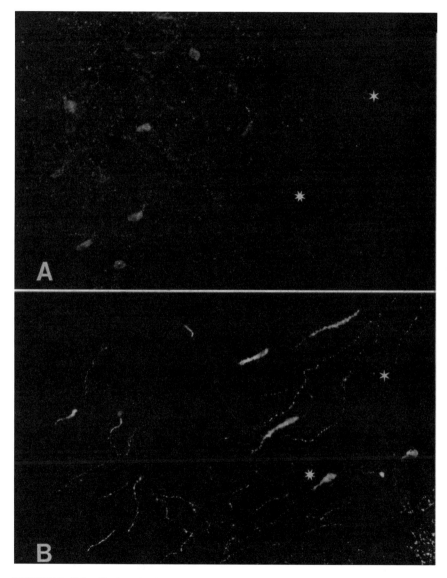

FIGURE 2. Colocalization of galanin (**A**) and LHRH (**B**) with double-labeling immunocytochemistry. In this section of a male rat, none of the cells colocalizes both peptides. Galanin-IR perikarya are round and located more laterally than the smaller, fusiform LHRH-IR cells. *Stars* and *asterisks* label identical vessels.

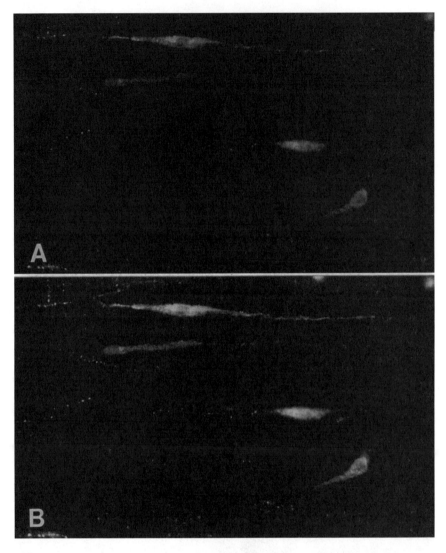

FIGURE 3. Colocalization of galanin (**A**) and LHRH (**B**) with double-labeling immunocytochemistry, utilizing fluorescent dye-labeled secondary antibodies (Texas red vs FITC) raised in two different species. In this section of a female rat, each LHRH perikaryon is immunoreactive for galanin.

ization is slightly lower during diestrus and proestrus compared with the high degree of colocalization in estrus. Interestingly, although the number of colocalizing neurons changes during the cycle, the number of LHRH-IR neurons remains unchanged.[13] These observations correlate well with the levels of GAL in the hypophysial portal blood, that is, these levels are the highest in estrus.[14] In addition to the changes in GAL peptide levels detected by immunocytochemistry and radioimmunoassay during the estrous cycle, similar changes were also noted within individual LHRH neurons at the mRNA level. Between 1200 and 1800 hours of estrus, a large increase in GAL mRNA can be detected with *in situ* hybridization histochemistry.[7] The levels of GAL mRNA in LHRH neurons remain elevated until 1800 hours of estrus, after which they return to nadir levels within 42 hours after the proestrous rise (1,000 hours on diestrus). Although these changes occur only in LHRH/GAL colocalizing cells, no changes in GAL mRNA levels can be seen in neurons that express galanin alone.[7] Interestingly, the group which reported the changes in galanin mRNA levels seen during the estrous cycle did not report accompanying changes in LHRH mRNA levels within individual LHRH/GAL coexpressing cells.[7] Others,[15–18] however, did measure an elevation in cellular LHRH mRNA levels during late proestrus. The observations of these immunocytochemical and *in situ* hybridization experiments suggest that the cosynthesis of GAL in LHRH-IR cells in intact female rats is estrogen dependent.

COLOCALIZATION OF LHRH AND GALANIN AT SUBMICROSCOPIC LEVEL: REGULATION BY ESTROGEN

LHRH- and GAL-IR axons overlap heavily in the lateral part of the median eminence, suggesting that the two peptides are also colocalized in the nerve terminals. Our electron microscopic immunocytochemical studies, utilizing dual colloidal gold immunolabeling, showed that LHRH and GAL are located in the same secretory vesicles (FIG. 4). The incidence of colocalization in the vesicles is high in the female (45%) and low in the male (3%) rat. Ovariectomy results in a dramatic decline in the numbers of LHRH/GAL coexpressing vesicles (23%) which was reversed by administration of estradiol (55%).[19] The extremely low rate of LHRH vesicles carrying GAL in the male (3%) indicates modest expression of the GAL gene and suggests that the synchrony of GAL and LHRH discharge is probably not a crucial mechanism in the maintenance of gonadotroph cell functions. With almost half the LHRH vesicles containing GAL in the female, the co-released GAL appears uniquely poised to potentiate the effect of LHRH. These observations indicate a sex-related difference in the synthesis and packaging of LHRH and GAL and suggest that the events are estrogen dependent.

The implication of this coexistence is that the LHRH and GAL prohormones are synthesized synchronously and undergo a similar sorting process that finally results in packaging of the structurally distinct peptides into the same neurosecretory vesicles. The processing of LHRH seems to be completed in the neurosecretory vesicles,[20] whereas the route of GAL maturation awaits elucidation. The assumption that the two peptides are co-released from the hybrid vesicles has been substantiated by our recent demonstration of a pulsatile secretory pattern of GAL with coincident LHRH pulse episodes.[14] Furthermore, the simultaneous release of GAL and LHRH from the colocalizing vesicles provides a mechanism whereby GAL may potentiate the effect of LHRH in the anterior pituitary (see below).

IS GALANIN A MARKER FOR SEXUAL DIMORPHISM?

The sexual differentiation of the brain is thought to be inherently female unless male determining signals, androgens, are present during the critical period of brain develop-

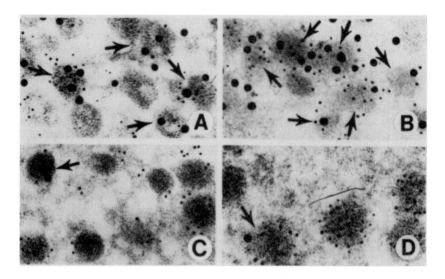

FIGURE 4. Colocalization of LHRH (labeled with 5 nm colloidal gold particles) and galanin (labeled with 15 nm gold particles) in nerve terminals of the median eminence in the male (**A**), female (**B**), ovariectomized (**C**), and ovariectomized-estrogen-treated (**D**) rat. *Arrows* point to secretory granules where both peptides are present. (Magnification: ×150,000.)

ment. The assumption that female sexual differentiation in the rat brain would proceed in the absence of gonadal steroids is based on the early observations that ovariectomy of newborn female rats did not interfere with female differentiation of the brain.[21-23] According to the classic "androgen theory," the organizational effect of androgens is believed to be mediated by intracellular conversion of androgens in certain brain areas to estrogens.[24] Sexual differentiation of the brain is mediated by the epigenetic action of gonadal steroids during the critical period of development (last few days of neonatal and first 5–8 days of postnatal life in rodents). When adult, orchidectomized animals are treated with estradiol, the number of LHRH/GAL colocalizing neurons remains low.[13] Interestingly, however, when neonatally gonadectomized male rats are treated with estrogen or testosterone in their adult life, the number of colocalizing neurons almost reaches the level seen in female rats.[15,26] These observations indicate that estrogen and/or testosterone, when present during the time of imprinting (critical period), is capable of suppressing GAL gene expression throughout the life of the animal. When neonatal male rats are orchidectomized, their LHRH neurons are not masculinized, but remain feminized, and when they are exposed to estrogen in adulthood, they synthesize GAL. The significance of these findings is that they clearly show that although one phenotype of the LHRH neurons, that is, their number, and the level of LHRH expression are not sexually dimorphic, the other phenotype, that is, GAL expression, is sexually dimorphic. In addition, these observations clearly demonstrate that different subpopulations of LHRH neurons exist in the rat hypothalamus. A small population of LHRH neurons (5–10%) express GAL in both sexes which is estrogen independent. Another small population of LHRH neurons do not express GAL under any steroidal condition. The third and largest group of LHRH neurons responds to estrogen and express GAL. Although it is not known how LHRH neurons in the third group acquire the potential to respond to estrogen by expressing GAL, it is clear that the absence of androgenic imprinting during the critical period of differentiation provides a permissive environment for them to retain estrogen responsiveness in adulthood. The colocalization of LHRH and GAL as an indicator of sexual dimorphism provides an example of the interdependence of "organizational" and "activational" effects of hormones.[27]

Although only a few, if any, LHRH neurons contain estrogen receptors,[28] they are sensitive to changes in estradiol levels during the critical period of brain differentiation and in adulthood. It is possible that estrogen receptors within LHRH neurons, similar to those in the cerebral cortex,[29] are expressed only transitionally during the perinatal period, or the actions of estrogens are mediated through complex connections among LHRH neurons and other peptidergic or aminergic neuronal systems. However, similar to other peptidergic neurons in the hypothalamus, estradiol may exert membrane effects on LHRH neurons which may lead to changes in membrane conductivity, the activation of second messenger systems, and the like, resulting in changes in LHRH synthesis and secretion (for a review see ref. 30).

PHYSIOLOGIC SIGNIFICANCE OF COLOCALIZATION OF LHRH WITH GALANIN

Colocalization of neurotransmitters, including neuropeptides, within the same neurons in certain areas of the central and peripheral nervous systems appears now to be the rule rather than the exception.[31] Galanin is one of the most frequently detected peptides which is colocalized with other neurotransmitter/neuromodulators. In this sense, GAL has been colocalized with catecholamines and several neurotransmitter-related enzymes such as choline acetyltransferase, glutamic acid decarboxylase, and tyrosine hydroxylase as well as with several neuropeptides (for a review see ref. 32). To establish the functional significance of coexistence it is necessary: (1) to demonstrate that the coexisting molecules are actually released; (2) to show that receptors for both molecules are present on target tissues; (3) to demonstrate that target tissues respond to both transmitters under physiologic conditions, and (4) to determine that the combined effect of both transmitters results in a modified physiologic effect. In the case of GAL and LHRH as colocalized transmitters, it was shown that: (1) both peptides are released into the hypophysial portal blood;[2,32–34] (2) LHRH receptors and GAL receptors are present in the anterior pituitary (LHRH-receptors in gonadotroph cells[25,26] while galanin receptors in as yet unidentified anterior pituitary cells);[26] (3) LH release is stimulated by both LHRH and GAL;[3,14] and (4) GAL potentiates the effect of LHRH from dispersed anterior pituitary cells in culture.[33,34] Galanin secreted into the hypophysial portal vasculature stimulates not only LH but also growth hormone and prolactin secretion (for a review see ref. 32). These effects are exerted at concentrations of GAL similar to those observed in portal blood,[14,22] suggesting that the actions of GAL at the pituitary level are mediated by specific GAL receptors. In fact, the cloning of pituitary[37] GAL receptors supports this hypothesis.

ROLE OF GALANIN IN THE GENERATION OF GONADOTROPIN SURGE: EFFECT OF ESTROGEN AND PROGESTERONE

The effects of estrogen and progesterone on GAL gene expression in LHRH neurons parallel the action of these steroids on the generation of an LH surge: estrogen induces the LH surge which is enhanced by progesterone, whereas progesterone itself is ineffective. More importantly, any conditions that lead to an LH surge also induce GAL gene expression in LHRH neurons, whereas conditions that block the LH surge prevent this induction.[5,8,10] For example, blockade of the LH surge by either pentobarbital, a specific α-adrenergic blocking agent, or an NMDA antagonist, prevents the induction of GAL gene expression in LHRH neurons, even in the presence of high levels of ovarian steroids.[10,16] The mechanism by which ovarian steroids act on LHRH/GAL neurons to activate the release of LHRH and GAL is unknown. Inasmuch as the LHRH neurons do not appear to contain steroid receptors,[28] it is likely that the neurons expressing the estrogen receptor act as transducers. These transducer neurons then transmit the steroid information to the LHRH/GAL neurons transynaptically. The observations that regardless of the nature of a stimulus, once the LHRH neurons are activated, the changes in GAL mRNA levels are strikingly higher than those of LHRH, suggest that GAL plays a pivotal role in the regulation of the activity of LHRH neurons. One of the most likely sites of GAL action is the median eminence where GAL, cosecreted into the hypophysial portal blood with LHRH, acts presynaptically on LHRH nerve terminals. The presence of GAL binding sites in the median eminence[39,40] and the fact that GAL stimulates LHRH release from hypothalamic fragments[33] and that pharmacologic blockade of GAL receptors in the hypothalamus inhibits LH secretion[41] support this notion. However, when GAL is colocalized with other neurotransmitters, such as with acetylcholine in the hippocampus,[42] it inhibits the release of acetylcholine. In cholinergic neurons, GAL appears to act in an autoinhibitory manner by imposing an ultrashort feedback restraint on acetylcholine release following a secretory burst. On the basis of the role of GAL in the cholinergic system in the hippocampus, Steiner's group[4,8,9] proposed an intriguing mechanism by which GAL regulates LHRH release in the median eminence. Although this proposal is attractive, it needs further experimental support. According to this group, GAL released from nerve terminals of LHRH/GAL neurons acts presynaptically and minimizes leakage of LHRH between large LHRH secretory bursts. As a result, the readily releasable stores of LHRH are augmented between pulses, so that LHRH output during the next secretory episode is maximal. This creates high amplitude LHRH pulses followed by a profound nadir as a reflection of the action of GAL on LHRH neurons. Thus, by shaping LHRH release into distinct, large amplitude pulses, GAL paradoxically increases the subsequent LH secretion. According to this hypothesis, without the presence of GAL in LHRH neurons, as seen during pregnancy, lactation, the prepubertal period, and aging when there is little demand for LH action, LHRH drains continuously in an unregulated, nonpulsatile fashion into the hypophysial portal circulation. On the contrary, during the proestrus LH surge, GAL acts not only by shaping LHRH in distinct pulses, but also possibly by amplifying the effects of LHRH postsynaptically, at the level of the gonadotrophs. The stimulatory action of GAL on LH secretion has been shown both under basal[33,34] and LHRH-induced conditions.[14] Because the intracellular levels of GAL mRNA within LHRH neurons and the number of LHRH/GAL-colocalizing neurons are higher in the adult female versus the male, this may be related to some unique function of GAL in LHRH neurons of female animals. As just mentioned, the ability of estrogen to generate an LH surge is sexually differentiated. Estrogen stimulates the preovulatory LHRH surge only in the female, and this mechanism may be based on the ability of estrogen to induce the expression of GAL in LHRH neurons.

THE ROLE OF CHRONICALLY ELEVATED LEVELS OF PROGESTERONE ON THE INCIDENCE OF COLOCALIZATION OF LHRH AND GALANIN

Although progesterone stimulates estrogen-induced GAL expression within LHRH neurons during the proestrous LH surge,[9,42] several observations indicated that chronically elevated levels of progesterone may blunt the stimulatory action of estrogen. This notion was first observed when ovariectomized rats were treated with estrogen or testosterone. Not only did these hormones restore the number of perikarya colocalizing LHRH and GAL, but also the number of colocalizing cells was slightly higher than that seen in cycling female rats. Moreover, estrogen increased the intensity of GAL immunostaining in colocalizing cells.[2] Because the number of "LHRH-like" galanin-IR perikarya was higher in ovariectomized estrogen-treated and prepubertal rats than in intact cycling animals, these observations raised the possibility that an ovarian factor(s) (e.g., progesterone) or a factor in the pituitary-gonadal axis (e.g., prolactin) is/are capable of blunting the effect of estrogen. The inhibitory effect of progesterone seemed to be supported by our recent observations in animals exhibiting high progesterone levels, such as pregnant and lactating[43] and aged rats.[44] In these models, the incidence of colocalization is low, almost undetectable. Although estrogen levels in some of these animals models is reduced (e.g., aging and lactation), estrogen administration to such animals does not result in elevation in the number of neurons colocalizing the two peptides. However, if these animals are ovariectomized, estradiol does increase the incidence of colocalization.[43,44] The blunting effect of lactation GAL gene expression in LHRH neurons, although not proven to be due to progesterone, has been confirmed at the mRNA level. A 60% reduction in signal (silver grains per cell) has been reported during lactation utilizing *in situ* hybridization histochemistry and autoradiography.[6]

Additional support for a potential blunting effect of progesterone on GAL expression in LHRH neurons derives from prepubertal animals. Before the twenty-fifth to thirtieth day of postnatal life, no "LHRH-like" galanin-IR perikarya can be seen. However, a few days before vaginal opening, the number of colocalizing cells dramatically increases and reaches a maximum at the time of first ovulation. The number of cells cosynthesizing these peptides at this age is higher than that seen in adult female rats. An even higher number can be seen in prepubertal animals that were treated with estradiol.[13] In the absence of corpora lutea, which are the major source of progesterone synthesis, progesterone levels are low in prepubertal animals. Thus, based on the observations that in aged, pregnant, and lactating animals the incidence of colocalization of LHRH and GAL is low, it seems likely that chronically elevated levels of progesterone blunt estradiol-induced GAL gene expression within LHRH neurons.

Although several of the studies just described suggested that chronically elevated progesterone levels may blunt the effect of estrogen in inducing GAL expression within LHRH neurons, our recent studies do not support this hypothesis. When ovariectomized rats were treated with estrogen or estrogen/progesterone, the combined treatment did not reduce the number of cells expressing both peptides.

As already mentioned, the levels of prolactin are also elevated in pregnant, lactating, and aged rats. However, our unpublished data do not support a blunting action of prolactin on the incidence of colocalization between LHRH and GAL. In female rats treated with haloperidol or domperidone, prolactin levels are elevated and yet the number of LHRH/ GAL colocalizing cells is similar to those seen in intact, cycling animals (Merchenthaler,

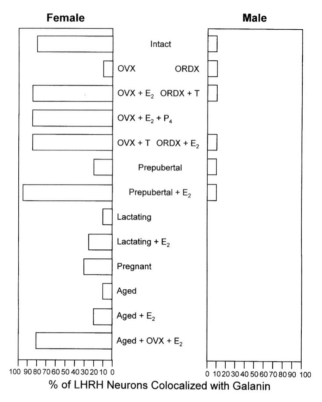

FIGURE 5. Effect of steroid milieu on the incidence of colocalization of LHRH and galanin in adult rats. For details, see text.

unpublished observations). FIGURES 5 and 6 summarize schematically the effect of endocrine milieu on the incidence of colocalization of GAL with LHRH in neonatally intact (FIG. 5) and manipulated (FIG. 6) animals.

CONCLUSIONS

The coexpression of GAL in a subset of LHRH neurons suggests that GAL may be essential for the activity of LHRH neurons and therefore for reproduction. The pattern of expression is sexually dimorphic, with much greater GAL expression in the LHRH neurons of females than of males, suggesting that GAL may be important in reproductive processes characteristic for the female, such as ovulation. The expression of GAL in LHRH neurons is regulated by sex steroids; estrogen supports the basal expression of GAL mRNA in LHRH neurons but also increases GAL gene expression in conjunction with progesterone during the estrous cycle. Because LHRH neurons do not seem to synthesize estrogen and progesterone receptors and the action of these steroid hormones requires an

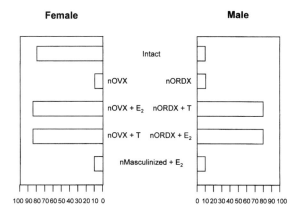

% of LHRH Neurons Colocalized with Galanin

FIGURE 6. Schematic representation of the effect of hormonal milieu on the incidence of colocalization of LHRH and galanin in rats that were manipulated neonatally.

intact synaptic transmission, it is likely that estrogen and progesterone act via interneurons on GAL gene expression in LHRH neurons. Although the current evidence collectively suggests that GAL gene expression within LHRH neurons represents a pivotal signal for activation of the entire reproductive axis, this notion is based on observations collected from only one species, the rat. Whether GAL plays a similar pivotal role or any role in humans remains to be established.

REFERENCES

1. CHARNAY, Y., C. BOURAS, P.G. VALLET, J. GOLAZ, R. GUNTERN & J. CONSTANTINIDIS. 1989. Immunohistochemical colocalization of delta sleep-inducing peptide and luteinizing hormone-releasing hormone in rabbit brain neurons. Neuroscience **31:** 495–505.
2. MERCHENTHALER, I., F.J. LÓPEZ & A. NEGRO-VILAR. 1990. Colocalization of galanin and luteinizing hormone-releasing hormone in a subset of preoptic hypothalamic neurons: Anatomical and functional correlates. Proc. Natl. Acad. Sci. USA **87:** 6326–6330.
3. COEN, C.W., C. MONTAGNESE & J.J. OPACKA. 1990. Coexistence of gonadotropin-releasing hormone and galanin: Immunohistochemical and functional studies. J. Neuroendocrinol. **2:** 107–111.
4. GRAFSTEIN-DUNN, E., D.K. CLIFTON & R.A. STEINER. 1994. Regulation of galanin and gonadotropin-releasing hormone gene expression in the hypothalamus and basal forebrain of the rat. Horm. Behav. **28:** 417–423.
5. MARKS, D.L., K.L. LENT, W.G. ROSSMANITH, D.K. CLIFTON & R.A. STEINER. 1994. Activation-dependent regulation of galanin gene expression in gonadotropin-releasing hormone neurons in the female rat. Endocrinology **134:** 1991–1998.
6. MARKS, D.L., M.S. SMITH, D.K. CLIFTON & R.A. STEINER. 1993. Regulation of GnRH and galanin gene expression in GnRH neurons during lactation in the rat. Endocrinology **133:** 1450–1458.

7. MARKS, D.L., M.S. SMITH, M. VRONTAKIS, D.K. CLIFTON & R.A. STEINER. 1993. Regulation of the galanin gene expression in gonadotropin-releasing hormone neurons during the estrous cycle of the rat. Endocrinology **132:** 1836–1844.
8. ROSSMANITH, W.G., D. L. MARKS, D.K. CLIFTON & R.A. STEINER. 1994. Induction of galanin gene expression in gonadotropin-releasing hormone neurons with puberty in the rat. Endocrinology **135:** 1401–1408.
9. ROSSMANITH, W.G., D.L. MARKS, D.K. CLIFTON & R.A. STEINER. 1996. Induction of galanin mRNA in GnRH neurons by estradiol and its facilitation by progesterone. J. Neuroendocrinol. **8:** 185–191.
10. ROSSMANITH, W.G., D.L. MARKS, R.A. STEINER & D.K. CLIFTON. 1996. Inhibition of steroid-induced galanin mRNA expression in GnRH neurons by specific NMDA-receptor blockade. J. Neuroendocrinol. **8:** 179–184.
11. KAPLAN, L.M., S.C. HOOI, D.R. ABRACZINSKAS, R.M. STRAUSS, M.B. DAVIDSON, D.W. HSU & J.I. KOENIG. 1990. Neuroendocrine Regulation of Galanin Gene Expression. Galanin: A Multifunctional Peptide in the Neuro-endocrine System. Macmillan Press. New York.
12. VRONTAKIS, M.E., L.M. PEDEN, M.L. DUCKWORTH & H.G. FRIESEN. 1987. Isolation and characterization of a complementary DNA (galanin) clone from estrogen-induced pituitary tumor messenger RNA. J. Biol. Chem. **262:** 16755–16758.
13. MERCHENTHALER, I., F.J. LÓPEZ, D.E. LENNARD & A. NEGRO-VILAR. 1991. Sexual differences in the distribution of neurons coexpressing galanin and luteinizing hormone-releasing hormone in the rat brain. Endocrinology **129:** 1977–1984.
14. LÓPEZ, F.J., I. MERCHENTHALER, M. CHING, M.G. WISNIEWSKI & A. NEGRO-VILAR. 1991. Galanin: A hypothalamic-hypophysiotrophic hormone modulating reproductive functions. Proc. Natl. Acad. Sci. USA **88:** 4508–4512.
15. PETERSON, S.L., S. MCCRONE, M. KELLER & E. GARDNER. 1991. Rapid increase in LHRH mRNA levels following NMDA. Endocrinology **129:** 1679–1681.
16. PETERSON, S.S., S. MCCRONE, M. KELLER & S. SHORES. 1995. Effects of estrogen and progesterone on luteinizing hormone-releasing hormone messenger ribonucleic acid levels: Consideration of temporal and neuroanatomical variables. Endocrinology **136:** 3604–3610.
17. ROBERTS, J.L., C.M. DUTLOW, M. JAKUBOWSKI, M. BLUM & R.P. MILLAR. 1989. Estradiol stimulates preoptic area-anterior hypothalamic proGnRH-GAP gene expression in ovariectomized rats. Brain Res. Mol. Brain Res. **6:** 127–134.
18. ROSIE, R., E. THOMPSON & G. FINK. 1990. Oestrogen positive feedback stimulates the synthesis of LHRH mRNA in neurons of the rostral diencephalon of the rat. J. Endocrinol. **124:** 285–289.
19. LIPOSITS, Z., J.J. REID, A. NEGRO-VILAR & I. MERCHENTHALER. 1995. Sexual dimorphism in copackaging of luteinizing hormone-releasing hormone and galanin into neurosecretory vesicles of hypophysiotropic neurons: Estrogen dependency. Endocrinology **136:** 1987–1992.
20. LIPOSITS, Z., I. MERCHENTHALER, W.C. WETSEL, J.J. REID, P.L. MELON, R.I. WEINER & A. NEGRO-VILAR. 1991. Morphological characteristics of immortalized hypothalamic neurons synthesizing luteinizing hormone-releasing hormone. Endocrinology **129:** 1575–1583.
21. DÖHLER, K.D. 1991. The pre- and postnatal influence of hormones and neurotransmitters on sexual differentiation of the mammalian hypothalamus. Int. Rev. Cytol. **131:** 1–57.
22. DE VRIES, G.J. 1990. Sex differences in neurotransmitter systems. J. Neuroendocrinol. **2:** 1–13.
23. RAISMAN, G. & P.M. FIELD. 1973. Sexual dimorphism in the neuropil of the preoptic area and its dependence on neonatal androgen. Brain Res. **54:** 1–29.
24. NAFTOLIN, F., K.J. RYAN, I.J. DAVIES, V.V. REDDY, F. FLORES, Z. PETRO & M. KUHN. 1975. The formation of estrogens by central neuroendocrine tissue. Recent Progress in Hormone Research. Academic Press. New York.
25. FINN, P.D., T.B. MCFALL, D.K. CLIFTON & R.A. STEINER. 1996. Sexual differentiation of galanin gene expression in gonadotropin-releasing hormone neurons. Endocrinology **137:** 4767–4772.
26. MERCHENTHALER, I., D.E. LENNARD, F.J. LÓPEZ & A. NEGRO-VILAR. 1993. Neonatal imprinting predetermines the sexually dimorphic, estrogen-dependent expression of galanin in luteinizing hormone-releasing hormone neurons. Proc. Natl. Acad. Sci. USA **90:** 10479–10483.
27. MCEWEN, B.S. 1991. Non-genomic and genomic effects of steroids on neural activity. Trends Neurosci. **12:** 141–147.

28. SHIVERS, B.D., R.E. HARLAN, J.I. MORRELL & D.W. PFAFF. 1983. Absence of oestradiol concentration in cell nuclei of LHRH immunoreactive neurons. Nature **304:** 345–347.

29. SHUGHRUE, P.J., W.E. STUMPF, N.J. MACLUSKY, J.E. ZIELINSKI & R.B. HOCHBERG. 1990. Developmental changes in estrogen receptors in mouse cerebral cortex between birth and postweaning: Studied by autoradiography with 11β-methoxy-16α-[^{125}I] iodoestradiol. Endocrinology **126:** 1112–1124.

30. BAULIEU, E.E. & P. ROBEL. 1995. Non-genomic mechanisms of action of steroid hormones. Ciba Found. Symp. **191:** 24–42.

31. HÖKFELT, T., Y. TSURUO, B. MEISTER, T. MELANDER, M. SCHALLING & B. EVERITT. 1987. Localization of nueroactive substances in the hypothalamus with special reference to coexistence of messenger molecules. Adv. Exp. Biol. **219:** 21–45.

32. MERCHENTHALER, I., F.J. LÓPEZ & A. NEGRO-VILAR. 1993. Anatomy and physiology of central galanin-containing pathways. Prog. Neurobiol. **40:** 711–769.

33. LÓPEZ, F.J., E.H. MEADE & A. NEGRO-VILAR. 1990. Development and characterization of a specific and sensitive radioimmunoassay for rat galanin: Measurement in rat brain tissue, hypophyseal portal and peripheral serum. Brain Res. Bull. **24:** 395–399.

34. LÓPEZ, F.J. & A. NEGRO-VILAR. 1990. Galanin stimulates luteinizing hormone-releasing hormone secretion from arcuate nucleus-median eminence fragments *in vitro*: Involvement of an alpha-adrenergic mechanism. Endocrinology **127:** 2431–2436.

35. CLAYTON, R.N. & K.J. KATT. 1981. Gonadotropin-releasing hormone receptors: Characterization, physiological regulation and relationship to reproductive function. Endocrinol. Rev. **2:** 186–209.

36. CONN, P.M., J. MARIAN, M. MCMILLIAN, J. STERN, D. ROGERS, M. HAMBY, A. PENNA & E. GRANT. 1981. Gonadotropin-releasing hormone action in the pituitary: A three step mechanism. Endocrinol. Rev. **2:** 174–185.

37. WYNICK, D., D.M. SMITH, M.A. GHATEI, K.O. AKINSANYA, R. BHOGAL, P. PURKISS, P. BYFIELD, N. YANAIHARA & S.R. BLOOM. 1993. Characterization of a high-affinity galanin receptor in the rat anterior pituitary. Proc. Natl. Acad. Sci. USA **90:** 4231–4235.

38. BRANN, D.W., L.P. CHORICH & V.B. MAHESH. 1993. Effect of progesterone on galanin mRNA levels in the hypothalamus and the pituitary: Correlation with the gonadatropin surge. Neuroendocrinology **58:** 531–538.

39. LAGNY-POURMIR, I. & I. EPELBAUM. 1992. Regional stimulatory and inhibitory effects of guanine nucleotides on [^{125}I]galanin binding in rat brain: Relationship with the rate of occupancy of galanin receptors by endogenous galanin. Neuroscience **49:** 829–847.

40. MELANDER, T., C. KOHLER, S. NILSSON, T. HOKFELT, E. BRODIN, E. THEODORSSON & T. BARTFAI. 1988. Autoradiographic quantitation and anatomical mapping of ^{125}I-galanin binding sites in the rat central nervous system. J. Chem. Neuroanat. **1:** 213–233.

41. SAHU, A., B. XU & S.P. KALRA. 1994. Role of galanin in stimulation of pituitary lutenizing hormone secretion as revealed by a specific receptor antagonist, galantide. Endocrinology **134:** 529–536.

42. FISONE, G., C.F. WU, S. CONSOLO, O. NORDSTROM, N. BRYNNE, T. BARTFAI, T. MELANDER & T. HOKFELT. 1987. Galanin inhibits acetylcholine release in the ventral hippocampus of the rat: Histochemical, autoradiographical, *in vivo* and *in vitro* studies. Proc. Natl. Acad. Sci. USA **84:** 7339–7343.

43. MERCHENTHALER, I. 1992. The expression of galanin in LHRH neurons is inhibited in pregnant and lactating rats. (Abstr.). 21st Annual Meeting of the Society for Neuroscience. 1086. Society for Neuroscience, Washington, DC.

44. CERESINI, G., A. MERCHENTHLAER, A. NEGRO-VILAR & I. MERCHENTHALER. 1994. Aging impairs galanin expression in luteinizing hormone-releasing hormone neurons: Effect of ovariectomy and /or estradiol treatment. Endocrinology **134:** 324–330.

Gonadal Steroid-Dependent GAL-IR Cells within the Medial Preoptic Nucleus (MPN) and the Stimulatory Effects of GAL within the MPN on Sexual Behaviors[a]

G.J. BLOCH,[b,c] P.C. BUTLER,[b] C.B. ECKERSELL,[d] AND R.H. MILLS[b]

[b]Department of Psychology, 1120 SWKT, Brigham Young University, Provo, Utah 84602, USA

[d]Department of Neurobiology, UCLA Center of Health Sciences, Los Angeles, California 90024, USA

ABSTRACT: More GAL-I cells exist within sexually dimorphic cell groups of the medial preoptic nucleus (MPN) in male rats than females, a large percentage of estrogen-concentrating cells within MPN cell groups are also GAL-immunoreactive (GAL-IR), and significantly more GAL-IR cells are visible with estrogen or its precursor, testosterone. Gonadal steroids also increase the size (diameter) of MPN GAL-IR cells and the number of GAL-IR cell processes within a portion of the MPN called the "GAL-IR MPOA plexus," which exists in males only. GAL microinjected into the MPN stimulated male-typical sexual behaviors, with more testosterone required in females than males. Immunoneutralization with anti-GAL serum inhibited male-typical sexual behavior, indicating a role for endogenous GAL within the MPN. Microinjection of GAL into the MPN also stimulated female-typical sexual behaviors in estrogen-treated females and males, and GAL within the MPN dramatically overrode an inhibition of lordosis by dihydrotestosterone in rats of both sexes.

Gonadal steroids act within the medial preoptic area (MPOA) to regulate sexual behaviors as well as anterior pituitary hormone secretion in the rat and other species.[1–9] Neural substrates within the MPOA participate in the regulation of both female-typical (lordosis)[1,7,8,10–13] and male-typical (mounting, intromission)[2,9,14–17] sexual behaviors. The MPOA contains many cytoarchitectonically distinct components,[18–20] and some of these, including the sexually dimorphic nucleus of the MPOA (SDN-POA),[21] which is within the medial and central divisions (MPNm and MPNc) of the medial preoptic nucleus (MPN),[19,20] are sexually dimorphic and contain large numbers of cells that concentrate gonadal steroids and have gonadal steroid receptors.[22–27] Although one study reported that lesions of the SDN-POA did not affect male-typical sexual behavior in male rats,[28] some studies support a role of the SDN-POA in male-typical sexual behaviors in both males and females.[29–32] We began studying galanin (GAL) within the MPN after reading early reports indicating that GAL was widely distributed within the rat CNS including the MPOA[33–38] and that GAL immunoreactivity and GAL mRNA levels within the pituitary and GAL immunoreactivity within the median eminence were increased by estrogen treatment in rats of both sexes.[39–42] Later studies of the paraventricular nucleus of the hypothalamus and of

[a]This work was supported by National Institutes of Health Grant HD-27334.

[c]Author to whom correspondence should be addressed. Phone, 801/378-2532; fax, 801/378-7862; e-mail, george_bloch@byu.edu

part of the MPOA rostral to the MPN also reported increased GAL immunoreactivity after estrogen treatment.[43,44] We patterned our study of GAL on our work indicating that gonadal steroid-sensitive sex differences exist in the distribution of CCK-immunoreactive cells within sexually dimorphic cell groups of the MPN and that microinjection of CCK-8 within the MPN affects sexual behavior in gonadal steroid-treated rats.[11,45]

COEXISTENCE OF GALANIN IMMUNOREACTIVITY AND ESTROGEN ACCUMULATION WITHIN MPN CELLS

Using radiolabeled estradiol, we determined that an average of 20% of estrogen-concentrating cells within the MPNc, 13% within the MPNm, and 7% within the lateral division (MPNl) were also GAL-positive (GAL-immunoreactive, GAL-IR).[22] Although the numbers studied were too small for statistical inferences, the percentage of estrogen-concentrating cells that were GAL-IR within MPN cell groups appeared to be equivalent between males and females (overall, 13.7% and 12.0%, respectively), but a higher percentage of GAL-IR cells concentrated estrogen within MPN cell groups of females than males (21.8% vs 3.3%).[22] A possible explanation for the sex difference is that the MPN cell groups contain many more GAL-IR cells in males than females (see below), but many of these do not concentrate estrogen. That GAL and estrogen interact within the same cell was also shown by Horvath *et al.*,[46] who recently reported the existence of estradiol receptors in GAL-producing neurons within the mediobasal hypothalamus. It is of interest that since GnRH (LHRH) neurons in the rat do not appear to concentrate estrogen or to contain estrogen receptors, these GAL-IR cells within the MPN are almost certainly not GnRH neurons, as was reported for a small population of galaninergic/GnRH cells located more rostrally in the MPOA.[44]

DISTRIBUTION OF GAL-IR CELLS WITHIN THE MPN AND RESPONSE TO GONADAL STEROIDS

We assessed the effects of estrogen on the distribution and number of GAL-IR cells in females and males, and because the aromatization of androgens to estrogens is very high in the male MPOA,[47,48] we assessed whether estrogenic effects on GAL-IR in males could be replicated with testosterone. FIGURE 1 illustrates the distribution of GAL-IR cells within the MPN and their response to gonadal steroids.[49,50] Concerning sex differences, 68% more GAL-IR cells were present within the MPNc of the gonadectomized (Gx) male than the Gx female and 79%–100% more GAL-IR cells within the MPNc of the gonadally intact, estrogen- and testosterone-treated male than the estrogen-treated female; this sex difference was also apparent for the MPNm and MPNl.[49] No sex differences were noted in the *density* of GAL-IR cells within the MPNc, MPNm, or MPNl of rats receiving similar treatments (i.e., between Gx males and Gx females or between estrogen-treated females and estrogen- or testosterone-treated males;[49] TABLE 1), indicating that sex differences in the number of GAL-IR cells were related to the larger size of these cell groups in males rather than to an increase in the concentration of GAL-IR cells within these cell groups. Concerning the response to gonadal steroids, GAL-IR cell numbers and densities within the MPNc were increased 60%–63% in estrogen-treated versus Gx females and by 74%–

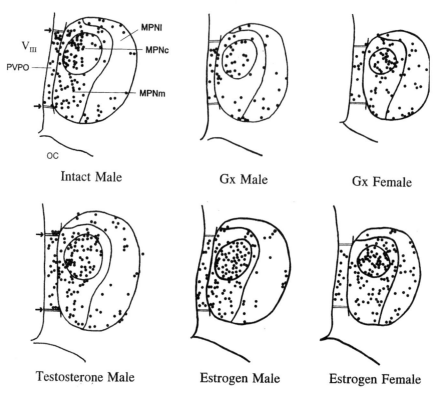

FIGURE 1. Drawings of 40-μm sections showing GAL-IR cells (*dark circles*) in the periventricular preoptic nucleus (PVPO) and the MPN. Animals were gonadally intact or gonadectomized (Gx) and received subcutaneously 1.57 mm id Silastic capsules filled with testosterone (9 mm/100 g BW, which results in testosterone levels normal for gonadally intact males),[49] or estradiol (60%, mixed with cholesterol, 2.3–2.5 mm/100 g BW, which results in high proestrus estrogen levels);[49] the capsules remained in the animals until sacrifice 9 days later. Two days before sacrifice animals received icv. colchicine, and after brain fixation sections were incubated sequentially in normal goat serum with 0.3% Triton X-100 and rabbit anti-GAL serum (Peninsula Labs, 48 hours at 4°C), and GAL-IR cells were visualized using a Vectastain ABC Elite Kit (Vector Labs) and diaminobenzidine tetrahydrochloride (DAB). Immunostaining in lightly thionin-counterstained sections was enhanced with 0.4% osmium tetroxide. (Reproduced with permission from Bloch *et al.*[49])

94% in gonadally intact, testosterone- and estrogen-treated males versus Gx males; similar results were observed within the MPNm[49] (TABLE 1).

When the fraction representing the number of GAL-IR cells out of the total number of cells was calculated for the MPNc, this fraction was 57% greater in gonadal steroid-treated males than in Gx males.[49] As there were no apparent differences between testosterone-treated and Gx males in the *total* numbers of cells (396.2 ± 15.7 and 423.6 ± 20.7 cells/mm^2 × 10^{-3}, respectively), it is likely that the increase in GAL-IR with gonadal steroids occurred within already existing cells.[49] This could be accomplished through increased GAL synthesis via a gonadal-steroid–induced increase in the expression of GAL

TABLE 1. Density of GAL-IR Cells (mean number of GAL-IR cells/mm^2 × 10^{-1} ± SEM), Diameters of GAL-IR Cell Bodies (μm), and Density of GAL-IR Cell Processes (number of processes/mm) within Sexually Dimorphic Cell Groups of the MPN in 40-μm Sections Obtained from Male and Female Rats under Various Gonadal Steroid Conditions (see legend to FIG. 1)

MPN Region	Gx Females (3)[d]	Gx Males (4)[d]	Est. Females (4)[d]	Est. Males (3)[d]	Test. Males (3)[d]	Intact Males (4)[d]
Cell Density[a]						
SDN-POA	58.4 ± 13.5	58.9 ± 7.6	95.2 ± 16.2[e]	118.4 ± 1.1[e]	86.7 ± 6.6[f]	87.5 ± 6.4[f]
MPOA GAL-IR Plexus	16.1 ± 2.0[g]	64.2 ± 7.8	37.1 ± 3.7[f,g]	102.5 ± 3.1[e]	87.4 ± 9.3[e]	85.3 ± 3.7[e]
MPNc[i]	44.8 ± 5.9	35.8 ± 3.9	71.8 ± 5.3[e]	75.5 ± 10.7[e]	58.7 ± 4.4[f]	52.4 ± 9.7[f]
MPNm[i]	16.0 ± 0.5	15.5 ± 0.5	21.5 ± 0.8[f]	29.3 ± 3.2[f]	23.6 ± 2.1[f]	22.1 ± 4.4[f]
MPNl[i]	13.3 ± 0.9	8.0 ± 1.5	16.1 ± 2.1	9.9 ± 1.4	9.8 ± 0.9	10.2 ± 3.1
Cell Diameter[b]						
MPNc	10.7 ± 0.4	10.1 ± 0.4	11.9 ± 0.4[e]	12.0 ± 0.5[e]	14.1 ± 0.6[e]	14.0 ± 0.5[e]
Process Density[c]						
MPOA GAL-IR Plexus	11.9 ± 1.9[g]	23.6 ± 1.1[h]	13.8 ± 1.9[g]	43.0 ± 6.8[e]	37.6 ± 0.5[e]	42.5 ± 3.5[e]

[a]GAL-IR cells with a visible nucleus were counted within each MPN region and the area quantified using a digitizing bit pad (Bioquant II). Three to eight sections were averaged for each rat (the size of MPN cell groups is smaller in females than males[19–21]).

[b]For each rat, cell diameters were obtained using an ocular micrometer for 20 GAL-IR cells with distinct nuclei, 10 from each of 2 sections separated by at least 80 μm. An average was taken from 2 diametric measurements of lines perpendicular to each other.

[c]Process density was determined for each section by counting the number of GAL-IR cell processes that crossed a line drawn through the middle of the outlined plexus (see FIG. 3) along its longest extent and a second line that crossed perpendicularly through the middle of the first, and dividing this number by the total line length.

[d]Number of animals.

[e]$p < 0.01$, [f]$p < 0.05$ vs Gx females and Gx males (Duncan's post-hoc tests).

[g]Although the MPOA GAL-IR plexus is not visible in females, the density of GAL-IR cells and GAL-IR cell processes within an area equivalent to males is given for comparison.

[h]$p < 0.01$ vs Gx and Est. females (Duncan's post-hoc tests).

[i]Adapted from Bloch et al.[49]

mRNA[39,51–54] and/or a variety of other cellular mechanisms. To determine whether gonadal steroids affected the size of GAL-IR cells, the diameters of GAL-IR cells were measured within the MPNc. GAL-IR cell sizes were very similar between Gx males and females, but these were clearly smaller than those in gonadally intact males or gonadal steroid-treated animals of both sexes (TABLE 1). Further research is needed to determine whether the increased cell size with gonadal steroids may reflect increased synthetic activity in GAL-IR cells or some other process.

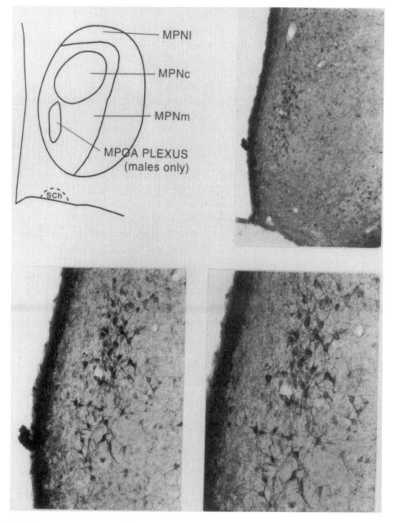

FIGURE 2. Drawing and photomicrographs of a 40-µm section illustrating the "MPOA GAL-IR plexus" at different magnifications in a gonadally intact male. Note the high density of GAL-IR cells and GAL-IR cell-process interdigitation.

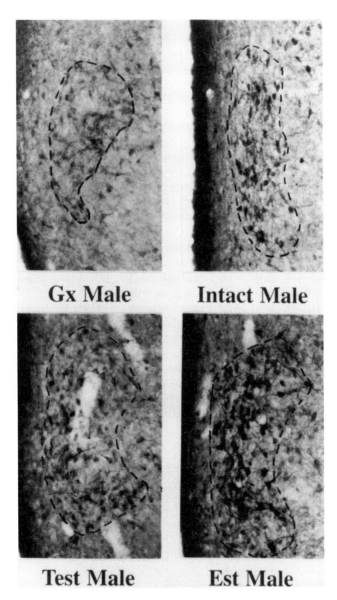

FIGURE 3. Photomicrographs illustrating the MPOA GAL-IR plexus in 40-μm sections obtained from males that were gonadectomized (Gx Male), gonadally intact (Intact Male), or Gx and received Silastic capsules filled with testosterone (Test Male) or estrogen (Est Male), as described in the legend to FIGURE 1. Outlines were used to obtain density measurements.

Interestingly, inspection of the MPNm revealed a highly GAL-IR region below the MPNc that extended anteriorly for about 120–200 μm. This region, which we called the "MPOA GAL-IR plexus,"[55] is illustrated in FIGURE 2. The MPOA GAL-IR plexus was evident in males only and was composed of a dense network of magnocellular-shaped, seemingly interconnected GAL-IR cells (FIG. 2). The total number of visibly GAL-IR cells located in the MPOA GAL-IR plexus was much higher in gonadally intact and gonadal steroid-treated males than in Gx males: 306 ± 67(SEM) vs 82 ± 18, $p < 0.01$, Duncan's *post-hoc* test (total cell counts corrected using a modification of the Abercrombie method).[49] As illustrated in FIGURE 3 and indicated in TABLE 1, the density of GAL-IR cells within the GAL-IR plexus was also much higher in gonadally intact and gonadal steroid-treated males than in Gx males ($F_{3,11} = 4.88$, $p < 0.002$; see TABLE 1 for *post-hoc p* values). The number of GAL-IR cell processes was affected as well ($F_{5,16} = 20.72$, $p < 0.001$); TABLE 1 indicates the large effect of gonadal steroids on the number of GAL-IR cell processes within the MPOA GAL-IR plexus.

The SDN-POA is a composite structure within the MPNm that includes most of the MPNc in males and a portion below the MPNc.[19] Importantly, as with the MPOA GAL-IR plexus, this ventral portion of the SDN-POA is evident in males only.[19] As the MPOA GAL-IR plexus was located in the same region of the MPNm as this ventral portion of the SDN-POA, we compared the distribution and steroid response of GAL-IR cells within the SDN-POA to those in other MPNm cell groups. Significant differences were noted among the groups in GAL-IR cell densities within the SDN-POA ($F_{5,16} = 6.32$, $p = 0.003$). As indicated in TABLE 1, compared to Gx animals the density of GAL-IR cells was very high within the SDN-POA of gonadally intact males and gonadal steroid-treated females and males. In the male the density of GAL-IR cells within the MPOA GAL-IR plexus was comparable to that within the SDN-POA as a whole, a result that suggests that the distribution of GAL-IR cells closely follows that of the SDN-POA. The density of GAL-IR cells within the MPNc and SDN-POA of the female was quite similar, and this also suggests that the distribution of GAL-IR cells closely follows that of the SDN-POA, because the SDN-POA of the female only includes the MPNc and an area that immediately surrounds it.[19] Importantly, unlike the female, the density of GAL-IR cells within the MPNc of the male averaged only .63 times that within the SDN-POA (TABLE 1); this also suggests that the distribution of GAL-IR cells within the MPN closely follows that of the SDN-POA, because approximately 40% of the MPNc of the male is not part of the SDN-POA.[19]

EFFECTS OF GALANIN WITHIN THE MPN ON MALE- AND FEMALE-TYPICAL SEXUAL BEHAVIORS IN RATS OF BOTH SEXES

Our discovery that GAL is distributed differentially within sexually dimorphic MPN cell groups, that a significant percentage of estrogen-concentrating cells within MPN cell groups also stain positively for GAL, that GAL-IR cell diameters and the number of processes increase in the presence of estrogen or testosterone, and that the number of visibly GAL-IR cells within MPN cell groups falls dramatically following castration suggested a possible role for GAL within the MPN in the regulation of sexually dimorphic, gonadal-steroid–sensitive functions. In the rat, sexual behaviors are precisely such functions, because not only are male- and female-typical behaviors very different from each other, but also the male is much more sensitive to the mount- and intromission-stimulating effects of testosterone than the female[56–59] and the female is much more sensitive to the lordosis-stimulating effect of estrogen than the male.[22,57] However, the differences are not absolute, because testosterone is aromatized to estrogen and many of the actions of testosterone on male-typical sexual behaviors can be replicated in the male with estrogen,[60–62] testosterone in high doses over a prolonged period will increase mounting behaviors in females,[57,63] and estrogen in high doses over a prolonged period[64] or in a pulsatile manner[65,66] can dramatically increase lordosis in the male. Thus, inasmuch as early[67–70] and subsequent[71,72] studies indicated that GAL receptors exist within the hypothalamus and other brain regions and that GAL binding was apparent within the MPOA,[34,72,73] we assessed the effects of GAL within the MPN on male- and female-typical sexual behaviors in both male and female rats.

Male-Typical Sexual Behaviors

In an initial experiment,[14] males with proven copulatory ability were Gx, implanted subcutaneously with 1.57 mm id Silastic capsules containing 2 mm crystalline testosterone, and received unilaterally a 22-gauge guide cannula aimed at a site 1.0 mm above the portion of the MPN that contains the MPNc and SDN-POA. (The 2-mm testosterone-filled capsules produce approximately 0.2 ng testosterone/ml plasma,[74,75] which allows for observation of behavioral effects that otherwise may not be apparent in maximally stimulated gonadally intact males or males treated with higher doses of the androgen.[74]) Starting 2 weeks later, these rats were tested for male-typical sexual behavior 10 minutes after microinjection of a 0.3-µl solution containing 0 (saline vehicle), 10, 50, 100, or 500 ng rat GAL (Peninsula Labs) using a 29-gauge injector that extended 1 mm beyond the guide.[14] GAL microinjected into the MPN significantly increased the percentage of males that displayed sexual behavior and decreased mount and intromission latencies; the facilitation of male-typical sexual behavior occurred in a dose-responsive fashion.[14] GAL microinjection into the MPN did not affect other measures, that is, mount and intromission frequencies to ejaculation, ejaculatory latencies, postejaculatory and intercopulatory intervals, and copulatory efficiency,[14] suggesting that the facilitation by GAL concerned sexual arousal rather than performance after copulation onset.[16,17] The stimulating effects of GAL within the MPN were not observed in males that were Gx *without* testosterone replacement, indicating that the effect required the presence of gonadal steroids.[14] Because there was no effect on open-field behaviors, the effect was not due to general arousal but was behaviorally specific.[14]

To assess endogenously released GAL we used anti-GAL serum to block GAL using the technique of passive immunoneutralization.[76,77] FIGURE 4 shows mount and intromission latencies as Kaplan-Meier curves; these illustrate the accumulative percentage of rats that mounted (or intromitted) at various latencies up to 1800 seconds, which was the time after which the test was terminated if there were no intromissions.[14] As indicated in FIGURE 4, the anti-GAL serum within the MPN significantly increased mount and intromission latencies compared to vehicle (normal sheep serum, NSS) controls: mount latencies of 464 ± 219 seconds (mean $\pm$ SEM) for 8 anti-GAL rats (8 of 10 mounted) versus 16 ± 3 seconds for 11 NSS controls (11 of 11 mounted); intromission latencies of 403 ± 273 seconds for 6 anti-GAL rats (6 of 10 males intromitted) versus 178 ± 92 seconds for 11 NSS controls (10 of 11 intromitted). All of the males that intromitted also ejaculated,

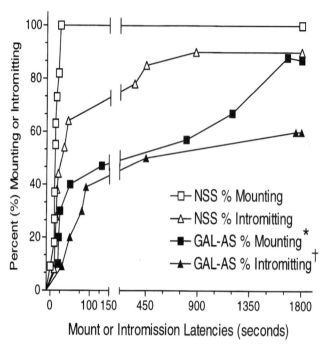

FIGURE 4. Kaplan-Meier curves illustrating Mount and Intromission Latency scores in male rats that received GAL antiserum (GAL-AS, 10 rats) or vehicle (normal sheep serum, NSS, 11 rats) bilaterally into the MPN. Males with proven ability (copulation to ejaculation in 2 preliminary tests) were Gx, implanted with capsules containing 2 mm crystalline testosterone, and received 26 gauge guide cannulas aimed 1 mm above the MPNc and SDN-POA.[14] Ten days later, these rats were tested for male-typical sexual behavior 1.5 hours after bilateral microinjection of 1 μl undiluted GAL antiserum (GAL-AS, lot #FMS-FJL 17-5, kindly provided by F. Lopez) or NSS, starting about 2 hours after lights off in the 14L:10D schedule (lights off 9 AM). A 32-gauge injector that extended 1 mm beyond the guide was used for each microinjection, which took 3 minutes; an additional minute was allowed for diffusion. At the end of the experiment, animals were given an overdose of anesthetic, perfused transcardially with formalin, and injection sites were verified by viewing 100-μm thionin-stained sections with a microscope. $^{*}p < 0.001$, $^{\dagger}p < 0.05$ vs NSS-microinjected males, Mantel-Haenzel tests[22] ("log-rank" tests in SAS).

and the anti-GAL serum did not inhibit other aspects of male-typical sexual behavior. (This supports the earlier study indicating that GAL acts within the MPN to increase sexual arousal rather than performance after copulation onset.) Interestingly, anti-GAL serum microinjected into the MPN did not inhibit sexual behavior in 23 males implanted with 4-mm testosterone-filled capsules. Gonadal steroids affect sexual behavior in concert with many neurochemicals acting in many brain regions. Thus, it is possible that by doubling the amount of testosterone, the immunoneutralization of GAL within the MPN was no longer sufficient to overcome stimulating effects originating perhaps within other brain regions and/or involving other neuroactive chemicals. Microinjection of anti-GAL serum into the MPN unilaterally or into sites that missed the MPN bilaterally were ineffective. (A total of 33 males fell into these latter categories.)

In a separate series of experiments, GAL microinjected into the MPN also facilitated male-typical sexual behavior dose-responsively in female rats.[63] Mount latencies decreased significantly after GAL microinjection within the MPN, while mount frequencies and the percentage of females that mounted increased significantly.[63] Since the females displayed no ejaculatory behaviors, the increase in mount frequencies also was a measurement of sexual arousal, not of performance.[63,64] Interestingly, the stimulation of male-typical sexual behavior by GAL within the MPN was evident in Gx females that received 22-mm testosterone-filled capsules but not in Gx females that received 4-mm testosterone-filled capsules, whereas a 2-mm testosterone-filled capsule was all that was needed to show a stimulating effect by GAL in Gx males.[14,63] Thus, larger amounts of testosterone were required in females than males to observe the behavioral effects of GAL, a result in keeping with the fact that male-typical sexual behaviors are more readily stimulated by testosterone in male rats than in females.

Others have reported that GAL injection into the lateral ventricle (icv) inhibits[78] and that icv injection of the GAL antagonist Galantide stimulates[79] male-typical sexual behavior in the gonadally intact male rat. As discussed by Benelli *et al.*,[79] a likely explanation for the discrepancy with our results is that the icv injection was acting in a different region (or regions) of the brain than the MPN, producing effects not unlike the opposite effects observed with male-typical sexual behavior after medial preoptic versus systemic administration of naloxone (see Benelli *et al.*[79]) and the different results obtained with female-typical sexual behavior after MPN versus icv (or ventromedial hypothalamic) administration of CCK[11,80,81] or after MPN versus icv administration of LHRH in the 5α-dihydrotestosterone-treated rat.[82,83] Support for this hypothesis comes from a series of experiments in gonadally intact males in which we observed no inhibitory effects on any parameter of male-typical sexual behavior after microinjection of either 50 or 500 ng GAL into the MPN.[63] (These gonadally intact males were too stimulated by the normally high circulating levels of testosterone to observe a facilitatory effect.)

Female-Typical Sexual Behaviors

In an initial experiment females were Gx and received unilaterally a 22-gauge guide cannula aimed at a site 1.0 mm above the portion of the MPN that contains the MPNc and SDN-POA.[63] Starting 1 week later these rats received 3 μg estradiol benzoate (EB)/day for 2 days, and behavior testing began 10 minutes after unilateral microinjection of a 0.3 μl solution containing 0 (saline vehicle), 10, 50, 100, or 500 ng rat GAL (Peninsula Labs) using a 29-gauge injector that extended 1 mm beyond the guide.[63] Lordosis behavior increased significantly after microinjection of GAL into the MPN. All doses of GAL were equally effective: lordosis quotient (LQ) scores ranged from 50.0 ± 12 (mean $\pm$ SEM) after 10 ng GAL to 60.0 ± 10.9 after 500 ng GAL versus 30.0 ± 11.0 for saline-microinjected controls.[63] This result was not due to nonspecific behavioral arousal, because general locomotor activity was not significantly different among groups.[63] Microinjection of GAL into the MPN did not affect proceptive behaviors (darting, hopping, and ear wiggling); these were low in all groups, probably because animals were estrogen primed but received no progesterone.[63]

The androgen 5α-dihydrotestosterone (DHT) is a known potent inhibitor of lordosis in EB-primed female rats,[84] and we recently reported the same for male rats.[85] In females the inhibition of lordosis by DHT appears to involve its metabolites,[86] but it may also involve peptides because DHT does interfere with the estrogen-induced LH surge.[87] Thus, we determined whether GAL microinjected within the MPN affects lordosis in the male and also whether GAL within the MPN affects lordosis in DHT-treated rats of both sexes. The results and methodologic details are presented in FIGURES 5 and 6 and TABLE 2. For the longitudinal analysis we used the General Estimating Equations (GEE) method (GENMOD Procedure, SAS computer program, 1997) to account for the correlations inherent to repeated weekly measurement of lordosis and the binomial nature of lordosis scores[88] (the lordosis quotient [LQ] is a ratio computed by dividing the number of lordotic responses by the number of mounts by the stimulus male [10 in the present studies] and multiplying by 100). As expected, LQ scores were lower in control (saline-microinjected) females treated with DHT than with no DHT (BK) and higher in BK-treated females microinjected with GAL than with saline: Zs = −6.00 and 3.21, respectively; $p < 0.0001$ and $p = 0.001$, GEE; see FIG. 5 and TABLE 2. The same result was obtained in males: LQ scores were lower in saline-microinjected animals with DHT capsules than with nothing (BK), and higher in BK-treated animals microinjected with GAL than with saline: Zs = −3.41 and 4.80, ps < 0.001, GEE; see FIG. 6 and TABLE 2. A significant steroid (BK versus DHT) X Week interaction in the saline-microinjected females (Z = −3.53, $p < 0.0001$, GEE) was due to

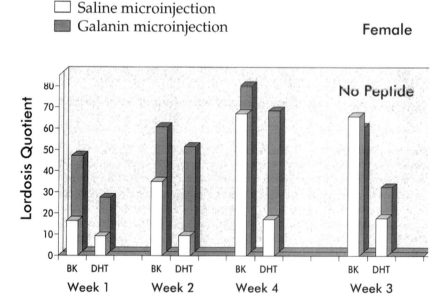

FIGURE 5. Mean lordosis quotient (LQ) scores in BK- and DHT-treated female rats after GAL microinjection into the MPN for 3 sessions (weeks 1, 2, and 4; see TABLE 2 for details). As indicated in the figure, no GAL was administered during week 3.

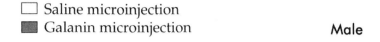

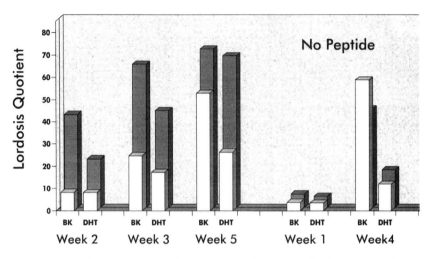

FIGURE 6. Mean lordosis quotient (LQ) scores in BK- and DHT-treated male rats after GAL micro-injection into the MPN for 3 sessions (weeks 2, 3, and 5; see TABLE 2). As indicated in the figure, no GAL was administered during weeks 1 and 4.

LQ scores that remained low across sessions (weeks) in DHT-treated saline controls, while they rose in animals that received no DHT. (It is well known that if LQ scores start at low levels in normal, Gx rats, they will increase over time with repeated estrogen priming.[80]) Although not as dramatic, this effect was evident also in males ($Z = -1.56$, $p = 0.12$, GEE; FIG. 6).

GAL microinjections into the MPN completely overrode the DHT-induced inhibition; as is evident in FIGURES 5 and 6 and TABLE 2, GAL dramatically increased LQ scores in DHT-treated females and males ($Z = 7.66$ and 7.69, GAL vs saline, $ps < 0.0001$, GEE). The GAL-induced increase in LQ scores was less in DHT- than in BK-treated females during the first session (Chi-square = 16.45, $p < 0.001$, "Proc Insight" in SAS, binomial distribution, Logit link function), but during the last two sessions there was no difference between DHT- and BK-treated females microinjected with GAL ($Z = 0.06$, $p = 0.95$, GEE; FIG. 5). With males, the GAL-induced increase in LQ scores was less in DHT- than in BK-treated animals during the first two sessions ($Z = -2.83$, $p < 0.01$, GEE), but by the third session any difference between DHT- and BK-treated males microinjected with GAL was no longer apparent (FIG. 6). Importantly, during weeks when GAL was not microinjected in DHT-treated rats, LQ scores were low in both "saline" and "GAL" groups (see FIGURES 5 and 6), indicating that the lordosis-stimulating effect of GAL in DHT-treated rats was reversible.

TABLE 2. Mean LQ Scores ± SEM in Females and Males Implanted with Silastic Capsules Filled with DHT or Nothing (BK) and Microinjected with Saline (Vehicle) or GAL into the MPN[a] (results illustrated in FIGURES 5 and 6)

Steroid Group	Sex[b]	Peptide Group	N[c]	Session 1[d]	Session 2[d]	Session 3[d]
BK	F	Saline	20	16.5 ±4.9	35.0 ±4.6	67.0 ±3.6
BK	M	Saline	11	3.6 ±2.0	23.6 ±3.6	58.2 ±5.4
DHT	F	Saline	22	9.1 ±2.9	9.6 ±3.0	17.3 ±3.9
DHT	M	Saline	11	8.2 ±3.8	17.3 ±4.1	26.4 ±7.3
BK	F	GAL	17	45.3 ±6.9	58.8 ±7.5	78.2 ±3.5
BK	M	GAL	12	44.2 ±7.2	65.8 ±6.5	72.5 ±6.3
DHT	F	GAL	22	25.5 ±4.5	49.6 ±6.8	66.4 ±4.5
DHT	M	GAL	11	21.8 ±5.2	43.6 ±7.3	68.2 ±6.1

[a]Animals underwent gonadectomy, insertion of 1.57 mm id BK capsules or capsules containing 11.5 mm DHT/100 g BW (these produced 1.63 ±.27 ng DHT/ml plasma), and unilateral implantation of a 22-gauge guide cannula aimed at a site 1.0 mm above the portion of the MPN that contains the MPNc and SDN-POA.[14] Starting 1 week later, females received 1 µg estradiol benzoate (EB)/day for 2 days and males received 6 µg EB/day for 3 days. Behavior testing began 10 minutes after microinjection of a 0.3-µl solution containing 50 ng rat GAL (Peninsula Labs), 50–53 hours (females) or 74–77 hours (males) after the first EB injection. A 29-gauge injector was used to inject over a 1-minute period, with an additional minute allowed for diffusion. Injection sites were verified microscopically as described in the legend for FIGURE 4.

[b]F, females; M, males.

[c]Number of animals that received microinjections into the MPN.

[d]Sessions 1, 2, and 3 were, respectively, weeks 1, 2, and 4 for females (FIG. 5) and weeks 2, 3, and 5 for males (FIG. 6).

SUMMARY

More GAL-IR cells exist within sexually dimorphic cell groups of the MPN in male rats than in females, a large percentage of estrogen-concentrating cells within MPN cell groups are also GAL-IR, and significantly more GAL-IR cells are visible with estrogen or its precursor, testosterone. Gonadal steroids also increased the size (diameter) of Mpnc GAL-IR cells and the number of GAL-IR cell processes within a portion of the MPN called the "GAL-IR MPOA plexus," which existed in males only. Microinjection of GAL into the MPN stimulated the arousal component of male-typical sexual behaviors (mount, intromission latencies, and percentage of animals mounting or intromitting) in both males and females; immunoneutralization with anti-GAL serum inhibited the behavior, indicating a role for endogenous GAL. Microinjection of GAL into the MPN also stimulated female-typical sexual behavior (lordosis) in estrogen-treated females and males, and GAL within the MPN dramatically overrode an inhibition of lordosis by dihydrotestosterone (DHT) in rats of both sexes. Because the stimulating effects of GAL on male-typical sexual behavior were not observed in males that were Gx *without* testosterone and much larger amounts of testosterone were required in females than males, it appears that GAL's effect was dependent on the gonadal steroid environment and that GAL within the MPN acted on neural systems less dominant than those responsible for sex differences. By contrast, as the lordosis-stimulating action of GAL was sufficient to eliminate a DHT-induced inhibition, it appears in this case that GAL acted on neural systems within the MPN that are more dominant than those responsible for the inhibition.

REFERENCES

1. BARFIELD, R.J. & J.J. CHEN. 1977. Activation of estrous behavior in ovariectomized rats by intracerebral implants of estradiol benzoate. Endocrinology **101:** 1716–1725.
2. DAVIDSON, J.M. 1966. Activation of the male rat's sexual behavior by intracerebral implantation of androgen. Endocrinology **79:** 783–794.
3. GORSKI, R.A. 1985. Sexual dimorphisms of the brain. J. Animal Sci. **61:** 38–61.
4. GUNNET, J.W. & M.E. FREEMAN. 1982. Sexual differences in regulation of prolactin secretion by two hypothalamic areas. Endocrinology **110:** 697–702.
5. JAKUBOWSKI, M. & J. TERKEL. 1986. Female reproductive function and sexually dimorphicprolactin secretion in rats with lesions in the medial preoptic-anterior hypothalamic continuum. Neuroendocrinology **43:** 696–705.
6. NEILL, J.D. 1972. Sexual differences in the hypothalamic regulation of prolactin secretion. Endocrinology **90:** 1154–1159.
7. PFAFF, D.W. 1981. Impact of estrogens on hypothalamic nerve cells: Ultrastructural, chemical, and electrical effects. Rec. Prog. Horm. Res. **39:** 127–179.
8. POWERS, B. & E.S. VALENSTEIN. 1972. Sexual receptivity: Facilitation by medial preoptic lesions in female rats. Science **175:** 1003–1005.
9. RYAN, E L. & A.I. FRANKEL. 1978. Studies on the role of the medial preoptic area in sexual behavior and hormonal response to sexual behavior in the mature male laboratory rat. Biol. Reprod. **19:** 971–983.
10. BAST, J.D., C. HUNTS, K.J. RENNER, R.K. MORRIS & D.M. QUADAGNO. 1987. Lesions in the preoptic area suppressed sexual receptivity in ovariectomized rats with estrogen implants in the ventromedial hypothalamus. Brain Res. Bull. **18:** 153–158.
11. DORNAN, W.A., G.J. BLOCH, C.A. PRIEST & P.E. MICEVYCH. 1989. Microinjection of cholecystokinin into the medial preoptic nucleus facilitates lordosis behavior in the female rat. Physiol. Behav. **45:** 969–974.

12. PFAFF, D.W. & D. MODIANOS. 1985. Neural mechanisms of female reproductive behavior. *In* Handbook of Behavioral Neurobiology: Reproduction. N. Adler, D. Pfaff, & R.W. Goy, Eds.: 423–480. Plenum Press. New York.

13. PFAFF, D.W. & Y. SAKUMA. 1979. Facilitation of the lordosis reflex of female rats from the ventromedial nucleus of the hypothalamus. J. Physiol. **288:** 189–202.

14. BLOCH, G.J., P.C. BUTLER, J.G. KOHLERT & D.A. BLOCH. 1993. Microinjection of galanin into the medial preoptic nucleus facilitates copulatory behavior in the male rat. Physiol. Behav. **54:** 615–624.

15. CHRISTENSON, L.W., D.M. NANCE & R.A. GORSKI. 1977. Effects of hypothalamic and preoptic lesions on reproductive behavior in male rats. Brain Res. Bull. **2:** 137–141.

16. MEISEL, R.L. & B.D. SACHS. 1994. The physiology of male sexual behavior. *In* The Physiology of Reproduction. E. Knobil & J.D. Neill, Eds. :3–105. Raven Press. New York.

17. SACHS, B.D. & R.L. MEISEL. 1988. The physiology of male sexual behavior. *In* The Physiology of Reproduction. E. Knobile & J. Neill, Eds. :1393–1485. Raven Press. New York.

18. BLEIER, R., W. BYNE & I. SIGGELKOW. 1982. Cytoarchitectonic sexual dimorphisms of the medial preoptic and anterior hypothalamic areas in guinea pig, rat, hamster, and mouse. J. Comp. Neurol. **212:** 118–130.

19. BLOCH, G.J. & R.A. GORSKI. 1988. Cytoarchitectonic analysis of the SDN-POA of the intact and gonadectomized rat. J. Comp. Neurol. **275:** 604–612.

20. SIMERLY, R.B., L.W. SWANSON & R.A. GORSKI. 1984. Demonstration of a sexual dimorphism in the distribution of serotonin-immunoreactive fibers in the medial preoptic nucleus of the rat. J. Comp. Neurol. **225:** 151–166.

21. GORSKI, R.A., J.H. GORDON, J.E. SHRYNE & A.M. SOUTHAM. 1978. Evidence for a morphological sex difference within the medial preoptic area of the rat brain. Brain Res. **148:** 333–346.

22. BLOCH, G.J., S.M. KURTH, T.R. AKESSON. & P.E. MICEVYCH. 1992. Estrogen- concentrating cells within cell groups of the medial preoptic area: Sex differences and colocalization with galanin-immunoreactive cells. Brain Res. **595:** 301–308.

23. JACOBSON, C.D., A.P. ARNOLD & R.A. GORSKI. 1987. Steroid autoradiography of the sexually dimorphic nucleus of the preoptic area. Brain Res. **414:** 349–356.

24. PFAFF, D.W. & M. KEINER. 1974. Atlas of estradiol-concentrating cells in the central nervous system of the female rat. J. Comp. Neurol. **151:** 121–158.

25. SAR, M. & W.E. STUMPF. 1975. Distribution of androgen-concentrating neurons in rat brain. *In* Anatomical Neuroendocrinology. W.E. Stumpf & L.D. Grant, Eds. :120–133. Karger. Basel.

26. SAR, M. & W.E. STUMPF. 1977. Distribution of androgen target cells in rat forebrain and pituitary after 3H-dihydrotestosterone administration. J. Steroid Biochem. **8:** 1131–1135.

27. SIMERLY, R.B., C. CHANG, M. MURAMATSU & L.W. SWANSON. 1990. Distribution of androgen and estrogen receptor mRNA-containing cells in the rat brain: An in situ hybridization study. J. Comp. Neurol. **294:** 76–95.

28. ARENDASH, G.W. & R.A. GORSKI. 1983. Effects of discrete lesions of the sexually dimorphic nucleus of the preoptic area or other medial preoptic regions on the sexual behavior of male rats. Brain Res. Bull. **10:** 147–154.

29. ANDERSON, R.H., D.E. FLEMING, R.W. RHEES & E. KINGHORN. 1986. Relationships between sexual activity, plasma testosterone, and the volume of the sexually dimorphic nucleus of the preoptic area in prenatally stressed and nonstressed rats. Brain Res. **370:** 1–10.

30. ARENDASH, G.W. & R.A. GORSKI. 1984. Brain tissue transplants and reproductive function. *In* Neural Transplants. J.R. Sladeck & D.M. Gash, Eds. :223–241. Plenum Publishing Corp. New York.

31. COMMINS, D. & P. YAHR. 1984. Lesions of the sexually dimorphic area disrupt mating and marking in male gerbils. Brain Res. Bull. **13:** 185–193.

32. TURKENBURG, J.L., D.F. SWAAB, E. ENDERT, A.L. LOUWERSE & N.E. VAN DE POLL. 1988. Effects of lesions of the sexually dimorphic nucleus on sexual behavior of testosterone-treated female Wistar rats. Brain Res. Bull. **21:** 215–224.

33. CH'NG, J.LC., N.D. CHRISTOFIDES, P. ANAND, S.J. GIBSON, Y.S. ALLEN, H.C. SU & K. TATEMOTO. 1985. Distribution of galanin immunoreactivity in the central nervous system and the responses of galanin-containing neuronal pathways to injury. Neuroscience **16:** 343–354.

34. MELANDER, T., T. HOKFELT & A. ROKAEUS. 1986. Distribution of galaninlike immuno-reactivity in the rat central nervous system. J. Comp. Neurol. **248:** 475–517.

35. PALKOVITS, M., A. ROKAEUS, F.A. ANTONI & A. KISS. 1987. Galanin in the hypothalamo-hypophyseal system. Neuroendocrinology 46: 417–423.
36. ROKAEUS, A., T. MELANDER, T. HOKFELT, J.M. LUNDBERG, K. TATEMOTO, M. CARLQUIST & V. MUTT. 1984. A galanin-like peptide in the central nervous system and intestine of the rat. Neurosci. Lett. 47: 161–166.
37. SKOFITSCH, G. & D.M. JACOBOWITZ. 1985. Immunohistochemical mapping of galanin-like neurons in the rat central nervous system. Peptides 6: 509–546.
38. SKOFITSCH, G. & D.M. JACOBOWITZ. 1986. Quantitative distribution of galanin-like immunoreactivity in the rat central nervous system. Peptides 7: 609–613.
39. GABRIEL, S.M., J.I. KOENIG & L.M. KAPLAN. 1990. Galanin-like immunoreactivity is influenced by estrogen in peripubertal and adult rats. Neuroendocrinology 51: 168–173.
40. KAPLAN, L.M., S.M. GABRIEL, J.I. KOENIG, M.E. SUNDAY, E.R. SPINDEL, J.B. MARTIN & W.W. CHIN. 1988. Galanin is an estrogen-inducible, secretory product of the rat anterior pituitary. Proc. Natl. Acad. Sci. USA 85: 7408–7412.
41. VRONTAKIS, M.E., L.M. PEDEN, M.L. DUCKWORTH & H.G. FRIESEN. 1987. Isolation and characterization of a complementary DNA (galanin) clone from estrogen-induced pituitary tumor messenger RNA. J. Biol. Chem. 262: 16755–16758.
42. VRONTAKIS, M.E., T. YAMAMOTO, I.C. SCHROEDTER, J.I. NAGY & H.G. FRIESEN. 1989. Estrogen induction of galanin synthesis in the rat anterior pituitary gland demonstrated by in situ hybridization and immunohistochemistry. Neurosci. Lett. 100: 59–64.
43. LEVIN, M.C. & P.E. SAWCHENKO. 1993. Neuropeptide co-expression in the magnocellular neurosecretory system of the female rat: Evidence for differential modulation by estrogen. Neuroscience 54: 1001–1018.
44. MERCHENTHALER, I., D.E. LENNARD, F.J. LOPEZ & A. NEGRO-VILAR. 1993. Neonatal imprinting predetermines the sexually dimorphic, estrogen-dependent expression of galanin in luteinizing hormone-releasing hormone neurons. Proc. Natl. Acad. Sci. USA 90: 10479–10483.
45. MICEVYCH, P.E. & G.J. BLOCH. 1989. Estrogen regulation of a reproductively relevant cholecystokinin circuit in the hypothalamus and limbic system of rat. In The Neuropeptide Cholecystokinin. J. Hughes, G. Dockray & G. Woodruff, Eds. :68–73. E. Horwood Ltd. Chichester, England.
46. HORVATH, T.L., C. LERANTH, S.P. KALRA & F. NAFTOLIN. 1995. Galanin neurons exhibit estrogen receptor immunoreactivity in the female rat mediobasal hypothalamus. Brain Res. 675: 321–324.
47. ROSELLI, C.E., L.E. HORTON & J.A. RESKO. 1985. Distribution and regulation of aromatase activity in the rat hypothalamus and limbic system. Endocrinology 117: 2471–2477.
48. SELMANOFF, M.K., L.D. BRODKIN, R.I. WEINER & P.K. SIITERI. 1977. Aromatization and 5α-reduction of androgens in discrete hypothalamic and limbic regions of the male and female rat. Endocrinology 101: 841–848.
49. BLOCH, G.J., C. ECKERSELL & R. MILLS. 1993. Distribution of galanin-immunoreactive cells within sexually dimorphic components of the medial preoptic area of the male and female rat. Brain Res. 620: 259–268.
50. ECKERSELL, C.B., R. MILLS, B. PADGETT & G.J. BLOCH. 1991. Soc. Neurosci. Abstr. 17: 497.
51. MILLER, M.A., P.E. KOLB & M.A. RASKIND. 1993. Testosterone regulates galanin gene expression in the bed nucleus of the stria terminalis. Brain Res. 611: 338–341.
52. PLANAS, B., P.E. KOLB, M.A. RASKIND & M.A. MILLER. 1994. Activation of galanin pathways across puberty in the male rat: Galanin gene expression in the bed nucleus of the stria terminalis and medial amygdala. Neuroscience 63: 851–858.
53. ROSSMANITH, W.G., D.K. CLIFTON & R.A. STEINER. 1996. Galanin gene expression in hypothalamic GnRH-containing neurons of the rat: A model for autocrine regulation. Horm. Metab. Res. 28: 257–266.
54. ROSSMANITH, W.G., D.L. MARKS, D.K. CLIFTON & R.A. STEINER. 1994. Induction of galanin gene expression in gonadotropin-releasing hormone neurons with puberty in the rat. Endocrinology 135: 1401–1408.
55. ECKERSELL, C.B., R. MILLS & G.J. BLOCH. 1992. Sex steroids and galanin-immunoreactive (GAL- IR) cells in the medial preoptic area (MPOA): Cell size and male-specific plexus. Soc. Neurosci. Abstr. 18: 818.

56. BLOCH., G.J. & R. MILLS. 1995. Prepubertal testosterone treatment of neonatally gonadecto-mized male rats: Defeminization and masculinization of behavioral and endocrine function in adulthood. Neurosci. Biobehav. Rev. **19:** 187–200.

57. BLOCH, G.J., R. MILLS & S. GALE. 1995. Prepubertal testosterone treatment of female rats: Defeminization of behavioral and endocrine function in adulthood. Neurosci. Biobehav. Rev. **19:** 177–186.

58. PFAFF, D.W. & R.E. ZIGMOND. 1971. Neonatal androgen effects on sexual and non-sexual behavior of adult rats tested under various hormone regimes. Neuroendocrinology **7:** 129–145.

59. YOUNG, W.C. 1961. The hormones and mating behavior. *In* Sex and Internal Secretions. W.C.Young, Ed. :1193–1199. Williams & Wilkins Co. Baltimore.

60. DAVIDSON, J.M. 1969. Effects of estrogen on the sexual behavior of male rats. Endocrinology **84:** 1365–1372.

61. GORZALKA, B.B., D.L. REZEK & R.E. WHALEN. 1975. Adrenal mediation of estrogen-induced ejaculatory behavior in the male rat. Physiol. Behav. **14:** 373–376.

62. SODERSTEN, P. 1973. Estrogen-activated sexual behavior in male rats. Horm. Behav. **4:** 247–256.

63. BLOCH, G.J., P.C. BUTLER & J.G. KOHLERT. 1996. Galanin microinjected into the medial preoptic nucleus facilitates female- and male-typical sexual behaviors in the female rat. Physiol. Behav. **59:** 1147–1154.

64. DAVIDSON, J.M. & G.J. BLOCH. 1969. Neuroendocrine aspects of male reproduction. Biol. Reprod. **1:** 67–92.

65. OLSTER, D.H. & J.D. BLAUSTEIN. 1988. Progesterone facilitation of lordosis in male and female Sprague-Dawley rats following priming with estradiol pulses. Horm. Behav. **22:** 294–304.

66. SODERSTEN, P., A. PETTERSSON & P. ENEROTH. 1983. Pulse administration of estradiol-17 cancels sex difference in behavioral estrogen sensitivity. Endocrinology **112:** 1883–1885.

67. CRAWLEY, J.N., M.C. AUSTIN, S.M. FISKE, B. MARTIN, S. CONSOLO, M. BERTHOLD, U. LANGEL & T. BARTFAI. 1990. Activity of centrally administered galanin fragments on stimulation of feeding behavior and on galanin receptor binding in the rat hypothalamus. J. Neurosci. **10:** 3695–3700.

68. FISONE, G., U. LANGEL, M. CARLQUIST, T. BERGMAN, S. CONSOLO, T. HOKFELT, A. UNDEN & T. BARTFAI. 1989. Galanin receptor and its ligands in the rat hippocampus. Eur. J. Biochem. **181:** 269–276.

69. LAND, T., U. LANGEL, M. LOW, M. BERTHOLD, A. UNDEN & T. BARTFAI. 1991. Linear and cyclic N-terminal galanin fragments and analogs as ligands at the hypothalamic galanin receptor. Int. J. Peptide Protein Res. **38:** 267–272.

70. SERVIN, A.L., B. AMIRANOFF, C. ROUYER-FESSARD, K. TATEMOTO & M. LABURTHE. 1987. Identification and molecular characterization of galanin receptor sites in rat brain. Biochem. Biophys. Res. Commun. **144:** 298–306.

71. BARTFAI, T. 1995. A neuropeptide with important central nervous system actions. *In* Psychopharmacology: The Fourth Generation of Progress. F.E. Bloom & D.J. Kupfer, Eds. :563–571. Raven Press. New York.

72. PLANAS, B., P.E. KOLB, M.A. RASKIND & M.A. MILLER. 1995. Galanin-binding sites in the female rat brain are regulated across puberty yet similar to the male pattern in adulthood. Neuroendocrinology **61:** 646–654.

73. SKOFITSCH, G., M.A. SILLS & D.M. JACOBOWITZ. 1986. Autoradiographic distribution of ^{125}I-galanin binding sites in the rat central nervous system. Peptides **7:** 1029–1042.

74. DAMASSA, D.A., E.R. SMITH, B. TENNENT & J.M. DAVIDSON. 1977. The relationship between circulating testosterone levels and male sexual behavior in rats. Horm. Behav. **8:** 275–286.

75. SMITH, E.R., D.A. DAMASSA & J.M. DAVIDSON. 1977. Hormone administration: Peripheral and intracranial implants. *In* Methods in Psychobiology. R.D. Myer, Ed. :259–279. Academic Press. New York.

76. BLOCH, G.J., B. JOHNSON, J. BETHEA, J. KOHLERT, E. DESPAIN, F. GRIMMER, M. CLINGER, S. HUBER, D. HAVENS, R. SMITH & P. BUTLER. 1993. Antigalanin(GAL) serum microinjected into the medial preoptic nucleus (MPN) inhibits copulatory behavior in the male rat. Neurosci. Abstr. **19:** 584.

77. LOPEZ, F.J., E.H. MEADE & A. NEGRO-VILAR. 1993. Endogenous galanin modulates the gonadotropin and prolactin surges in the rat. Endocrinology **132:** 795–800.

78. POGGIOLI, R., E. RASORI & A. BERTOLINI. 1992. Galanin inhibits sexual behavior in male rats. Eur. J. Pharmacol. **213:** 87–90.

79. BENELLI, A., R. ARLETTI, A. BERTOLINI, B. MENOZZI, R. BASAGLIA & R. POGGIOLI. 1994. Galantide stimulates sexual behavior in male rats. Eur. J. Pharmacol. **260:** 279–282.

80. BLOCH, G.J., A.M. BABCOCK, R.A. GORSKI & P.E. MICEVYCH. 1987. Cholecystokinin stimulates and inhibits lordosis behavior in female rats. Physiol. Behav. **39:** 217–224.

81. BABCOCK, A.M., G.J. BLOCH & P.E. MICEVYCH. 1988. Injections of cholecystokinin into the ventromedial hypothalamic nucleus inhibit lordosis behavior in the rat. Physiol. Behav. **43:** 195–199.

82. BUTLER, P.C., R.H. MILLS, M.A. MALSTROM, P. OLSON, S. GARRARD, P. WONG, R. HILL & G.J. BLOCH. 1998. Microinjection of luteinizing hormone-releasing hormone (LHRH) within the medial preoptic nucleus (MPN) stimulates lordosis in the dihydrotestosterone-treated female and male rat. Soc. Neurosci. Abstr. **24:** in press.

83. ERSKINE, M.S. 1989. Effect of 5α-dihydrotestosterone and flutamide on the facilitation of lordosis by LHRH and naloxone in estrogen-primed female rats. Physiol. Behav. **45:** 753–759.

84. BAUM, M.J., P. SODERSTEN & J.T.M. VREEBURG. 1974. Mounting and receptive behavior in the ovariectomized female rat: influence of estradiol, dihydrotestosterone, and genital anesthetization. Horm. Behav. **5:** 175–1 90.

85. BUTLER, P.C. S.E. HUBER & G.J. BLOCH. 1995. Effects of testosterone (T), progesterone (P), and dihydrotestosterone (DHT) on the inhibition of lordotic behavior in the male rat. Soc. Neurosci. Abstr. **21:** 1463.

86. FRYE, C.A., K.R. VAN KEUREN & M.S. ERSKINE. 1996. Behavioral effects of 3α-androstanediol I: Modulation of sexual receptivity and promotion of GABA-stimulated chloride flux. Behav. Brain Res. **79:** 109–118.

87. KRAULIS, I., S.J. NAISH, D. GRAVENOR & K.B. RUF. 1981. 5-androstane-3, 17-diol: inhibitor of sexual maturation in the female rat. Biol. Reprod. **24:** 445–453.

88. DIGGLE, P.J., K.-Y. LIANG & S.L. ZEGER. 1995. Analysis of Longitudinal Data. Clarendon Press. Oxford.

Differential Functions of Hypothalamic Galanin Cell Grows in the Regulation of Eating and Body Weight[a]

SARAH F. LEIBOWITZ[b]

The Rockefeller University, New York, New York 10021, USA

ABSTRACT: Evidence suggests that hypothalamic galanin (GAL) has a variety of functions related to energy and nutrient balance, reproduction, water balance, and neuroendocrine regulation. The focus of this chapter is the role of GAL in eating and body weight regulation. Findings described herein demonstrate that GAL, in a cell group of the anterior region of the paraventricular nucleus (aPVN) that projects to the median eminence, has a role in the control of fat intake, fat metabolism, and body fat. This function of aPVN GAL neurons is carried out in close relation to circulating insulin and glucose. Galanin-expressing perikarya in the medial preoptic area (MPOA) have a similar function, although GAL here operates in association with the female steroids estrogen and progesterone. These GAL cell groups of the aPVN and MPOA contrast with those in the arcuate nucleus as well as the magnocellular vasopressin-containing neurons of the PVN and supraoptic nucleus, which show no relation to fat balance. This evidence reveals differential functions for the distinct GAL neuronal cell groups of the hypothalamus.

The 29-amino acid peptide galanin (GAL) has been implicated in various neuronal processes involved in controlling different behaviors related to food ingestion and reproduction as well as endocrine and metabolic functions.[12,59,78] These functions are believed to be mediated by GAL-containing neurons in the hypothalamus. Within this structure, GAL-like immunoreactivity (ir) and GAL receptor binding are particularly dense.[12,20,75,78] Furthermore, GAL is colocalized and perhaps coreleased with a variety of other neuropeptides. These include corticotropin-releasing factor (CRF), thyrotropin-releasing hormone (TRH), gonadotropin-releasing hormone (GnRH), growth hormone-releasing hormone (GHRH), vasopressin (AVP), and oxytocin (OT), which have known functions, respectively, in activation of stress, energy metabolism, reproduction, growth, water balance, and lactation.[28,43,58,71,74,78,81] Moreover, GAL has a role in controlling the secretion of hormones from the pituitary or peripheral organs that contribute directly or indirectly to these functions. These hormones, in turn, feed back to regulate, possibly through transcriptional mechanisms, the expression of the GAL gene in the hypothalamus and pituitary.[12,75,78]

There are different GAL-expressing neuronal populations within the hypothalamus that may have different functions and therefore need to be examined individually (TABLE 1). Dense clusters of GAL-containing perikarya are found in different sections of the paraventricular nucleus (PVN), medial preoptic nucleus (MPOA), arcuate nucleus (ARC), and supraoptic nucleus (SON), amongst other areas. Each of these cell groups is known to

[a]This research was supported by US Public Health Service Grant MH43422.

[b]Address for correspondence: Dr. Sarah F. Leibowitz, The Rockefeller University, 1230 York Avenue, New York, N.Y. 10021. Phone, 212-327-8378; fax, 212-327-8447.

TABLE 1. Hypothalamic Galanin-Expressing Cell Groups

---

1. Anterior Paraventricular Nucleus (aPVN)
   - Parvocellular neurons
   - Colocalizes with corticotropin-releasing, thyrotropin-releasing hormones
   - Responsive to fat intake and fat metabolism
   - Responsive to insulin and glucose
   - Function in body fat regulation

   Posterior Paraventricular Nucleus
   - Magnocellular neurons
   - Colocalizes with vasopressin
   - Function in water balance

2. Medial Preoptic Nucleus (MPOA)
   - Colocalizes with gonadotropin-releasing hormone
   - Responsive to dietary fat
   - Responsive to progesterone and estrogen
   - Function in body fat regulation

3. Arcuate Nucleus (ARC)
   - Colocalizes with growth hormone-releasing hormone
   - Responsive to growth hormone
   - Function in growth

4. Supraoptic Nucleus (SON)
   - Magnocellular neurons
   - Colocalizes with vasopressin
   - Function in water balance

---

project fibers to the median eminence (ME), which are well situated to control pituitary function.[20,75,83] They also exhibit different patterns of peptide colocalization, with examples given in TABLE 1.

This chapter describes evidence that argues for diverse roles of these different hypothalamic cell groups in eating and body weight regulation. The focus is on the GAL subgroups in the PVN and MPOA, which are closely related to energy and nutrient balance, both its behavioral and its metabolic aspects. The effects of GAL on these functions, and the feedback of certain hormones on GAL production, are reviewed. Changes in GAL, hormones, and eating behavior are also considered in relation to natural biologic rhythms, as well as in pathologic states of obesity and diabetes. Evidence is described suggesting a specific role for GAL, synthesized in PVN and MPOA perikarya that project to the ME, in processes related to fat intake, fat metabolism, and body fat (TABLE 1).

POSITIVE FEEDBACK LOOP BETWEEN GALANIN AND FAT INTAKE

Pharmacologic studies provided the first evidence that GAL has a role in energy and nutrient balance. Injections of GAL into the hypothalamus stimulate feeding behavior[34,56,93] and specifically the consumption of fat and carbohydrate.[29,108] They also reduce energy expenditure[76] and sympathetic nervous system activity.[80] Whereas the stimulatory effect of GAL is particularly strong in the medial hypothalamus,[57] other sites in the brain, including the hindbrain, are also responsive to this peptide.[33,55]

Further studies of endogenous GAL support a close relation between GAL and dietary fat. In rats given a free choice of pure macronutrient diets, GAL gene expression in the PVN and GAL fiber density in the ME are positively related to the animals' natural preference for fat.[2,61] In fat-preferring rats, levels of GAL mRNA and peptide immunoreactivity (ir) are considerably higher specifically in the anterior parvocellular region of the PVN (aPVN) as opposed to other hypothalamic sites such as the MPOA or ARC. These functional studies, together with anatomic evidence,[75,78] support the existence of a parvocellular aPVN cell group that projects to the external zone of the ME and functions in close relation to dietary fat. This contrasts with the magnocellular GAL-containing neurons, in a more posterior region of the PVN, that send projections to the internal zone of the ME on their course to the posterior pituitary.[75] This cell group has a known function in water balance[101] but appears unrelated to dietary fat.[61,125]

This projection from the aPVN to the ME, related to a rat's natural selection of fat in a choice situation, is also stimulated in rats with no opportunity to choose but maintained, instead, on a single diet rich in fat.[61] This indicates that the relation between GAL and fat reflects, in part, an effect of the diet itself on this GAL projection. The precise amount of fat is clearly important in this response. Whereas a 30% fat diet compared to a 10% fat diet stimulates GAL gene expression but not peptide production, a further rise in dietary fat above 30% increases the synthesis as well as release of GAL.[61]

Pharmacologic studies suggest that exogenous GAL may, in turn, affect fat ingestion. In rats given a choice of macronutrient diets, hypothalamic injection of GAL in satiated animals stimulates the ingestion of both fat and carbohydrate, while having no impact on protein intake.[29,103,108] Whereas the effect of GAL may shift in relation to the rats' natural preference for these two macronutrients,[103] a preferential change in fat intake is suggested by a number of findings. In particular, GAL produces a stronger and more prolonged feeding response in subgroups or strains of rats that naturally prefer fat, and it has a greater effect in rats tested on a high-fat compared to a low-fat diet.[13,67,110] Moreover, hypothalamic injections of a GAL receptor antagonist[33,62] or of antisense oligonucleotides to GAL mRNA which reduce GAL levels in the PVN[2] produce a marked suppression of spontaneous fat ingestion. The intestinal peptide enterostatin, which is synthesized in proportion to the amount of fat ingested and selectively reduces fat intake,[35] has a potent inhibitory effect on GAL-stimulated feeding.[66] This pentapeptide, however, has relatively little impact on the feeding response elicited by neuropeptide Y (NPY), which in contrast to GAL preferentially stimulates the intake of carbohydrate.[104]

This biochemical and pharmacologic evidence indicates that endogenous GAL, specifically in the aPVN and ME, is part of a positive feedback loop related to dietary fat. In this loop, GAL stimulates the ingestion of a nutrient which further enhances the endogenous activity of this peptide. The possibility exists that this feedback loop mediates the stimulatory effect of dietary fat on total caloric intake.[85,113] The introduction of a diet with increasing fat content produces hyperphagia during the initial 7–10 days of diet presentation,[61,119] and it increases the size of individual meals.[99,122] This response, possibly due to increased diet palatability[88] and reduced satiating capacity of fat,[99,122] may involve GAL neurons in the PVN. This idea is supported by the finding that the range of fat critical to the hyperphagia, above 30%, is the same as that needed to potentiate GAL peptide synthesis and release in the PVN, along with GAL peptide-ir in the ME.[61]

CIRCULATING HORMONES AND GLUCOSE IN RELATION TO GALANIN

The enhanced activity of the aPVN-ME GAL projection produced by a fat-rich diet may be attributed, in part, to associated changes in circulating hormones or glucose. For example, levels of insulin and CORT are generally lower on a high-fat diet.[19,32,61,119] This endocrine pattern may contribute to the overexpression of GAL, because both hormones are known to reduce GAL gene expression in the PVN.[42,107,120] Their endogenous levels are also inversely related to PVN GAL in diabetic as well as intact rats.[2,6,107,120]

The inhibitory effect observed with insulin is particularly potent and evident in the PVN. When centrally injected, this hormone markedly suppresses GAL mRNA and peptide production in intact rats, and when given peripherally, it effectively reverses the enhanced GAL activity observed in diabetic rats.[107,120] *In vitro*, insulin also reduces K^+-evoked GAL release from a mediodorsal hypothalamic section containing the PVN, and it suppresses basal GAL release from cultures of neonatal rat hypothalamic cells.[120] Thus, insulin may act directly on PVN GAL neurons, perhaps through the relatively high concentration of insulin receptor binding sites in this hypothalamic nucleus.[95,114]

Disturbances in circulating glucose levels may also contribute to the diet-induced enhancement of PVN GAL, possibly through glucose-sensitive neurons in the PVN.[82] When animals are on a 60% fat diet compared to a 30% one, glucose levels rise significantly, along with GAL.[19,54,61] Moreover, a strong positive correlation is readily detected between blood glucose, PVN GAL gene expression, and the amount of fat ingested.[61,119] This change in glucose may reflect either the development of insulin resistance, commonly associated with a high-fat diet,[94] or a change in circulating levels of the glucoregulatory hormones insulin or glucagon. Consistent with their lower concentration in a high-fat diet condition as just described, insulin levels are reduced by GAL injection in the PVN,[109] similar to its effect in the pancreas,[68] whereas insulin is enhanced by PVN injection of antisense oligonucleotides to GAL mRNA.[2] Moreover, pancreatic GAL stimulates the release of glucagon, which itself raises glucose levels in the blood.[1] Thus, the increase in hypothalamic GAL associated with a high-fat diet, in addition to being a consequence of endocrine changes and disturbances in glucose metabolism, may also serve to exacerbate the physiologic as well as the behavioral effects of dietary fat.

This association between PVN GAL neurons and circulating insulin may reflect their opposing functions in relation to nutrient consumption and metabolism. As just indicated, GAL is a stimulant of feeding and an inhibitor of metabolism; it increases the ingestion of fat and reduces energy expenditure as well as sympathetic nerve activity in brown adipose tissue.[62,76,80] Conversely, insulin acts centrally to inhibit food intake, preferentially fat consumption, and to enhance energy expenditure.[31,95] Analyses of freely feeding animals on macronutrient diets support this opposing relation, revealing an inverse correlation between these parameters across the natural diurnal cycle, specifically at the onset of spontaneous eating,[2,6] and a positive relation between PVN GAL mRNA or peptide-ir and the ingestion of fat.[61]

A disturbance of this balance in diabetic animals, resulting in enhanced GAL production,[107,120] may contribute to these animals' strong preference for fat-rich foods to avoid carbohydrates.[50] A similar imbalance may exist in genetically obese rats, which exhibit increased hypothalamic GAL mRNA[77] and PVN GAL peptide levels,[15] reduced responsiveness to insulin,[95] and a strong preference for dietary fat.[27,89] Whereas the direct cause of these disturbances in hypothalamic GAL remains to be determined, the findings that circulating glucose is a close correlate of aPVN GAL mRNA or peptide-ir[61] specifically on a high-fat diet, and that this correlation is also evident in relation to body fat,[61,119] argues for the responsiveness of aPVN GAL neurons to fat-induced changes in glucose metabolism in peripheral tissue and perhaps within the PVN itself.

DIURNAL RHYTHMS OF GALANIN, HORMONES, AND SPONTANEOUS EATING BEHAVIOR

In relation to the light/dark cycle, there exists a rhythm of nutrient intake and metabolism.[8,59,100,110] Subsequent to a period of little eating resulting in low carbohydrate stores, the early hours of the feeding cycle are characterized by a strong preference for carbohydrate; they are then followed by a rise in fat consumption 3–4 hours later. This behavioral shift, from carbohydrate-rich meals to fat-rich meals, is accompanied by metabolic shifts. These involve gluconeogenesis, glycogenolysis and then increased respiratory quotient early in the feeding cycle, followed by reduced insulin sensitivity and increased fat deposition during the later hours of the cycle.

In association with these rhythms of behavioral and physiologic responses are diurnal rhythms in the hypothalamic peptides that are distinct and anatomically localized. For GAL, levels of this peptide rise towards the middle of the nocturnal feeding cycle, between the 3rd and 6th hours, and this rise is detected specifically in the PVN.[6] This delayed peak occurs around the same time as the spontaneous increase in the animals' ingestion of fat.[100] It is also associated with a gradual decline in insulin levels and insulin sensitivity that occurs over the course of the feeding cycle.[65] In two separate studies, an inverse relation is found to exist between PVN GAL and insulin levels, seen across the light/dark cycle[6] and in animals on macronutrient diets.[2]

This pattern for endogenous GAL is very different from that observed with the feeding-stimulatory peptide NPY, which is expressed in neurons of the ARC.[9] In contrast to GAL, this peptide preferentially increases the ingestion of carbohydrate rather than fat.[104] In the hypothalamus, a rise in NPY mRNA occurs in the ARC, but not other sites, a few hours before feeding onset; this is followed by increased peptide synthesis and peptide levels at the start of the feeding cycle, specifically in the PVN to which the ARC neurons project.[3,44] This peak in NPY gene expression and peptide-ir, seen earlier than that of GAL, occurs at a time when carbohydrate is the preferred macronutrient[3,100] and insulin levels and sensitivity to insulin are greatest.[65] This carbohydrate preference, along with the rise in NPY, is closely linked to circulating levels of CORT.[3,110] This steroid stimulates the gene expression and production of NPY.[5,59,73,110] However, it has only a weak inhibitory effect on GAL in the PVN,[4,42] underscoring the differences between these peptides.

HYPOTHALAMIC GALANIN IN RELATION TO FAT METABOLISM

Information on the metabolic mechanisms controlling GAL production should help to elucidate the functional role of this peptide in eating and body weight regulation. Recent results[118] demonstrate that hypothalamic GAL is responsive to injection of the antimetabolite mercaptoacetate (MA), a selective inhibitor of fatty acid oxidation.[14] The expression and production of GAL, specifically in the PVN, are suppressed by MA but are unaffected by another antimetabolite, 2-deoxy-D-glucose (2-DG), which blocks glucose utilization.[25]

The reduction in GAL after MA injection suggests that this peptide may be activated, under normal conditions, by signals related to fatty acid oxidation. This idea is consistent with the finding that GAL gene expression and peptide-ir are stimulated by consumption of a high-fat diet,[61] which enhances the oxidation of fatty acids.[36,112,121] Whereas the signal of fatty acid oxidation may originate in peripheral tissues,[86] metabolic events within the hypothalamus, perhaps having direct impact on local GAL neurons, may also be involved.[121]

The importance of fat metabolism to PVN GAL expression is underscored by the finding that GAL shows no change in response to injections of 2-DG.[118] This is diametrically opposite to the pattern observed with NPY in the ARC-PVN projection, which is potentiated by 2-DG injection but not affected by MA.[7,79] The NPY system, opposite to that observed with GAL, shows greatest activity in animals consuming a high-carbohydrate diet and can actually be suppressed by the ingestion of dietary fat.[39,45,117] Thus, the signals controlling these two peptide systems are clearly different, suggesting that their physiologic functions may also differ.

With GAL, an effect opposite to that of MA is observed in animals exposed to food deprivation, which enhances GAL gene expression and peptide production in the PVN.[118] This effect is highly localized, it is detected specifically in the aPVN, and it may be attributed to a deprivation-induced increase in fatty acid metabolism in the brain.[53] In addition to being anatomically localized, the change in GAL is relatively small, a 10–30% increase in peptide level, possibly explaining the inconclusive results obtained to date in food-deprived rats.[7,11,15,22,24,46] This response can, once again, be contrasted with that observed with NPY in the ARC-PVN projection, which is more dramatically increased by food deprivation.[49,96] This result underscores the differences between these two peptide systems and the metabolic and hormonal signals to which they respond.[59]

Additional investigations suggest that the changes in endogenous GAL, produced by blockade of fatty acid metabolism and by food deprivation,[118] have functional consequences in relation to nutrient ingestion. Behavioral analyses show that MA injection causes a reduction in fat intake,[118] possibly resulting from the animals' inability to metabolize fat. This effect may be mediated by the associated reduction in GAL mRNA and peptide levels in the aPVN,[118] and it is in direct contrast to the stimulatory effect of 2-DG on the ingestion of carbohydrate, linked to an increase in NPY.[7,51,79,118] These behavioral and biochemical effects of MA can be likened to those of insulin, which reduces fat ingestion and GAL activity in the PVN.[31,107,120] Moreover, they can be contrasted to those observed in diabetic animals, which involve an increase in GAL activity along with a strong preference for fat-rich foods.[50,107,120]

Whereas the deprivation-induced stimulation of GAL and NPY may result, in part, from a reduction in insulin levels,[91,95,107,120,123] the marked difference in the magnitude of their response to food deprivation is very likely attributed to fundamental differences in their relation to fat and carbohydrate metabolism, respectively. Carbohydrate stores are the first to be depleted by deprivation, declining rapidly within hours; this is in contrast to fat stores, which are much larger in capacity and are affected in a more gradual manner.[37] Thus, the greater enhancement of NPY seen with deprivation is very likely related to this peptide's responsiveness to disturbances in carbohydrate metabolism.[7,79,117] The smaller GAL response, in contrast, may reflect changes in fat stores and fat metabolism.[61,118] It is likely that the rise in GAL and NPY in the PVN after deprivation may contribute to the compensatory feeding, of fat more than of carbohydrate, observed when the macronutrient diets are restored.[17,98,111]

HYPOTHALAMIC GALANIN AND ADIPOSITY

In addition to their association with fat intake and fat metabolism, the aPVN-ME GAL projection may contribute to the increase in body weight and adiposity that is invariably produced by a high-fat diet.[21,92] This is supported by pharmacologic studies showing GAL injections to reduce energy expenditure[76] and sympathetic nervous system activity.[80] Moreover, repeated PVN injections of GAL antisense oligonucleotides, which suppress GAL production, reduce body weight.[2] Whereas one report with repeated ventricular injections of GAL failed to demonstrate an increase in body weight,[102] a recent study demonstrated that injections of GAL directly into the PVN can increase both food intake and body fat, while causing little change in body weight.[126] This effect is evident with daily GAL injections during the natural feeding cycle and only in rats maintained on a high-fat diet (> 30% fat).

Analyses of endogenous GAL provide further support for a close relation between this peptide and body fat. Hypothalamic expression of GAL is enhanced in genetically obese rats.[15,46,77] It is also increased in normal-weight rats that have a greater propensity to gain weight and show greater adiposity with the macronutrient diets.[61] The dual stimulatory effect of a high-fat diet on body fat and GAL production suggests that these parameters may be closely linked specifically under conditions of high dietary fat. With a high-fat diet, but not a low-fat diet, strong positive correlations can be detected between GAL and body fat pad weights and also between GAL and glucose levels which, in turn, are closely reflective of adiposity as well as insulin resistance.[40,61] With measurements of circulating peptides, a recent clinical study reported higher concentrations of GAL, as well as NPY, in the plasma of women with moderate and severe obesity.[10]

In light of this relation between hypothalamic GAL and body fat, it is not surprising that GAL neurons are also a target for circulating leptin. This hormone, a product of the *ob* gene, is synthesized in adipose tissue and believed to act directly on leptin receptors in the PVN, ARC, and other hypothalamic areas.[41] This hormone, which reduces eating behavior and body weight,[26,84,127] was first shown to decrease NPY gene expression in obese and lean mice.[87,106] In subsequent studies, a similar effect of leptin on GAL was observed with measurements of GAL expression and production in the whole hypothalamus[90] or specifically the PVN.[63] As with insulin (see above), this leptin-induced reduction in GAL and NPY may be involved in the inhibitory effect of this hormone on fat and carbohydrate ingestion.[16]

RHYTHMS OF GALANIN, STEROIDS, AND EATING BEHAVIOR
ACROSS THE ESTROUS CYCLE

Recent studies in adult female rats reveal similarities and differences to male rats in the GAL system as it relates to eating patterns and body weight. This is demonstrated through analyses across the estrous cycle which, along with the gonadal steroids and eating behavior, reveal clear shifts in GAL in three specific areas. These are the aPVN and ME, which are functional in the male as well as female rat, and the MPOA, which is responsive only in females.

Several studies have demonstrated cycle-related changes in GAL within specific areas, with peaks during the proestrous period.[48,60,69,72,78] This pattern is seen in the MPOA and ME and, more recently, was detected in the aPVN.[60] As expected based on published studies,[48] the gonadal steroids E_2 and PROG also rise during proestrous, and correlational analyses reveal significant associations with GAL.[60] In particular, a consistent positive relation is seen between circulating PROG and levels of GAL in the MPOA, PVN, and ME. Interestingly, this association is evident primarily during the proestrous period, when both the steroid and peptide are most active and are likely to functionally interact. Whereas E_2 is known to stimulate GAL in several areas, including the MPOA, PVN, and ME, in addition to the anterior pituitary,[18,38,52,70,72] PROG in E_2-primed rats produces a further enhancement of GAL in the hypothalamus and pituitary[23] and specifically the MPOA.[64] Gonadal steroid receptors and GAL neurons are concentrated and possibly coexist in these areas.[78]

Considerable evidence exists for a shift in eating behavior across the female cycle, showing a decline during the estrous phase.[60,116,124] This has been confirmed in a recent report which additionally reveals, with macronutrient diets, a specific reduction in fat ingestion during estrous.[60] This effect may be attributed, in part, to the sharp decline in GAL levels in the PVN, in addition to the MPOA which may also have a role in feeding and energy metabolism.[47,59] During the proestrous stage, in contrast, the rats' preference for dietary fat increases, followed by a rise in fat pad weights before the start of estrous.[60] In prior studies, measures of body weight have revealed greatest weight gain during diestrous and proestrous.[115,116]

RELATION OF GALANIN AND STEROIDS TO FAT INTAKE
AND BODY FAT IN FEMALES

As just described, investigations in male rats have demonstrated a strong relation between fat intake or body fat and GAL specifically in the aPVN and ME, but not in any other hypothalamic area. In female rats as in males, GAL in the aPVN and ME is also related to the ingestion of fat.[60] This is seen in analyses of rats showing differential preferences for dietary fat and also across the estrous cycle which temporally links GAL and fat ingestion with simultaneous peaks during proestrous. Of particular note, however, are the results obtained in the MPOA. In females, this area is similar to the aPVN in its relation to fat ingestion; however, this pattern is not seen in males.[2,61,63] Similar to the aPVN, levels of the peptide in the MPOA are positively correlated with fat consumption, and they exhibit a rise during proestrous when dietary fat is naturally preferred.[60]

The additional involvement of the gonadal steroids, in particular PROG, in this relationship between hypothalamic GAL, fat intake, and adiposity is indicated by several findings.[60,64] Injections of PROG in E_2-primed ovariectomized (OVX) rats stimulate GAL gene expression in the MPOA,[78] suggesting that PROG may mediate the rise in GAL in this area observed in fat-preferring rats. This is supported by the additional evidence that PROG has a stimulatory effect on food intake in E_2-primed OVX rats.[105,116] Comparisons between female rats of differential body weight show that the heavier subjects with greater body fat, compared to lean rats, have higher circulating levels of PROG, despite similar patterns of fat intake.[60] These heavier rats also have higher levels of GAL in the MPOA, which are positively correlated with body fat. Thus, in addition to the behavioral process of fat ingestion, peptide level in the MPOA is related to adiposity in female subjects but not in males. The involvement of PROG in this relationship is supported by published evidence showing its stimulatory effect on lipogenesis and body fat and an inhibitory effect on fat oxidation.[97,105,116] This steroid, through its impact on GAL projections, may be involved in the normal shift in eating and body weight across the estrous cycle. It may also have a role in the development of obesity in female subjects consuming a high-fat diet.

DIFFERENTIAL FUNCTIONS OF HYPOTHALAMIC GALANIN-EXPRESSING CELL GROUPS

The evidence described herein clearly differentiates certain GAL cell groups in the hypothalamus, suggesting that they have different functions in eating and body weight regulation (TABLE 1). The GAL neurons in the aPVN clearly differ from the magnocellular neurons in the more posterior region of the PVN and exhibit both similarities and differences when compared to the GAL-containing neurons of the MPOA. These cell groups are differentiated in relation to their biologic rhythms, which presumably reflect their different responses to peptide and steroid hormones, diet, metabolic challenges, and body fat.

Other areas of the hypothalamus have dense concentrations of GAL-containing cell groups and fibers (TABLE 1). These include the ARC and SON.[12,20,75,78] These two areas in the male rat show weaker effects or no change in response to injections of MA, insulin, or gonadal steroids and are unaffected by the consumption of a high-fat diet or by food deprivation.[2,60,61,107,118,120] One possible explanation is that these areas are less accessible to circulating hormones and nutrients, or they may contain lower concentrations of receptors responsive to these hormones or metabolic signals.

This evidence underscores the anatomic specificity of GAL's action in the hypothalamus (TABLE 1). It converges on the aPVN as being uniquely responsive to signals related to fat intake and fat metabolism, working in conjunction with circulating insulin, glucose, and perhaps CORT. This is in contrast to the MPOA, where GAL functions predominantly in female rats, along with E_2 and PROG, to control fat balance and adiposity. Galanin in the ARC, which is unaffected by fat diet or manipulations of fat metabolism,[61,118] is known to coexist with GHRH in GAL-synthesizing neurons[81] and to be stimulated by GH administration,[30] suggesting its possible role in controlling body growth. Finally, PVN and SON magnocellular neurons, that express GAL together with AVP,[58] may have a function in relation to water balance.[43,101]

ACKNOWLEDGMENTS

I am grateful to Laurie Castellanos for her excellent technical assistance in the preparation of this manuscript.

REFERENCES

1. AHREN, B. & S. LINDSKOG. 1992. Galanin and the regulation of islet hormone secretion. Int. J. Pancreatol. **11:** 147–160.
2. AKABAYASHI, A., J.I. KOENIG, Y. WATANABE, J.T. ALEXANDER & S.F. LEIBOWITZ. 1994. Galanin-containing neurons in the paraventricular nucleus: A neurochemical marker for fat ingestion and body weight gain. Proc. Natl. Acad. Sci. USA **91:** 10375–10379.
3. AKABAYASHI, A., N. LEVIN, X. PAEZ, J.T. ALEXANDER & S.F. LEIBOWITZ. 1994. Hypothalamic neuropeptide Y and its gene expression: Relation to light/dark cycle and circulating corticosterone. Molec. & Cell. Neurosci. **5:** 210–218.
4. AKABAYASHI, A., Y. WATANABE, S.M. GABRIEL, H.J. CHAE & S.F. LEIBOWITZ. 1994. Hypothalamic galanin-like immunoreactivity and its gene expression in relation to circulating corticosterone. Molec. Brain Res. **25:** 305–312.
5. AKABAYASHI, A., Y. WATANABE, C. WAHLESTEDT, B.S. MCEWEN, X. PAEZ & S.F. LEIBOWITZ. 1994. Hypothalamic neuropeptide Y, its gene expression and receptor activity: Relation to circulating corticosterone in adrenalectomized rats. Brain Res. **665:** 201–212.
6. AKABAYASHI, A., C.T. ZAIA, J.I. KOENIG, S.M. GABRIEL, I. SILVA & S.F. LEIBOWITZ. 1994. Diurnal rhythm of galanin-like immunoreactivity in the paraventricular and suprachiasmatic nuclei and other hypothalamic areas. Peptides **15:** 1437–1444.
7. AKABAYASHI, A., C.T. ZAIA, I. SILVA, H.J. CHAE & S.F. LEIBOWITZ. 1993. Neuropeptide Y in the arcuate nucleus is modulated by alterations in glucose utilization. Brain Res. **621:** 343–348.
8. ARMSTRONG, S.A. 1980. A chronometric approach to the study of feeding behavior. Neurosci. Biobehav. Rev. **4:** 27–53.
9. BAI, F.L., M. YAMANO, Y. SHIOTANI, P.C. EMSON, A.D. SMITH, J.F. POWELL & M. TOHYAMA. 1985. An arcuato-paraventricular and -dorsomedial hypothalamic neuropeptide Y-containing system which lacks noradrenaline in the rat. Brain Res. **331:** 172–175.
10. BARANOWSKA, B., E. WASILEWSKA-DZIUBINSKA, M. RADZIKOWSKA, A. PTONOWSKI & K. ROGUSKI. 1997. Neuropeptide Y, galanin, and leptin release in obese women and in women with anorexia nervosa. Metabolism **46:** 1384–1389.
11. BARKER-GIBB, M.L. & I.J. CLARKE. 1996. Increased galanin and neuropeptide-Y immunoreactivity within the hypothalamus of ovariectomised ewes following a prolonged period of reduced body weight is associated with changes in plasma growth hormone but not gonadotropin levels. Neuroendocrinology **64:** 194–207.
12. BARTFAI, T., T. HOKFELT & U. LANGEL. 1993. Galanin—a neuroendocrine peptide. Crit. Rev. Neurobiol. **7:** 229–274.
13. BARTON, C., L. LIN, D.A. YORK & G.A. BRAY. 1995. Differential effects of enterostatin, galanin and opioids on high-fat diet consumption. Brain Res. **702:** 55–60.
14. BAUCHE, F., D. SABOURAULT, Y. GIUDICELLI, J. NORDMANN & R. NORDMANN. 1983. Inhibition in vitro of acyl-CoA dehydrogenases by 2-mercaptoacetate in rat liver mitochondria. Biochem. J. **215:** 457–464.
15. BECK, B., A. BURLET, J.P. NICOLAS & C. BURLET. 1993. Galanin in the hypothalamus of fed and fasted lean and obese Zucker rats. Brain Res. **623:** 124–130.
16. BEDRIN, Z.U., J.T. ALEXANDER, A. MANITIU, R. YUN, & S.F. LEIBOWITZ. 1996. Relationship between leptin and ingestion of macronutrients. Obes. Res. **4:** 42S (Abstract).
17. BERNARDINI, J., K. KAMARA & T.W. CASTONGUAY. 1993. Macronutrient choice following food deprivation: Effect of dietary fat dilution. Brain Res. Bull. **32:** 543–548.
18. BLOCH, G.J., C. ECKERSELL & R. MILLS. 1993. Distribution of galanin-immunoreactive cells within sexually dimorphic components of the medial preoptic area of the male and female rat. Brain Res. **620:** 259–268.
19. BOIVIN, A. & Y. DESHAIES. 1995. Dietary rat models in which the development of hypertriglyceridemia and that of insulin resistance are dissociated. Metabolism **44:** 1540–1547.
20. BONNEFOND, C., J.M. PALACIOS, A. PROBST & G. MENGOD. 1997. Distribution of galanin mRNA containing cells and galanin receptor binding sites in human and rat hypothalamus. Eur. J. Neurosci. **2:** 629–637.
21. BOOZER, C.N., G. SCHOENBACH & R.L. ATKINSON. 1995. Dietary fat and adiposity: A dose-response relationship in adult male rats fed isocalorically. Am. J. Physiol. **268:** (Pt 1): E546–550.

22. BRADY, L.S., M.A. SMITH, P.W. GOLD & M. HERKENHAM. 1990. Altered expression of hypotha-lamic neuropeptide mRNAs in food-restricted and food-deprived rats. Neuroendocrinology **52:** 441–447.
23. BRANN, D.W., L.P. CHORICH & V.B. MAHESH. 1993. Effect of progesterone on galanin mRNA levels in the hypothalamus and the pituitary: Correlation with the gonadotropin surge. Neu-roendocrinology **58:** 531–538.
24. BROGAN, R.S., S.K. FIFE, L.K. CONLEY, A. GIUSTINA & W.B. WEHRENBERG. 1997. Effects of food deprivation on the GH axis: Immunocytochemical and molecular analysis. Neuroendocrinol-ogy **65:** 129–135.
25. BROWN, J. 1962. Effects of 2-deoxy-D-glucose on carbohydrate metabolism: Review of the liter-ature and studies in the rat. Metabolism **11:** 1098–1112.
26. CAMPFIELD, L.A., F.J. SMITH, Y. GUISEZ, R. DEVOS & P. BURN. 1995. Recombinant mouse OB pro-tein: Evidence for a peripheral signal linking adiposity and central neural networks. Science **269:** 546–549.
27. CASTONGUAY, T.W., W.J. HARTMAN, E.A. FITZPATRICK & J.S. STERN. 1982. Dietary self-selection and the Zucker rat. J. Nutr. **112:** 796–800.
28. CECCATELLI, S., L. GIARDINO & L. CALZA. 1992. Response of hypothalamic peptide mRNAs to thyroidectomy. Neuroendocrinology **56:** 694–703.
29. CHAE, H.J., B.G. HOEBEL, D.L. TEMPEL, M. PAREDES & S.F. LEIBOWITZ. 1995. Neuropeptide-Y, galanin and opiate agonists have differential effects on nutrient ingestion. Soc. Neurosci. Abstr. **21:** 696.
30. CHAN, Y.Y., E. GRAFSTEIN-DUNN, H.A. DELEMARRE-VAN DE WAAL, K.A. BURTON, D.K. CLIFTON & R.A. STEINER. 1996. The role of galanin and its receptor in the feedback regulation of growth hormone secretion. Endocrinology **137:** 5303–5310.
31. CHAVEZ, M., C.A. RIEDY, G. VAN DIJK & S.C. WOODS. 1996. Central insulin and macronutrient intake in the rat. Am. J. Physiol. **271:** R727–731.
32. CHICCO, A., M.E. D'ALESSANDRO, L. KARABATAS, R. GUTMAN & Y.B. LOMBARDO. 1996. Effect of moderate levels of dietary fish oil on insulin secretion and sensitivity, and pancreas insulin content in normal rats. Ann. Nutr. Metab. **40:** 61–70.
33. CORWIN, R.L., J.K. ROBINSON & J.N. CRAWLEY. 1993. Galanin antagonists block galanin-induced feeding in the hypothalamus and amygdala of the rat. Eur. J. Neurosci. **5:** 1528–1533.
34. CRAWLEY, J.N., M.C. AUSTIN, S.M. FISKE, B. MARTIN, S. CONSOLO, M. BERTHOLD, U. LANGEL, G. FISONE & T. BARTFAI. 1990. Activity of centrally administered galanin fragments on stimula-tion of feeding behavior and on galanin receptor binding in the rat hypothalamus. J. Neurosci. **10:** 3695–3700.
35. ERLANSON-ALBERTSSON, C. & D. YORK. 1997. Enterostatin - A peptide regulating fat intake. Obes. Res. **5:** 360–372.
36. FLATT, J.P. 1987. The difference in the storage capacities for carbohydrate and for fat, and its implications in the regulation of body weight. Ann. N.Y. Acad. Sci. **499:** 104–123.
37. FLATT, J.P. 1996. The RQ/FQ concept and weight maintenance. *In* Progress in Obesity Research. A. Angel, H. Anderson, C. Bouchard D. Lau, L. Leiter & R. Mendelson, Eds.: 49–66. John Libbey & Co. London.
38. GABRIEL, S.M., J.I. KOENIG & D.L. WASHTON. 1993. Estrogen stimulation of galanin gene expres-sion and galanin-like immunoreactivity in the rat and its blockade by the estrogen antagonist keoxifene (LY156758). Regul. Pept. **45:** 407–419.
39. GIRAUDO, S.Q., C.M. KOTZ, M.K. GRACE, A.S. LEVINE & C.J. BILLINGTON. 1994. Rat hypotha-lamic NPY mRNA and brown fat uncoupling protein mRNA after high-carbohydrate or high-fat diets. Am. J. Physiol. **266:** R1578–1583.
40. GOLAY, A. & E. BOBBIONI. 1998. The role of dietary fat in obesity. Int. J. Obesity **21:** S2–S11.
41. HAKANSSON, M., H. BROWN, N. GHILARDI, R.C. SKODA & B. MEISTER. 1998. Leptin receptor immunoreactivity in chemically defined target neurons of the hypothalamus. J. Neurosci. **18:** 559–572.
42. HEDLUND, P.B., J.I. KOENIG & K. FUXE. 1994. Adrenalectomy alters discrete galanin mRNA lev-els in the hypothalamus and mesencephalon of the rat. Neurosci. Lett. **170:** 77–82.
43. HOKFELT, T., T. BARTFAI, D.M. JACOBOWITZ & D. OTTOSON. 1991. Galanin- A New Multifunc-tional Peptide in the Neuro-endocrine System. Macmillan Academic and Professional LTD. Houndsmills, Basingstoke, Hampshire.

44. JHANWAR-UNIYAL, M., B. BECK, C. BURLET & S.F. LEIBOWITZ. 1990. Diurnal rhythm of neuropeptide Y-like immunoreactivity in the suprachiasmatic, arcuate and paraventricular nuclei and other hypothalamic sites. Brain Res. **536:** 331–334.

45. JHANWAR-UNIYAL, M., B. BECK, Y.S. JHANWAR, C. BURLET & S.F. LEIBOWITZ. 1993. Neuropeptide Y projection from arcuate nucleus to parvocellular division of paraventricular nucleus: Specific relation to the ingestion of carbohydrate. Brain Res. **631:** 97–106.

46. JHANWAR-UNIYAL, M. & S.C. CHUA, JR. 1993. Critical effects of aging and nutritional state on hypothalamic neuropeptide Y and galanin gene expression in lean and genetically obese Zucker rats. Molec. Brain Res. **19:** 195–202.

47. JOLICOEUR, F.B., S.M. BOUALI, A. FOURNIER & S. ST-PIERRE. 1995. Mapping of hypothalamic sites involved in the effects of NPY on body temperature and food intake. Brain Res. Bull. **36:** 125–129.

48. KALRA, S.P. & W.R. CROWLEY. 1992. Neuropeptide Y: A novel neuroendocrine peptide in the control of pituitary hormone secretion, and its relation to luteinizing hormone. Front. Neuroendocrinol. **13:** 1–46.

49. KALRA, S.P. & P.S. KALRA. 1997. Neuropeptide Y - A novel peptidergic signal for the control of feeding behavior. *In* Current Topics in Neuroendocriology. D.W. Pfaff and D. Ganten, Eds. :192–217. Springer-Verlag. Berlin.

50. KANAREK, R.B. & L. HO. 1984. Patterns of nutrient selection in rats with streptozotocin-induced diabetes. Physiol. Behav. **32:** 639–645.

51. KANAREK, R.B., R. MARKS-KAUFMAN, R. RUTHAZER & L. GUALTIERI. 1983. Increased carbohydrate consumption by rats as a function of 2-deoxy-D-glucose administration. Pharmacol. Biochem. Behav. **18:** 47–50.

52. KAPLAN, L.M., S.M. GABRIEL, J.I. KOENIG, M.E. SUNDAY, E.R. SPINDEL, J.B. MARTIN & W.W. CHIN. 1988. Galanin is an estrogen-inducible, secretory product of the rat anterior pituitary. Proc. Natl. Acad. Sci. USA **85:** 7408–7412.

53. KASSER, T.R., R.B. HARRIS & R.J. MARTIN. 1989. Level of satiety: In vitro energy metabolism in brain during hypophagic and hyperphagic body weight recovery. Am. J. Physiol. **257:** R1322–1327.

54. KIM, Y., S. IWASHITA, T. TAMURA, K. TOKUYAMA & M. SUZUKI. 1995. Effect of high-fat diet on the gene expression of pancreatic GLUT2 and glucokinase in rats. Biochem. Biophys. Res. Commun. **208:** 1092–1098.

55 KOEGLER, F.H. & S. RITTER. 1996. Feeding induced by pharmacological blockade of fatty acid metabolism is selectively attenuated by hindbrain injections of the galanin receptor antagonist, M40. Obes. Res. **4:** 329–336.

56. KYRKOULI, S.E., B.G. STANLEY & S.F. LEIBOWITZ. 1986. Galanin: Stimulation of feeding induced by medial hypothalamic injection of this novel peptide. Eur. J. Pharmacol. **122:** 159–160.

57. KYRKOULI, S.E., B.G. STANLEY, R.D. SEIRAFI & S.F. LEIBOWITZ. 1990. Stimulation of feeding by galanin: Anatomical localization and behavioral specificity of this peptide's effects in the brain. Peptides **11:** 995–1001.

58. LANDRY, M., D. ROCHE, E. ANGELOVA & A. CALAS. 1997. Expression of galanin in the hypothalamic magnocellular neurones of lactating rats: co-existence with vasopressin and oxytocin. J. Endocrinol. **155:** 467–481.

59. LEIBOWITZ, S.F. 1995. Brain peptides and obesity: Pharmacologic treatment. Obes. Res. 3 (Suppl 4): 573S–589S.

60. LEIBOWITZ, S.F., A. AKABAYASHI, J.T. ALEXANDER & J. WANG. 1998. Gonadal steroids and hypothalamic galanin and neuropeptide Y: Role in eating behavior and body weight control in female rats. Endocrinology **139:** 1771–1780.

61. LEIBOWITZ, S.F., A. AKABAYASHI & J. WANG. 1998. Obesity on a high-fat diet: role of hypothalamic galanin in neurons of the anterior paraventricular nucleus projecting to the median eminence. J. Neurosci. **18:** 2709–2719.

62. LEIBOWITZ, S.F. & T. KIM. 1992. Impact of a galanin antagonist on exogenous galanin and natural patterns of fat ingestion. Brain Res. **599:** 148–152.

63. LEIBOWITZ, S.F. & J. WANG. 1996. Circulating leptin: Specific effects on brain peptides involved in eating and body weight regulation. Obes. Res. **4:** 1S.

64. LEIBOWITZ, S.F., J. WANG, J.T. DOURMASHKIN & H. YU. 1997. Galanin gene expression in medial preoptic nucleus of female rats: relation to high-fat diet and gonadal steroids (abstr.). Soc. Neurosci Abstr. **23:** 1075.
65. LEIGHTON, B., J.M. KOWALCHUK, R.A. CHALLISS & E.A. NEWSHOLME. 1988. Circadian rhythm in sensitivity of glucose metabolism to insulin in rat soleus muscle. Am. J. Physiol. **255:** E41–45.
66. LIN, L., D.R. GEHLERT, D.A. YORK & G.A. BRAY. 1993. Effect of enterostatin on the feeding response to galanin and NPY. Obes. Res. **1** (3).
67. LIN, L., D.A. YORK & G.A. BRAY. 1996. Comparison of Osborne-Mendel and S5B/PL strains of rat: Central effects of galanin, NPY, beta-casomorphin and CRH on intake of high-fat and low-fat diets. Obes. Res. **4:** 117–124.
68. LINDSKOG, S. & B. AHREN. 1992. Effects of galanin and norepinephrine on insulin secretion in the mouse. Pancreas **7:** 636–641.
69. LOPEZ, F.J., I. MERCHENTHALER, M. CHING, M.G. WISNIEWSKI & A. NEGRO-VILAR. 1991. Galanin: A hypothalamic-hypophysiotropic hormone modulating reproductive functions. Proc. Natl. Acad. Sci. USA **88:** 4508–4512.
70. MARKS, D.L., K.L. LENT, W.G. ROSSMANITH, D.K. CLIFTON & R.A. STEINER. 1994. Activation-dependent regulation of galanin gene expression in gonadotropin-releasing hormone neurons in the female rat. Endocrinology **134:** 1991–1998.
71. MARKS, D.L., M.S. SMITH, D.K. CLIFTON & R.A. STEINER. 1993. Regulation of gonadotropin-releasing hormone (GnRH) and galanin gene expression in GnRH neurons during lactation in the rat (published erratum appears in Endocrinology, 1994. 134: 498). Endocrinology **133:** 1450–1458.
72. MARKS, D.L., M.S. SMITH, M. VRONTAKIS, D.K. CLIFTON & R.A. STEINER. 1993. Regulation of galanin gene expression in gonadotropin-releasing hormone neurons during the estrous cycle of the rat. Endocrinology **132:** 1836–1844.
73. MCKIBBIN, P.E., S.J. COTTON, H.D. MCCARTHY & G. WILLIAMS. 1992. The effect of dexamethasone on neuropeptide Y concentrations in specific hypothalamic regions. Life Sci. **51:** 1301–1307.
74. MEISTER, B., S. CECCATELLI, M.J. VILLAR & T. HOKFELT. 1990. Localization of chemical messengers in magnocellular neurons of the hypothalamic supraoptic and paraventricular nuclei: An immunohistochemical study using experimental manipulations. Neuroscience **37:** 603–633.
75. MELANDER, T., T. HOKFELT & A. ROKAEUS. 1986. Distribution of galanin-like immunoreactivity in the rat central nervous system. J. Comp. Neurol. **248:** 475–517.
76. MENENDEZ, J.A., D.M. ATRENS & S.F. LEIBOWITZ. 1992. Metabolic effects of galanin injections into the paraventricular nucleus of the hypothalamus. Peptides **13:** 323–327.
77. MERCER, J.G., C.B. LAWRENCE & T. ATKINSON. 1996. Regulation of galanin gene expression in the hypothalamic paraventricular nucleus of the obese Zucker rat by manipulation of dietary macronutrients. Mol. Brain Res. **43:** 202–208.
78. MERCHENTHALER, I., F.J. LOPEZ & A. NEGRO-VILAR. 1993. Anatomy and physiology of central galanin-containing pathways. Prog. Neurobiol. **40:** 711–769.
79. MINAMI, S., J. KAMEGAI, H. SUGIHARA, N. SUZUKI, H. HIGUCHI & I. WAKABAYASHI. 1995. Central glucoprivation evoked by administration of 2-deoxy-D-glucose induces expression of the c-fos gene in a subpopulation of neuropeptide Y neurons in the rat hypothalamus. Mol. Brain Res. **33:** 305–310.
80. NAGASE, H., G.A. BRAY & D.A. YORK. 1996. Effect of galanin and enterostatin on sympathetic nerve activity to interscapular brown adipose tissue. Brain Res. **709:** 44–50.
81. NIIMI, M., J. TAKAHARA, M. SATO & K. KAWANISHI. 1990. Immunohistochemical identification of galanin and growth hormone-releasing factor-containing neurons projecting to the median eminence of the rat. Neuroendocrinology **51:** 572–575.
82. OOMURA, Y. 1983. Glucose as a regulator of neuronal activity. Advan. Metab. Dis. **10:** 31–65.
83. PALKOVITS, M., A. ROKAEUS, F.A. ANTONI & A. KISS. 1987. Galanin in the hypothalamo-hypophyseal system. Neuroendocrinology **46:** 417–423.
84. PELLEYMOUNTER, M.A., M.J. CULLEN, M.B. BAKER, R. HECHT, D. WINTERS, T. BOONE & F. COLLINS. 1995. Effects of the obese gene product on body weight regulation in ob/ob mice. Science **269:** 540–543.

85. RAMIREZ, I. & M.I. FRIEDMAN. 1990. Dietary hyperphagia in rats: Role of fat, carbohydrate, and energy content. Physiol. Behav. **47:** 1157–1163.

86. RITTER, S. & J.S. TAYLOR. 1990. Vagal sensory neurons are required for lipoprivic but not glucoprivic feeding in rats. Am. J. Physiol. **258:** R1395–1401.

87. ROHNER-JEANRENAUD, F., I. CUSIN, A. SAINSBURY, K.E. ZAKRZEWSKA & B. JEAURENAUD. 1996. The loop system between neuropeptide Y and leptin in normal and obese rodents. Horm. Metab. Res. **28:** 642–648.

88. ROLLS, B.J. & D.J. SHIDE. 1992. The influence of dietary fat on food intake and body weight (published erratum appears in Nutr. Rev. 1993. **51:** 31), Nutr. Rev. **50:** 283–290.

89. ROMSOS, D.R. & D. FERGUSON. 1982. Self-selected intake of carbohydrate, fat, and protein by obese (ob/ob) and lean mice. Physiol. Behav. **28:** 301–305.

90. SAHU, A. 1998. Evidence suggesting that galanin (GAL), melanin-concentrating hormone (MCH), neurotensin (NT), proopiomelanocortin (POMC) and neuropeptide Y (NPY) are targets of leptin signaling in the hypothalamus. Endocrinology **139:** 795–798.

91. SAHU, A., C.A. SNINSKY, C.P. PHELPS, M.G. DUBE, P.S. KALRA & S.P. KALRA. 1992. Neuropeptide Y release from the paraventricular nucleus increases in association with hyperphagia in streptozotocin-induced diabetic rats. Endocrinology **131:** 2979–2985.

92. SALMON, D.M. & J.P. FLATT. 1995. Effect of dietary fat content on the incidence of obesity among ad libitum fed mice. Int. J. Obes. **9:** 443–449.

93. SCHICK, R.R., S. SAMSAMI, J.P. ZIMMERMANN, T. EBERL, C. ENDRES, SCHUSDZIARRA, V. & M. CLASSEN. 1993. Effect of galanin on food intake in rats: involvement of lateral and ventromedial hypothalamic sites. Am. J. Physiol. **264:** R355–361.

94. SCHREZENMEIR, J. 1996. Hyperinsulinemia, hyperproinsulinemia and insulin resistance in the metabolic syndrome. Experientia **52:** 426–432.

95. SCHWARTZ, M.W. & R.J. SEELEY. 1997. The new biology of body weight regulation. J. Am. Diet. Assoc. **97:** 54–58.

96. SCHWARTZ, M.W., A.J. SIPOLS, C.E. GRUBIN & D.G. BASKIN. 1993. Differential effect of fasting on hypothalamic expression of genes encoding neuropeptide Y, galanin, and glutamic acid decarboxylase. Brain Res. Bull. **31:** 361–367.

97. SHIRLING, D., J.P. ASHBY & J.D. BAIRD. 1983. A direct anabolic effect of progesterone in the intact female rat. J. Endocrinol. **99:** 47–50.

98. SHOR-POSNER, G., A.P. AZAR, M. JHANWAR-UNIYAL, R. FILART & S.F. LEIBOWITZ. 1986. Destruction of noradrenergic innervation to the paraventricular nucleus: Deficits in food intake, macronutrient selection, and compensatory eating after food deprivation. Pharmacol. Biochem. Behav. **25:** 381–392.

99. SHOR-POSNER, G., G. BRENNAN, C. IAN, R. JASAITIS, K. MADHU & S.F. LEIBOWITZ. 1994. Meal patterns of macronutrient intake in rats with particular dietary preferences. Am. J Physiol. **266:** R1395–1402.

100. SHOR-POSNER, G., C. IAN, G. BRENNAN, T. COHN, H. MOY, A. NING & S.F. LEIBOWITZ. 1991. Self-selecting albino rats exhibit differential preferences for pure macronutrient diets: characterization of three subpopulations. Physiol. Behav. **50:** 1187–1195.

101. SKOFITSCH, G., D.M. JACOBOWITZ, R. AMANN & F. LEMBECK. 1989. Galanin and vasopressin coexist in the rat hypothalamo-neurohypophyseal system. Neuroendocrinology **49:** 419–427.

102. SMITH, B.K., D.A. YORK & G.A. BRAY. 1994. Chronic cerebroventricular galanin does not induce sustained hyperphagia or obesity. Peptides **15:** 1267–1272.

103. SMITH, B.K., D.A. YORK & G.A. BRAY. 1996. Effects of dietary preference and galanin administration in the paraventricular or amygdaloid nucleus on diet self-selection. Brain Res. Bull. **39:** 149–154.

104. STANLEY, B.G., K.C. ANDERSON, M.H. GRAYSON & S.F. LEIBOWITZ. 1989. Repeated hypothalamic stimulation with neuropeptide Y increases daily carbohydrate and fat intake and body weight gain in female rats. Physiol. Behav. **46:** 173–177.

105. STEINGRIMSDOTTIR, L., J. BRASEL & M.R. GREENWOOD. 1980. Hormonal modulation of adipose tissue lipoprotein lipase may alter food intake in rats. Am. J. Physiol. **239:** E162–167.

106. STEPHENS, T.W., M. BASINSKI, P.K. BRISTOW, J.M. BUE-VALLESKEY, S.G. BURGETT, L. CRAFT, J. HALE, J. HOFFMANN, H.M. HSINNG, A. KRIAUCINNAS et al. 1995. The role of neuropeptide Y in the antiobesity action of the obese gene product. Nature **377:** 530–532.

107. TANG, C., A. AKABAYASHI, A. MANITIU & S.F. LEIBOWITZ. 1997. Hypothalamic galanin gene expression and peptide levels in relation to circulating insulin: Possible role in energy balance. Neuroendocrinology 65: 265–275.
108. TEMPEL, D.L., K.J. LEIBOWITZ & S.F. LEIBOWITZ. 1988. Effects of PVN galanin on macronutrient selection. Peptides 9: 309–314.
109. TEMPEL, D.L. & S.F. LEIBOWITZ. 1990. Galanin inhibits insulin and corticosterone release after injection into the PVN. Brain Res. 536: 353–357.
110. TEMPEL, D.L. & S.F. LEIBOWITZ. 1994. Adrenal steroid receptors: Interactions with brain neuropeptide systems in relation to nutrient intake and metabolism. J. Neuroendocrinol. 6: 479–501.
111. TEMPEL, D.L., G. SHOR-POSNER, D. DWYER & S.F. LEIBOWITZ. 1989. Nocturnal patterns of macronutrient intake in freely feeding and food-deprived rats. Am. J. Physiol. 256: R541–548.
112. THOMAS, C.D., J.C. PETERS, G.W. REED, N.N. ABUMRAD, M. SUN & J.O. HILL. 1992. Nutrient balance and energy expenditure during ad libitum feeding of high-fat and high-carbohydrate diets in humans. Am. J. Clin. Nutr. 55: 934–942.
113. TREMBLAY, A. 1995. Nutritional determinants of the insulin resistance syndrome. Int. J. Obes. Relat. Metab. Disord. 19: S60–68.
114. UNGER, J.W., J.N. LIVINGSTON & A.M. MOSS. 1991. Insulin receptors in the central nervous system: Localization, signalling mechanisms and functional aspects. Prog. Neurobiol. 36: 343–362.
115. WADE, G.N. 1972. Gonadal hormones and behavioral regulation of body weight. Physiol. Behav. 8: 523–534.
116. WADE, G.N. & J.E. SCHNEIDER. 1992. Metabolic fuels and reproduction in female mammals. Neurosci. Biobehav. Rev. 16: 235–272.
117. WANG, J., A. AKABAYASHI, J. DOURMASHKIN, H. YU, J.T. ALEXANDER, H.J. CHAE & S.F. LEIBOWITZ. 1998. Neuropeptide Y in relation to carbohydrate intake, corticosterone and dietary obesity. Brain Res. 802: 75–88.
118. WANG, J., A. AKABAYASHI, H. YU, J. DOURMASHKIN, I. SILVA, J. LIGHTER & S.F. LEIBOWITZ. 1998. Hypothalamic galanin: Control by signals of fat metabolism. Brain Res. 804: 7–20.
119. WANG, J., J.T. ALEXANDER, P. ZHENG, H. YU, J. DOURMASHKIN & S.F. LEIBOWITZ. 1998. Behavioral and endocrine traits of obesity-prone and obesity-resistant rats on macronutrient diets. Am. J. Physiol. 274: E1057–E1066.
120. WANG, J. & K.L. LEIBOWITZ. 1997. Central insulin inhibits hypothalamic galanin and neuropeptide Y gene expression and peptide release in intact rats. Brain Res. 777: 231–236.
121. WANG, S.W., M. WANG, B.M. GROSSMAN & R.J. MARTIN. 1994. Effects of dietary fat on food intake and brain uptake and oxidation of fatty acids. Physiol. Behav. 56: 517–522.
122. WARWICK, Z.S. 1996. Probing the causes of high-fat diet hyperphagia: A mechanistic and behavioral dissection. Neurosci. Biobehav. Rev. 20: 155–161.
123. WOODS, S.C., M. CHAVEZ, C.R. PARK, C. RIEDY, K. KAIYALA, R.D. RICHARDSON, D.P. FIGLEWICZ, M.W. SCHWARTZ, D. PORTE, JR. & R.J. SEELEY. 1996. The evaluation of insulin as a metabolic signal influencing behavior via the brain. Neurosci. Biobehav. Rev. 20: 139–144.
124. WURTMAN, J.J. & M.J. BAUM. 1980. Estrogen reduces total food and carbohydrate intake, but not protein intake, in female rats. Physiol. Behav. 24: 823–827.
125. YU, H.J., J. WANG, H.J. CHAE, Z.U. BEDRIN & S.F. LEIBOWITZ. 1996. Pituitary galanin (GAL) and vasopressin (AVP) in relation to high-fat diet in female rats. Soc. Neurosci. Abstr. 22: 397.
126. YUN, R., J. DOURMASHKIN, J.T. ALEXANDER, R. SPIRO & S.F. LEIBOWITZ. 1998. Chronic hypothalamic galanin injection increases amount of body fat while enhancing food intake during the first half of the 12-hr feeding cycle. Soc. Neurosci. Abstr. 24: 447.
127. ZHANG, Y., R. PROENCA, M. MAFFEI, M. BARONE, L. LEOPOLD & J.M. FRIEDMAN. 1994. Positional cloning of the mouse obese gene and its human homologue (published erratum appears in Nature 1995 Mar 30; 374 [6521]:479). Nature 372: 425–432.

Galanin: Analysis of Its Coexpression in Gonadotropin-Releasing Hormone and Growth Hormone-Releasing Hormone Neurons

JOHN G. HOHMANN,[a] DONALD K. CLIFTON,[b] AND ROBERT A. STEINER[b-e]

[a]*Program for Neurobiology and Behavior,* [b]*Departments of Obstetrics and Gynecology,* [c]*Physiology and Biophysics, and* [d]*Zoology, University of Washington, Seattle, Washington 98195, USA*

ABSTRACT: Galanin is coexpressed in a subset of gonadotropin-releasing hormone (GnRH) and growth hormone-releasing hormone (GHRH) neurons in the brain and has an important role in the neuroendocrine regulation of gonadotropin and growth hormone secretion. Our overall goal has been to understand the functional significance of galanin as a cotransmitter with GnRH and GHRH in the regulation of these important physiologic processes. To this end, we studied the regulation of galanin's expression in GnRH and GHRH neurons under a variety of physiologic and experimental conditions. Using double-label *in situ* hybridization and computerized image analysis, we observed that in GnRH neurons, galanin's expression is increased over the course of development in both sexes. Galanin achieves a higher basal expression in GnRH neurons in females, and it is sexually differentiated in the adult as a result of the differential exposure to testosterone during the neonatal critical period. Galanin is induced in GnRH neurons coincident with and subsequent to the proestrous luteinizing hormone surge (reflecting the combined action of estradiol and progesterone) acting indirectly on GnRH neurons through a synaptic relay. Galanin's expression in GnRH neurons is inhibited during lactation, when the neuroendocrine reproductive axis is relatively quiescent. In GHRH neurons, the expression of galanin is also induced over the course of development in both sexes. Galanin's expression in GHRH neurons in the adult is sexually differentiated, but in this case, its expression is higher in males than females, reflecting the stimulatory effect of testosterone on galanin in the male. Galanin's expression in GHRH neurons is induced by growth hormone (GH), whereas the absence of GH leads to a reduction of galanin mRNA in these same cells. On the basis of these observations, we conclude that galanin is an important target for regulation by many hormones, and we postulate that as a cotransmitter, galanin acts presynaptically to modulate the secretion of GnRH and GHRH, possibly by altering their pulsatile release patterns, which in turn influences the release of the gonadotropins and GH from the pituitary.

Galanin plays an important role in the regulation of both the hypothalamic-pituitary-gonadal-axis and the somatotropic axis. Early evidence for galanin's influence on reproductive function was the finding that injection of galanin into the cerebral ventricle (ICV) of ovariectomized (OVX) rats increases plasma levels of luteinizing hormone (LH).[1] Galanin also induces the release of gonadotropin-releasing hormone (GnRH) from isolated arcuate nucleus-median eminence fragments *in vitro.*[2] Conversely, administration of either galanin antiserum[3] or the galanin receptor antagonist galantide[4] significantly blunts basal

---

[e]Address for correspondence: Dr. Robert Steiner, Department of Physiology and Biophysics, Box 357290, University of Washington, Seattle, WA 98195. Phone, 206/543-8712; fax, 206/543-3915; e-mail, steiner@u.washington.edu

LH release and the LH surge. The distribution of galanin in areas of the hypothalamus known to be involved in reproductive regulation[5] and the localization of galanin receptor sub-types in the hypothalamus[6–8] lend credence to galanin's putative role as a peptide acting directly in the brain to facilitate the coordinated release of gonadotropins.

Galanin may also play a direct role in the regulation of pituitary hormone secretion. Galanin levels are high in the portal circulation,[9] presumably reflecting its release from hypothalamic neurosecretory cells at the median eminence, and galanin mRNA is expressed in the pituitary, with message levels being highest on diestrus.[10] Both galanin mRNA and peptide content in the pituitary are increased following estrogen treatment,[11,12] and galanin concentrations are decreased in OVX animals.[13] Although galanin has not been colocalized in gonadotropes, it has a stimulatory effect on LH release. When galanin is introduced to the medium of dispersed pituitary cells, it induces a dose-dependent increase in LH content and potentiates the stimulation of LH secretion by GnRH.[9] Together, these observations suggest that galanin may act directly on the pituitary to regulate LH secretion.

The argument for a functional relationship between galanin and GnRH is strengthened by the anatomic proximity of neurons containing these neuropeptides. A subset of GnRH neurons in the medial preoptic area (MPOA) and diagonal band of Broca are surrounded by galanin-containing nerve terminals, suggesting that galanin exerts a postsynaptic effect on these GnRH cells.[14] The location of cell bodies that are the source of this galanin is unknown, but they could reside in other areas of the forebrain or even the brainstem, where the noradrenergic neurons that coexpress galanin and project to the hypothalamus are located. A clue that there may be a functional link between galanin and GnRH secretion is the finding that galanin is coexpressed in many GnRH neurons.[14–16] This colocalization is sexually dimorphic, with up to 65% of GnRH cells in female rats showing double-labeling for GnRH and galanin, whereas only 10-15% of cells are double-labeled in males.[16,17] This finding suggests that galanin expression in GnRH neurons is more important in the female than the male, perhaps helping to shape the unique temporal pattern of LH release characteristic of the female. The secretion of GnRH and galanin into the portal circulation is pulsatile and remarkably coincident,[9] and both hormones are present in the same secretory vesicles in axon terminals at the median eminence.[18] Galanin could theoretically act presynaptically on GnRH nerve terminals or postsynaptically as a hypophysiotropic factor to control gonadotrope activity in the pituitary.

Galanin also has an important role in the regulation of the somatotropic axis, acting as a mediator of growth hormone-releasing hormone (GHRH) and growth hormone (GH) release. Administration of galanin evokes the release of GH in rats and humans,[19,20] and in rats, treatment with galanin antiserum inhibits GH secretion.[21] Galanin immunoneutralization also changes the pattern of GH pulses in male rats,[22] reducing pulse height, increasing pulse frequency, and changing its profile to resemble GH release patterns unique to the female. Incubation of median eminence fragments with galanin increases GHRH concentrations in the medium,[23] suggesting that galanin stimulates GH activity by regulating GHRH release into the portal circulation. Infusions of galanin potentiate GHRH release in humans,[24] and, interestingly, appear to normalize the impaired response of somatotropes to GHRH treatment in elderly humans.[25] Further evidence for a direct action of galanin on GHRH activity is the observation that antisera to GHRH blocks the galanin-induced stimulation of GH in rats.[26] The possible direct effects of galanin on the pituitary are controversial, as several studies reported that galanin has a positive,[27,28] negative,[29] or lack of effect[20,21] on GH release in cultured or dispersed pituitary cells.

The source of galanin involved in the regulation of the GH axis is uncertain. Galanin is produced in cell bodies located in several hypothalamic areas that project to the median eminence. These include the arcuate nucleus (Arc), periventricular nucleus (PeN), and medial preoptic area (MPOA)[5], but galanin is also produced in the pituitary and brainstem. Galanin, made in GHRH neurons in the Arc, is obviously well placed to play a direct role in the regulation of GHRH and GH secretion, and has been the subject of intense investigation. Double-label immunostaining has revealed that both galanin and GHRH peptides coexist in many Arc cells,[30] and retrograde transport studies from the median eminence show abundant labeling of neurons that contain both galanin and GHRH.[31] Galanin may be acting presynaptically to shape GHRH pulses, and it may also function as a regulator of its own release, as many Arc galanin-positive neurons receive synaptic input from galanin-containing fibers.[32]

APPROACH

Recent work on galanin in our laboratory has focused on learning how this peptide is regulated in GnRH and GHRH neurons in a variety of different physiologic conditions. Our approach has been to measure relative levels of galanin mRNA in GnRH or GHRH neurons with the use of double-label *in situ* hybridization. GnRH and GHRH mRNA-containing neurons are visualized by the use of antisense RNAs labeled with the hapten digoxigenin, which appears as a purple precipitate in labeled cells. Galanin antisense RNA is labeled with ^{35}S, and it appears as silver grains clustered over galanin mRNA-expressing neurons. Relative concentrations of galanin mRNA, represented by silver grains overlying digoxigenin-labeled cells, are counted under dark-field illumination with a computerized image processor.[16] Although measurements of cellular mRNA content do not necessarily reflect a commensurate synthesis of bioactive peptides, considerable evidence would suggest that cellular levels of mRNA are indicative of a cell's capacity to synthesize proteins at a particular time. This method offers a sensitive and specific way to achieve quantitative cellular resolution of expressed genes in phenotypically identified neurons.

GALANIN AND GnRH COEXPRESSION

Development and Sexual Dimorphism

The transition from the prepubertal to the adult state is accompanied by the orderly reshaping and amplifying of GnRH secretion, transforming it from a constant basal release mode to a pattern of discrete quantal pulses that activate the reproductive system. If galanin, as a cotransmitter, plays a role in shaping the GnRH release mechanism, we hypothesized that galanin gene expression may increase during the pubertal period as a reflection of its role in this process. To study this, we compared levels of galanin mRNA between prepubertal 25-day-old male and female rats with their 70-day-old counterparts.[33] We found that in GnRH neurons, galanin mRNA was upregulated over development and that this increase was much greater in females than males. In prepubertal animals, levels of galanin mRNA in GnRH neurons were indistinguishable between sexes, but in adults mRNA levels in these cells were about 300% higher in females. This agrees with earlier studies reporting sexual dimorphism in galanin peptide levels[17] and an increase over puberty in galanin content in the median eminence.[34] This further suggests that galanin has a unique role in the female reproductive axis. To extend these findings, we examined whether this developmental pattern was dependent on gonadal hormones. We compared levels of galanin mRNA in GnRH neurons between castrated and intact rats at 25 and 70 days of age. Neither male nor female animals that were prepubertally castrated had increased coexpression of galanin and GnRH, in marked contrast to the dramatic increase seen in the intact rats. These studies show that both the sexual dimorphism and adult patterns of galanin gene expression depend on hormonal input from the gonads.

Perhaps the increase seen in galanin mRNA levels in the adult female represents a role for the peptide in the generation of the LH surge, an event not seen in males. If this were the case, it might be expected that, as with the ability to produce an LH surge, galanin expression might be altered by exposure to high levels of testosterone (T) during the neonatal "critical period." To test this hypothesis, we measured galanin mRNA in adult rats that had received one of four treatments neonatally: intact or castrated males and intact or testosterone-exposed females.[35] When the animals attained adulthood, they were all gonadectomized to remove the influence of endogenous steroid sex hormones and were given a dose of estrogen (E) and progesterone (P) that reliably generates an LH surge. We reconfirmed the classic observation that the E/P induced LH surge was suppressed in females that were treated neonatally with T[36] and was present in males castrated soon after birth.

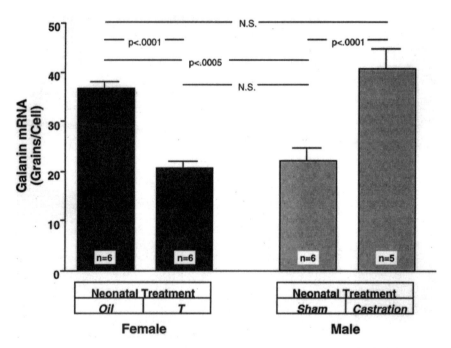

FIGURE 1. Relative levels of galanin mRNA in GnRH neurons throughout the forebrain in groups of adult, gonadectomized, estradiol- and progesterone-primed male and female rats under different neonatal treatment regimens. (Reprinted from Finn et al.[35])

We found that neonatally castrated males, which presumably experienced very little T during the critical period of sexual differentiation, had levels of galanin mRNA as adults that were indistinguishable from those normal adult females (FIG. 1). Even more striking was the profound reduction of galanin message levels in GnRH neurons of females that were neonatally exposed to T; their levels of galanin mRNA were now identical to those of normal adult males. These results demonstrate that galanin gene expression is sexually differentiated neonatally and suggest that this peptide may have a role in regulating the female-specific pattern of LH release.

ESTROUS CYCLE REGULATION

One hallmark of the rat estrous cycle is the changing level of LH secretion, with a large preovulatory rise in plasma levels of LH during the afternoon of proestrus. This burst of secretory activity is temporally preceded by an increase in GnRH release into the portal circulation.[37] If one of galanin's functions is to enhance or sharpen pulsatile GnRH release, we hypothesized that galanin mRNA might be regulated across the estrous cycle and that increased message levels could be associated with induction of the LH surge. To examine this idea, we measured galanin gene expression in GnRH neurons and assayed GnRH mRNA at various times during the cycle.[38] We found that levels of galanin mRNA were low during diestrus, and rose dramatically on proestrus, with a twofold increase in message levels from noon to 6 pm on that day. Curiously, the galanin mRNA signal remained high for at least 24 hours after the LH surge, suggesting that either galanin plays a continuing or different role subsequent to ovulation or transcription is ramped-up to replenish the stores of galanin depleted during the surge itself. In contrast to this clear and unequivocal regulation of galanin mRNA, we found no changes in GnRH mRNA during the estrous cycle, in agreement with our previous studies that showed a stubborn resistance by the GnRH gene to regulation in any physiologic paradigm.[38–43]

The initiation of the LH surge is directly dependent on the positive feedback effect of increasing levels of E originating in the ovary. If galanin has a stimulatory role in the surge-generating mechanism, its expression and synthesis should also be responsive to high levels of E. To test this, we ovariectomized female rats and compared coexpression of galanin and GnRH in two groups of rats: those with and those without estrogen implants.[38] We found that rats treated with E had levels of galanin mRNA significantly higher than those of rats without E, suggesting that the presence of E stimulates the production of galanin. Also, E-treated animals had galanin message levels similar to those seen in the intact controls. To elucidate the relative control of galanin expression by E and/or P, we examined the regulation of galanin mRNA when animals were given E, E/P, or P alone.[38,42] Galanin mRNA levels responded robustly to a steroid-priming regimen, with a 400% increase in message in GnRH neurons during the E/P-induced LH surge. This compares to a modest increase in galanin mRNA seen with E treatment alone (accompanied by a modest increase in plasma LH) and no increase with P treatment alone (with no increase in LH release induced by this treatment). Although it can be reasonably argued that changes in galanin gene expression are only associated with general GnRH activation and are not necessarily causal to the LH surge, the fact that levels of galanin mRNA increase significantly during proestrus while GnRH gene expression remains relatively constant, regardless of the treatment or surgical manipulation, suggests that galanin is a physiologic regulator of gonadotropin release.

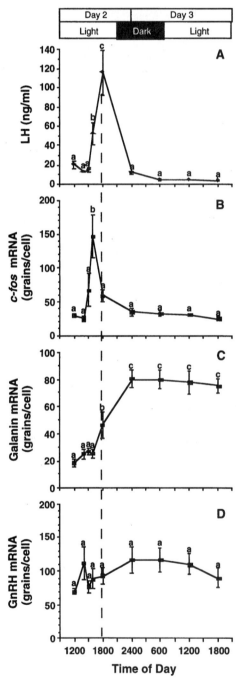

FIGURE 2. Time course of **(A)** serum LH concentrations; **(B)** relative levels of *c-fos* mRNA; **(C)** relative levels of galanin mRNA; and **(D)** relative levels of GnRH mRNA in estrogen- and progesterone-primed ovariectomized rats during a 30-hour period bracketing the time of the expected LH surge. Values with different letters are significantly different from one another, $p < 0.05$. Values with the same letter are not significantly different from one another, $p > 0.05$. *Dashed line* indicates the time and peak of the LH surge. (Reprinted from Finn *et al.*[47])

It is now well established that the presence of the neuronal marker Fos in GnRH neurons indicates activation of these cells.[44,45] Cellular levels of *c-fos* mRNA levels increase in GnRH neurons on the day of proestrus, and triple-labeling studies show that Fos, GnRH, and galanin are all produced in the same neurons.[46] To further our knowledge of the relationship between galanin and GnRH and to assess the possible role of *c-fos* in GnRH neurons, we studied the temporal patterns of expression for each of these peptides during the 30-hour period surrounding the LH surge.[47] Rats were ovariectomized and treated with E/P to induce an LH surge and were then sacrificed at several time points before and during peak LH release and for 24 hours after the peak. We found *c-fos* mRNA to be elevated 2 hours before the surge, with message levels increased to 300% over basal levels (FIG. 2). This increase was followed 2 hours later (coincident with the peak of LH release) by an upregulation of galanin mRNA. This agrees with the notion that galanin is somehow involved in the regulation of gonadotropin secretion and that transcription of the galanin gene may result from an increase in Fos activity. The galanin gene has an AP-1 response element, the DNA sequence where the Fos-Jun dimer binds,[48] so it is plausible that galanin expression should be responsive to Fos regulation. The GnRH promoter also has an AP-1 site[49]; however, we could adduce no evidence of changes in GnRH message over the course of the LH surge, suggesting once again that the GnRH gene is transcribed at a relatively constant pace and that the critical aspect of its secretory control is at the nerve terminal. We also reconfirmed our earlier observation[38] that galanin mRNA levels remain high for at least 24 hours following the surge, well after LH levels (and *c-fos* message) have returned to basal states. This indicates that although galanin may be involved in events during the period of highest gonadotropin release, it may also have a role in subsequent activities, perhaps as a tonic inhibitor of GnRH release during the quiescent estrous period.

COEXPRESSION CONSTRAINTS

If galanin induction in GnRH neurons depends on synaptic activation of these cells, then agents that block afferent signals should also inhibit the increase in galanin message seen concurrently with high gonadotropin secretion. Several neurotransmitter antagonists are effective in blocking the GnRH-induced proestrous surge, including the α-adrenergic receptor blocker phenoxybenzamine and the NMDA receptor antagonist MK801. We studied the effects of these agents and the general anesthetic pentobarbital on galanin coexpression in GnRH cells.[41,43] We observed that MK801 and pentobarbital completely blocked LH surge activity, whereas the attempted blockade of the α-adrenergic receptor was only partially effective in suppressing the E/P-induced rise in LH levels. In parallel to these findings was the discovery that galanin message levels in GnRH neurons were not elevated in the surge-blocked animals regardless of the mode of blockade. When galanin message was quantified in non-GnRH neurons, no changes in mRNA levels were seen with any treatment, suggesting that the galanin induction phenomenon is specific to those cells that coexpress both GnRH and galanin. These results also support the idea that the induction of galanin in GnRH cells is blocked by any event that inhibits LH surge activity. Enhancement of galanin gene expression may well derive from the E/P-induced activation of GnRH cells, either directly or transsynaptically via other cells that make contact with GnRH neurons.

Are there any physiologic circumstances in which galanin message levels drop to below basal amounts in GnRH cells? If the induction of galanin has a positive effect on gonadotropin release, then periods when GnRH secretion is low or nonpulsatile should also be times when coexpression is minimal. To test this hypothesis, we measured cellular levels of GnRH and galanin mRNAs during lactation,[40] a time when GnRH release is at a secretory nadir. In agreement with our earlier work, we found no differences in either GnRH mRNA or GnRH peptide between lactating and cycling animals. However, significant decreases were seen in amounts of galanin mRNA within GnRH cells. Compared to diestrus, when galanin mRNA in GnRH cells is lowest in cycling rats, lactating animals had 60% lower levels of galanin in these neurons. This possibly reflects a reduced need for galanin during a period when reproductive axis activity is relatively quiescent.

GALANIN AND GHRH COEXPRESSION

Development of Sexual Dimorphism

The sexually dimorphic pattern of GH secretion from the pituitary has been well characterized.[50] Males have a dramatically rhythmic pattern of GH release that consists of high amplitude pulses every 3–4 hours, with low basal release in the intervals. In contrast, females have a higher level of basal secretory activity, with lower amplitude, less regular peaks. The characteristic patterns of secretion are controlled by the actions of somatostatin and GHRH in the hypothalamus, which again have pronounced sexually dimorphic neuronal actions.[51,52] As we know that galanin is colocalized with GHRH[30] and affects both GHRH and GH release, it is reasonable to postulate that galanin has an important role in the gender-related differences in somatotrope activity. To explore this idea, we performed a series of experiments that had three objectives.[53] Our initial aim was to establish that galanin mRNA was actually being made in GHRH cells and to confirm the earlier reported colocalization of these peptides. The second goal was to ascertain whether galanin mRNA is sexually dimorphic in these cells, and if so, to determine when during postnatal development this difference becomes manifest. Our final objective in this series of studies was to determine if manipulation of sex steroids could alter the coexpression patterns of galanin and GHRH as a possible mechanism for sexual differentiation. We first examined groups of rats at several ages: 5- and 10-day-old neonates, 25-day-old juveniles, and 70-day-old adult animals. We found galanin mRNA to be robustly coexpressed in all areas where GHRH neurons are located, including the Arc, the periarcuate area, and the ventromedial hypothalamus. Quantitative analysis of galanin message in GHRH cells revealed significant differences at all ages from 10 days to adult (FIG. 3). In the neonates, galanin mRNA levels were higher in females than males in all areas examined. The significance of this observation is not known and may or may not be critical, as overall levels of galanin message are very low in GHRH cells of both males and females at this age. Levels of galanin mRNA in GHRH neurons were upregulated in both sexes in the 25-day-old juveniles compared to neonates. Galanin message levels were higher overall in the female rats, but only in the Arc, with lower mRNA levels in the female periarcuate area. In adult animals, the trend was reversed, with males having greater galanin mRNA in GHRH cells than did females in all areas. Galanin message levels in adult females were not different from those

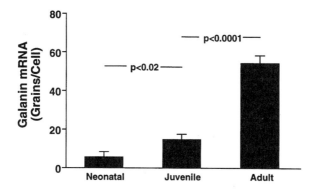

FIGURE 3. Galanin mRNA levels in GHRH neurons of the male rat throughout development. The ages of rats are as follows: neonatal, 10 days; juveniles, 25 days; and adult, 70 days. Values are presented as the mean ± SEM. (Reprinted from Delamarre-Van De Waal *et al.*[53])

in juvenile females. Levels of galanin mRNA in adult males were higher in the Arc (380%) and in the periarcuate area (350%) than in their juvenile counterparts. The dramatic increases seen in galanin mRNA in GHRH neurons in the Arc and periarcuate area suggest that these are important areas for the male-specific episodic pattern of GHRH and GH release. The observation that galanin message levels in females do not differ between prepubertal and adult rats also girds the idea that it is the change from low to high levels of galanin mRNA that triggers the male pattern that becomes evident during this period. These results support the hypothesis that galanin may be helping to shape the pattern of GHRH and GH secretion, which also both show a corresponding change over development. It should be noted that basal and peak amounts of GH release are similar in male and female juvenile rats and do not begin to differentiate until after day 22.[54]

Does the rise in T that accompanies the transition through puberty also regulate the coexpression of galanin and GHRH in male rats? Earlier studies from our laboratory have revealed that treatment with T stimulates both somatostatin and GHRH in castrated rats[51,55] and that neonatal castration of male rats produces a pattern of GH pulsatility similar to that of females.[56] From these observations it is reasonable to posit that changing T levels may influence the expression of galanin in GHRH neurons. To test this hypothesis, we castrated or sham-castrated adult male rats, then treated the castrated animals with T. We found that galanin message levels in GHRH cells were 21% lower in castrated rats than in intact animals and that T-replacement treatment for 5 days resulted in a 33% increase in galanin mRNA over that of the castrated group. The changes were seen only in the Arc, further strengthening the argument that this region of the hypothalamus may be a control center for the galanin-induced, male pattern of GH release. Because galanin is known to have effects presynaptically at the median eminence[57] and galanin-containing terminals make contact with other galanin-positive perikarya in the Arc,[32] galanin may be acting to shape the release pattern of GHRH and possibly acts as a regulator of its own rate of transcription.

REGULATION OF COEXPRESSION BY GH

GH controls its own release by acting in a short-feedback loop on both GHRH and somatostatin neurons to stimulate and inhibit their activity, respectively, in a coordinated reciprocal manner. High levels of GH stimulate somatostatin synthesis and inhibit GHRH, whereas low levels of GH inhibit somatostatin and stimulate GHRH synthesis. The mechanisms for this feedback control are now being clarified; however, the role of galanin in this process is still a mystery. If galanin has a positive effect on GHRH release, it is conceivable that galanin mRNA in these cells might be upregulated by GH during periods preceding a GH pulse. It is also possible that physiologic states wherein plasma GH levels are low could be reflected by minimal coexpression of galanin and GHRH. To study these questions, we measured galanin message levels in GHRH cells of animals that had either high or low circulating levels of GH.[58] In one experiment, we assayed galanin mRNA in GHRH neurons in normal Lewis rats and in Lewis dwarf rats that have a congenital GH deficiency. We found that dwarf rats had 47% lower galanin levels in GHRH neurons than did control animals, which was almost paralleled by a 40% decrease in insulin-like growth factor (IGF-1) concentrations. Since IGF-1 levels are a good indicator of plasma GH values, these nearly equal decreases suggest that galanin may, in fact, be regulated by changes in circulating levels of GH. Subsequently, we performed another study in which GH levels were experimentally manipulated to determine if alterations in GH could affect changes in galanin mRNA in GHRH neurons. Three groups of rats were examined: an intact group, a hypophysectomized group (to remove endogenous GH), and a hypophysectomized group with replacement GH. Analysis of message levels between the groups revealed a precipitous (92%) drop in galanin mRNA in the hypophysectomized group compared to the intact group (FIG. 4). Plasma levels of GH in the hypophysectomized group also were reduced by more than 90%, implying again that galanin is extremely sensitive to changes in circulating levels of GH. This agrees with a report by Selvais *et al.*[59] who showed that total hypothalamic galanin RNA as measured by Northern blot is significantly lower in hypophysectomized rats relative to intact controls. These investigators also reported that

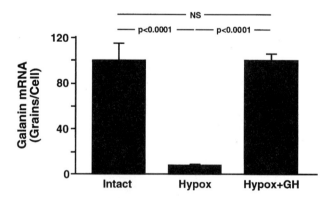

FIGURE 4. Relative levels of galanin mRNA in the Arc GHRH neurons of intact/vehicle, hypox/vehicle, and hypox/rGH groups. Values presented are the mean grains per cell ± SEM. (Reprinted from Chan *et al.*[58])

GH replacement therapy did not cause an overall increase in *hypothalamic* galanin; however, they did not measure galanin message *specifically in* GHRH cells. In our study, when hypophysectomized rats were infused with GH via the Alzet-mini pump for 3 days, galanin message in GHRH cells increased to levels that were indistinguishable from those of intact controls. These results lend credence to the idea that galanin, along with somatostatin and GHRH, is a target for GH feedback regulation in the hypothalamus.

Increasing levels of GH consistently inhibit GHRH release, and galanin is thought to stimulate GHRH release. How can these observations be reconciled with the apparent induction of galanin after GH administration? It may be that GH acts through some other, time-delayed pathway to regulate galanin levels in a negative direction, changing the positive stimulus to an inhibitory one. This, in turn, could lead to changes in GHRH secretion as galanin activity is altered. One candidate for involvement in this pathway is the population of somatostatin neurons in the PeN. These cells express the GH receptor, their nerve terminals are thought to make synaptic contact with GHRH neurons,[60] and presumably have an inhibitory influence. Other possible mediators of GH actions on GHRH (and galanin) activity are the neuropeptide Y (NPY)-containing neurons in the Arc. These cells express the GH receptor[61] and may convey the inhibitory signal resulting from increased GH levels to GHRH/galanin cells. It also is conceivable that galanin is involved in its own regulation, a hypothesis that makes sense in a system that depends on reciprocal, pulsatile activity among the various components of a neuronal circuit. To determine the site of galanin's actions in this hypothalamic network, we studied expression of the galanin (GAL-R1) receptor in both somatostatin and GHRH neuronal populations in the rat brain.[58] Using computerized image analysis, we counted the relative number of GAL-R1 mRNA-dependent silver grains over somatostatin- or GHRH-labeled cells (signal) and compared this to background readings (noise) for each assay. Using a signal-to-noise ratio of 6, we found that about 40% of PeN somatostatin neurons express GAL-R1, thus implicating this neuronal group as a probable mediator of galanin's (and perhaps GH's) modulation of GHRH release. Using the same signal-to-background noise criteria of 6, we were unable to find convincing evidence for GAL-R1 expression in any other somatostatin neuronal population in the forebrain or in *any* GHRH neurons. The source of the galanin acting on somatostatin cells through GAL-R1 as a neurotransmitter is unknown, but it could be coming from the population of galanin/GHRH coexpressing cells in the Arc. GHRH cells make synaptic contact with somatostatin neurons,[60] but there is no evidence of GHRH receptors in these cells. This implicates galanin, working as a cotransmitter within GHRH cells, as a potential modulator of somatostatin, GHRH, and thus GH activity. Galanin may function as an inhibitor of somatostatin release to allow maximal GHRH secretion when somatostatin activity is low, contributing to the ultradian rhythm of GH secretion. Alternatively, galanin may function to upregulate the somatostatin cellular machinery, acting as a dampener of GHRH release after a burst of secretory activity; this would serve to sharpen the pulsatile nature of GH release.

PERSPECTIVES

Despite what we have learned thus far about galanin's role as a cotransmitter with GnRH and GHRH (FIG. 5), many questions remain. For example, does galanin work in a similar way in these two systems and perhaps in others? Studies of the interaction between

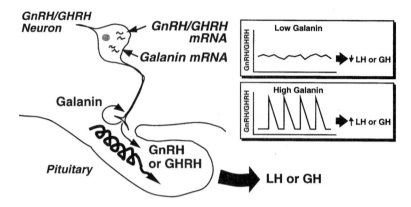

FIGURE 5. A model for the function of galanin in GnRH and GHRH neurons. Galanin is coexpressed with these hormones in the hypothalamus and is coreleased with GnRH or GHRH at the nerve terminal. It may act presynaptically at the median eminence and/or travel through the portal circulation to act directly on the pituitary. High levels of galanin are associated with increases in LH or GH release, but continued high galanin levels may be inhibitory to hormone secretion. Low levels of galanin are associated with decreases in plasma LH or GH.

galanin and acetylcholine[62] imply that galanin acts in the hippocampal cholinergic pathway as an inhibitor of acetylcholine release immediately following a secretory event. One can imagine that the continued high levels of galanin mRNA seen in GnRH neurons after the LH surge might serve as a tonic inhibitory clamp against further pulsatile hormone release. Regarding the growth axis, the positive effect of galanin on GHRH and GH secretion may be the result of an inhibitory action of galanin on somatostatin neurons, allowing maximal pulses of GHRH and GH. Alternatively, galanin could be working presynaptically to shape GHRH pulses. If galanin and GHRH are cosecreted in the same vesicles, galanin might act on its own receptor at the median eminence to inhibit GHRH release for discrete periods, allowing a repetitive pattern of pulse, no-pulse, pulse, etc. and ultimately having the same effect on somatotrope activity.

Another major question revolves around the sites of galanin's actions as a regulator of neuroendocrine function. Although no coexpression of galanin receptors by either GnRH or GHRH neurons has yet been reported, the recent cloning of the GAL-R2 and GAL-R3 receptors could provide insights into the anatomic localization of galanin activity. Galanin-containing terminals surround MPOA GnRH neurons in the same general area as GnRH/galanin cells,[14] and the same is apparently true for galanin-containing varicosities making synaptic contact with cells in the Arc close to where GHRH (and by inference galanin/GHRH) neurons reside.[32] Galanin also directly modulates both GnRH and GHRH release when applied directly to nerve terminals at the median eminence.[2,23] Clarifying whether galanin acts pre- or postsynaptically, or both, will greatly enhance our understanding of how this neuropeptide exerts its influence on these complex neuroendocrine systems.

REFERENCES

1. SAHU, A. *et al.* 1987. Effects of neuropeptide Y, NPY analogue (norleucine[4]-NPY), galanin and neuropeptide K on LH release in ovariectomized (ovx) and ovx estrogen, progesterone-treated rats. Peptides **8:** 921–926.

2. LOPEZ, F.J. & A. NEGRO-VILAR. 1990. Galanin stimulates luteinizing hormone-releasing hormone secretion from arcuate nuceus-median eminence fragments in vitro: Involvement of an alpha-adrenergic mechanism. Endocrinology **127:** 2431–2436.

3. LOPEZ, F.J., E.H. MEADE & A. NEGRO-VILAR. 1993. Endogenous galanin modulates the gonadotropin and prolactin proestrous surges in the rat. Endocrinology **132:** 795–800.

4. SAHU, A., B. XU & S.P. KALRA. 1994. Role of galanin in stimulation of pituitary luteinizing hormone secretion as revealed by a specific receptor anatogonist, galantide. Endocrinology **134:** 529–536.

5. SKOFITSCH, G., M.A. SILLS & D.M. JACOBOWITZ. 1986. Autoradiographic distribution of ^{125}I-galanin binding sites in the rat central nervous system. Peptides **7:** 1029–1042.

6. BURGEVIN, M. *et al.* 1995. Cloning, pharmacological characterization, and anatomical distribution of a rat cDNA encoding for a galanin receptor. J. Mol. Neurosci. **6:** 33–41.

7. GUSTAFSON, E.L. *et al.* 1996. Distribution of a rat galanin receptor mRNA in rat brain. Neuroreport **7:** 953–957.

8. FATHI, Z. *et al.* 1997. Cloning, pharmalogical characterization and distribution of a novel galanin receptor. Molec. Brain Res. **51**(1–2): 49–59.

9. LOPEZ, F.J. *et al.* 1991. Galanin: A hypothalamic-hypophysiotrophic hormone modulating reproductive functions. Proc. Natl. Acad. Sci. USA **88:** 4508–4512.

10. KAPLAN, L.M. *et al.* 1988. Tissue-specific expression of the rat galanin gene. Proc. Natl. Acad. Sci. USA **85:** 1065–1069.

11. KAPLAN, L.M. *et al.* 1988. Galanin is an estrogen-inducible, secretory product of the rat anterior pituitary. Proc. Natl. Acad. Sci. USA **85:** 7408–7412.

12. GABRIEL, S.M., J.I. KOENIG & L.M. KAPLAN. 1990. Galanin-like immunoreactivity is influenced by estrogen in peripubertal and adult rats. Neuroendocrinology **51:** 168–173.

13. O'HALLORAN, D. *et al.* 1990. Effect of endocrine manipulation on anterior pituitary galanin in the rat. Endocrinology **127:** 467–475.

14. MERCHENTHALER, I., F.J. LOPEZ & A. NEGRO-VILAR. 1990. Colocalization of galanin and luteinizing hormone-releasing hormone in a subset of preoptic hypothalamic neurons: Anatomical and functional correlates. Proc. Natl. Acad. Sci. USA **87:** 6326–6330.

15. COEN, C., C. MONTAGNESE & J. OPACKA-JUFFRY. 1990. Coexistence of gonadotropin-releasing hormone and galanin: Immunohistochemical and functional studies. J. Neuroendocrinol. **2:** 107–111.

16. MARKS, D.L. *et al.* 1992. Simultaneous visualization of two cellular mRNA species in individual neurons by use of a new double *in situ* hybridization method. Mol. Cell. Neurosci. **3:** 395–405.

17. MERCHENTHALER, I. *et al.* 1991. Sexual differences in the distribution of neurons coexpressing galanin and luteinizing hormone-releasing hormone in the rat brain. Endocrinology **129:** 1977–1986.

18. LIPOSITS, Z. *et al.* 1995. Sexual dimorphism in copackaging of luteinizing hormone-releasing hormone and galanin into neurosecretory vesicles of hypophysiotrophic neurons: estrogen dependency. Endocrinology **136:** 1987–1992.

19. BAUER, F.E. *et al.* 1986. Growth hormone release in man induced by galanin, a new hypothalamic peptide. Lancet **2** (8500): 192–195.

20. OTTLECZ, A., W.K. SAMSON & S.M. MCCANN. 1986. Galanin: Evidence for a hypothalamic site of action to release growth hormone. Peptides **7:** 51–53.

21. OTTLECZ, A., G.D. SNYDER & S.M. MCCANN. 1988. Regulatory role of galanin in control of hypothalamic-anterior pituitary function. Proc. Natl. Acad. Sci. USA **85:** 9861–9865.

22. MAITER, D.M. *et al.* 1990. Sexual differentiation of growth hormone feedback effects on hypothalamic growth hormone-releasing hormone and somatostatin. Neuroendocrinology **51:** 174–180.

23. AGUILA, M., U. MARUBAYASHI & S. McCANN. 1992. The effect of galanin on growth hormone-releasing factor and somatostatin release from median eminence fragments in vitro. Neuroendocrinology **56:** 889–894.

24. DAVIS, T.M., J.M. BURRIN & S.R. BLOOM. 1987. Growth hormone (GH) release in response to GH-releasing hormone in man is 3-fold inhanced by galanin. J. Clin. Endocrinol. Metab. **65**(6): 1248–1252.

25. CREMAGNANI, L. *et al.* 1996. Potentiating effect of galanin on GHRH-induced GH release. Comparison between old and young subjects. Horm. Metab. Res. **28**(2): 101–104.

26. MURAKAMI, Y. *et al.* 1987. Galanin stimulates growth hormone (GH) secretion via GH-releasing factor (GRF) in conscious rats. Eur. J. Pharmacol. **136:** 415–418.

27. GABRIEL, S.M. *et al.* 1988. Galanin stimulates rat pituitary growth hormone secretion *in vitro.* Life Sci. **42:** 1981–1986.

28. SATO, M. *et al.* 1991. Characterization of the stimulatory effect of galanin on growth hormone release from the rat anterior pituitary. Life Sci. **48:** 1639–1644.

29. GUISTINA, A. *et al.* 1997. Inhibitory effects of galanin on growth hormone (GH) release in cultured GH-secreting adenoma cells: Comparative study with octreotide, GH-releasing hormone, and thyrotropin-releasing hormone. Metabolism-Clin. Exp. **46:** 425–430.

30. MEISTER, B. & T. HOKFELT. 1988. Peptide- and transmitter-containing neurons in the mediobasal hypothalamus and their relation to GABAnergic systems: Possible roles in control of prolactin and growth hormone secretion. Synapse **2:** 585–605.

31. NIIMI, M. *et al.* 1990. Immunohistochemical identification of galanin and growth hormone-releasing factor-containing neurons projecting to the median eminence of the rat. Neuroendocrinology **51:** 572–575.

32. LOPEZ, F.J., Z. LIPOSITS & I. MERCHENTHALER. 1992. Evidence for a negative ultrashort loop feedback regulating galanin release from the arcuate nuleus-median eminence functional unit. Endocrinology **130**(3): 1499–1507.

33. ROSSMANITH, W.G. *et al.* 1994. Induction of galanin gene expression in gonadotropin-releasing hormone neurons with puberty in the rat. Endocrinology **135:** 1401–1408.

34. GABRIEL, S.M. *et al.* 1989. Tissue specific sex differences in galanin-like immunoreactivity and galanin mRNA during development in the rat. Peptides **10**(2): 369–374.

35. FINN, P.D. *et al.* 1996. Sexual differentiation of galanin gene expression in gonadotropin-releasing hormone neurons. Endocrinology **137:** 4767–4772.

36. HANDA, R.J. & R.A. GORSKI. 1985. Alterations in the onset of ovulatory failure and gonadotropin secretion following steroid administration to lightly androgenized female rats. Biol. Reprod. **32:** 248–256.

37. SARKAR, D.K. *et al.* 1976. Gonadotropin-releasing hormone surge in pro-oestrous rats. Nature **264:** 461–463.

38. MARKS, D.L. *et al.* 1993. Regulation of galanin gene expression in gondadotropin-releasing homrone neurons during the estrous cycle of the rat. Endocrinology **132:** 1836–1844.

39. WIEMANN, J.N., D.K. CLIFTON & R.A. STEINER. 1990. Gonadotropin-releasing hormone messenger ribonucleic acid levels are unaltered with changes in the gonadal hormone milieu of the adult male rat. Endocrinology **127:** 523–532.

40. MARKS, D.L. *et al.* 1993. Regulation of gonadotropin-releasing hormone (GnRH) and galanin gene expression in GnRH neurons during lactation in the rat. Endocrinology **133:** 1450–1458.

41. MARKS, D.L. *et al.* 1994. Activation-dependent regulation of galanin gene expression in gonadotropin-releasing hormone neurons in the female rat. Endocrinology **134:** 1991–1998.

42. ROSSMANITH, W.G. *et al.* 1996. Induction of galanin mRNA in GnRH neurons by estradiol and its facilitation by progesterone. J. Neuroendocrinol. **8:** 185–191.

43. ROSSMANITH, W.G. *et al.* 1996. Inhibition of steroid-induced galanin mRNA expression in GnRH neurons by specific NMDA-receptor blockade. J. Neuroendocrinol. **8:** 179–184.

44. LEE, W.S., M.S. SMITH & G.E. HOFFMAN. 1990. Luteinizing hormone-releasing hormone neurons express Fos protein during the proestrous surge of luteinizing hormone. Proc. Natl. Acad. Sci. USA **87:** 5163–5167.

45. LEE, W.S., M.S. SMITH. & G.E. HOFFMAN. 1992. C-Fos activity identifies recruitment of luteinizing hormone releasing hormone neurons during the ascending phase of the proestrous luteinizing hormone surge. J Neuroendocrinol. **4:** 161–166.

46. HRABOVSZKY, E., M.E. VRONTAKIS & S.L. PETERSON. 1995. Triple-labeling method combining immunocytochemistry and in situ hybridization histochemistry: Demonstration of overlap between Fos-immunoreactive and galanin mRNA-expressing subpopulations of luteinizing hormone-releasing hormone neurons in female rats. J. Histochem. Cytochem. **43:** 363–370.

47. FINN, P.D., R.A. STEINER & D.K. CLIFTON. 1998. Temporal patterns of gonadotropin-releasing hormone (GnRH), c-fos, and galanin gene expression in GnRH neurons relative to the luteinizing hormone surge. J. Neurosci. **18:** 713–719.

48. ANOUAR, Y. *et al.* 1994. Identification of a TPA-responsive element mediating preferential trans-activation of the galanin gene promoter in chromaffin cells. J. Biol. Chem. **269:** 6823–6831.

49. BOND, C., T *et al.* 1989. The rat gonadotropin-releasing hormone: SH locus: structure and hypothalamic expression. Mol. Endocrinol. **3:** 1257–1262.

50. JANSSON, J.O., S. EDEN & O. ISAKSSON. 1985. Sexual dimorphism in the control of growth hormone secretion. Endocrinol. Rev. **6:** 128–149.

51. CHOWEN-BREED, J.A., R.A. STEINER & D.K. CLIFTON. 1989. Sexual dimorphism and testosterone dependent regulation of somatostatin gene expression in the periventricular nucleus of the rat brain. Endocrinology **125:** 357–362.

52. ARGENTE, J. *et al.* 1991. Sexual dimorphism of growth hormone-releasing hormone and somatostatin gene expression in the hypothalamus of the rat during development. Endocrinology **128:** 2369–2375.

53. DELEMARRE-VAN DE WAAL, H.A. *et al.* 1994. Expression and sexual dimorphism of galanin messenger ribonucleic acid in growth hormone-releasing hormone neurons of the rat during development. Endocrinology **134:** 665–671.

54. EDÉN, S. 1979. Age- and sex-related differences in episodic growth hormone secretion in the rat. Endocrinology **105:** 155–160.

55. ZEITLER, P. *et al.* 1990. Growth hormone-releasing hormone messenger ribonucleic acid in the hypothalamus of the adult male rat is increased by testosterone. Endocrinology **127:** 1362–1368.

56. JANSSON, J.-O. *et al.* 1984. Influence of gonadal steroids on age- and sex-related secretory patterns of growth hormone in the rat. Endocrinology **114:** 1287–1294.

57. ARAI, R. & A. CALAS. 1991. Ultrastructural localization of galanin immunoreactivity in the rat median eminence. Brain Res. **562:** 339–343.

58. CHAN, Y.Y. *et al.* 1996. The role of galanin and its receptor in the feedback regulation of growth hormone secretion. Endocrinology **137:** 5303–5310.

59. SELVAIS, P.L. *et al.* 1993. Effects of hypophysectomy on galaninergic neurons in the rat hypothalamus. Neuroendocrinology **58:** 539–547.

60. HORVATH, S. *et al.* 1989. Electron microscopic immunocytochemical evidence for the existence of bidirectional synaptic connections between growth hormone-releasing hormone- and somatostatin-containing neurons in the hypothalamus of the rat. Brain Res. **481:** 8–15.

61. CHAN, Y.Y., R.A. STEINER & D.K. CLIFTON. 1996. Regulation of hypothalamic neuropeptide-Y neurons by growth hormone in the rat. Endocrinology **137:** 1319–1325.

62. CRAWLEY, J.N. 1996. Galanin-acetylcholine interactions: Relevance to memory and Alzheimer's. disease. Life Sci. **58:** 2185–2199.

Neuroendocrine Interactions between Galanin, Opioids, and Neuropeptide Y in the Control of Reproduction and Appetite[a]

SATYA P. KALRA[b,d] AND TAMAS L. HORVATH[c]

[b]Department of Neuroscience, University of Florida College of Medicine, Gainesville, Florida 32610-0244, USA

[c]Department of Ob-Gyn, Yale School of Medicine, New Haven, Connecticut 36250, USA

ABSTRACT: Galanin is a pleiotropic neuroendocrine signal produced in discrete subpopulations of neurons distributed in several sites in the hypothalamus. Neuropeptide Y and β-endorphin also display pleiotropism, but they are produced by subpopulations of neurons located only in the arcuate nucleus of the hypothalamus. Each of these neuropeptides exerts a regulatory influence on reproduction and appetitive behavior. Experimental and morphologic evidence from our laboratory show direct contacts and interplay among these diverse signals. Seemingly, an interconnected network composed of these three neuropeptide-producing neurons provides precision and site specificity in the relay of information necessary to govern reproduction and appetite. Disruptions in this interplay are likely to manifest in untoward consequences such as infertility and obesity.

Research spanning the last two decades clearly documents that a host of regulatory peptides are involved in the hypothalamic control of pituitary function and appetitive behavior.[1–3] The study of these regulatory peptides has allowed a deeper understanding of the functional organization of the hypothalamus. Neuroanatomists not only have mapped the neuronal pathways containing these signals with great precision, but also have revealed intricate interconnections among them.[3,4] It is evident that these neurotransmitters/neuromodulators act in a site-specific manner in the hypothalamus. This new insight has also reinforced the existence of cross-talk and redundancy in their action.[5] In addition, these neuropeptides are pleiotropic and respond to the ever-changing internal milieu to elicit diverse neuroendocrine effects.[1,2,4,5]

The three peptidergic signals, galanin (GAL), neuropeptide Y (NPY), and the endogenous opioid peptide β-endorphin (β-END), produced locally in the hypothalamus, have been studied extensively.[1–6] Each of these messenger molecules has been shown to modulate the hypothalamic control of reproduction[1] and appetitive behavior.[2] A comparative analysis revealed the commonality of their actions in governing the two neuroendocrine mechanisms.[7] We have devoted our efforts to elucidating how these three peptidergic signals operate within the hypothalamic neural circuitry regulating reproduction and appetite.[7] In this article the recently identified mode of interactive communication among

[a]This work was supported in part by grants from the National Institutes of Health (HD08634 and DK37273).

[d]Address for correspondence: Satya P. Kalra, PhD, Department of Neuroscience, University of Florida, College of Medicine, Box 100244, 1600 SW Archer Road, Gainesville, FL 32610-0244. Phone, 352/392-2895; fax, 352/392-8347; e-mail, skalra@neocortex.health.ufl.edu

GAL, NPY, and β-END, as revealed by examination of their morphologic and functional relationships, is briefly summarized.

FUNCTIONAL AND MORPHOLOGIC RELATIONSHIP BETWEEN GAL AND NPY IN THE HYPOTHALAMIC REGULATION OF LHRH SECRETION

Role of Galanin. Luteinizing hormone-releasing hormone (LHRH) produced by a network of neurons in the hypothalamus is the primary signal stimulating release of the gonadotropins, luteinizing hormone, and follicle-stimulating hormone (FSH). Evidence suggests that a pulse generator network within the hypothalamus is responsible for LHRH secretion into the hypophyseal portal system. Generally, two basic oscillating patterns of LHRH secretion have been described. The basal secretion pattern is in the form of low amplitude pulses at regular intervals throughout the 24-hour period in males and through various stages of the estrous cycle in females. This pattern is interrupted by an abrupt acceleration in LHRH discharge frequency on proestrus, which in turn evokes the ovulatory surge of gonadotropins.[5]

A distinct excitatory component in the hypothalamic circuitry is apparently responsible for stimulating the basal and cyclic patterns of LHRH secretion. Our concerted efforts to dissect out the excitatory component of this circuitry revealed a causal role for GAL and NPY in the two patterns of LHRH output.[1,5] Administration of GAL into the third cerebroventricle (icv) of ovariectomized (ovx) rats pretreated with ovarian steroids rapidly stimulated the release of pituitary LH in a dose-dependent manner.[8] This excitatory effect on pituitary gonadotropin release was due primarily to neural activation in the hypothalamus, because GAL administration stimulated release of LHRH from the median eminence-arcuate nucleus (ME-ARC) of these rats, and a competitive GAL receptor antagonist, galantide [M-15], a chimeric peptide of 20 amino acids (GAL-[1-13]) and substance-P-[5-11], suppressed both basal and GAL-induced LHRH release.[9] That this stimulatory effect of GAL is physiologically relevant in modulating the two patterns of LH secretion was shown by a number of studies. GAL secretion into the hypophyseal portal vessels was pulsatile, and GAL pulses either preceded or coincided with LHRH episodes;[10] blockade of the effects of GAL secretory episodes by either passive immunoneutralization with GAL antibody (GAL-Ab) or by the GAL receptor antagonist, galantide, attenuated the basal episodic pattern of LH secretion.[9,11] Thus, these results clearly reinforced the views that GAL is an excitatory component of the LHRH pulse generator and that episodic secretion of GAL under the direction of the pulse generator played an excitatory role in synchronizing LHRH discharge into the hypophyseal portal system.

Further investigations revealed that GAL also participated in the preovulatory discharge of LHRH on proestrus. Central administration of galantide inhibited the LH surge on proestrus, blocked ovulation, and also inhibited the LH surge induced by ovarian steroids in ovx rats.[9] Thus, the neural signals responsible for the initiation and sustenance of LHRH hypersecretion necessary for the preovulatory LH surge on proestrus engage GAL receptors in the ME-ARC and possibly elsewhere in the hypothalamus. These findings together with the reports that GAL gene expression in the hypothalamus is upregulated in association with the LHRH surge[10] are clearly in agreement with our proposal that hypothalamic GAL is an important component of the neural circuitry involved in the two modalities of LHRH secretion in rats.

Role of Neuropeptide Y. NPY is another peptidergic signal shown to stimulate LH release in ovarian steroid-primed ovx rats and LHRH release from the ME-ARC.[1,12,13]

NPY-producing neurons located in the ARC apparently participated in stimulation of LHRH release. NPY released at both the LHRH perikaryal level in the medial preoptic area (MPOA) and the LHRH nerve terminals in the ME elicits LHRH release.[1] Like GAL, NPY participates in the basal and cyclic patterns of LHRH secretion in the rat. NPY secretion within the ME-ARC was pulsatile, with the peaks in NPY levels coinciding with the peaks in LHRH secretion,[14,15] and passive immunoneutralization with NPY-Ab or reduction of NPY availability by antisense oligodeoxynucleotides reduced LHRH pulsatility.[1,16] Thus, NPY is also an excitatory component of the neural network involved in elicitation of episodic LHRH secretion. Furthermore, NPY was critical in preovulatory LHRH secretion, because NPY production preceded the onset and secretion and thereafter closely paralleled the LHRH pattern.[1,17,18] Blockade of these neurosecretory events with antisense oligodeoxynucleotides extinguished the LH surge.[19]

Galanin-Neuropeptide Y Interaction in the Rat Hypothalamus. Experimental evidence: Whereas GAL and NPY are the two most abundant peptides in the rat hypothalamus,[1] each of them exciting LHRH release and participating in basal and cyclic discharge of LH, an important question is whether GAL and NPY act separately or in concert in synchronizing the two modalities of LHRH secretion.

Because both NPY and GAL are secreted in a pulsatile manner and evidence showed that each is capable of driving LHRH pulsatility, we undertook to investigate the physiologic role of each in governing basal LHRH secretion in ovx rats. Because our previous studies indicated that passive immunoneutralization of either NPY or GAL could not abolish the episodic LH secretion, it suggested that GAL and NPY together may be involved in the intermittent secretion of LHRH (LH) in ovx rats. To test this possibility, in a series of experiments we infused various combinations of GAL-Ab and NPY-Ab icv to discern the contribution of each in driving LH episodes.[11] The results showed that passive immunoneutralization of GAL and NPY, in concentrations that individually exerted no detectable impact on LH secretion, markedly suppressed LH pulsatility when infused together. Apparently, the characteristic LHRH episodic pattern in ovx rats is critically dependent on the combined excitatory action of NPY and GAL. These findings led us to propose that a distinct pulse generator located in the hypothalamus imparts intermittence to GAL and NPY secretion which, in turn, imposes a pulsatile LHRH secretion pattern.[5,11] Because evidence already exists of a considerable degree of concordance between GAL, NPY, LHRH, and LH episodes,[10,14,15] these experimental findings affirm the view that GAL and NPY are indeed responsible for the propagation and sustenance of LHRH pulsatility.[5,11]

Morphologic Evidence. Because of the striking similarities in the modulatory effects of GAL and NPY on LHRH secretion and the evidence that receptive elements for excitatory action reside in the basal hypothalamus, we explored the possibility that to provide a substrate for the excitatory information transfer necessary for the synchronous discharge of LHRH, GAL, and NPY may be anatomically linked in the hypothalamus. Indeed, examination of the morphologic relationships by light and electron microscopic double immunocytochemistry for GAL and NPY revealed that the NPY network is synaptically linked with GAL neurons in the diagonal band of Broca, MPOA, and ARC.[20] These revelations raised the possibility that NPY-dependent LHRH secretion may be mediated, in part, by GAL released in response to NPY. This is highly likely because the GAL-receptor antagonist galantide partially suppressed NPY-induced LH release.[20] Consequently, these results concur with the thesis that information transfer from the hypothalamic pulse generator to the LHRH network mobilizes a NPY→GAL line of communication in addition to the direct action of NPY and GAL on LHRH neurons.[1] The site of interaction presumably extends from the MPOA rostrally to the ME-ARC caudally.[1]

FUNCTIONAL AND MORPHOLOGIC RELATIONSHIPS BETWEEN GAL AND OPIOIDS IN THE HYPOTHALAMIC REGULATION OF FEEDING BEHAVIOR

A large body of evidence shows that GAL stimulates feeding in rats.[21,22] GAL injections into the cerebroventricular system or microinjection into various hypothalamic sites evoked food intake in satiated rats.[22] Opioids have also long been known to stimulate feeding.[23] Of the three endogenous opioid peptides, the feeding behavior induced by β-END resembles that elicited by GAL, and microinjection of GAL and β-END in similar hypothalamic sites stimulated feeding.[2,22,23] The morphologic and functional relationship between NPY and GAL in the regulation of hypothalamic LHRH secretion led us to explore the possibility that GAL and β-END may interact to evoke feeding behavior.

A correlated light and electron microscopic double immunostaining of the medial basal hypothalamus revealed GAL-immunoreactive boutons in close proximity to β-END perikarya and dendrites in the ARC, with most β-END–immunoreactive neurons apposed by GAL nerve terminals.[24] Electron microscopic examination showed that GAL boutons formed axosomatic and axodendritic synaptic connections with β-END neurons. Further investigations involving deafferentation of the ARC showed that the GAL boutons contacting β-END perikarya and dendrites were of local origin.[24] Thus, these morphologic links between GAL and β-END networks in the ARC suggested that GAL-induced feeding behavior may be mediated in part by stimulation of β-END release by GAL. If this is true, then we argued that it should be possible to decrease GAL-induced feeding by administration of opiate receptor antagonists. Indeed, nalaxone, an opiate receptor antagonist, administered immediately preceding GAL injection suppressed feeding in a dose-related manner.[25] Consequently, it is highly likely that a functional link between GAL and b-END exists in the hypothalamus and that stimulation of food intake by GAL may be mediated in part by increased β-END release.[25] However, because nalaxone was unable to completely suppress GAL-induced feeding, we concluded that GAL may elicit feeding both on its own and through the β-END system.

Thus, these diverse experimental and morphologic approaches demonstrate the existence of an interconnected network composed of at least three components—GAL, NPY, and β-END—in the hypothalamic regulation of reproduction and appetite. It is highly likely that this network operates similarly in a site-specific manner to regulate other hypothalamic hormones important in the secretion of several pituitary hormones.

ACKNOWLEDGMENT

Dawn Stewart's secretarial assistance is appreciated.

REFERENCES

1. KALRA, S.P. 1993. Mandatory neuropeptide-steroid signaling for the preovulatory luteinizing hormone-releasing hormone discharge. Endocrinol. Rev. **14:** 507–538.
2. KALRA, S.P., B. XU, M.G. DUBE, S. PU, T.L. HORVATH & P.S. KALRA. 1999. Interacting appetite regulating pathways in the hypothalamic regulation of body weight. Endocr. Rev. In press.

3. LERANTH, C., F. NAFTOLIN, M. SHANBROUGH & T.L. HORVATH. 1992. Neuronal circuits regulating gonadotropin release. *In* The Neurobiology of Puberty. T.M. Plant & P.A. Lee, Eds. J. Endocrinol. Ltd. Bristol. UK. 55–73.

4. HÖKFELT, R., O. JOHANSSON & M. GOLDSTEIN. 1984. Chemical anatomy of the brain. Science **225:** 1326–1334.

5. KALRA, S.P., T.L. HORVATH, F. NAFTOLIN, B. XU, S. PU & P.S. KALRA. 1997. The interactive language of the gonadotropin releasing hormone (GnRH) system. J. Neuroendocrinol. **9:** 569–576.

6. MOTTA, M. 1991. Brain Endocrinology: 1–483. Raven Press. New York.

7. KALRA, S.P. & P.S. KALRA. 1996. Nutritional infertility: The role of the interconnected hypothalamic neuropeptide Y-galanin-opioid network. Front. Neuroendocrinology **17:** 371–401.

8. SAHU, A., W.R. CROWLEY, K. TATEMOTO, A. BALASUBRAMANIAN & S.P. KALRA. 1987. Effects of neuropeptide Y, NPY analog (norleucine4-NPY), galanin and neuropeptide K on LH release in ovariectomized (ovx) and ovx estrogen, progesterone-treated rats. Peptides **8:** 921–926.

9. SAHU, A., B. XU & S.P. KALRA. 1994. Role of galanin in stimulation of pituitary luteinizing hormone secretion as revealed by a specific receptor antagonist, galantide. Endocrinology **134:** 529–536.

10. MERCHENTHALER, I., F.J. LOPEZ & A. NEGRO-VILAR. 1993. Anatomy and physiology of central galanin-containing pathways. Prog. Neurobiol. **40:** 711–769.

11. XU, B., P.S. KALRA, J.F. HYDE, W.R. CROWLEY & S.P. KALRA. 1996. An interactive physiological role of neuropeptide Y and galanin in pulsatile luteinizing hormone secretion. Endocrinology **137:** 5297–5302.

12. KALRA, S.P. & W.R. CROWLEY. 1984. Norepinephrine-like effects of neuropeptide Y on LH release in the rat. Life Sci. **35:** 1173–1176.

13. CROWLEY, W.R. & S.P. KALRA. 1987. Neuropeptide Y stimulates the release of luteinizing hormone-releasing hormone from medial basal hypothalamus *in vitro*: Modulation by ovarian steroids. Neuroendocrinology **46:** 97–103.

14. TERASAWA, E. 1995. Control of luteinizing hormone-releasing hormone pulse generation in nonhuman primates. Cell. Molec. Neurobiol. **14:** 141–163.

15. SAHU, A., C. PHELPS, J.D. WHITE, S.P. KALRA & P.S. KALRA. 1992. Steroidal regulation of hypothalamic neuropeptide Y release and gene expression. Endocrinology **130:** 3331–3336.

16. XU, B., A. SAHU, W.R. CROWLEY, T.L. HORVATH & S.P. KALRA. 1993. Role of neuropeptide Y in episodic LH release in ovariectomized rats: An excitatory component and opioid involvement. Endocrinology **133:** 747–754.

17. SAHU, A., W. JACOBSON, W.R. CROWLEY & S.P. KALRA. 1989. Dynamic changes in neuropeptide Y concentrations in the median-eminence in association with preovulatory luteinizing hormone (LH) release in the rat. J. Neuroendocrinol. **1:** 83–87.

18. SAHU, A., W.R. CROWLEY & S.P. KALRA. 1995. Evidence that hypothalamic neuropeptide Y gene expression increases before the onset of the preovulatory LH surge. J. Neuroendocrinol. **7:** 291–296.

19. KALRA, P.S., J.J. BONAVERA & S.P. KALRA. 1995. Central administration of anti-sense oligodeoxynucleotides to neuropeptide Y (NPY) mRNA reveals the critical role of newly synthesized NPY in regulation of LHRH release. Reg. Pept. **59:** 215–220.

20. HORVATH, T.L., F. NAFTOLIN, C. LERANTH, A. SAHU & S.P. KALRA. 1996. Morphological and pharmacological evidence for neuropeptide Y-galanin interaction in the rat hypothalamus. Endocrinology **137:** 3069–3071.

21. CRAWLEY, J.N. 1995. Biological actions of galanin. Reg. Pept. **59:** 1–6.

22. LEIBOWITZ, S.F. 1995. Brain peptides and obesity: Pharmacologic treatment. Obesity Res. **3:** 573S–589S.

23. MORELY, J.E. 1987. Neuropeptide regulation of appetite and weight. Endocrinol. Rev. **8:** 256–287.

24. HORVATH, T.L., S.P. KALRA, F. NAFTOLIN & C. LERANTH. 1995. Morphological evidence for a galanin-opiate interaction in the rat mediobasal hypothalamus. J. Neuroendocrinol. **7:** 579–588.

25. DUBE, M.G., T.L. HORVATH, C. LERANTH, P.S. KALRA & S.P. KALRA. 1994. Nalaxone reduces the feeding evoked by intracerebroventricular galanin injection. Physiol. Behav. **56:** 811–813.

Galanin–Galanin Receptor Systems in the Hypothalamic Paraventricular and Supraoptic Nuclei

Some Recent Findings and Future Challenges[a]

ANDREW L. GUNDLACH[b] AND TANYA C.D. BURAZIN

The University of Melbourne, Clinical Pharmacology and Therapeutics Unit, Department of Medicine, Austin & Repatriation Medical Centre, Heidelberg, Victoria 3084, Australia

ABSTRACT: Galanin and galanin receptors are widely distributed within the central nervous system, but historically much research has been focused on hypothalamic galanin systems including those in the preoptic area, paraventricular nucleus (PVN), supraoptic nucleus (SON), and median eminence. In early studies, galanin mRNA, immunoreactivity, and binding sites were detected in neurons of the SON and both the magnocellular and parvocellular regions of the PVN, all of which also contain vasopressin, oxytocin, and several other peptides. This article briefly reviews some important recent studies of the electrophysiologic effects of galanin on magnocellular neurons *in vitro*; regulation of galanin expression by the physiologic stimulus of lactation; the role of parvocellular galanin systems in energy balance, body weight, and obesity; and the regional and cellular localization of galanin and galanin receptor mRNAs in the PVN/SON. In relation to the latter issue, two distinct galanin receptor subtypes, GalR1 and GalR2, have now been cloned and characterized. *In situ* hybridization histochemical studies of rat brain by several groups have consistently demonstrated GalR1 mRNA in the SON and PVN, in the magnocellular and parvocellular regions. By contrast, our recent experiments using [^{35}S]-labeled oligonucleotide probes detected GalR2 mRNA enriched in the parvocellular, *not* the magnocellular regions of the PVN, and the transcripts were not detected in the SON, whereas studies by others using a digoxigenin-labeled RNA probe *have* detected GalR2 mRNA in the SON (and PVN). Nonetheless, given the known effects of hyperosmotic stimuli, changes in metabolic status, and various hormones on galanin synthesis and release and the ability of galanin to regulate the electrical and secretory activity of magnocellular neurons, it will be of interest to determine any possible (differential) regulation of galanin receptor subtype expression and the pre- and postsynaptic roles of GalR1 and GalR2 receptors in magnocellular and parvocellular neurons.

G alanin, a 29-30 amino acid neuropeptide, is widely distributed throughout the peripheral and central nervous systems and has been ascribed a number of physiologic effects that are thought to be mediated by distinct galanin receptor subtypes.[1–3] However, as recently as 1996-1997, the likely existence of multiple galanin receptors was largely

[a]Research in the authors' laboratory is supported by grants from the National Health and Medical Research Council of Australia and by the Austin Hospital Medical Research Foundation and the Sylvia and Charles Viertel Charitable Foundation.

[b]Address for correspondence: Dr. A.L. Gundlach, Clinical Pharmacology and Therapeutics Unit, Department of Medicine, Austin & Repatriation Medical Centre, Heidelberg, Victoria 3084, Australia. Phone, 61-3-9496-5495; fax, 61-3-9459-3510; e-mail, agund@austin.unimelb.edu.au

based on pharmacologic studies using truncated galanin analogs and chimeric peptide antagonists in various tissues including brain (in particular hippocampus), anterior pituitary gland, and peripheral tissues such as pancreas and small intestine (for a review see Kask *et al.*[4]).

Currently, however, two galanin receptors, GalR1 and GalR2, have been cloned and characterized in several species including rat and man, and their primary structure and other characteristics have been elucidated using receptor expression systems.[5–12] These studies have revealed the differences in the GalR1 and GalR2 receptor amino acid sequence (*only* 35–40% identity), pharmacology, and second messenger signaling systems. Thus, both galanin receptors are G-protein–coupled proteins located in the cell membrane, but GalR1 is coupled to inhibition of adenylate cyclase, whereas GalR2 is coupled to stimulation of phospholipase C.[7,8,10,11,13] Various detection methods have shown GalR1 and GalR2 mRNAs to be differentially distributed in rat brain, and GalR2 mRNA is reported to be more widespread than GalR1 mRNA, which has only been detected in significant levels in brain and spinal cord and not in peripheral tissues.[7,8,10,14] (For further descriptions of the molecular characteristics of galanin receptors, including their structure and binding properties, and signal transduction including the effects on K^+- and Ca^{2+}-channels, coupling to inhibition of adenylate cyclase, and stimulation of phosphatidyl inositol production, see refs. 4, 6–11, and 13).

In this article we review studies that highlight some of the most recent advances in our understanding of galanin systems in the magnocellular (and parvocellular) neurons of the paraventricular nucleus (PVN) and supraoptic nucleus (SON) and briefly discuss some important issues for future research.

PHYSIOLOGIC EFFECTS OF GALANIN ON MAGNOCELLULAR NEUROSECRETORY CELLS *IN VITRO*

In a recent electrophysiologic study using superfused hypothalamic explants, the cellular basis of the action of galanin as a central neuromodulator of magnocellular neurosecretory cells was investigated in identified neurons of this type in the SON.[15] Application of full-length galanin-(1-29) or the NH_2-terminal fragment galanin-(1-16) produced a dose-dependent and reversible membrane hyperpolarization with an IC_{50} of ~10 nM. These effects were tetrodotoxin-insensitive, indicating that the receptors responsible were located postsynaptically. Changes in the external chloride and potassium concentrations indicated that the effects of galanin were not mediated by modulation of chloride conductances, but probably involved a potassium conductance, as described in other types of neurons. Hyperpolarizing effects of galanin were associated with suppression of firing of both continuously active and phasically active neurons. Inhibition of phasic bursts was mediated through inhibitory effects of hyperpolarization and through galanin-mediated inhibition of the depolarizing potential that is responsible for the production of individual bursts.[15] The authors suggested that because the phasic pattern of activity maximizes peptide hormone release from the pituitary, the regulation of its expression by modulation of the depolarizing afterpotential amplitude represents a potentially important cellular mechanism for regulating humoral output, under different physiologic and pathologic conditions. Previous immunohistochemical studies have shown that approximately equal numbers of oxytocin- and vasopressin-containing neurosecretory neurons are present in the SON of the rat, and as most cells studied in this *in vitro* preparation were affected by galanin-like ligands, it is probable that both types of cells express galanin receptors (see below) and could potentially be regulated by endogenously released galanin *in vivo*. Thus, reported effects of intraventricularly administered galanin on oxytocin[16] and vasopressin[17] release *in vivo* might have been mediated by direct inhibition of action potential discharge at the magnocellular neuron somata.

Although the source of galanin fibers innervating magnocellular neurons in the SON remains to be established, previous studies have demonstrated the presence of galanin-containing neurons in a wide variety of areas known to send projections to the SON, including the preoptic-periventricular area around the third ventricle[18] which is known to play an important role in the regulation of magnocellular neurons.[19] Importantly, however, magnocellular neurons express high levels of galanin,[20,21] and it is possible that these cells may secrete physiologically relevant concentrations of galanin along with vasopressin and oxytocin from somatodendritic sites, with galanin providing inhibitory feedback regulation of spike discharge in vasopressin- and oxytocin-releasing cells. It will be of interest to learn more about the pharmacology of these acute electrophysiologic effects and to determine which of the currently identified galanin receptors[6–11,22] is responsible for the acute actions of galanin (see ref. 23).

Another recent finding that may assist the *in vitro* study of the physiologic effects of galanin (and vasopressin/oxytocin systems) in the PVN/SON, particularly in relation to galanin's possible role in regenerative processes, is the use of cultured magnocellular neurons isolated from the rat SON, which were recently found to express galanin immunoreactivity after 7–18 days in culture.[24] By contrast, freshly dispersed cells that were round-shaped and lacked neurite processes as a consequence of dispersion did not contain significant levels of galanin (or cholecystokinin) immunoreactivity, providing further support for the theory that galanin is important in the regenerative processes occurring during the first days in culture and during similar regeneration *in vivo*, following pituitary stalk transection[25] or hypophysectomy.[26,27]

REGULATION OF GALANIN mRNA AND IMMUNOREACTIVITY IN MAGNOCELLULAR NEURONS BY LACTATION

Earlier studies extensively investigated the regulation of galanin mRNA and galanin immunoreactivity in PVN and SON following various experimental manipulations, including salt-loading and hypophysectomy.[25–28]

In recent articles by Eriksson *et al.*[29] and Landry *et al.*,[30] the pattern of changes in galanin mRNA and galanin immunoreactivity in the SON and PVN were examined during lactation. Both galanin peptide and mRNA concentrations decreased in magnocellular neurons in the early stages of lactation (3–7 days). After 14 days of lactation, galanin mRNA expression had increased and attained control levels again. Thus, levels of galanin mRNA were altered in the opposite direction to those of oxytocin and vasopressin mRNA.[29,30] During 14 days of lactation, cellular galanin immunoreactivity was just detectable in the magnocellular somata, although the number of galanin-containing neurons possibly increased in the SON. In lactating rats galanin was homogeneously distributed throughout the cytoplasm of PVN and SON cells.

Several mechanisms may be involved in producing these effects including a decrease in galanin synthesis in the cell bodies or changes in galanin processing, sorting, or both. Galanin gene expression in magnocellular neurons is increased by estrogen,[31] so the decrease in galanin mRNA seen in lactating rats may be due to the decrease in estrogen concentrations reported during lactation.[29] Alternatively, changes in mRNA stability may play a part in the altered galanin content during lactation with increased degradation causing the rapid decrease in expression. In addition, galanin may be present in magnocellular neurons, but not in an immunoreactive form (see Ryan and Gundlach[32]), and lactation might alter galanin processing, making the peptide detectable. Alternatively, stimulation of neuronal activity might induce galanin mis-sorting and modify galanin distribution by diverting some peptide from the secretory pathway.[30]

These studies provide strong evidence that lactation represents a physiologic condition that stimulates the expression of galanin in oxytocinergic magnocellular neurons. The functional role of galanin is not yet established, although as just discussed, it was proposed to have an inhibitory effect on neurohormone expression in magnocellular neurons— injections of galanin decrease plasma concentrations of oxytocin; thus, the inhibitory effect on the expression of oxytocin could be attenuated by downregulation of galanin production.[30]

INVOLVEMENT OF PARVOCELLULAR GALANIN SYSTEMS IN ENERGY BALANCE, EATING BEHAVIOR, AND WEIGHT CONTROL

In several recent articles, Leibowitz and colleagues[33,34] provided strong evidence for the involvement of galanin neurons in the anterior parvocellular region of the PVN in the regulation of body weight and obesity in both male and female rats. Rats were tested in different feeding paradigms with diets containing fat, carbohydrate, or protein, and using a range of techniques these studies identified a specifically responsive group of galanin neurons in the anterior parvocellular PVN and galanin-containing nerve terminals in the external zone of the median eminence that underwent changes in galanin expression and/or release in close relation to dietary fat, circulating glucose, and body fat.[34] Correlative and other histochemical data support the existence of an anterior PVN to median eminence projection related to fat intake and deposition. Changes were also seen in the activity of this pathway during the estrous cycle, with a peak in galanin levels during proestrous.[33]

Given the documented importance of particular populations of galanin-positive neurons in the physiology of nutritional intake and metabolism, it is of interest to determine the relative involvement of the different galanin receptor subtypes (see below) in these processes, as there are exciting therapeutic implications for agents that might selectively block the activation of these hypothalamic galanin systems that stimulate, and are stimulated by, high fat intake. Initial studies towards this aim might examine the response of the GalR1 and GalR2 receptors in the PVN to food restriction[35,36] or other dietary alterations.[34]

In another important study with implications for the regulation of body weight and feeding/drinking behavior in rats, Håkansson et al.[37] described the presence of leptin receptor immunoreactivity in galanin/corticotropin-releasing hormone-containing parvocellular neurons and both vasopressin- and oxytocin-containing magnocellular neurons. Leptin is a recently identified cytokine-like molecule that is produced by adipocytes and regulates body weight homeostasis. Experimentally, leptin induces weight reduction in mice with diet-induced obesity and in normal mice by decreasing food intake and increasing energy expenditure.[38] Leptin is thought to act centrally, and although the arcuate nucleus is possibly the major site of action,[38] the presence of leptin receptors on parvocellular and magnocellular neurons suggests a potentially important link with the hypothalamo-pituitary-adrenal axis and even with the processes of fluid balance and dietary changes during reproduction and lactation.[33,37]

REGIONAL AND SUBCELLULAR LOCALIZATION OF GALANIN mRNA IN MAGNOCELLULAR AND PARVOCELLULAR NEURONS

The distribution of galanin mRNA throughout the CNS and specifically within the hypothalamus was reported by several groups,[26,32,39,40] and galanin transcripts are known to be present in high abundance in the PVN and SON and to coexist with vasopressin, oxytocin, and other peptides under normal or pathophysiologic conditions.[20,21,26,28]

In a recent study using nonradioactive in situ hybridization and immunohistochemistry at the light and electron microscopic levels, the localization of galanin mRNA in the hypothalamo-hypophyseal system was further investigated in normal and salt-loaded rats.[41] After salt loading, galanin transcripts were found throughout the perikaryal cytoplasm and in the perinuclear area. Galanin immunoreactivity was also found in the perinuclear area of control rats, suggesting that galanin synthesis may occur in this cytoplasmic domain. Galanin mRNA was also clustered in dendrites containing rough endoplasmic reticulum and segregated in axonal projections coursing through the internal layer of the median eminence after salt loading. These studies provide evidence that the exportation of mRNAs into axons in the magnocellular system is not limited to the two principal hormone mRNAs, vasopressin and oxytocin.[42–44] Peptide mRNA targeting to dendrites could lead to dendritic synthesis and release of the peptide product. The presence of synaptic contacts close to the translation sites has been reported in dendrites and could, in the case of galanin, provide for the local rapid regulation of galanin mRNA translation by synaptic inputs, although at this time the exact functional significance of axonal mRNAs remains unclear.[41]

LOCALIZATION OF GALANIN RECEPTOR mRNAS IN MAGNOCELLULAR AND PARVOCELLULAR NEURONS

The distribution of galanin receptors in hypothalamus and other regions of the CNS was initially determined by autoradiographic mapping of $[^{125}I]$galanin binding.[45–47] Subsequent to the molecular cloning of the GalR1 receptor, several reports appeared describing the distribution of GalR1 mRNA in various brain areas containing $[^{125}I]$galanin binding sites and galanin immunoreactivity, including the hypothalamus.[7,14]

Recently a detailed study of the distribution of mRNA encoding the GalR1 receptor in the hypothalamus described high levels of expression in the medial preoptic area and the PVN and SON.[48] Numerous expressing neurons were widely distributed throughout the rostrocaudal extent of the PVN, including the anterior and caudal parts of the medial subdivision. The highest number and density of GalR1 mRNA-positive cells were present in the posterior magnocellular division and the medial part of the parvocellular subdivision. The dorsal parvocellular and posterior parvocellular subdivisions were nearly devoid of labeled cells. The SON also contained numerous GalR1 mRNA-expressing cells with dense labeling present in the ventromedial and dorsal parts of this nucleus.[48] The high levels of hypothalamic GalR1 mRNA expression corresponded to high levels of [^{125}I]galanin binding reported previously[45–47] and are consistent with the expression of GalR1 receptors by neurons secreting vasopressin, oxytocin, and other peptides such as corticotropin-releasing hormone.

Until recently, only preliminary reports existed on the distribution of GalR2 mRNA in the adult rat brain[8] (but see Depczynski et al., this volume). In these studies using a digoxigenin-labeled RNA probe, GalR2 mRNA was reported to be present in the PVN (subdivision not stipulated) and the dorsal and ventral portions of the SON. However, in recent studies in our laboratory we used multiple oligonucleotide probes directed against GalR1 and GalR2 mRNAs to localize their expression in the hypothalamus and other brain areas of adult rats and postnatal rats of different ages. Thus, three GalR1- and three GalR2-DNA oligonucleotide probes were synthesized complimentary to distinct, nonoverlapping nucleotide sequences of their respective cDNAs.[7,9] Screening of these sequences against available gene databases revealed homology (78–100%) only with appropriate galanin receptor cDNAs of the rat and other species. For *in situ* hybridization histochemistry, sections were incubated overnight at 42°C with [^{35}S]-labeled probes in 50% formamide—4 × SSC hybridization buffer, containing 10% dextran sulfate and 200 mM dithiothreitol. Slides were washed in 1 × SSC at 55°C, rinsed, then dehydrated, before being apposed to x-ray film for 1–4 weeks and then nuclear emulsion for 6–20 weeks. (For further methodologic details, see Burazin and Gundlach.[49])

In mapping studies in the forebrain, GalR1 mRNA was detected in the glomerular and mitral cell layers of the olfactory bulb, the tenia tecta, and various hypothalamic and thalamic nuclei of rat brain (data not shown), consistent with previous reports.[6,14] Similarly, GalR2 mRNA was present in the dentate gyrus, ventral CA3 field of hippocampus, and arcuate hypothalamic nucleus (data not shown) as previously described.[8] Specific hybridization signal was effectively eliminated by incubation in the presence of a 100-fold excess of unlabeled probes (data not shown).

In the anterior hypothalamus, GalR1 mRNA was present in the magnocellular and parvocellular regions of the PVN (FIG. 1B) and in the dorsal and ventral parts of the SON (FIG. 1E). GalR2 mRNA was detectable in neurons of the parvocellular and medial subdivisions of the PVN (FIG. 1C), but GalR2 mRNA was not detected within the SON (FIG. 1F). In studies of the expression of GalR1 and GalR2 in hypothalamus from rats 4–

FIGURE 1. Distribution of GalR1 and GalR2 mRNAs in the paraventricular and supraoptic nuclei of the adult rat, detected using [^{35}S]-labeled oligonucleotides. (A) High-power brightfield micrograph of the ipsilateral paraventricular nucleus (PVN). (B,C) Darkfield micrographs of GalR1 and GalR2 mRNAs in near-adjacent sections of the PVN. Note the enrichment of GalR1 in the magnocellular and parvocellular divisions. The third ventricle (V) is marked (*) as a landmark. (D) High-power brightfield micrograph of the ipsilateral supraoptic nucleus (SON). (E,F) Darkfield micrographs of GalR1 and GalR2 mRNAs in near-adjacent sections of the SON. GalR1 mRNA is readily detected, whereas GalR2 mRNA is undetectable. Silver grains over the optic nerve (**) are the result of "nonspecific binding" of oligonucleotides to this myelinated tract. Abbreviations: dp, dorsal parvocellular division PVN; mmp, medial dorsal parvocellular division PVN; oc, optic chiasm; PaMC, magnocellular division PVN; PaPC, parvocellular subdivision PVN. Scale bar = 10 μm.

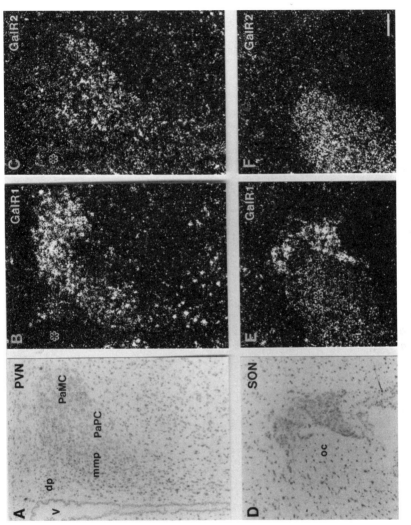

FIGURE 1. *See legend in facing page.*

70 days old, GalR1 mRNA was expressed in the PVN and SON as early as postnatal days 4–7 at levels approximately similar to those at postnatal days 14–28, but slightly lower than adult levels (Burazin, Ryan and Gundlach, unpublished observations). In the limited material examined, GalR2 mRNA was detected in the PVN at postnatal days 7–14 and through to adulthood (day 70), but was not detected in the SON (Burazin and Gundlach, unpublished observations).

Thus, these and some previous findings suggest a differential expression (or level of expression) of galanin receptor subtypes in different hypothalamic and other neuronal types and the possibility of a differential response of these receptors in situations where the amount of galanin peptide is increased, predicting complex adaptive mechanisms in various galanin systems throughout the CNS (see Burazin, Ryan and Gundlach[49]).

FUTURE STUDIES OF GALANIN SYSTEMS IN THE HYPOTHALAMUS

With the ability to now assess the level of GalR1 *and* GalR2 mRNA in a semiquantitative and anatomic context, it will be interesting to examine the regulation of GalR1 and GalR2 transcripts within the hypothalamus and particularly the magnocellular system by experimental manipulations that were shown to alter the secretory activity of these neurons and the expression of vasopressin, oxytocin, and galanin.[25–28] It will also be important to determine if both ligand *and* receptor(s) are affected by particular hormones and modulatory factors relevant to the galanin system such as estrogen,[31,33] corticosterone,[50] insulin,[51] or even leukemia inhibitory factor.[52] Information currently available indicates that the two galanin receptor subtypes exhibit distinct, yet overlapping, patterns of distribution in the rat CNS, but future double-labeling *in situ* hybridization or immunohistochemical studies are required to definitively determine potential colocalization of GalR1 and GalR2 receptors.

The development of high affinity ligands that specifically recognize the GalR1 or GalR2 receptor would assist in determining if any changes in galanin receptor mRNA levels are directly related to an increase in receptor protein expression. Although most galanin analogs display similar binding affinities for rat GalR1 and GalR2 receptors, the affinity of galanin-(2-29) for GalR2 is 42-fold higher than that for GalR1 in receptor expression systems,[11] and [D-Trp^2]galanin-(1-29) can also distinguish the two receptor subtypes.[10] Thus, studies are in progress in our laboratory to develop suitable radioligands to label GalR2 receptors in brain and explore the level and localization of GalR1 and GalR2 receptor protein in various paradigms of altered hypothalamic function.

More generally, it is of interest to determine if the localization and actions of both GalR1 and GalR2 receptors account for all the physiologic effects of galanin and galanin-like ligands within the CNS, as recent evidence indicates the existence of at least one additional subtype of galanin receptor, the GalR3,[22] although its presence in the CNS, and the hypothalamus in particular, has not yet been demonstrated. However importantly, the GalR3 receptor was cloned from a hypothalamic cDNA library and so it is presumed to be expressed in this area, even if only at low levels.[22]

Clearly, specific antagonists or antibodies for galanin receptor subtypes, or targeted disruption of each receptor gene by receptor antisense studies, or the development of receptor knockout models will be required to determine the exact role of each galanin receptor in mediating the many biologic effects of galanin described to date and potential new functions as well.

ACKNOWLEDGMENTS

The authors gratefully acknowledge the contribution of Dr. Mary C. Ryan to early studies on the distribution of galanin-R1 receptor mRNA.

Note added in proof: In a recent article (Landry, M., K. Åman, & T. Hökfelt. 1998. Galanin-R1 receptor in anterior and mid-hypothalamus: Distribution and regulation. J. Comp. Neurol. **399:** 321–340), Hökfelt and colleagues describe the regulation of GalR1 mRNA in the PVN and SON by physiologic and experimental stimuli. They observed a marked increase after salt loading and a moderate decrease during lactation, parallel to galanin mRNA, and a decrease following hypophysectomy, in the opposite direction to galanin mRNA levels (see comments in text).

REFERENCES

1. SKOFITSCH, G. & D.M. JACOBOWITZ. 1990. Galanin in the central nervous system: A review. In Current Aspects of the Neurosciences. N.N. Osborne, Ed.: 1–64. Macmillan Press. London.
2. MERCHENTHALER, I., F.J. LÓPEZ & A. NEGRO-VILAR. 1993. Anatomy and physiology of central galanin-containing pathways. Prog. Neurobiol. **40:** 711–769.
3. CRAWLEY, J.N. 1995. Biological actions of galanin. Regul. Pept. **59:** 1–16.
4. KASK, K., M. BERTHOLD & T. BARTFAI. 1997. Galanin receptors: Involvement in feeding, pain, depression and Alzheimer's disease. Life Sci. **60:** 1523–1533.
5. HABERT-ORTOLI, E., B. AMIRANOFF, I. LOQUET, M. LABURTHE & J.-F. MAYAUX. 1994. Molecular cloning of a functional human galanin receptor. Proc. Natl. Acad. Sci. USA **91:** 9780–9783.
6. BURGEVIN, M.-C., I. LOQUET, D. QUARTERONET & E. HABERT-ORTOLI. 1995. Cloning, pharmacological characterization, and anatomical distribution of a rat cDNA encoding for a galanin receptor. J. Mol. Neurosci. **6:** 33–41.
7. PARKER, E.M., D.G. IZZARELLI, H.P. NOWAK, C.D. MAHLE, L.G. IBEN, J. WANG & M.E. GOLDSTEIN. 1995. Cloning and characterization of the rat GALR1 galanin receptor from Rin14B insulinoma cells. Mol. Brain Res. **34:** 179–189.
8. FATHI, Z., A.M. CUNNINGHAM, L.G. IBEN, P.B. BATTAGLINO, S.A. WARD, K.A. NICHOL, K.A. PINE, J. WANG, M.E. GOLDSTEIN, T.P. IISMAA & I.A. ZIMANYI. 1997. Cloning, pharmacological characterization and distribution of a novel galanin receptor. Mol. Brain Res. **51:** 49–59.
9. HOWARD, A.D., C. TAN, L.-L. SHIAO, O.C. PALYHA, K.K. MCKEE, D.H. WEINBERG, S.D. FEIGHNER, M.A. CASCIERI, R.G. SMITH, L.H.T. VAN DER PLOEG & K.A. SULLIVAN. 1997. Molecular cloning and characterization of a new receptor for galanin. FEBS Lett. **405:** 285–290.
10. SMITH, K.E., C. FORRAY, M.W. WALKER, K.A. JONES, J.A. TAMM, J. BARD, T.A. BRANCHEK, D.L. LINEMEYER & C. GERALD. 1997. Expression cloning of a rat hypothalamic galanin receptor coupled to phosphoinositide turnover. J. Biol. Chem. **39:** 24612–24616.
11. WANG, S., T. HASHEMI, C. HE, C. STRADER & M. BAYNE. 1997. Molecular cloning and pharmacological characterization of a new galanin receptor subtype. Mol. Pharmacol. **52:** 337–343.
12. BLOOMQUIST, B.T., M.R. BEAUCHAMP, L. ZHELNIN, S.-E. BROWN, A.R. GORE-WILLSE, P. GREGOR & L.J. CORNFIELD. 1998. Cloning and expression of the human galanin receptor GalR2. Biochem. Biophys. Res. Commun. **243:** 474–479.
13. WANG, S., T. HASHEMI, S. FRIED, A.L. CLEMMONS & B.E. HAWES. 1998. Differential intracellular signaling of the GalR1 and GalR2 galanin receptor subtypes. Biochemistry **37:** 6711–6717.
14. GUSTAFSON, E.L., K.E. SMITH, M.M. DURKIN, C. GERALD & T.A. BRANCHEK. 1996. Distribution of a rat galanin receptor mRNA in rat brain. NeuroReport **7:** 953–957.

15. PAPAS, S. & C.W. BOURQUE. 1997. Galanin inhibits continuous and phasic firing in rat hypothalamic magnocellular neurosecretory cells. J. Neurosci. **17:** 6048–6056.

16. BJÖRKSTRAND, E., A.-L. HULTING, B. MEISTER & K. UVNÄS-MÖBERG. 1993. Effect of galanin on plasma levels of oxytocin and cholecystokinin. NeuroReport **4:** 10–12.

17. KONDO, K., T. MURASE, K. OTAKE, M. ITO, F. KURIMOTO & Y. OISO. 1993. Galanin as a physiological neurotransmitter in hemodynamic control of arginine vasopressin release in rats. Neuroendocrinology **57:** 224–229.

18. MELANDER, T., T. HÖKFELT & Å. RÖKAEUS. 1986. Distribution of galaninlike immunoreactivity in the rat central nervous system. J. Comp. Neurol. **248:** 475–517.

19. BOURQUE, C.W., S.H.R. OLIET & D. RICHARD. 1994. Osmoreceptors, osmoreception and osmoregulation. Front. Neuroendocrinol. **15:** 231–274.

20. RÖKAEUS, Å., W.S. YOUNG, III & E. MEZEY. 1988. Galanin coexists with vasopressin in the normal rat hypothalamus and galanin's synthesis is increased in the Brattleboro (diabetes insipidus) rat. Neurosci. Lett. **90:** 45–50.

21. SKOFITSCH, G., D.M. JACOBOWITZ, R. AMANN & F. LEMBECK. 1989. Galanin and vasopressin coexist in the rat hypothalamo-neurohypophyseal system. Neuroendocrinology **49:** 419–427.

22. WANG, S., C. HE, T. HASHEMI & M. BAYNE. 1997. Cloning and expressional characterization of a novel galanin receptor. Identification of different pharmacophores within galanin for the three galanin receptor subtypes. J. Biol. Chem. **272:** 31949–31952.

23. KINNEY, G.A., P.J. EMMERSON & R.J. MILLER. 1998. Galanin receptor-mediated inhibition of glutamate release in the arcuate nucleus of the hypothalamus. J. Neurosci. **18:** 3489–3500.

24. SANCHEZ, A., M. BILINSKI, V. GONZALEZ NICOLINI, M.J. VILLAR & J.H. TRAMEZZANI. 1997. Galanin and cholecystokinin in cultured magnocellular neurons isolated from adult rat supraoptic nuclei: A correlative light and scanning electron microscopical study. Histochem. J. **29:** 631–638.

25. YOUNG, W.S. III, S. HORVÁTH & M. PALKOVITS. 1990. The influences of hyperosmolality and synaptic inputs on galanin and vasopressin expression in the hypothalamus. Neuroscience **39:** 115–125.

26. MEISTER, B., R. CÓRTES, M.J. VILLAR, M. SCHALLING & T. HÖKFELT. 1990. Peptides and transmitter enzymes in hypothalamic magnocellular neurons after administration of hyperosmotic stimuli: Comparison between messenger RNA and peptide/protein levels. Cell Tissue Res. **260:** 279–297.

27. VILLAR, M.J., B. MEISTER, R. CORTÉS, M. SCHALLING, M. MORRIS & T. HÖKFELT. 1990. Neuropeptide gene expression in hypothalamic magnocellular neurons of normal and hypophysectomized rats: A combined immunohistochemical and *in situ* hybridization study. Neuroscience **36:** 181–199.

28. MEISTER, B., M.J. VILLAR, S. CECCATELLI & T. HÖKFELT. 1990. Localization of chemical messengers in magnocellular neurons of the hypothalamic supraoptic and paraventricular nuclei: An immunohistochemical study using experimental manipulations. Neuroscience **37:** 603–633.

29. ERIKSSON, M., S. CECCATELLI, K. UVNÄS-MÖBERG, M. IADAROLA & T. HÖKFELT. 1996. Expression of Fos-related antigens, oxytocin, dynorphin and galanin in the paraventricular and supraoptic nucleus of lactating rats. Neuroendocrinology **63:** 356–367.

30. LANDRY, M., D. ROCHE, E. ANGELOVA & A. CALAS. 1997. Expression of galanin in hypothalamic magnocellular neurones of lactating rats: Co-existence with vasopressin and oxytocin. J. Endocrinol. **155:** 467–481.

31. LEVIN, M.C. & P.E. SAWCHENKO. 1993. Neuropeptide co-expression in the magnocellular neurosecretory system of the female rat: Evidence for differential modulation by estrogen. Neuroscience **54:** 1001–1018.

32. RYAN, M.C. & A.L. GUNDLACH. 1996. Localization of preprogalanin messenger RNA in rat brain: Identification of transcripts in a subpopulation of cerebellar Purkinje cells. Neuroscience **70:** 709–728.

33. LEIBOWITZ, S.F., A. AKABAYASHI, J.T. ALEXANDER & J. WANG. 1998. Gonadal steroids and hypothalamic galanin and neuropeptide Y: Role in eating behavior and body weight control in female rats. Endocrinology **139:** 1771–1780.

34. LEIBOWITZ, S.F., A. AKABAYASHI & J. WANG. 1998. Obesity on a high-fat diet: Role of hypothalamic galanin in neurons of the anterior paraventricular nucleus projecting to the median eminence. J. Neurosci. **18:** 2709–2719.

35. O'SHEA, R.D. & A.L. GUNDLACH. 1993. Regulation of cholecystokinin receptors in the hypothalamus of the rat: Reciprocal changes in magnocellular nuclei induced by food deprivation and dehydration. J. Neuroendocrinol. **5:** 697–704.

36. O'SHEA, R.D. & A.L. GUNDLACH. 1995. Activity-linked alterations in cholecystokinin$_B$ receptor messenger RNA levels in magnocellular hypothalamic neurones by food and water deprivation in the rat. Neurosci. Lett. **194:** 189–192.

37. HÅKANSSON, M.-L., H. BROWN, N. GHILARDI, R.C. SKODA & B. MEISTER. 1998. Leptin receptor immunoreactivity in chemically defined target neurons of the hypothalamus. J. Neurosci. **18:** 559–572.

38. CAMPFIELD, L.A., F.J. SMITH, Y. GUISEZ, R. DEVOS & P. BURN. 1995. Recombinant mouse OB protein: Evidence for a peripheral signal linking adiposity and central neural networks. Science **269:** 546–549.

39. GUNDLACH, A.L., W. WISDEN, B.J. MORRIS & S.P. HUNT. 1990. Localization of preprogalanin mRNA in rat brain: *In situ* hybridization study with a synthetic oligonucleotide probe. Neurosci. Lett. **114:** 241–247.

40. JACOBOWITZ, D.M. & G. SKOFITSCH. 1991. Localization of galanin cell bodies in the brain by imunocytochemistry and *in situ* hybridization histochemistry. *In* Galanin: A New Multifunctional Peptide in the Neuroendocrine System. T. Hökfelt, T. Bartfai, D. Jacobowitz & D. Ottoson, Eds.: 69–92. Macmillan Press, London.

41. LANDRY, M. & T. HÖKFELT. 1998. Subcellular localization of preprogalanin messenger RNA in perikarya and axons of hypothalamo-posthypophyseal magnocellular neurons: An *in situ* hybridization study. Neuroscience **84:** 897–912.

42. JIRIKOWSKI, G.F., P.P. SANNA & F.E. BLOOM. 1990. mRNA coding oxytocin is present in axons of the hypothalamo-hypophyseal tract. Proc. Natl. Acad. Sci. USA. **87:** 7400–7404.

43. MOHR, E. & D. RICHTER. 1992. Diversity of mRNAs in the axonal compartment of peptidergic neurons in the rat. Eur. J. Neurosci. **4:** 870–876.

44. TREMBLEAU, A., M. MORALES & F.E. BLOOM. 1994. Aggregation of vasopressin mRNA in a subset of axonal swellings of the median eminence and posterior pituitary: Light and electron microscopic evidence. J. Neurosci. **14:** 39–53.

45. SKOFITSCH, G., M.A. SILLS & D.M. JACOBOWITZ. 1986. Autoradiographic distribution of [^{125}I]-galanin binding sites in the rat central nervous system. Peptides **7:** 1029–1042.

46. MELANDER, T., C. KÖHLER, S. NILSSON, T. HÖKFELT, E. BRODIN, E. THEODORSSON & T. BARTFAI. 1988. Autoradiographic quantitation and anatomical mapping of ^{125}I-galanin binding sites in the rat central nervous system. J. Chem. Neuroanat. **1:** 213–233.

47. LAGNY-POURMIR, I. & J. EPELBAUM. 1992. Regional stimulatory and inhibitory effects of guanine nucleotides on [^{125}I]galanin binding in rat brain: Relationship with the rate of occupancy of galanin receptors by endogenous galanin. Neuroscience **49:** 829–847.

48. MITCHELL, V., E. HABERT-ORTOLI, J. EPELBAUM, J.-P. AUBERT & J.-C. BEAUVILLAIN. 1997. Semiquantitative distribution of galanin-receptor (GAL-R1) mRNA-containing cells in the male rat hypothalamus. Neuroendocrinology **66:** 160–172.

49. BURAZIN, T.C.D. & A.L. GUNDLACH. 1998. Inducible galanin and GalR2 receptor system in motor neuron injury and regeneration. J. Neurochem. **71.** In press.

50. HEDLUND, P.B., J.I. KOENIG & K. FUXE. 1994. Adrenalectomy alters discrete galanin mRNA levels in the hypothalamus and mesencephalon of the rat. Neurosci. Lett. **170:** 77–82.

51. TANG, C., A. AKABAYASHI, A. MANITIU & S.F. LEIBOWITZ. 1997. Hypothalamic galanin gene expression and peptide levels in relation to circulating insulin: Possible role in energy balance. Neuroendocrinology **65:** 265–275.

52. Sun, Y. & R.E. Zigmond. 1996. Involvement of leukemia inhibitory factor in the increases in galanin and vasoactive intestinal peptide mRNA and the decreases in neuropeptide Y and tyrosine hydroxylase mRNA in sympathetic neurons after axotomy. J. Neurochem. **67:** 1751–1760.

Galanin in Ascending Systems

Focus on Coexistence with 5-Hydroxytryptamine and Noradrenaline[a]

TOMAS HÖKFELT,[b] ZHI-QING DAVID XU, TIE-JUN SHI,
KRISTINA HOLMBERG, AND XU ZHANG

Department of Neuroscience, Karolinska Institutet, S-171 77 Stockholm, Sweden

ABSTRACT: Galanin can be synthesized in several ascending systems including cholinergic forebrain neurons, serotonergic dorsal raphe neurons, and the noradrenergic locus coeruleus system. Recent immunohistochemical studies suggest that of these three systems, the locus coeruleus neurons express the highest levels of galanin and that in cortex and hippocampus galanin peptide can only be detected in the noradrenergic projections. Electrophysiologic studies show that galanin hyperpolarizes both serotonergic dorsal raphe neurons and noradrenergic locus coeruleus neurons at fairly high concentrations (10^6–10^{-7} M). In addition, galanin at low concentrations (10^{-9} M) enhances the 5-HT- and noradrenaline-induced hyperpolarization. Consequently, a galanin antagonist could attenuate an inhibitory tone on both dorsal raphe and locus coeruleus neurons and thus perhaps exert antidepressant activity.

The early histochemical studies on the neuropeptide galanin[1] revealed a wide distribution in the central nervous system.[2–4] It was also clear that in many cases galanin coexisted with a classic transmitter. Thus, among others, several of the ascending, highly divergent systems in the brain stem have the capacity to synthesize galanin, including the cholinergic basal forebrain neurons,[5] serotonergic dorsal raphe neurons,[6] tuberomamillary magnocellular neurons,[6,7] and, finally, noradrenergic locus coeruleus neurons in the pons.[6,8] It was apparent early that the levels of galanin in most of these systems under normal circumstances were very low (see also ref. 6); in fact, they were in some cases undetectable. However, after intraventricular colchicine treatment, distinct galanin-like immunoreactivity could be observed in all these cell groups, although noradrenergic locus coeruleus neurons had detectable galanin levels also under normal circumstances. Furthermore, it was believed that this effect of colchicine merely represented an inhibition of centrifugal transport due to microtuble breakdown.[9–11] It was subsequently recognized that colchicine can increase mRNA levels for various peptides including galanin.[12,13]

It was not surprising against this background that it was difficult to visualize galanin in the projection areas of these four cell groups which all are known to send projections to many parts of the brain, including cortex and hippocampal formation. However, evidence indicated that some of the weakly immunoreactive galanin fibers in cortex were noradrenergic,[14] and biochemical analyses combined with lesion experiments strongly supported that view.[15] Using an improved immunohistochemical technique galanin was recently demonstrated in fibers in cortex and hippocampus, and most of them were positive for

[a]This study was supported by the Swedish MRC (04X-2887), Astra Arcus AB and Marianne och Marcus Wallenbergs Stiftelse.

[b]Author to whom correspondence should be addressed. Phone, 46 8-7287070; fax, 46 8-331692; e-mail, Tomas.Hokfelt@neuro.ki.se

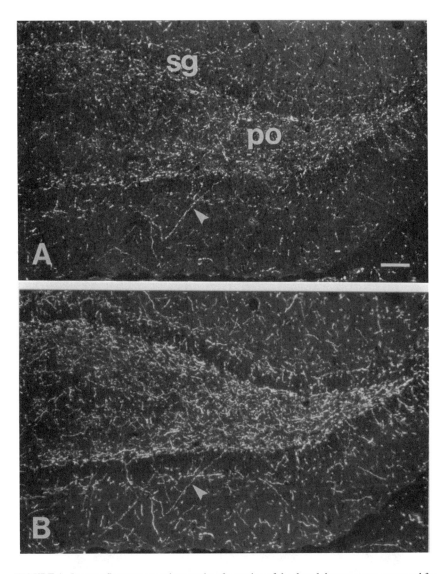

FIGURE 1. Immunofluorescence micrographs of a section of the dorsal dentate gyrus processed for double labeling with antiserum/antibodies to galanin **(A)** and dopamine β-hydroxylase (DBH) **(B)**. Note close overlap between galanin and DBH staining patterns, although in most cases DBH staining appears stronger. Note high degree of coexistence of galanin and DBH in all layers, with the highest density in the polymorph layer (po), especially along the granule cell layer (sg). *Arrowheads* denote galanin- and DBH-positive fiber. Bar indicates 80 μm.

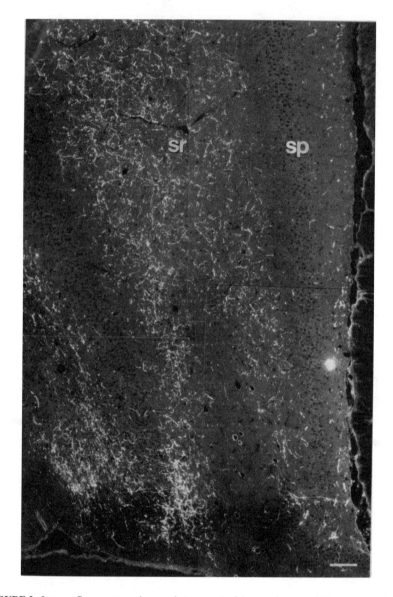

FIGURE 2. Immunofluorescence micrograph (montage) of the anterior ventral hippocampus of a 6-hydroxydopamine-treated rat after incubation with antiserum to galanin. Note that numerous galanin-positive fibers remain after 6-hydroxydopamine treatment, which removes all DBH-positive fibers (not shown). Bar indicates 100 μm.

dopamine β-hydroxylase (DBH) (FIG. 1A and B),[16] the enzyme converting dopamine to noradrenaline. In agreement, treatment with 6-hydroxydopamine, a neurotoxin that destroys catecholamine neurons,[17] caused disappearance of almost all galanin-positive fibers in the dorsal hippocampus and most of them in the ventral hippocampus, although distinct galanin-positive, DBH-negative networks could be detected, especially in its anterior, ventral parts (FIG. 2).[16]

The colchicine-induced upregulation of galanin is not confined to neurons; evidence indicates that this also can occur in glial cells.[18] Thus, after intraventricular or intracerebral colchicine injections, numerous galanin-positive cells can be seen around the injection site, such as the striatum and cortex. These cells are also present in white matter structures such as the anterior commissure. Double-labeling experiments suggest that these cells are not astrocytes, because they do not stain for glial fibrillary acidic protein. However, their exact nature has not been defined. Calzà *et al.* (this volume) demonstrated

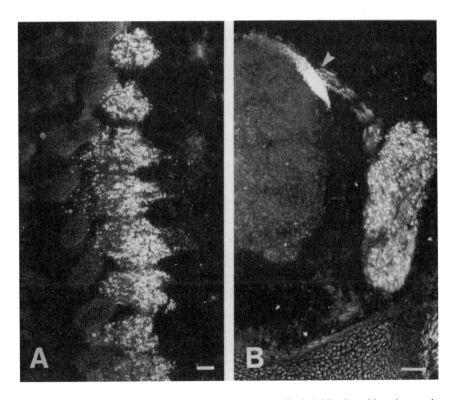

FIGURE 3. Darkfield micrograph of dorsal root ganglia (**A**) after hybridization with probe complementary to prepro-galanin mRNA, and fluorescence micrograph of dorsal root ganglion and spinal cord after incubation with galanin message-associated peptide antiserum (**B**). Note distinct prepro-galanin mRNA (**A**) and galanin message-associated peptide (**B**) expression in dorsal root ganglia. Immunoreactive fibers run in the dorsal roots and form a dense fiber plexus in the dorsal horn (*arrowhead*) (**B**). Bars indicate 100 μm.

that this upregulation does not occur in hypothyroid rats, suggesting a steroid hormone dependence of this phenomenon. The role of galanin in these presumptive glial cells has not been defined.

Studies on galanin and other peptides suggest that peptide systems can be divided in three categories depending on the mode of expression of the peptide.[19,20] Thus, there are neurons that have a robust expression of peptide under normal circumstances. The peptide can then easily be detected in nerve endings, suggesting that the peptide is available for release. In the second category the rate of expression is very low, so low that the peptide often cannot be detected with current histochemical techniques. However, after certain manipulations, such as colchicine injection or nerve injury, a distinct increase in synthesis occurs. This may represent induction, but it is also possible that a low rate of synthesis occurs but the levels are not sufficiently high to be detected. A third category includes peptides that are transiently expressed during embryogenesis. It is important to note that one and the same peptide can be expressed according to all three modes, and this is true also for galanin. For example, galanin in several hypothalamic systems can easily be detected under normal circumstances, whereas in several central systems, as just discussed, as well as in sensory systems the normal rate of synthesis is low, but upregulation occurs after, for example, nerve injury. Galanin is also transiently expressed at high levels during embryogenesis in several sensory systems including dorsal root ganglia (FIG. 3A and B), sensory epithelia in the eye and ear, olfactory epithelium, and even bone.[21]

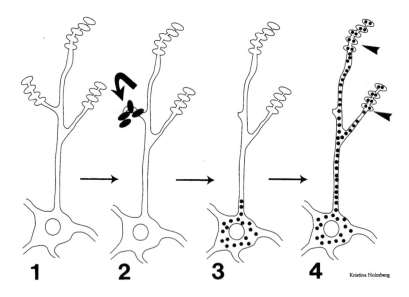

Kristina Holmberg

FIGURE 4. Hypothetical sequence of events during degeneration of cholinergic basal forebrain neurons. Under normal circumstances a basal cholinergic forebrain neuron does not express detectable levels of galanin (**1**). If one of its collateral branches degenerates (*curved arrow*) (**2**), this is a stimulus to upregulate galanin (**3**), which is transported centrifugally to the remaining collateral systems (**4**). Galanin could then inhibit acetylcholine release from these nerve terminals (*arrowheads*).

BASAL CHOLINERGIC FOREBRAIN NEURONS

The capacity of cholinergic forebrain neurons to synthesize galanin evoked an early interest in a possible involvement of galanin in Alzheimer's disease. Thus, on the basis of the colchicine/lesion-induced upregulation of galanin in these neurons[12,22] and the demonstration of galanin-induced inhibition of acetylcholine release,[23] it was hypothesized that degeneration of a collateral network may lead to upregulation of galanin synthesis in the lesioned neuron.[24] This in turn may be followed by centrifugal transport of galanin to the remaining, "healthy" nerve terminals, where galanin could inhibit acetylcholine release and thus worsen Alzheimer symptoms (FIG. 4). It was consequently suggested that a galanin antagonist could attenuate Alzheimer symptoms.[24] Furthermore, the interesting demonstration of galaninergic hyperinnervation of remaining cholinergic forebrain neurons in Alzheimer's disease[25–27] ignited further interest in this problem. It now seems clear that galanin expression in cholinergic forebrain neurons of man and apes is low, whereas monkey cholinergic forebrain neurons have high galanin levels.[28] Nevertheless, it still remains to be excluded that low-expressing cholinergic forebrain neurons can upregulate galanin in the early phase of Alzheimer's disease.

Galanin binding sites seem to be widespread in cortical regions of monkeys and man.[29–31] Changes in putative galanin receptors in Alzheimer brains have been reported.[32] The relation between galanin and cholinergic neurons as well as a possible involvement of galanin in learning and memory and in Alzheimer's disease will not be further discussed here, but we refer to chapters in this volume by Mufson *et al.*, Crawley *et al.*, Miller *et al.*, and Ögren *et al.*

SEROTONERGIC DORSAL RAPHE NEURONS

Dorsal raphe nuclei harbor several large groups of 5-HT neurons, first visualized with the Falck-Hillarp formaldehyde-induced fluorescence technique[33] and subsequently with autoradiography[34] and immunohistochemistry.[35] These neurons send projections to many forebrain areas and are involved in numerous central functions (for a review see ref. 36). With regard to galanin expression these neurons assume an intermediate position between the very low-expressing cholinergic forebrain neurons (see above) and the high-expressing noradrenergic locus coeruleus neurons (see below). Thus, under normal circumstances they have clearly detectable prepro-galanin mRNA levels, but galanin peptide cannot be visualized with immunohistochemistry. After colchicine treatment galanin peptide can be detected in most of these 5-HT neurons[6] and prepro-galanin mRNA levels are increased.[12] The comparatively low synthesis rate of galanin in these neurons is further supported by the fact that so far galanin has not been shown to coexist with 5-HT in forebrain nerve endings.[37,38] At the light microscopic level, 5-HT dorsal raphe neurons are surrounded by galanin-positive nerve endings which apparently do not express 5-HT, as also confirmed in the electron microscope.[38] Thus, they represent an input to the dorsal raphe of unknown origin, and their putative classic transmitter has not been identified. At the ultrastructural level it could be established that dendrites sometimes contain not only 5-HT but also galanin, suggesting a higher sensitivity of electron microscopic analysis.[38] Synapses could be seen between galanin-alone nerve endings and 5-HT and 5-HT/galanin dendrites.[38] These findings suggest that dorsal raphe galanin/5-HT neurons are innervated by galanin nerve endings.

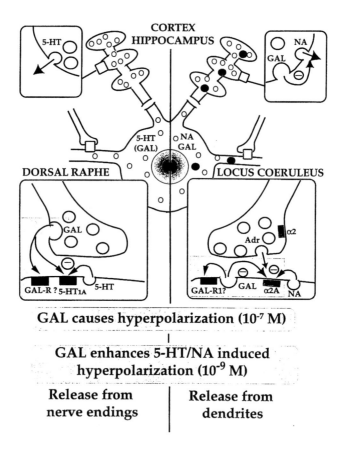

FIGURE 5. Schematic illustration of effects of galanin on a serotoninergic dorsal raphe neuron (**left panel**) and a noradrenergic locus coeruleus neuron (**right panel**). Under normal circumstances the 5-HT neuron expresses low levels of galanin and the peptide cannot be detected in cell bodies or forebrain nerve terminals. By contrast, the noradrenergic neuron has a robust galanin synthesis, and galanin can be detected in cell bodies as well as in cortical and hippocampal nerve terminals. The 5-HT neurons are innervated by non-serotonergic galanin-containing boutons of unknown origin. There are comparatively few galanin nerve endings surrounding and synapsing on locus coeruleus neurons. Therefore, under normal circumstances galanin acting on 5-HT neurons may mainly originate from synaptic nerve endings in the dorsal raphe, but from dendrites and soma in the locus coeruleus. Especially under conditions when galanin synthesis is upregulated in 5-HT neurons, galanin may also in this region be released from dendrites and soma. The effect of galanin on 5-HT and noradrenaline neurons is similar, causing hyperpolarization via a direct action on a galanin receptor of not yet defined type. Somewhat higher concentrations are needed in the dorsal raphe than in the locus coeruleus. In addition, galanin at low concentrations (10^{-9} M) enhances the inhibitory effect of 5-HT on the $5-HT_{1A}$ receptor on the 5-HT neurons and of the α_{2A} receptor on the noradrenaline neurons. These effects, obtained at low peptide concentrations, may in fact be in the physiologic range.

As discussed by Pieribone *et al.* (this volume), galanin induces hyperpolarization accompanied by a decrease in membrane resistance in most 5-HT–sensitive neurons at a concentration of 10^{-6}–10^{-7} M.[38] More importantly, at a much lower concentration (10^{-9} M) galanin enhances and prolongs the 5-HT–induced outward current exerted at the 5-HT$_{1A}$ receptor.[38] The galanin receptor(s) involved has not been defined. However, *in situ* hybridization studies of the dorsal raphe reveals numerous strongly GAL-R1 mRNA-positive neurons in the ventral aspects of the periacqueductal grey, but they are not concentrated in the midline as the 5-HT neurons are. It is thus unlikely that they represent 5-HT neurons. However, double-labeling experiments have to be performed to exclude the occurrence of GAL-R1 receptors in dorsal raphe 5-HT neurons. For further discussion see FIGURE 5 and below. Further aspects on galanin–5-HT interactions will be discussed in this volume by Fuxe *et al.* (see also ref. 39).

NORADRENERGIC LOCUS COERULEUS NEURONS

The noradrenergic locus coeruleus cell group, first described by Dahlström and Fuxe,[33] in contrast to 5-HT dorsal raphe neurons, has a robust expression of galanin also under normal circumstances.[16] Thus, galanin can be seen with both the routine immunofluorescence method and the more sensitive tyramide signal amplification method. Also, galanin mRNA levels are readily detectable. However, it is obvious that the number of distinct galanin-positive nerve endings surrounding locus coeruleus neurons appears much lower than that in the dorsal raphe, and ultrastructural analysis revealed few galanin-positive boutons making synaptic contact with noradrenergic dendrites.[40] We have therefore proposed that galanin in the locus coeruleus may mainly be released from dendrites and soma of noradrenergic cell bodies. Evidence for peptide release from dendrites was obtained from studies of magnocellular hypothalamic neurons.[41,42] This contrasts to the situation in the dorsal raphe nucleus, where we assume that galanin under normal circumstances is mainly released from non-serotonergic boutons synapsing on 5-HT neurons, particularly because the somatic galanin levels are so low.

Electrophysiologic analysis of the locus coeruleus reveals results similar to those seen in the dorsal raphe (see ref. 40 and Pieribone *et al.*, this volume). Thus, galanin causes an outward current presumably via a potassium channel, but somewhat lower concentrations of galanin are needed to cause this effect (10^{-7}–10^{-8} M) than in the dorsal raphe. Also, in the locus coeruleus galanin has a sensitizing effect at low concentrations (10^{-9} M) and enhances the hypopolarization induced by noradrenaline and adrenaline at α_{2A} receptors (unpublished results). These results are summarized in FIGURE 5.

The receptor present in locus coeruleus neurons has been studied by several groups. Parker *et al.*[43] described the presence of GAL-R1 in the locus coeruleus, and this was confirmed by Walker *et al.* (this volume). In the study by Xu *et al.*,[16] only low galanin R1 mRNA levels were observed in the locus coeruleus, whereas the adjacent Barrington nucleus expressed high levels of this transcript. The more sensitive riboprobe technique used by the former two groups, as compared to our oligonucleotide approach, may explain why we did not detect GAL-R1 mRNA in the locus coeruleus. The GAL-R1 receptor could then be responsible for the direct inhibitory effect seen with the comparatively high concentrations of galanin in the locus coeruleus.

CORTICAL GALANIN TERMINALS

The role of galanin in the cortical and hippocampal noradrenergic nerve endings remains to be studied. Interestingly, a single dose of reserpine causes marked depletion of galanin, strongly suggesting that galanin in these fibers is in a releasable form and can be released by reflex activation of the locus coeruleus.[16] It was previously shown that galanin mRNA levels are increased in the locus coeruleus following reserpine treatment,[44,45] presumably representing an increase in synthesis to compensate for galanin release. Functionally it was shown that galanin can inhibit noradrenaline release in cortex[46] via α_2 receptors. Furthermore, galanin inhibits the noradrenaline-induced accumulation of cyclic AMP in rat cortex.[47,48]

The double-staining experiments with DBH and galanin antibodies as well as the 6-hydroxydopamine experiments clearly show that there are non-noradrenergic galanin-positive fiber systems in the hippocampus, particularly in its ventral, anterior portion (FIG. 2). They have been described in detail by Xu et al.,[16] but their classic transmitter(s) and their origin(s) have so far not been established.

CONCLUDING REMARKS

In the present review we focus on the ascending serotonin and noradrenaline systems originating in the dorsal raphe and locus coeruleus, respectively. Whereas galanin synthesis and levels in the noradrenergic neurons appear robust, leading to detectable peptide levels in cortical and hippocampal nerve terminals, galanin peptide could not be detected in 5-HT dorsal raphe neurons, although galanin mRNA can be visualized in 5-HT cell bodies under normal circumstances. The noradrenergic nature of the cortical and hippocampal galanin nerve terminals was confirmed by double-staining experiments with antibodies to the noradrenaline synthesizing enzyme DBH and with 6-hydroxydopamine treatment, a neurotoxin that leads to degeneration of several central catecholamine systems including noradrenergic forebrain fibers. These findings suggest that under normal circumstances coexisting galanin may influence serotonergic mechanisms to a more limited extent, whereas galanin may act at both the cell body and the nerve terminal level of noradrenergic neurons. Electrophysiologic analysis shows that the effects of galanin in both the dorsal raphe and locus coeruleus are at least twofold: one is to directly depolarize 5-HT and noradrenaline neurons, but this occurs at fairly high concentrations. Another is to sensitize the 5-HT- and noradrenaline-induced inhibition via, respectively, 5-HT_{1A} and α_{2A} receptors, and this occurs at lower concentrations. In fact, in view of the generally low concentrations of peptides in brain (it has been calculated that peptides are present at 100–1,000 times lower concentrations than are classic transmitters), it is possible that only the sensitizing effect is of physiologic importance. Also, that a coexisting peptide sensitizes the effect of its classic transmitter seems to represent a logical mechanism.

REFERENCES

1. TATEMOTO, K., Å. RÖKAEUS, H. JÖRNVALL, T.J. McDONALD & V. MUTT. 1983. Galanin: A novel biologically active peptide from porcine intestine. FEBS Lett. **164:** 124–128.

2. RÖKAEUS, Å., T. MELANDER, T. HÖKFELT, J.M. LUNDBERG, K. TATEMOTO, M. CARLQUIST & V. MUTT. 1984. A galanin-like peptide in the central nervous system and intestine of the rat. Neurosci. Lett. **47:** 161–166.

3. SKOFITSCH, G. & D.M. JACOBOWITZ. 1985. Immunohistochemical mapping of galanin-like neurons in the rat central nervous system. Peptides. **6:** 509–546.

4. MELANDER, T., T. HÖKFELT & Å. RÖKAEUS. 1986. Distribution of galanin-like immunoreactivity in the rat central nervous system. J. Comp. Neurol. **248:** 475–517.

5. MELANDER, T., W.A. STAINES, T. HÖKFELT, Å. RÖKAEUS, F. ECKENSTEIN, P.M. SALVATERRA & B.H. WAINER. 1985. Galanin-like immunoreactivity in cholinergic neurons of the septum-basal forebrain complex projecting to the hippocampus of the rat. Brain Res. **360:** 130–138.

6. MELANDER, T., T. HÖKFELT, Å. RÖKAEUS, A.C. CUELLO, W.H. OERTEL, A. VERHOFSTAD & M. GOLDSTEIN. 1986. Coexistence of galanin-like immunoreactivity with catecholamines, 5-hydroxytryptamine, GABA and neuropeptides in the rat CNS. J. Neurosci. **6:** 3640–3654.

7. KÖHLER, C., H. ERICSON, T. WATANABE, J. POLAK, S.L. PALAY & V. CHAN-PALAY. 1986. Galanin immunoreactivity in hypothalamic histamine neurons: Further evidence for multiple chemical messengers in the tuberomammillary nucleus. J. Comp. Neurol. **250:** 58–64.

8. HOLETS, V.R., T. HÖKFELT, Å. RÖKAEUS, L. TERENIUS & M. GOLDSTEIN. 1988. Locus coeruleus neurons in the rat containing neuropeptide Y, tyrosine hydroxylase or galanin and their efferent projections to the spinal cord, cerebral cortex and hypothalamus. Neuroscience **24:** 893–906.

9. DAHLSTRÖM, A. 1968. Effect of colchicine on transport of amine storage granules in sympathetic nerves of rat. Eur. J. Pharmacol. **5:** 111–113.

10. KREUTZBERG, G.W. 1969. Neuronal dynamics and axonal flow. IV. Blockage of intra-axonal enzyme transport by colchicine. Proc. Natl. Acad. Sci. USA **62:** 722–728.

11. LJUNGDAHL, Å., T. HÖKFELT, G. NILSSON & M. GOLDSTEIN. 1978. DISTRIBUTION of substance P-like immunoreactivity in the central nervous system of the rat. II. Light microscopic localization in relation to catecholamine-containing neurons. Neuroscience **3:** 945–976.

12. CORTÉS, R., S. CECCATELLI, M. SCHALLING & T. HÖKFELT. 1990. Differential effects of intracerebroventricular colchicine administration on the expression of mRNAs for neuropeptides and neurotransmitter enzymes, with special emphasis on galanin: An in situ hybridization study. Synapse **6:** 369–391.

13. RETHELYI, M., A. FÜST & T. BARTFAI. 1989. Effect of nerve injury on the structure and peptide content of primary sensory neurons. International Union of Pysiology and Sciences Abstr. 198, Helsinki.

14. MELANDER, T. & W.A. STAINES. 1986. A galanin-like peptide coexists in putative cholinergic somata of the septum-basal forebrain complex and in acetylcholinesterase containing fibers and varicosities within the hippocampus in the owl monkey (*Aoutus trivirgatus*). Neurosci. Lett. **68:** 17–22.

15. GABRIEL, S.M., P.J. KNOTT & V. HAROUTUNIAN. 1995. Alterations in cerebral cortical galanin concentrations following neurotransmitter-specific subcortical lesions in the rat. J. Neurosci. **15:** 5526–5534.

16. XU, Z.-Q.D., T.-J.S. SHI & T. HÖKFELT. 1998. Galanin/GMAP- and NPY-like immunoreactivities in locus coeruleus and noradrenergic nerve terminals in the hippocampal formation and cortex with notes on the galanin-R1 and -R2 receptors. J. Comp. Neurol. **392:** 227–251.

17. TRANZER, J.P. & H. THOENEN. 1967. Ultramorphologische Veränderungen der sympatischen Nervendigungen der Katze nach Vorbehandlung mit 5- und 6-HydroxyDopamin. Arch. Pharmak. exp. Path. **257:** 343–344.

18. ZHANG, X., R. CORTÉS, M. VILLAR, P. MORINO, M.-N. CASTEL & T. HÖKFELT. 1992. Evidence for upregulation of galanin synthesis in rat glial cells in vivo after colchicine treatment. Neurosci. Lett. **145:** 185–188.

19. HÖKFELT, T., X. ZHANG, Z.Q. XU, R.R. JI, T. SHI, J. CORNESS, N. KEREKES, M. LANDRY, M. RYDH-RINDER, J. KOPP, K. HOLMBERG & C. BROBERGER. 1997. The ups and downs of neuropeptides. *In* Neuroendocrinology. Retrospect and Perspectives. H.W. Korf & K.-H. Usadel, Eds.: 5–23. Springer. Berlin.

20. TOHYAMA, M. 1992. An overview of the ontogeny of neurotransmitters and neuromodulators in the central nervous system. *In* Handbook of Chemical Neuroanatomy. Ontogeny of Transmit-

ters and Peptides in the CNS. A. Björklund, T. Hökfelt & M. Tohyama, Eds.: 647–650. Elsevier Science Publishers. Amsterdam.

21. XU, Z.-Q., T.-J. SHI & T. HÖKFELT. 1996. Expression of galanin and a galanin receptor in several sensory systems and bone anlage of rat embryos. Proc. Natl. Acad. Sci. USA 93: 14901–14905.

22. BRECHT, S., T. BUSCHMANN, S. GRIMM, M. ZIMMERMANN & T. HERDEGEN. 1997. Persisting expression of galanin in axotomized mammillary and septal neurons of adult rats labeled for c-Jun and NADPH-diaphorase. Mol. Brain Res. 48: 7–16.

23. FISONE, G., C.F. WU, S. CONSOLO, O. NORDSTRÖM, N. BRYNNE, T. BARTFAI, T. MELANDER & T. HÖFELT. 1987. Galanin inhibits acetylcholine release in the ventral hippocampus of the rat: Histochemical, autoradiographic, in vivo, and in vitro studies. Proc. Natl. Acad. Sci. USA 84: 7339–7343.

24. HÖKFELT, T., D. MILLHORN, K. SEROOGY, Y. TSURUO, S. CECCATELLI, B. LINDH, B. MEISTER, T. MELANDER, M. SCHALLING & L. TERENIUS. 1987. Coexistence of peptides with classical neurotransmitters. Experientia 43: 768–780.

25. CHAN-PALAY, V. 1988. Neurons with galanin innervate cholinergic cells in the human basal forebrain and galanin and acetylcholine coexists. Brain Res. Bull. 21: 465.

26. CHAN-PALAY, V. 1988. Galanin hyperinnervates surviving neurons of the human basal nucleus of Meynert in dementias of Alzheimer's and Parkinson's disease: A hypothesis for the role of galanin in accentuating cholinergic dysfunction in dementia. J. Comp. Neurol. 273: 543.

27. MUFSON, E.J., E. COCHRAN, W. BENZING & J.H. KORDOWER. 1993. Galaninergic innervation of the cholinergic vertical limb of the diagonal band (Ch2) and bed nucleus of the stria terminalis in aging, Alzheimer's disease and Down's syndrome. Dementia 4: 237–250.

28. BENZING, W.C., J.H. KORDOWER & E.J. MUFSON. 1993. Galanin immunoreactivity within the primate basal forebrain: Evolutionary change between monkeys and apes. J. Comp. Neurol. 336: 31–39.

29. KÖHLER, C. & V. CHAN-PALAY. 1990. Galanin receptors in the post-mortem human brain. Regional distribution of ^{125}I-galanin binding sites using the method of in vitro receptor autoradiography. Neurosci. Lett. 120: 179–182.

30. KÖHLER, C., H. HALLMAN, T. MELANDER, T. HÖKFELT & E. NORHEIM. 1989. Autoradiographic mapping of galanin receptors in the monkey brain. J. Chem. Neuroanat. 2: 269–284.

31. KÖHLER, C., A. PERSSON, T. MELANDER, E. THEODORSSON, G. SEDVALL & T. HÖKFELT. 1989. Distribution of galanin-binding sites in the monkey and human telencephalon: Preliminary observations. Exp. Brain Res. 75: 375.

32. RODRIGUEZ-PUERTAS, R., S. NILSSON, J. PASCUAL, A. PAZOS & T. HÖKFELT. 1997. ^{125}I-galanin binding sites in Alzheimer's disease: Increases in hippocampal subfields and a decrease in the caudate nucleus. J. Neurochem. 68: 1106–1113.

33. DAHLSTRÖM, A. & K. FUXE. 1964. Evidence for the existence of monoamine neurons in the central nervous system. I. Demonstration of monoamines in the cell bodies of brainstem neurons. Acta Physiol. Scand. 62: 1–55.

34. CHAN-PALAY, V. 1977. Indoleamine neurons and their processes in the normal rat brain and in chronic diet-induced thiamine deficiency demonstrated by uptake of ^{3}H-serotonin. J. Comp. Neurol. 176: 467–493.

35. STEINBUSCH, H.W.M. 1981. Distribution of serotonin-immunoreactivity in the central nervous system of the rat: Cell bodies and terminals. Neuroscience 6: 557–618.

36. WHITAKER-AZMITIA, P.M. & S.J. PEROUTKA. (Eds.) 1990. The Neuropharmacology of Serotonin. Ann. N.Y. Acad. Sci. 600.

37. XU, Z.-Q.D. & T. HÖKFELT. 1997. Expression of galanin and nitric oxide synthase in subpopulations of serotonin neurons of the rat dorsal raphe nucleus. J. Chem. Neuroanat. 13: 169–187.

38. XU, Z.-Q.D., X. ZHANG, V.A. PIERIBONE, S. GRILLNER & T. HÖKFELT. 1998. Galanin-5-hydroxytryptamine interactions: Electrophysiological, immunohistochemical and in situ hybridization studies on rat dorsal raphe neurons with a note on galanin R1 and R2 receptors. Neuroscience 87: 79–94.

39. HEDLUND, P. & K. FUXE. 1996. Galanin and 5-HT$_{1A}$ receptor interactions as an integrative mechanism in 5-HT neurotransmission in the brain. Ann. N.Y. Acad. Sci. 780: 193–212.

40. PIERIBONE, V., Z.-Q. XU, X. ZHANG, S. GRILLNER, T. BARTFAI & T. HÖKFELT. 1995. Galanin induces a hyperpolarization of norepinephrine-containing locus coeruleus neurons in the brainstem slice. Neuroscience **64:** 861–874.

41. MORRIS, J.F., D.V. POW, H.W. SOKOL & A. WARD. 1993. Dendritic release of peptides from magnocellular neurons in normal rats, Brattleboro rats and mice with hereditary nephrogenic diabetes insipidus. *In* Vasopressin. P. Gross, D. Richter & G.L. Robertson, Eds.: 171–182. John Libbey Eurotext. Paris.

42. ZAIDI, Z.F. & M.R. MATTHEWS. 1997. Exocytotic release from neuronal cell bodies, dendrites and nerve terminals in sympathetic ganglia of the rat, and its differential regulation. Neuroscience **80:** 861–891.

43. PARKER, E.M., D.G. IZZARELLI, H.P. NOWAK, C.D. MAHLE, L.G. IBEN, J. WANG & M.E. GOLDSTEIN. 1995. Cloning and characterization of the rat GALR1 galanin receptor from Rin 14B insulinoma cells. Mol. Brain Res. **34:** 179–189.

44. GUNDLACH, A.L., S.D. RUTHERFURD & W.J. LOUIS. 1990. Increase in galanin and neuropeptide Y mRNA in locus coeruleus following acute reserpine treatment. Eur. J. Pharmacol. **184:** 163–167.

45. AUSTIN, M.C., S.L. COTTINGHAM, S.M. PAUL & J.N. CRAWLEY. 1990. Tyrosine hydroxylase and galanin mRNA levels in locus coeruleus neurons are increased following reserpine administration. Synapse **6:** 351–357.

46. TSUDA, K., H. YOKOO & M. GOLDSTEIN. 1989. Neuropeptide Y and galanin in norepinephrine release in hypothalamic slices. Hypertension **14:** 81–86.

47. NISHIBORI, M., R. OISHI, Y. ITOH & K. SAEKI. 1988. Galanin inhibits noradrenaline-induced accumulation of cyclic AMP in the rat cerebral cortex. J. Neurochem. **51:** 1953–1955.

48. KARELSON, E., J. LASIK & R. SILLARD. 1995. Regulation of adenylate cyclase by galanin, neuropeptide Y, secretin and vasoactive intestinal polypeptide in rat frontal cortex, hippocampus and hypothalamus. Neuropeptides **28:** 21–28.

Electrophysiologic Effects of Galanin on Neurons of the Central Nervous System[a]

VINCENT A. PIERIBONE,[b–d] ZHI-QING DAVID XU,[c] XU ZHANG,[c]
AND TOMAS HÖKFELT[c]

[b]The John B. Pierce Laboratory, Department of Cellular and Molecular Physiology,
Yale University School of Medicine, New Haven, Connecticut 06519, USA

[c]The Department of Neuroscience, Karolinska Institutet, Stockholm, Sweden S-171 77

ABSTRACT: The neuropeptide galanin is found in a large number of neurons and
nerve terminals throughout the nervous system. In nerve terminals, galanin is contained in large dense-core vesicles and is released upon electrical stimulation. A variety of electrophysiologic studies have examined the effects of galanin application onto
neurons of the central nervous system. Overall, galanin appears to have inhibitory
effects in the central nervous system, causing in most cases a potassium-mediated
hyperpolarization accompanied by a decrease in input resistance. Other actions
include a reduction in presynaptic excitatory inputs and an interaction with other
applied neurotransmitters. These effects are robust and long lasting in most cases.
Differences in the responses mediated by the various receptor subtypes have not been
explored electrophysiologically. More complete analysis awaits the availability of
more potent and specific receptor anatagonists.

G alanin (GAL) is a 29 amino acid peptide first isolated from the gut by Tatemoto et al.[1] Subsequently, GAL was found in the central nervous system (CNS), almost exclusively in neurons throughout the brain and spinal cord, highly concentrated in nerve termi-
nals and large dense-core vesicles.[2–10] There is also evidence for GAL release in vivo after
electrical stimulation.[11] These studies have led to the proposal that GAL has a neurotrans-
mitter/neuromodulator role. GAL acts on a variety of G-protein–linked membrane receptors, some of which were recently cloned. These receptors activate a variety of
intracellular cascades via the G_i/G_0 GTP-binding proteins. The molecular and pharmacologic characteristics of these receptors are described in several chapters in this volume (Iismaa et al., Branchek et al., and Walker et al.).

Since the first GAL symposium in 1990, several studies have examined the effects of
GAL application on CNS neurons.[12–18] (For further information on electrophysiologic
studies with GAL, see Parsons et al., this volume.) In summary, these studies have shown
that in the CNS GAL produces predominantly inhibitory effects. This inhibition is in the
form of hyperpolarization via an outward potassium current, inhibition of excitatory
inputs, and depression of a sustained (plateau) depolarizing current. However, a presynaptic action of GAL has been proposed in several studies.[17,19] In all cases GAL's potency
appears similar to that of other studied neuropeptides.

[a]This study was supported by the Swedish MRC (04X-2887), Marianne och Marcus Wallenbergs
Stiftelse (VAP, ZQX, XZ, TH), Astra Arcus AB, a Fogarty International Center grant (F20 TWO
1586-01; VAP), and a National Science Foundation grant (INT-8908720; VAP).

[d]Author for correspondence: The John B. Pierce Laboratory; Cellular and Molecular Physiology;
Yale University School of Medicine, 290 Congress Avenue, New Haven, CT 06519. Phone, 203/562-
9901, ext. 214; fax, 203/562-9901, ext 285.

The effect of GAL on insulin secretion from the pancreas[20] involves nucleotide-sensitive potassium channels.[21-25] The hypoglycemic effects of circulating GAL may in part arise from its actions on these cells. In the CNS, however, there is no evidence that GAL mediates its effects on neurons via such channels. In fact, GAL exerts strong effects on neurons that are unresponsive to classic activators of such channels, and the effects of GAL are not inhibited by blockers of nucleotide-sensitive potassium channels.[14,18] Nonetheless, GAL expression is dramatically upregulated by CNS cellular damage,[26-30] and it is tantalizing to speculate that GAL may act in times of hypoxia, a condition in which nucleotide-sensitive potassium channels[31] are believed to be active in the CNS.[32-36]

We review major studies to date describing the electrophysiologic effects of GAL application on CNS neurons (see also Parsons *et al.*, this volume).

LOCUS COERULEUS

Most noradrenergic neurons of the locus coeruleus (LC) coexpress GAL.[37,38] Terminals from the LC, which contain both messengers (noradrenaline and GAL), are found in cortical areas and hippocampus.[38] Apart from robust GAL-immunoreactive (IR) cell bodies, there are fairly few GAL-IR fibers in the LC cell body area and within the major LC dendritic field in the surrounding gray matter.[38] These GAL-IR fibers form axodendritic and axosomatic synapses with LC neurons.[14] Previous anatomic studies indicated that LC neurons make dendrodendritic autosynapses,[39,40] and electrophysiologic evidence also indicates that LC neurons may receive recurrent axon collateral innervation from adjacent LC neurons.[41] It is therefore possible that at least some of the GAL innervation in the LC arises from recurrent collaterals from other LC neurons. In addition, some afferents to the LC arising from the ventrolateral and dorsomedial medulla[42-44] could potentially contain GAL.

Radioactive GAL binds to brain sections containing the LC.[45,46] In addition, GAL-R1 receptor mRNA has been localized to LC neurons using *in situ* hybridization (see Depzynski *et al.*, this volume).

Iontophoretic pressure or bath application of GAL onto LC neurons *in vitro* consistently causes a slowly developing inhibition of spontaneous activity in electrophysiologic studies with both extra- and intracellular recordings.[12-14,47] Hyperpolarization and a decrease in membrane resistance accompany this inhibition.[12,14] The reversal potential for this effect shifts to a more positive level with increasing concentrations of extracellular potassium.[14] Whereas GAL's actions in the pancreas are mediated by the opening of nucleotide-sensitive potassium channels (see above), this does not seem to be the case in the LC, because the actions of GAL are blocked by the addition of tetraethylammonium chloride (TEA) but not by glibenclamide.[14] In addition, agonists (diazoxide) of these channels have little effect on the resting membrane properties of LC neurons.[14]

When co-applied to LC neurons during extracellular recording from a brain slice, inhibition of spontaneous LC discharge by GAL is enhanced by the mu-opioid receptor antagonists naloxone and beta-funaltrexamine.[13] However, the actions of noradrenaline or (Met5)-enkephalin were unaffected by the presence of GAL.[13] GAL may exert a concerted effect on the excitability of LC neurons by augmenting the effects of opioids.[13]

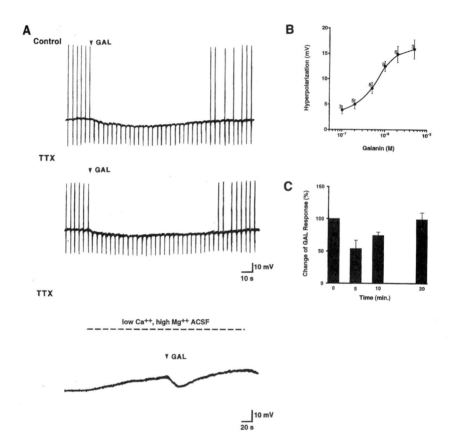

FIGURE 1. (A) Galanin-induced hyperpolarization is present in tetrodotoxin (TTX) and TTX/low Ca^{2+}, high Mg^{2+} containing artificial cerebrospinal fluid (ACSF). (*Upper trace*) galanin (20 pmol, applied at the *arrowhead*) induces hyperpolarization of a dorsal raphe neuron in normal ACSF. (*Middle trace*) In media-containing TTX, the cell continues to discharge (Ca^{2+} action potentials) upon activation, and galanin still induces hyperpolarization. (*Lower trace*) When the medium switches to TTX/ low Ca^{2+}, high Mg^{2+}, the cell stops discharging Ca^{2+} action potentials and becomes depolarized. Galanin, applied at the same concentration, causes strong hyperpolarization. The resting potential was −61 mV. **(B)** Dose response curve of dorsal raphe neurons to galanin. The amplitude of the hyperpolarization was plotted as a function of the logarithmic concentration of galanin applied by superfusion. Numbers adjacent to each point indicate the number of cells tested at that concentration. In all cells, membrane potential was set to −60 mV prior to galanin application. At least three concentrations of galanin were tested on each neuron. **(C)** Tachyphylaxis of the hyperpolarization evoked by galanin. Hyperpolarizations obtained from 8 cells were normalized to that elicited by the first application of galanin. A given cell was superfused with the same concentration for the same length of time. The concentration of galanin in the bath was 10^{-7} M. The duration of application was about 2 minutes. Intervals between application are illustrated above. Vertical lines are ± SEM. (From ref. 18, with permission.)

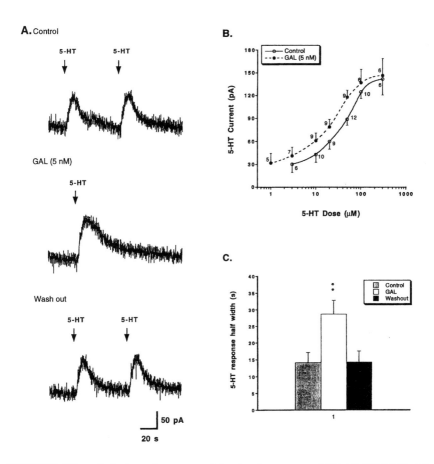

FIGURE 2. Effect of galanin on the response of dorsal raphe neurons to 5-HT. (**A**) 5-HT (100 mM, applied from a pipette at the *arrowhead*) induced a persistent outward current (*upper trace*). When galanin (5 nM) was present, the 5-HT–induced outward current was enhanced and the duration was prolonged (*middle trace*). The resting current is the same as that in **A.** After washout of galanin, the amplitude and duration of the 5-HT response were similar as before galanin administration (*lower trace*). The holding potential in all cases was −62 mV. (**B**) Effect of galanin on dose response of 5-HT in the dorsal raphe. The amplitude of hyperpolarization was plotted as a function of the concentration of 5-HT applied by superfusion. The 5-HT dose response curve was shifted to the left, when galanin (5 nM) was present. The numbers beside each point indicate the number of cells tested at each concentration. (**C**) The duration of the 5-HT–induced current was increased in the presence of galanin. (From ref. 18, with permission.)

It is likely that the endogeneous source of a significant portion of GAL input to LC neurons arises from the noradrenaline-containing neurons themselves, thereby representing at least in part a feedback mechanism.

DORSAL RAPHE NUCLEUS

There is a dense GAL-IR fiber plexus within the dorsal raphe nucleus (DR).[3,4,18,48] In untreated animals, few GAL-IR neurons are detected in the midline DR cell groups. However, following colchicine pretreatment, several GAL-IR neurons become evident.[3,4,18,37] With immunoelectron microscopy, GAL-IR dendrites are seen in the medial DR in untreated animals, indicating a higher sensitivity of the electron microscopic technique.[18] In all cases in which double labeling is performed, GAL-IR neurons are also serotonin (5-hydroxytryptamine, 5-HT)-IR and, conversely, approximately 60% of 5-HT neurons are GAL-IR.[48] GAL-positive, 5-HT–negative axon terminals make synaptic contacts with 5-HT–positive dendrites in the DR. No double-labeled (GAL-IR plus 5-HT-IR) axon terminals are seen in the DR.[18] Taken together, these findings imply that, unlike the situation in the LC, GAL acting on DR neurons may under normal circumstances, at least not mainly, originate from the 5-HT DR neurons.

Using in situ hybridization with probes for the GAL-R1 receptor mRNA, positive neuronal somata are found in the ventrolateral area of the DR, but only a few positive somata are seen within the midline region, where the majority of 5-HT neurons are present.[18] It is likely that the GAL receptor(s) present on 5-HT–containing neurons in the DR are not of the GAL-R1 type or, alternatively, GAL-R1 receptors are expressed at very low levels.

Most neurons in the DR contain 5-HT and respond to exogenously applied 5-HT.[18,49,50] Of the 5-HT-responsive neurons examined, 73% were hyperpolarized by the application of GAL (FIG. 1A), 4% were depolarized, and 22% were unresponsive to even high concentrations of GAL (10 μM).[18] The hyperpolarizing response of DR neurons to GAL had an EC_{50} of around 600 nM (FIG. 1B). A minority of neurons in the DR do not contain 5-HT and are also not responsive to applied 5-HT.[18,49,50] Those neurons in the DR that did not respond to 5-HT were also unresponsive to GAL.[18] Many effects of GAL on DR neurons[18] were similar to those effects seen in LC,[14] namely, (1) the responses often desensitized with closely spaced applications, (2) hyperpolarization was accompanied by a decrease in membrane resistance (FIG. 1C), (3) the response was unaffected by the addition or removal of chloride ions from the recording pipette, (4) the reversal potential of the response was highly negative (−103 mV), and it became more positive with increasing concentrations of potassium in the bathing Ringer's solution, and (5) the hyperpolarization was blocked by TEA but was not affected by the blockade of synaptic input (with tetradotoxin [TTX], low Ca^{2+}/high Mg^{2+}) (FIG. 1A). It is therefore likely that a similar potassium channel is activated in LC and DR neurons in response to GAL.

When high concentrations of 5-HT are applied to DR neurons, a saturating level of hyperpolarization is evoked. During such 5-HT–induced hyperpolarization, GAL still produces hyperpolarization.[18] This observation likely indicates that two distinct intracellular pathways and/or potassium channels mediate these two responses. Interestingly, under voltage clamp conditions the response of DR neurons to 5-HT is distinctly enhanced (up to 1.5-fold) in the presence of low concentrations of GAL (1-5 nM) (FIG. 2).[18] These results indicate a postsynaptic modulatory role of GAL on the autoresponsiveness of 5-HT–containing neurons to 5-HT. Thus, release of GAL could enhance the effect of 5-HT released from nerve endings or cell soma/dendrites (see also Hökfelt *et al.*, this volume).

HYPOTHALAMUS

The actions of GAL on hypothalamic magnocellular neurons has been studied in the *in vitro* brain slice preparation.[16] Two apparently distinct actions were reported. One action, similar to the one reported for LC and DR neurons,[14,18] causes the activation of a potassium conductance, whereas the other action reduces an afterdepolarization current that serves to create a sustained burst of action potentials following a brief depolarizing stimulation.[16] Both of these effects were reported to have an IC_{50} of around 10 nM. The increased potassium conductance is not affected by removing synaptic inputs (i.e., during the application of TTX), suggesting involvement of a postsynaptic galanin receptor(s).[16]

By contrast, in the arcuate nucleus GAL inhibits glutamate release via a presynaptic action, as recently described by Kinney *et al.*[17] Thus, application of GAL resulted in inhibition of evoked glutamatergic excitatory postsynaptic potentials (EPSPs) in a dose-dependent manner and a decrease in paired-pulse depression, but it did not cause an outward current. The frequency of recorded spontaneous miniature EPSPs in the presence of TTX and Cd^{2+} was reduced during GAL application, whereas the amplitude distribution of miniature excitatory postsynaptic currents (EPSCs) was not affected by GAL under the same conditions.[17] These data suggest that GAL has an inhibitory effect on the vesicular release process at a site close to the final vesicle-fusion step.[17] Various GAL analogs were also tested, and it was found that GAL fragments 1-16 and 1-15 produce robust depression of synaptic transmission, whereas fragment 3-29 causes a lesser degree of depression.[17] Meanwhile, the chimeric peptides C7, M15, M32, and M40 (see Langel and Bartfai, this volume) also produce varying degrees of depression of evoked EPSCs, but in a few cases they antagonize the actions of GAL. Those data suggest that GAL acts via several subtypes of presynaptic receptors to depress synaptic transmission in the rat arcuate nucleus.[17]

HIPPOCAMPUS

GAL is highly expressed in axons and nerve terminals within the hippocampus.[38] Most dopamine beta-hydroxylase immunoreactive fibers in the hippocampus apparently co-contain GAL, indicating more widespread terminal distribution of GAL in noradrenergic terminals than previously thought.[38]

The effects of GAL on the membrane properties of hippocampal neurons were first studied by Dutar *et al.*[19] They found that bath application of GAL caused only slight hyperpolarization of CA1 neurons without an obvious change in membrane resistance. The most dramatic effects of GAL were on evoked responses. GAL affected synaptic activation of CA1 neurons in two ways: it slightly reduced the size of excitatory amino acid-mediated Schaffer-collateral activation and dramatically reduced an atropine-sensitive long-lasting depolarization evoked by train stimulation.[19] GAL did not affect the responsiveness of CA1 neurons to exogenously applied acetylcholine.[19] These results indicate a specific presynaptic action of GAL on acetylcholine-releasing nerve terminals on CA1 neurons.[19] These findings agree with several studies on GAL regulation of acetylcholine release and acetylcholine-dependent functions in the hippocampus[51–53] (see also chapters in this volume by Mufson *et al.*, Crawley *et al.*, Miller *et al.*, and Ögren *et al.*).

One recent report indicates that GAL specifically blocks the expression of long-term potentiation (LTP) in CA1 neurons in guinea pig hippocampal slices.[15] Contrary to the aforementioned studies on rat,[19] bath application of GAL did not affect the size of the evoked Schaffer collateral-CA1 synaptic potentials, but it caused a dose-dependent reduction in the magnitude of EPSP potentiation (LTP) following tetanic stimulation.[15] The site of this action of GAL is not clear, but it may represent a basis for some of the effects of GAL on acquisition and retention described in other chapters in this volume (see Crawley *et al.* and Ögren *et al.*).

CONCLUSIONS

Since the first meeting in 1990, a number of electrophysiologic studies have been published dealing with the effects of GAL in the CNS. Using intracellular recording technique, several types of actions have been described, mainly at postsynaptic sites causing hyperpolarization via a potassium channel. It therefore seems that GAL generally is an inhibitory messenger molecule, but other types of actions have been described. Of special interest is the "sensitizing" effect of GAL at low concentrations (nanomolar range) on 5-HT–induced inhibition of DR 5-HT neurons. It is, however, clear that further extensive studies are needed to understand the multiple mechanisms of action of GAL in the CNS. Although a series of peptide GAL analogs blocking the actions of exogenous GAL have been developed (see Langel and Bartfai, this volume), nonpeptide antagonists specific for the three, until now cloned GAL receptors (see Iismaa *et al.*, Branchek *et al.*, and Walker *et al.*, this volume) are urgently needed.

REFERENCES

1. TATEMOTO, K., Å. RÖKAEUS, H. JÖRNVALL, T.J. McDONALD & V. MUTT. 1983. Galanin: A novel biologically active peptide from porcine intestine. FEBS. Lett. **164:** 124–128.
2. RÖKAEUS, Å., T. MELANDER, T. HÖKFELT, J.M. LUNDBERG, K. TATEMOTO, M. CARLQUIST & V. MUTT. 1984. A galanin-like peptide in the central nervous system and intestine of the rat. Neurosci. Lett. **47:** 161–166.
3. SKOFITSCH, G. & D.M. JACOBOWITZ. 1985. Immunohistochemical mapping of galanin-like neurons in the rat central nervous system. Peptides **6:** 509–546.
4. MELANDER, T., T. HÖKFELT & Å. RÖKAEUS. 1986. Distribution of galanin-like immunoreactivity in the rat central nervous system. J. Comp. Neurol. **248:** 475–517.
5. RÖKAEUS, Å. 1987. Galanin: A newly isolated biologically active neuropeptide. TINS **10:** 158–164.
6. SKOFITSCH, G. & D.M. JACOBOWITZ. 1990. Galanin in the central nervous system: A review. Curr. Asp. Neurosci. **1:** 1–63.
7. HÖKFELT, T., T. BARTFAI, D. JACOBOWITZ & D. OTTOSON, EDS. 1991. Galanin: A New Multifunctional Peptide in the Neuro-Endocrine System. Wenner-Gren Center International Symposium Series, Vol. 58. MacMillan. London.
8. BARTFAI, T., T. HÖKFELT & Ü. LANGEL. 1993. Galanin: A neuroendocrine peptide. Current Rev. Neurobiol. **7:** 229–274.
9. MERCHENTHALER, I., F.J. LOPEZ & V.A. NEGRO. 1993. Anatomy and physiology of central galanin-containing pathways. Prog. Neurobiol. **40:** 711–769.

10. CRAWLEY, J.N. 1995. Biological actions of galanin. Reg. Pept. **59:** 1–16.
11. CONSOLO, S., G. BALDI, G. RUSSI, G. CIVENNI, T. BARTFAI & A.-M. VEZZANI. 1994. Impulse flow dependency of galanin release in vivo in the rat ventral hippocampus. Proc. Natl. Acad. Sci. USA **91:** 8047–8051.
12. BARTFAI, T., K. BEDECS, T. LAND, Ü. LANGEL, R. BERTORELLI, P. GIROTTI, S. CONSOLO, X. XU, Z. WIESENFELD-HALLIN, S. NILSSON, V. PIERIBONE & T. HÖKFELT. 1991. M-15: High-affinity chimeric peptide that blocks the neuronal actions of galanin in the hippocampus, locus coeruleus, and spinal cord. Proc. Natl. Acad. Sci. USA **88:** 10961–10965.
13. SEVCIK, J., E.P. FINTA & P. ILLES. 1993. Galanin receptors inhibit the spontaneous firing of locus coeruleus neurones and interact with μ-opioid receptors. Eur. J. Pharmacol. **230:** 223–230.
14. PIERIBONE, V., Z.-Q. XU, X. ZHANG, S. GRILLNER, T. BARTFAI & T. HÖKFELT. 1995. Galanin induces a hyperpolarization of norepinephrine-containing locus coeruleus neurons in the brainstem slice. Neuroscience **64:** 861–874.
15. SAKURAI, E., T. MAEDA, S. KANEKO, A. AKAIKE & M. SATOH. 1996. Galanin inhibits long-term potentiation at Schaffer collateral-CA1 synapses in guinea-pig hippocampal slices. Neurosci. Lett. **212:** 21–24.
16. PAPAS, S. & C.W. BOURQUE. 1997. Galanin inhibits continuous and phasic firing in rat hypothalamic magnocellular neurosecretory cells. J. Neurosci. **17:** 6048–6056.
17. KINNEY, G.A., P.J. EMMERSON & R.J. MILLER. 1998. Galanin receptor-mediated inhibition of glutamate release in the arcuate nucleus of the hypothalamus. J. Neurosci. **18:** 3489–3500.
18. XU, Z.-Q.D., X. ZHANG, V.A. PIERIBONE, S. GRILLNER & T. HÖKFELT. 1998. Galanin-5-hydroxytryptamine interactions: Electrophysiological, immunohistochemical and *in situ* hybridization studies on rat dorsal raphe neurons with a note on galanin R1 and R2 receptors. Neuroscience **87:** 79–94.
19. DUTAR, P., Y. LAMOUR & R.A. NICOLL. 1989. Galanin blocks the slow cholinergic EPSP in CA1 pyramidal neurons from ventral hippocampus. Eur. J. Pharmacol. **164:** 355–360.
20. MCDONALD, T.J., J. DUPRE, K. TATEMOTO, G.R. GREENBERG, J. RADZIUK & V. MUTT. 1985. Galanin inhibits insulin secretion and induces hyperglycemia in dogs. Diabetes **34:** 192–196.
21. AHRÉN, B., P. ARKHAMMAR, P.O. BERGGREN & T. NILSSON. 1986. Galanin inhibits glucose-stimulated insulin release by a mechanism involving hyperpolarization and lowering of cytoplasmic free Ca^{2+} concentration. Biochem. Biophys. Res. Commun. **140:** 1059–1063.
22. DE WEILLE, J., A.H. SCHMID, M. FOSSET & M. LAZDUNSKI. 1988. ATP-sensitive K^+ channels that are blocked by hypoglycemia-inducing sulfonylureas in insulin-secreting cells are activated by galanin, a hyperglycemia-inducing hormone. Proc. Natl. Acad. Sci. USA **85:** 1312–1316.
23. AHRÉN, B., P.O. BERGGREN, K. BOKVIST & P. RORSMAN. 1989. Does galanin inhibit insulin secretion by opening of the ATP-regulated K+ channel in the beta-cell? Peptides **10:** 453–457.
24. DUNNE, M.J., M.J. BULLETT, G.D. LI, C.B. WOLLHEIM & O.H. PETERSEN. 1989. Galanin activates nucleotide-dependent K^+ channels in insulin-secreting cells via a pertussis toxin-sensitive G-protein. EMBO. J. **8:** 413–420.
25. DREWS, G., A. DEBUYSER, M. NENQUIN & J.C. HENQUIN. 1990. Galanin and epinephrine act on distinct receptors to inhibit insulin release by the same mechanisms including an increase in K^+ permeability of the B-cell membrane. Endocrinology **126:** 1646–1653.
26. VILLAR, M.J., R. CORTÉS, E. THEODORSSON, Z. WIESENFELD-HALLIN, M. SCHALLING, J. FAHRENKRUG, P.C. EMSON & T. HÖKFELT. 1989. Neuropeptide expression in rat dorsal root ganglion cells and spinal cord after peripheral nerve injury with special reference to galanin. Neuroscience **33:** 587–604.
27. CORTÉS, R., S. CECCATELLI, M. SCHALLING & T. HÖKFELT. 1990. Differential effects of intracerebroventricular colchicine administration on the expression of mRNAs for neuropeptides and neurotransmitter enzymes, with special emphasis on galanin: an in situ hybridization study. Synapse **6:** 369–391.
28. CORTÉS, R., M.J. VILLAR, A. VERHOFSTAD & T. HÖKFELT. 1990. Effects of central nervous system lesions on the expression of galanin: A comparative in situ hybridization and immunohistochemical study. Proc. Natl. Acad. Sci. USA **87:** 7742–7746.
29. MEISTER, B., R. CORTÉS, M.J. VILLAR, M. SCHALLING & T. HÖKFELT. 1990. Peptides and transmitter enzymes in hypothalamic magnocellular neurons after administration of hyperosmotic stimuli: Comparison between messenger RNA and peptide/protein levels. Cell Tissue Res. **260:** 279–297.

30. VILLAR, M.J., B. MEISTER, R. CORTÉS, M. SCHALLING, M. MORRIS & T. HÖKFELT. 1990. Neuropeptide gene expression in hypothalamic magnocellular neurons of normal and hypophysectomized rats: A combined immunohistochemical and in situ hybridization study. Neuroscience 36: 181–199.

31. ASHCROFT, F.M. 1988. Adenosine 5'-triphosphate-sensitive potassium channels. Annu. Rev. Neurosci. 11: 97–118.

32. KRNJEVIĆ, K. & J. LEBLOND. 1988. Are there hippocampal ATP-sensitive K⁺ channels that are activated by anoxia? Eur. J. Physiol. 411: 2157–2161.

33. BEN-ARI, Y. 1990. Modulation of ATP sensitive K⁺ channels: A novel strategy to reduce the deleterious effects of anoxia. Adv. Exp. Med. Biol. 268: 481–489.

34. BEN-ARI, Y., K. KRNJEVIC & V. CRÉPEL. 1990. Activators of ATP-sensitive K⁺ channels reduce anoxic depolarization in CA3 hippocampal neurons. Neuroscience 37: 55–60.

35. MOURRE, C., C. WIDMANN & M. LAZDUNSKI. 1990. Sulfonylurea binding sites associated with ATP-regulated K⁺ channels in the central nervous system: Autoradiographic analysis of their distribution and ontogenesis, and of their localization in mutant mice cerebellum. Brain Res. 519: 29–43.

36. MOURRE, C., C. WIDMANN & M. LAZDUNSKI. 1991. Specific hippocampal lesions indicate the presence of sulfonylurea binding sites associated to ATP-sensitive K⁺ channels both postsynaptically and on mossy fibers. Brain Res. 540: 340–344.

37. MELANDER, T., T. HÖKFELT, Å. RÖKAEUS, A.C. CUELLO, W.H. OERTEL, A. VERHOFSTAD & M. GOLDSTEIN. 1986. Coexistence of galanin-like immunoreactivity with catecholamines, 5-hydroxytryptamine, GABA and neuropeptides in the rat CNS. J. Neurosci. 6: 3640–3654.

38. XU, Z.-Q.D., T.J. SHI & T. HÖKFELT. 1998. Galanin/GMAP- and NPY-like immunoreactivities in locus coeruleus and noradrenergic nerve terminals in the hippocampal formation and cortex with notes on the galanin-R1 and -R2 receptors. J. Comp. Neurol. 392: 227–251.

39. GROVES, P.M. & C.J. WILSON. 1980. Monoaminergic presynaptic axons and dendrites in rat locus coeruleus seen in reconstructions of serial sections. J. Comp. Neurol. 193: 853–862.

40. GROVES, P.M. & C.J. WILSON. 1980. Fine structure of rat locus coeruleus. J. Comp. Neurol. 193: 841–852.

41. ENNIS, M. & G. ASTON-JONES. 1986. Evidence for self- and neighbor-mediated postactivation inhibition of locus coeruleus neurons. Brain Res. 374: 299–305.

42. ASTON-JONES, G., M. ENNIS, V.A. PIERIBONE, W.T. NICKELL & M.T. SHIPLEY. 1986. The brain nucleus locus coeruleus: Restricted afferent control of a broad efferent network. Science 234: 734–737.

43. ASTON-JONES, G., M.T. SHIPLEY, M. ENNIS, V A. PIERIBONE, E.J. VAN BOCKSTAELE, B. ASTIER, G. CHOUVET, H. AKAOKA, P. CHARLÉTY, R. SHIEKATTAR & C. CHAING. 1990. Regulation of locus coeruleus by its major afferents: Anatomy, physiology and pharmacology. Eur. J. Neurosci. Suppl. 3: 9.

44. PIERIBONE, V.A. & G. ASTON-JONES. 1991. Adrenergic innervation of the rat nucleus locus coeruleus arises predominantly from the C1 adrenergic cell group in the rostral medulla. Neuroscience 41: 525–542.

45. SKOFITSCH, G., M.A. SILLS & M. JACOBOWITZ. 1986. Autoradiographic distribution of ¹²⁵I-galanin binding sites in the rat central nervous system. Peptides 7: 1029–1042.

46. MELANDER, T., C. KÖHLER, S. NILSSON, T. HÖKFELT, E. BRODIN, E. THEODORSSON & T. BARTFAI. 1988. Autoradiographic quantification and anatomical mapping of ¹²⁵I-galanin binding in the rat central nervous system. J. Chem. Neuroanat. 1: 213–233.

47. SEUTIN, V., P. VERBANCK, L. MASSOTTE & A. DRESSE. 1989. Galanin decreases the activity of locus coeruleus neurons in vitro. Eur. J. Pharmacol. 164: 373–376.

48. XU, Z.-Q.D. & T. HÖKFELT. 1997. Expression of galanin and nitric oxide synthase in subpopulations of serotonin neurons of the rat dorsal raphe nucleus. J. Chem. Neuroanat. 13: 169–187.

49. AGHAJANIAN, G.K., R.Y. WANG & J.M. BARABAN. 1978. Serotoninergic and non-serotoninergic neurons of the dorsal raphe: Reciprocal changes in firing induced by peripheral nerve stimulation. Brain Res. 153: 169–175.

50. WILLIAMS, J.T., W.F. COLMERS & Z.Z. PAN. 1988. Voltage- and ligand-activated inwardly rectifying currents in dorsal raphe neurons in vitro. J. Neurosci. 8: 3499–3506.

51. FISONE, G., C.F. WU, F. CONSOLO, Ö. NORDSTRÖM, N. BRYNNE, T. BARTFAI, T. MELANDER & T. HÖKFELT. 1987. Galanin inhibits acetylcholine release in the ventral hippocampus of the rat:

Histochemical, autoradiographic, in vivo and in vitro studies. Proc. Natl. Acad. Sci. USA **88:** 7339–7343.

52. PALAZZI, E., G. FISONE, T. HÖKFELT, T. BARTFAI & S. CONSOLO. 1988. Galanin inhibits the muscarinic stimulation of phosphoinositide turnover in rat ventral hippocampus. Eur. J. Pharmacol. **148:** 479–480.

53. PALAZZI, E., S. FELINSKA, M. ZAMBELLI, G. FISONE, T. BARTFAI & S. CONSOLO. 1991. Galanin reduces carbachol stimulation of phosphoinositide turnover in rat ventral hippocampus by lowering Ca^{2+} influx through voltage-sensitive Ca^{2+} channels. J. Neurochem. **56:** 739–747.

Galanin Modulates 5-Hydroxytryptamine Functions

Focus on Galanin and Galanin Fragment/ 5-Hydroxytryptamine$_{1A}$ Receptor Interactions in the Brain[a]

K. FUXE,[b] A. JANSSON, Z. DIAZ-CABIALE, A. ANDERSSON, B. TINNER, U.-B. FINNMAN, I. MISANE, H. RAZANI, F.-H. WANG, L.F. AGNATI, AND S.O. ÖGREN

Department of Neuroscience, Karolinska Institute, 171 77 Stockholm, Sweden

ABSTRACT: The reciprocal interactions between galanin and 5-HT$_{1A}$ receptors in the rat brain are presented. Galanin and its NH$_2$-terminal fragments antagonize 5-HT$_{1A}$ receptor-mediated transmission at the postjunctional level, whereas galanin receptor activation mimics the inhibitory action of 5-HT$_{1A}$ receptor activation at the soma-dendritic level, leading to reductions of 5-HT metabolism and release. These interactions have been shown in both receptor binding studies and functional studies. In view of the present findings, galanin antagonists may represent a new type of anti-depressant drug, based on the 5-HT hypothesis of depression, by enhancing 5-HT release and postjunctional 5-HT$_{1A}$-mediated transmission. Moreover, following intracerebroventricular injection galanin was found to be internalized in a popula-tion of hippocampal nerve cells mainly representing GABA, somatostatin, and/or NPY-immunoreactive nerve cells. The relevance of these findings is discussed in rela-tion to the concept of volume transmission.

In the late 1980s, evidence was first obtained that the neuropeptide galanin (GAL) can interact with central 5-hydroxytryptamine (5-HT) neurons at both the prejunctional and at the postjunctional level.[1,2] Thus, intraventricular injections of porcine GAL reduced 5-HT metabolism within the hippocampal formation, ventral limbic cortex, and the fronto-parietal cortex,[2] effects that were postulated to take place at the somadendritic level of the mesencephalic 5-HT neurons. Furthermore, in membrane preparations from the ventral limbic cortex, including especially the amygdaloid cortex, entorhinal cortex, and pyriform cortex, porcine GAL in the nanomolar range (10 nM) could reduce the affinity of the 5-HT$_{1A}$ agonist binding sites (^{3}H-8-OH-DPAT used as radioligand) associated with a small increase in the B$_{max}$ values. This finding suggested the existence of an intramembrane antagonistic GAL/5-HT$_{1A}$ receptor interaction at the postjunctional level.[1,3] In similar membrane preparations from the ventral limbic cortex GAL failed to modulate 5-HT$_2$ ago-nist and antagonist binding sites, suggesting a preferential interaction with the 5-HT$_{1A}$

[a]This work was supported by a grant (04X-715) from the Swedish Medical Research Council and a grant from the Marianne and Marcus Wallenberg Foundation.

[b]Address for correspondence: Professor Kjell Fuxe, Department of Neuroscience, Karolinska Institute, S-171 77 Stockholm, Sweden. Phone, +46-8-728 7078; fax, +46-8-33 79 41; e-mail, Kjell.Fuxe@neuro.ki.se

receptor subtype. Additional evidence later showed that NH_2-terminal GAL fragments can strongly modulate dorsal hippocampal 5-HT_{1A} receptors by reducing their affinity.[4,5] This development is reviewed in the present article with the focus on new observations, leading to the proposal that GAL and especially GAL fragment receptor antagonists may represent new types of antidepressant compounds based on their ability to enhance 5-HT neurotransmission, especially via the 5-HT_{1A} receptor subtype in limbic regions.

BIOCHEMICAL AND FUNCTIONAL EVIDENCE FOR ANTAGONISTIC POSTJUNCTIONAL INTRAMEMBRANE GAL/5-HT_{1A} AND GAL FRAGMENT/5-HT_{1A} RECEPTOR INTERACTIONS

The dorsal hippocampal formation in the rat contains a high density of 5-HT_{1A} receptor binding sites with a very low number of high affinity ^{125}I-GAL binding sites.[6] It was therefore assumed that GAL-(1-29), when incubated in membrane preparations of the dorsal hippocampal formation, would fail to modulate the affinity of the 5-HT_{1A} agonist binding sites in this region. This was in fact true when bacitracin was added to the incubation medium to prevent the breakdown of GAL by endopeptidases.[5,7] However, when GAL-(1-29) was added to the membrane preparation of the dorsal hippocampus without the addition of bacitracin, GAL-(1-29) (10 nM) markedly reduced the affinity of the 5-HT_{1A} binding sites, suggesting that GAL fragments may be formed capable of activating GAL fragment receptors antagonistically regulating 5-HT_{1A} receptors.[5] Evidence to support this view had previously been obtained in autoradiographic studies using ^{125}I-GAL-(1-15) as radioligand.[8] Thus, a large number of high affinity ^{125}I-GAL-(1-15) binding sites could *inter alia* be demonstrated in the frontoparietal cortex, dorsal hippocampus, and neostriatum, where very few ^{125}I-porcine GAL high affinity binding sites had been mapped out.[6,9] In addition, high affinity GAL fragment binding sites could be demonstrated in regions also rich in high affinity GAL-(1-29) binding sites such as the hypothalamus, ventral limbic cortex, and mesencephalic raphe nuclei. A substantial overlap was noted between the distribution of the high affinity NH_2-terminal GAL-(1-15) binding sites and the high affinity ^{3}H-8-OH-DPAT binding sites, for example in the dorsal hippocampus involving especially the dentate gyrus and the CA1 and CA2 regions. The overlap was strongest in the dendritic layers, that is, the stratum radiatum of the CA regions and the molecular layer of the dentate gyrus.

These studies showed that GAL-(1-15) strongly reduced the affinity of the 5-HT_{1A} receptors in membrane preparations of dorsal hippocampus in the concentration range 1–3 nM and that this action could be blocked by the GAL receptor antagonist M35 in a concentration of 1 nM.[5] Importantly, the ^{125}I-GAL-(1-15) binding sites do not label a low affinity GAL-(1-29) binding site in the dorsal hippocampus, because only 30% of the specific high affinity ^{125}I-GAL-(1-15) binding disappeared in the presence of 10 μM of porcine GAL-(1-29). Also, the distribution pattern of porcine ^{125}I-GAL-(1-29) binding sites was similar in a number of species.[10] This argues against the possibility of the existence of a rat GAL receptor subtype in the dorsal hippocampus and other regions,[8] which cannot bind porcine GAL in view of its different COOH-terminal ending from that of rat GAL.

Taken together, studies on the dorsal hippocampal formation give *in vitro* evidence for the existence of a GAL fragment receptor recognizing NH_2-terminal GAL fragments capable of strongly and antagonistically interacting with the 5-HT_{1A} receptors through intramembrane interactions leading to substantial increases of the K_D values.[4,5]

Recent evidence from studies on membrane preparations from the ventral limbic cortex of the rat in the presence of bacitracin also suggests that GAL-(1-16) of the rat and porcine type in concentrations from 1–100 nM can strongly and concentration dependently reduce the affinity of 5-HT$_{1A}$ agonist binding sites in the ventral limbic cortex, with porcine and rat GAL (1-29) being less potent and less effective than GAL (1-16) (FIG. 1). Note that GAL-(1-16) has about five times lower affinity than GAL-(1-29) at rostral hippocampal GAL receptors.[11] Thus, GAL fragment receptors may regulate 5-HT$_{1A}$ receptors also within the ventral limbic cortex together with the high affinity GAL-(1-29) receptors in this region[1] that are also activated by NH$_2$-terminal GAL fragments but with GAL-(1-29) being more potent.[12–14]

Functional evidence for the existence of antagonistic GAL/5-HT$_{1A}$ receptor interactions was obtained early in studies on thyroid-stimulating hormone (TSH) secretion in the

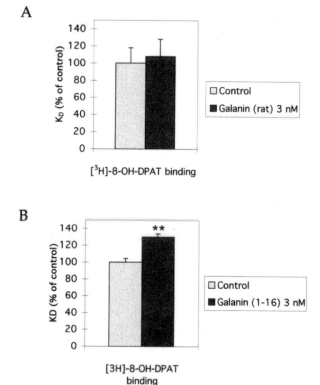

FIGURE 1. Effects of 3 nM of rat GAL-(1-29) and rat (porcine) GAL-(1-16) on the binding characteristics of ^{3}H-8-OH-DPAT (5-HT$_{1A}$) binding sites in rat membrane preparations of the ventral limbic cortex. For details, see Hedlund *et al.*[5] Saturation analysis with concentrations of 0.1–10 nM of ^{3}H-8-OH-DPAT. Means ± SEM are shown for five experiments in percentage of respective control group K_D mean value (100% = 1.212 nM). B_{max} values are unaltered by GAL-(1-29) and GAL-(1-16) in this experiment (100% [fmol/mg protein] = 274 ± 45). Mann-Whitney U-test. **$p < 0.01$.

normal rat. The 8-OH-DPAT-induced inhibition of serum TSH levels could be counteracted by the intraventricular injection of nanomolar amounts of porcine GAL, which by themselves did not change TSH levels.[3,15] Recently, it was possible to obtain the first indications that intraventricular GAL can antagonize a 5-HT$_{1A}$ receptor-mediated behavioral response in the rat, namely the impairment of passive avoidance retention caused by 5-HT$_{1A}$ receptor activation.[16,17] The passive avoidance impairment by a postjunctional dose of 8-OH-DPAT (0.2 mg/kg, sc) was dose dependently diminished by porcine GAL given intraventricularly with a significant attenuation at 3.0 nmol/rat. The postsynaptic 5-HT$_{1A}$ receptors mediating this response are probably located predominantly in the forebrain, especially in the dorsal and ventral hippocampus and in parts of the amygdala. It

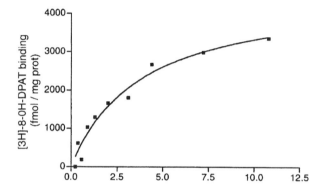

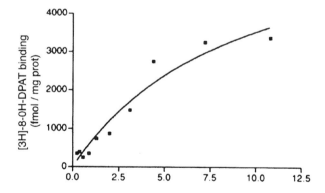

FIGURE 2. Effects of intraventricular injections of porcine GAL-(1-29) in awake male rat on ^{3}H-8-OH-DPAT binding sites in transverse brain sections at Bregma level: −3.6 mm. Saturation analysis with concentrations of ^{3}H-8-OH-DPAT ranging from 0.1–10 nM. Receptor autoradiographic analysis is illustrated in the molecular layer of the dentate gyrus with representative saturation curves. The upper curve is obtained from a CSF-treated rat (K_D = 3.166 nM; B_{max} = 4263 fmol/mg prot) and the lower curve is obtained from a rat GAL-(1-29) treated rat. (K_D = 9.250 nM; B_{max} = 6797 fmol/mg prot).

should be noted however that the signs of the 5-HT syndrome induced by the postjunctional dose of 8-OH-DPAT were not diminished by the intraventricular doses of GAL used. Thus, the antagonistic GAL/5-HT$_{1A}$ receptor interactions may be more strongly developed at some 5-HT$_{1A}$ receptors than at others.

Recently, in support of the functional findings, we also obtained preliminary observations suggesting that intraventricular injections of nanomolar amounts of porcine GAL in the rat sacrificed 10 minutes after administration can increase the K_D value for ^{3}H-8-OH-DPAT binding sites in the CA1 area and in the dentate gyrus of the dorsal hippocampus associated with increases in B_{max} values based on receptor autoradiographical studies (FIGS. 2 and 3). In view of the *in vitro* evidence just presented, it must be considered that NH$_2$-terminal GAL fragments formed *in vivo* from porcine GAL can contribute to the demonstrated attenuation of postjunctional 5-HT$_{1A}$ receptor transduction in these functional experiments. A GAL fragment receptor may be more strongly involved than GAL-(1-29) receptors in mediating the attenuation of 5-HT$_{1A}$ receptor activation by the 5-HT$_{1A}$ agonist in certain forebrain regions such as the hippocampus.

Signal transduction studies have also been performed on GAL/5-HT receptor interactions. It is known that noradrenaline-induced accumulation of cyclic AMP in the cortical regions of the rat is inhibited by GAL.[18] Of particular interest is the observation that GAL-(1-15) and GAL can exert inhibitory concentration-dependent actions on forskolin-stimulated adenylyl cyclase activity in membrane preparations from the hypothalamus

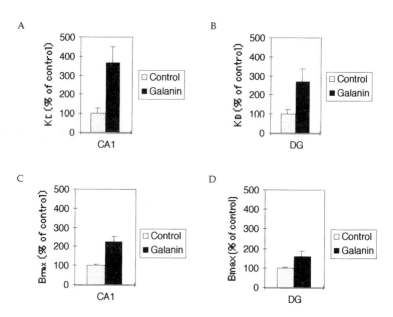

FIGURE 3. Effects of intraventricular injections of 3 nmol of porcine GAL-(1-29) in awake male rat on K_D and B_{max} values of ^{3}H-8-OH-DPAT binding sites in the dentate gyrus (molecular layer) and the CA1 area (stratum radiatum) using receptor autoradiography. Means ± SEM are shown for three rats. Statistical analysis was not performed because of the limited number of rats in this experiment. Dentate gyrus (DG): K_D (100%) = 3.783 nM; B_{max} (100%) = 4852 fmol/mg protein; CA1 area: K_D (100%) = 3.559 nM; B_{max} (100%) = 3408 fmol/mg protein.

and from the entorhinal cortex but not from the hippocampus.[19] The $5\text{-}HT_{1A}$ receptor agonist 8-OH-DPAT induced similar inhibitory effects on forskolin-stimulated adenylyl cyclase activity in hippocampal and entorhinal membrane preparations. However, when 5-HT or 8-OH-DPAT and GAL were incubated together, no synergistic interactions or antagonistic interactions were found. Instead, additive inhibitory actions were observed on forskolin-stimulated adenylyl cyclase activity, suggesting that the two receptors are linked to independent pools of G_i/G_o proteins. Thus, the demonstrated antagonistic intramembrane interactions between GAL and $5\text{-}HT_{1A}$ receptors do not lead to altered inhibitory coupling of the $5\text{-}HT_{1A}$ receptors to the adenylyl cyclase,[19] but may result in an altered coupling to other types of $5\text{-}HT_{1A}$ signal transduction pathways.

AUTORADIOGRAPHIC, BIOCHEMICAL, AND FUNCTIONAL EVIDENCE FOR THE EXISTENCE OF FACILITATORY $5\text{-}HT_{1A}$/GAL RECEPTOR INTERACTIONS

Activation of $5\text{-}HT_{1A}$ receptors by 8-OH-DPAT increases the affinity of the GAL receptor in many di- and telencephalic regions of the rat as shown by receptor autoradiography.[20] 8-OH-DPAT in a concentration of 10 nM reduced the IC50 values of porcine $^{125}I\text{-}GAL$ binding sites by about 55% in cryostat sections from the di- and telencephalon. This action was of a much smaller magnitude (20% reduction) and also required higher concentrations of 8-OH-DPAT (100 nM) in membrane preparations of the ventral di- and telencephalon. These results indicate the possible existence of an enhancing cytoplasmic factor that is not present within the membrane preparations used in the biochemical studies. Thus, a second messenger may contribute to the facilitatory intramembrane $5\text{-}HT_{1A}$/ GAL receptor interaction. This mechanism may represent in part an intramembrane rapid inhibitory feedback to control $5\text{-}HT_{1A}$ receptor affinity and efficacy in view of the results just reported on antagonistic GAL-GAL fragment/$5\text{-}HT_{1A}$ receptor interactions. This action involves $5\text{-}HT_{1A}$ receptors, because the $5\text{-}HT_{1A}$ antagonist NAN 190 was able to block the facilitatory effect of 8-OH-DPAT on GAL binding sites and this interaction appeared to be G protein independent, inasmuch as enhancement of the affinity was also demonstrated in the presence of GTP.[20]

The $5\text{-}HT_{1A}$/GAL receptor interactions could also be demonstrated by quantitative receptor autoradiography within the nucleus tractus solitarius and within the caudal raphe nuclei (raphe pallidus and obscurus nuclei).[21] These results are of particular interest because intracisternally coinjected GAL and $5\text{-}HT_{1A}$ agonist 8-OH-DPAT can act synergistically to cause vasodepressor actions in the rat. The $5\text{-}HT_{1A}$ receptors involved in this vasodepressor activity are probably located within the medullary raphe nuclei, reducing the neuronal firing rate.[22] In this analysis a threshold dose (1 nmol) of GAL enhanced the vasodepressor action of either an ED50 dose or a threshold dose of 8-OH-DPAT. Higher doses of GAL by itself will induce vasodepressor responses possibly by reducing the firing rate in the medullary raphe neurons.[4,23] It therefore seems likely that the interaction in the raphe nuclei, i.c. at the somadendritic level of the 5-HT neurons, encompasses the facilitatory $5\text{-}HT_{1A}$/GAL interactions enhancing GAL receptor affinity and efficacy (see below).

Taken together, these results indicate that the postjunctional $5\text{-}HT_{1A}$ receptors are antagonistically regulated by GAL and especially GAL fragment receptors through an

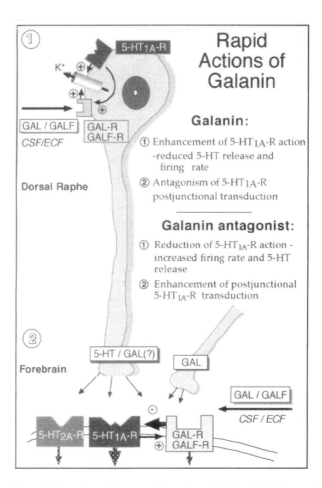

FIGURE 4. Schematic illustration of the synergistic actions of GAL and/or NH$_2$-terminal GAL fragments at the pre- and postjunctional level of the ascending 5-HT pathways to the tel- and diencephalon. GAL-(1-29) and/or GAL fragments (1-15; 1-16) will markedly reduce especially 5-HT$_{1A}$-mediated transmission both by acting at the cell body level to reduce 5-HT firing rate, 5-HT release, and 5-HT metabolism and by reducing the transduction of the postjunctional 5-HT$_{1A}$ receptors through the antagonistic GAL-GAL fragment/5-HT$_{1A}$ receptor interaction. Antagonists of GAL and GAL fragment receptors may therefore represent new types of antidepressant drugs.

intramembrane, probably G protein-independent, interaction. This interaction may in part represent an inhibitory feedback control of the 5-HT_{1A} receptor transduction, because activation of 5-HT_{1A} receptors induces an increase in the affinity of the GAL receptors and probably an enhancement of the GAL receptor transduction (FIG. 4). However, it is currently not known if the $^{125}\text{I-GAL-(1-15)}$ binding sites may become modulated by 5-HT_{1A} receptor activation.

PREJUNCTIONAL INTERACTIONS BETWEEN 5-HT_{1A} AND GAL RECEPTORS AT THE SOMADENDRITIC LEVEL OF THE 5-HT NEURONS

In 1988 it was shown that intraventricular injections of porcine GAL reduced 5-HT turnover within the frontoparietal cortex, hippocampal formation, and ventral limbic cortex of male rats,[2] and it was suggested that this action may reflect an effect of GAL on the 5-HT cell body regions of the mesencephalic raphe nuclei, many of which costore GAL immunoreactivity.[24] This interpretation was supported by the aforementioned cardiovascular studies[21] that coactivation of GAL and 5-HT_{1A} receptors at the level of the caudal raphe nuclei can lead to enhanced vasodepressor responses. GAL-(1-15) is not as effective in this respect and produces vasopressor effects by itself.[25] Furthermore, electrophysiological studies of Xu and Hökfelt[26] demonstrated that GAL can produce hyperpolarization of dorsal raphe neurons through opening of potassium channels. Thus, GAL mimics the actions of 5-HT_{1A} receptor activation, which strongly supports the foregoing interpretation. The fact that GAL also can prolong the outward current induced by 5-HT_{1A} receptor activation[26] may be in line with the finding that the 5-HT_{1A} receptor agonist 8-OH-DPAT could enhance the affinity and possibly the efficacy of the GAL receptor within the caudal raphe nuclei. Thus, it seems possible that the main interaction between the two receptors within the raphe nuclei is one of enhancement of GAL receptor transduction upon 5-HT_{1A} receptor activation, so that the 5-HT_{1A} receptors can recruit a stronger outward potassium current through enhancement of GAL receptor function, further prolonging the hyperpolarization episodes. The existence of such mechanisms at the somadendritic level of the 5-HT raphe neurons will then result in substantial reductions in the neuronal firing rate and in reduced 5-HT release and metabolism in terminal areas (FIG. 4).

LONG-TERM ACTIONS OF INTRAVENTRICULAR GAL

Recently, it was possible to demonstrate upon intraventricular injection of 1.5 nmol of porcine GAL at the 10-minute time interval, the appearance not only of a ventricular zone (100–200 μm wide) of diffuse GAL-immunoreactivity but also of GAL immunoreactive nerve cell bodies with dendrites within the dorsal and ventral hippocampus and within the ventricular parts of the striatum[16,27] (Jansson *et al.*, 1998, unpublished data). Also, the dendrites of these nerve cell bodies were strongly labeled, whereas the scattered GAL-immunoreactive nerve terminals, for example, those in the hippocampal formation, were not changed in their morphologic appearance or in their density upon the intraventricular GAL injection (FIGS. 5–7). It was of particular interest not only that cytoplasmic GAL immunoreactivity appeared but also that GAL immunoreactivity was present over the nucleus in some nerve cells. Within the hippocampal formation the strongly labeled nerve

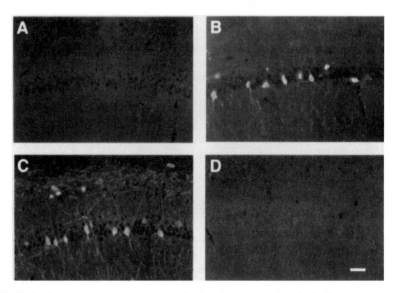

FIGURE 5. Time course for the appearance of galanin immunoreactivity in the dorsal hippocampus (CA1) following intraventricular injection of porcine galanin (1.5 nmol/rat). **(A)** The control injection of CSF (20 min) where only a few punctate galanin-immunoreactive terminals were found. At the 10- **(B)** and 20- **(C)** minute time intervals following galanin injection, galanin immunoreactivity was found in many small- to medium-sized rounded cell bodies and some pyramidal-like cells mainly in the pyramidal and stratum oriens layers. At the 60-minute time interval, very few if any cell bodies were found to be galanin immunoreactive. **(D)** Bregma = −3.6 mm. Scale bar = 50 μm.

cell bodies that appeared upon the exogenous GAL intraventricular injection were scattered all over the dorsal and ventral hippocampus as well as within the dentate gyrus and usually appeared as small to medium sized, rounded to oval nerve cells, but a few pyramidal-like cell bodies also accumulated GAL peptides. This unique nerve cell system with exogenous GAL immunoreactivity was shown in double immunolabeling experiments to mainly belong to GAD, NPY, and somatostatin-immunoreactive nerve cells (FIG. 7). These results indicate that a number of nerve cell bodies with dendrites exist capable of endocytotic uptake of diffusing exogenous GAL. These neurons represent in part GABA interneurons possibly costoring NPY and somatostatin with location in both the dendritic and cell body layers of the gyrus hippocampus and dentate gyrus. Similar types of nerve cell populations with their dendrites are labeled upon intrahippocampal injection of the same amount of porcine GAL in the ventral hippocampus.[27] This endocytotic uptake could partly be mediated via activation of the hippocampal GAL fragment receptors possibly located on these nerve cell body populations, because the process of accumulation is substantially reduced by coinjection of the GAL receptor antagonist M35.

These results open up *inter alia* the possibility that diffusing GAL peptides exert not only membrane actions via G protein-coupled GAL and GAL fragment receptors, but also

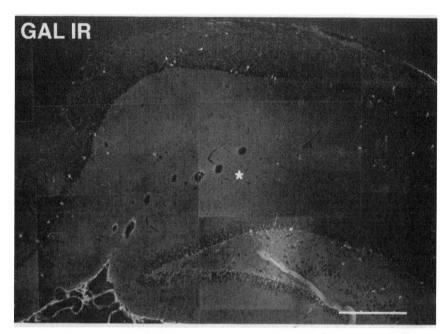

FIGURE 6. Galanin immunoreactivity (GAL-IR) in the dorsal hippocampus 10 minutes following intrahippocampal microinjection of porcine galanin (1.5 nmol/0.5 μl). Many nerve cell bodies spread over the dorsal hippocampus, mainly in the pyramidal layer and in the stratum oriens of CA1 and in the polyform layer of dentate gyrus, became galanin immunoreactive. Close to the injection site (*), a zone of diffuse galanin immunoreactivity in combination with a few galanin-immunoreactive cell bodies was observed. Bregma = −3.6 mm. Scale bar = 500 μm.

long-term actions via endocytotic uptake in the somadendritic regions and transport into the nucleus, where effects may be exerted on gene transcription. Also, AngII immunoreactivity was found located over nuclei and specifically over the transcriptionally active heterochromatin.[28] Previously, β-endorphin was also demonstrated on intraventricular injection to be accumulated in discrete nerve cell body populations within the hippocampal formation and paraventricular hypothalamic and preoptic regions.[29,30] It must therefore be emphasized that specific peri-paraventricular nerve cell populations in the core of the brain can accumulate neuropeptides and/or their fragments, such as β-endorphin and GAL and related peptides. These results open up the possibility that CSF peptides may directly influence gene expression of discrete peri-paraventricular nerve cell populations, leading to long-term actions. Previously, somatodendritic internalization and perinuclear targeting of neurotensin was also observed in brain slices.[31]

Another exciting possibility based on the present findings is that the accumulated GAL and NH$_2$-terminal GAL fragments act as false transmitters in these interneurons to become released via inverse endocytosis acting on GAL fragment receptors located on the same and adjacent neurons to regulate the activity at adjacent receptors, such as 5-HT$_{1A}$ receptors that can be reached by 5-HT diffusing from adjacent terminals. In this way the neu-

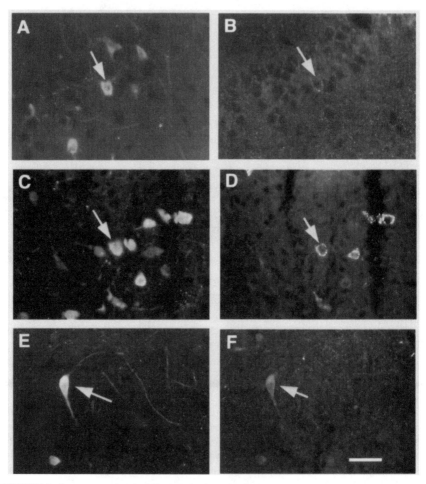

FIGURE 7. Immunocytochemical characterization of nerve cell bodies in the dorsal hippocampus, with the appearance of galanin immunoreactivity 10 minutes following intraventricular injection of porcine galanin (1.5 nmol/rat) using double-labeling immunocytochemistry. In the *left column* (**A**, **C**, and **E**), galanin immunoreactivity is shown, and in the *right column* the glutamic acid decarboxylase (GAD) in CA1 (**B**), somatostatin (SOM) in CA3 (**D**), and neuropeptide Y (NPY) in CA1 (**F**) immunoreactivities are shown. *Arrows* show corresponding cells. Many cells that exhibited galanin immunoreactivity 10 minutes following galanin injection were also GAD, SOM, or NPY immunoreactive, but there was no complete match between galanin-immunoreactive cell bodies and any of the other three demonstrated cell body populations. Bregma = −3.6 mm. Scale bar = 50 μm.

ronal activity of this unique nerve cell population would become strongly and preferentially affected by diffusing GAL and especially its NH_2-terminal GAL fragments, such as (1-15). This may be one mode of action of endogenous CSF GAL peptides and NH_2-terminal fragments.

Based on these observations the concept of the "opportunistic" neuron is introduced (Agnati, Jansson, Ögren, and Fuxe, to be published). It is proposed that peri-paraventricular neurons represent a "sink" for neuropeptides in the ECF and CSF that through neuronal uptake can integrate WT and VT via dendritic transport (WT) and peptide/peptide fragment release into the ECF (VT). The opportunistic neurons appear to be localized mainly to the brain core and may give a unitary frame to Nauta's model of the limbic system.

PATHOPHYSIOLOGIC ASPECTS ON INTRAMEMBRANE GAL AND GAL FRAGMENT RECEPTOR/5-HT$_{1A}$ RECEPTOR INTERACTIONS: FOCUS ON DEPRESSIVE ILLNESS

The 5-HT hypothesis of depression states that a reduction in central 5-HT neurotransmission in the limbic forebrain particularly via the postjunctional 5-HT$_{1A}$ receptors is involved with transduction over the 5-HT$_{2A}$ receptors becoming more dominant.[32–34] It is therefore of particular interest that the current findings indicate that synergistic actions of GAL and the GAL NH_2-terminal fragments exist at the cell body and postjunctional level, acting to reduce postjunctional 5-HT$_{1A}$-mediated transmission (FIG. 4). Thus, exaggerated enhancement of GAL and/or GAL fragment transmission may contribute to the development of depression. It is of interest that GAL does not antagonistically regulate forebrain 5-HT$_{2A}$ receptors[1,2] because they may in contrast favor the development of depression based on the fact that many classic antidepressants can block 5-HT$_{2A}$ receptors acutely and on chronic treatment produce downregulation of this 5-HT receptor subtype;[33–35] see review by Ögren and Fuxe.[32] Thus, based on the available evidence, GAL and the GAL fragment receptors may mimic 5-HT$_{1A}$ receptor action at the cell body-dendritic level by hyperpolarizing actions,[26] in this way reducing firing rate and 5-HT release and metabolism. Also, the facilitatory 5-HT$_{1A}$/GAL receptor action here appears to dominate. At the postjunctional level, GAL and GAL fragment peptides will instead antagonize 5-HT$_{1A}$ postjunctional transduction (FIG. 4).

GAL receptor and GAL fragment receptor antagonists may in contrast counteract the development of depression by increasing the 5-HT neuron firing rate and 5-HT release and at the postjunctional level by favoring postjunctional 5-HT$_{1A}$ receptor transduction.

GALANIN AND NH$_2$-TERMINAL FRAGMENTS AS VOLUME TRANSMISSION SIGNALS

Within the 5-HT cell body rich raphe regions, the GAL and GAL fragment signals may originate from the CSF, the GAL nerve terminals, and possibly the dendrites and the soma of the 5-HT neurons. Thus, one mode of regulation may involve volume transmission (VT), leading to an inhibitory GAL receptor tone on the ascending and descending 5-HT pathways reducing their firing rate. At the postjunctional level in several cortical regions the GAL signals appear to originate from the CSF and the sparse terminal plexa of the

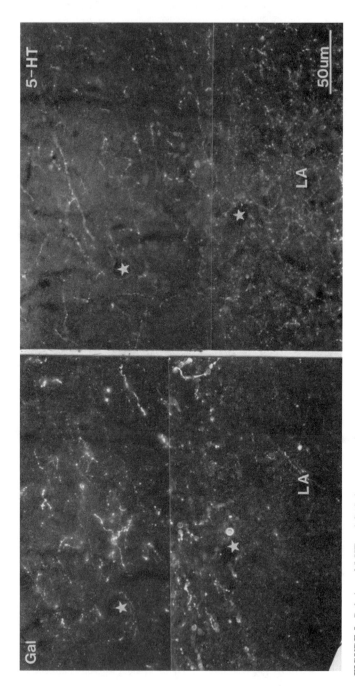

FIGURE 8. Relation of 5-HT and GAL-immunoreactive nerve terminal networks in the lateral amygdala (LA) and the region dorsal to the LA. Double immunofluorescence-labeling procedures with rabbit anti-GAL (porcine) antibody (Peninsula, IHC7153, lot no. 961028, diluted 1:800) and rabbit anti-5-HT antibody (dr. Steinbusch; 1:500). Two structurally independent GAL and 5-HT networks are formed. For orientation, *asterisks* indicate the same vessels in the two figures.

GAL-immunoreactive interneurons and GAL/NA costoring terminals[36] (see Hökfelt, this symposium) (transmitter/receptor mismatches), again leading to tonic activation of the GAL receptors and especially the GAL fragment receptors, exerting an inhibitory modulation of the 5-HT_{1A} receptor affinity and efficacy. Again, GAL signaling appears through VT to have wide access to the networks regulated by the 5-HT_{1A} receptors. Very few GAL/5-HT costoring terminals appear to exist in the tel- and diencephalon (FIG. 8). In the few GAL/5-HT costoring terminals of the forebrain,[37] where GAL appears to be core-leased with 5-HT, there may exist a demand for a phasic release of GAL in order to strongly regulate the 5-HT_{1A} receptor transduction through the GAL receptors. Thus, a frequency code of GAL receptor activation may here be essential for the appropriate regulation of the 5-HT_{1A} receptor-mediated cotransmission.

CONCLUSIONS

1. GAL and GAL fragment modulation of 5HT-1A receptors at the postjunctional level

A. Existence of intramembrane antagonistic postjunctional $GAL/5\text{-HT}_{1A}$ receptor interactions.

B. Existence of intramembrane antagonistic postjunctional GAL NH_2-terminal fragment/5-HT_{1A} receptor interactions.

The mechanism for these interactions is unknown, but it is not directly related to adenylyl cyclase (AC). Additive inhibitory effects of GAL and 8-OH-DPAT on stimulated AC activity have been observed.[19]

2. GAL modulation of 5HT neurons at the prejunctional level

A. Reduction of tel-diencephalic 5-HT metabolism by intraventricular GAL (action at rostral raphe level).

B. Hyperpolarizing actions of GAL on 5-HT nerve cell bodies.[26]

GAL action at the somadendritic level may dominate after ivt injections of GAL with regard to control of 5-HT release.

3. 5-HT modulation of GAL receptors at the postjunctional level

A. Increase of ^{125}I-GAL binding affinity in sections by 8-OH-DPAT in many tel-diencephalic regions and in the raphe nuclei.

B. This action is mimicked by chronic antidepressant treatment with imipramine, suggesting *in vivo* activation of 5-HT_{1A} receptors by imipramine through reduction of 5-HT reuptake.[38] After such *in vivo* treatment, 8-OH-DPAT can *in vitro* no longer enhance GAL receptor affinity, suggesting involvement of 5-HT_{1A} receptor activation after chronic imipramine treatment.

Besides the foregoing rapid membrane actions of GAL and GAL fragments, long-term actions of these GAL peptides may also develop.

4. Long-term actions of galanin

Intraventricular GAL is internalized into dendrites and soma of specific nerve cell populations of peri-paraventricular structures, in the hippocampus mainly representing GAD, NPY, and/or somatostatin positive nerve cells, opening up the possibility that GAL and its NH_2-terminal fragments can directly control gene expression or act as a false transmitter in these discrete nerve cell populations. The concept of opportunistic neuron is introduced on the basis of these observations.

5. Relevance for depression

GAL and/or GAL fragment antagonists may have potential in the treatment of depression by (1) increasing 5-HT neuronal activity and release and (2) removing intramembrane antagonistic postjunctional feedback on 5-HT_{1A} receptor transduction through GAL and especially GAL fragment receptors. The frequent failure of many antidepressants to produce a therapeutic action may be related in part to their ability to activate this negative intramembrane feedback through the facilitatory 5-HT_{1A} receptor/GAL receptor interaction at the postjunctional level.[3,15,21] The 5-HT_{1A}/GAL receptor interactions at the raphe level may also be activated by antidepressants, contributing to a reduction in 5-HT release, and may thus also reduce the therapeutic action of 5-HT reuptake blockade.

REFERENCES

1. FUXE, K., G. VON EULER, L.F. AGNATI & S.O. ÖGREN. 1988. Galanin selectively modulates 5-hydroxytryptamine 1A receptors in the rat ventral limbic cortex. Neurosci. Lett. **85:** 163–167.
2. FUXE, K., S. ÖGREN, A. JANSSON, A. CINTRA, A. HÄRFSTRAND & L. AGNATI. 1988. Intraventricular injections of galanin reduces 5-HT metabolism in the ventral limbic cortex, the hippocampal formation and the fronto-parietal cortex of the male rat. Acta Physiol. Scand. **133:** 579–581.
3. FUXE, K., L. AGNATI, G. VON EULER, K. LUNDGREN, M. ZOLI, B. BJELKE, P. ENEROTH & S. ÖGREN. 1990. Galanin/5-HT receptor interactions. A new integrative mechanism in the control of 5-HT neurotransmission in the central nervous system. *In* Serotonin from Cell Biology to Pharmacology and Therapeutics. R. Paoletti, P. Vanhoutte, N. Brunello & F. Maggi, Eds.: 169–185. Kluwer Academic Publ. Dordrecht.
4. HEDLUND, P. & K. FUXE. 1996. Galanin and 5-HT1A receptor interactions as an integrative mechanism in 5-HT neurotransmission in the brain. *In* Neuropeptides: Basic and Clinical Advances. J. Crawley & S. McLean, Eds. Ann. N.Y. Acad. Sci. **780:** 193–212.
5. HEDLUND, P., U.-B. FINNMAN, N. YAHAIHARA & K. FUXE. 1994. Galanin-(1-15), but not galanin-(1-29), modulates 5-HT1A receptors in the dorsal hippocampus of the rat brain: Possible existence of galanin receptor subtypes. Brain Res. **634:** 163–167.
6. MELANDER, T., C. KÖHLER, S. NILSSON, T. HÖKFELT, E. BRODIN, E. THEODORSSON & T. BARTFAI. 1988. Autoradiographical quantitation and anatomical mapping of ^{125}I-galanin binding sites in the rat central nervous system. J. Chem. Neuroanat. **1:** 213–233.
7. LAND, T., Ü. LANGEL & T. BARTFAI. 1991. Hypothalamic degradation of galanin(1-29) and galanin(1-16): Identification and characterization of the peptidolytic products. Brain Res. **558:** 245–250.
8. HEDLUND, P., N. YAHAIHARA & K. FUXE. 1992. Evidence for specific N-terminal galanin fragment binding sites in the rat brain. Eur. J. Pharmacol. **224:** 203–205.
9. SKOFITSCH, G., M. SILLS & D. JACOBOWITZ. 1986. Autoradiographic distribution of ^{125}I-galanin binding sites in the rat central nervous system. Peptides **7:** 1029–1042.
10. KÖHLER, C. & V. CHAN-PALAY. 1991. Brain galanin receptors: Anatomical localization and possible functional role. *In* Aspects of Synaptic Transmission: LTP, Galanin, Opioids, and 5-HT. T. W. Stone, Ed.: 65–85. Taylor & Francis. London.
11. FISONE, G., M. BERTHOLD, K. BEDECS, A. UNDEN, T. BARTFAI, R. BERTORELLI, S. CONSOLO, J. CRAWLEY, B. MARTIN, S. NILSON & T. HÖKFELT. 1989. N-terminal galanin-(16) fragment is an antagonist at the hippocampal galanin receptor. Proc. Natl. Acad. Sci. USA **86:** 9588–9591.
12. BEDECS, K., M. BERTHOLD & T. BARTFAI. 1995. Galanin—10 years with a neuroendocrine peptide. Int. J. Biochem. Cell Biol. **27:** 337–349.
13. BURGEVIN, M., I. LOQUET, D. QUARTERONET & E. HABERT-ORTOLI. 1995. Cloning, pharmacological characterization, and anatomical distribution of a rat cDNA encoding for a galanin receptor. J. Molec. Neurosci. **6:** 33–41.
14. HOWARD, A., C. TAN, L. SHIAO, O. PALYHA, K. MCKEE, D. WEINBERG, S. GEGHNER, M. CASCIERI, R. SMITH, L. VAN DER PLOEG & K. SULLIVAN. 1997. Molecular cloning and characterization of a new receptor for galanin. FEBS Lett. **405:** 285–290.
15. FUXE, K., P. HEDLUND, G. VON EULER, K. LUNDGREN, M. MARTIRE, S. ÖGREN, P. ENEROTH & L. AGNATI. 1991. Galanin/5-HT interactions in the rat central nervous system. Relevance for depression. *In* Galanin: A New Multifunctional Peptide in the Neuro-Endocrine System. Wen-

ner-Gren Center International Symposium Series, Vol. 58. T. Hökfelt, T. Bartfai, D. Jacobow-itz & D. Ottoson, Eds.: 221–235. MacMillan. London.

16. MISANE, I., H. RAZANI, F.-H. WANG, A. JANSSON, K. FUXE & S. ÖGREN. 1998. Intraventricular galanin modulates a 5-HT1A receptor mediated behavioural response in the rat. Eur. J. Neurosci. **10:** 1230–1240.

17. ÖGREN, S. 1985. Evidence for a role of brain serotonergic neurotransmission in avoidance learning. Acta Physiol. Scand. Suppl. **544:** 1–71.

18. NISHIBORI, M.R., Y. ITOH & K. SAEKI. 1988. Galanin inhibits noradrenaline-induced accumulation of cyclic AMP in the rat cerebral cortex. J. Neurochem. **51:** 1953–1955.

19. BILLECOCQ, A., P. HEDLUND, F. BOLANOS-JIMENEZ & G. FILLION. 1994. Characterization of galanin and 5-HT1A receptor coupling to adenylyl cyclase in discrete regions in the rat brain. Eur. J. Pharmacol. **269:** 209–217.

20. HEDLUND, P., G. VON EULER & K. FUXE. 1991. Activation of 5-hydroxytryptamine$_{1A}$ receptors increases the affinity of galanin receptors in di- and telencephalic areas of the rat. Brain Res. **560:** 251–259.

21. HEDLUND, P.B., J.A. AGUIRRE, J.A. NARVAEZ & K. FUXE. 1991. Centrally coinjected galanin and a 5-HT$_{1A}$ agonist act synergistically to produce vasodepressor responses in the rat. Eur. J. Pharmacol. **204:** 87–95.

22. CHALMERS, J., P. PILOWSKY, J. MINSON, V. KAPOOR, E. MILLS & M. WEST. 1988. Central serotonergic mechanisms in hypertension. Am. J. Hypertens. **1:** 79–83.

23. HÄRFSTRAND, A., K. FUXE, T. MELANDER, T. HÖKFELT & L. AGNATI. 1987. Evidence for a cardiovascular role of central galanin neurons: Focus on interactions with α2-adrenergic and neuropeptide Y mechanism. J. Cardiovasc. Pharmacol. **10 (Suppl 12):** 199–204.

24. XU, Z.-Q. & T. HÖKFELT. 1997. Expression of galanin and nitric oxide synthase in subpopulations of serotonin neurons of the rat dorsal raphe nucleus. J. Chem. Neuroanat. **13:** 169–187.

25. NARVÁEZ, J., Z. DIAZ, J. AGUIRRE, S. GONZÁLEZ-BARÓN, N. YAHAIHARA, K. FUXE & P. HEDLUND. 1994. Intracisternally injected galanin-(1–15) modulates the cardiovascular responses of galanin-(1–29) and the 5-HT$_{1A}$ receptor agonist 8-OH-DPAT. Eur. J. Pharmacol. **257:** 257–265.

26. XU, Z., X. ZHANG, V. PIERIBONE, S. GRILLNER & T. HÖKFELT. 1998. Galanin responses in rat dorsal raphe neurons: Electrophysiological and immunohistochemical studies with a note on galanin-R1 receptors. J. Neurosci. In press.

27. SCHÖTT, P., B. BJELKE & S. ÖGREN. 1998. Distribution and kinetics of galanin infused into the ventral hippocampus of the rat: Relationship to spatial learning. Neuroscience **83:** 123–136.

28. ERDMANN, B., K. FUXE & D. GANTEN. 1996. Subcellular localization of angiotensin II immunoreactivity in the rat cerebellar cortex. Hypertension **28:** 818–824.

29. AGNATI, L., B. BJELKE & K. FUXE. 1992. Volume transmission in the brain. Do brain cells communicate solely through synapses? A new theory proposes that information also flows in the extracellular space. Am. Sci. **80:** 362–374.

30. FUXE, K., X.M. LI, B. BJELKE, P. HEDLUND, G. BIAGINI & L. AGNATI. 1994. Possible mechanisms for the powerful actions of neuropeptides. Ann. N.Y. Acad. Sci. **739:** 42–59.

31. FAURE, M.-P., A. ALONSO, D. NOUEL, G. GAUDRIAULT, M. DENNIS, J.-P. VINCENT & A. BEAUDET. 1995. Somatodendritic internalization and perinuclear targeting of neurotensin in the mammalian brain. J. Neurosci. **15:** 4140–4147.

32. ÖGREN, S. & K. FUXE. 1985. Effects of antidepressant drugs on serotonin receptor mechanisms. *In* Neuropharmacology of Serotonin. A. R. Green, Ed.: 131–180. Oxford University Press. New York.

33. FUXE, K., S. ÖGREN, L. AGNATI, J.-Å. GUSTAFSSON & G. JONSSON. 1977. On the mechanism of action of the antidepressant drugs amitriptyline and nortriptyline. Evidence for 5-hydroxytryptamine receptor blocking activity. Neurosci. Lett. **6:** 339–343.

34. ÖGREN, S.-O., K. FUXE, L. F. AGNATI, J.-Å. GUSTAFSSON, G. JONSSON & A.C. HOLM. 1979. Reevaluation of the indoleamine hypothesis of depression. Evidence for a reduction of functional activity of central 5-HT systems by antidepressant drugs. J. Neural Transm. **46:** 85–103.

35. FUXE, K., S. ÖGREN, L. AGNATI, F. BENFENATI, B. FREDHOLM, K. ANDERSSON, I. ZINI & P. ENEROTH. 1983. Chronic antidepressant treatment and central 5-HT synapses. Neuropharmacology **22:** 389–400.

36. MELANDER, T., T. HÖKFELT & Å. RÖKAEUS. 1986. Distribution of galanin-like immunoreactivity in the rat central nervous system. J. Comp. Neurol. **248:** 475–517.

37. MELANDER, T., T. HÖKFELT, Å. RÖKAEUS, A.C. CUELLO, W.H. OERTEL, A. VERHOFSTAD & M. GOLD-STEIN. 1986. Coexistence of galanin-like immunoreactivity with catecholamines, 5-hydroxytryptamine, GABA and neuropeptides in the rat CNS. J. Neurosci. **6:** 3640–3654.
38. HEDLUND, P. & K. FUXE. 1991. Chronic imipramine treatment increases the affinity of [^{125}I]galanin binding sites in the tel- and diencephalon of the rat and alters the 5-HT1A/galanin receptor interaction. Acta Physiol. Scand. **141:** 137–138.

Galanin Expression within the Basal Forebrain in Alzheimer's Disease

Comments on Therapeutic Potential[a]

ELLIOTT J. MUFSON,[b,f] ULRIKA KAHL,[b] ROBERT BOWSER,[c] DEBORAH C. MASH,[d] JEFFREY H. KORDOWER,[b] AND DARLENE C. DEECHER[e]

[b]Department of Neurological Sciences and Rush Alzheimer's Disease Center, Rush Presbyterian/St. Lukes Medical Center, Chicago, Illinois 60612, USA

[c]Division of Neuropathology, University of Pittsburgh Medical Center, Pittsburgh, Pennsylvania, USA

[d]Department of Neurology, University of Miami School of Medicine, Miami, Florida, USA

[e]Molecular Biology, Women's Health Research Institute, Wyeth-Ayerst Research, Radnor, Pennsylvania 19087, USA

ABSTRACT: The inhibitory neuropeptide galanin has widespread distribution throughout the central nervous system. Studies indicate that galanin modulates cognition by regulating cholinergic basal forebrain (CBF) neuron function. The chemoanatomic organization of galanin within the mammalian CBF differs across species. In monkeys, all CBF neurons coexpress galanin, whereas in apes and humans galanin is found within a separate population of interneurons that are in close apposition to the CBF perikarya. Pharmacologic investigations revealed a low and high affinity galanin receptor within the basal forebrain in humans. *In vitro* autoradiographic investigations of the primate brain indicate that galanin receptors are concentrated within the anterior subfields of the CBF as well as the bed nucleus of the stria terminalis, amygdala, and entorhinal cortex. Galaninergic fibers hyperinnervate remaining CBF neurons in Alzheimer's disease. Because galanin inhibits the release of acetylcholine in the hippocampus, it has been suggested that the overexpression of galanin in Alzheimer's disease may downregulate the production of acetylcholine within CBF perikarya, further exacerbating cholinergic cellular dysfunction in this disorder. These observations suggest that the development of a potent galanin antagonist would be a useful step towards the successful pharmacologic treatment of Alzheimer's disease.

Over the last few years a wealth of data derived from behavioral, neurobiologic, and neuropathologic studies of patients with Alzheimer's disease (AD) has suggested that the neuropeptide galanin (GAL) plays a crucial role in the modulation of cholinergic basal forebrain (CBF) neurons (see review in ref. 1). These neurons provide the major cholinergic innervation of the cortex and hippocampus[2] and are associated with cognitive function.[3] In AD, CBF neurons undergo extensive degeneration that correlates with the

[a]This work was supported in part by AG10606, AG10668, AG09466, and the Medical Research Council of Sweden and the Wallenberg Foundation.

[f]Address for correspondence: Elliott J. Mufson, PhD, Department of Neurological Sciences, Rush Presbyterian Medical Center, 2242 West Harrison Street, Chicago Illinois 60612. Phone, 312/633-1550; fax, 312/633-1564; e-mail, emufson@rush.edu

duration of disease and degree of cognitive impairment.[4] The extensive galaninergic fiber network that courses through the basal forebrain in humans hyperinnervates the remaining CBF neurons in AD.[5,6] Inasmuch as GAL inhibits the release of acetylcholine in the hippocampus,[7] it was suggested that the overexpression of GAL may downregulate the function of the remaining CBF neurons, further exacerbating cholinergic dysfunction in AD.[5,6] These observations suggest that the development of a potent GAL antagonist would be a useful step towards successful pharmacologic treatment of AD. In view of these observations, the aims of the studies described here were to address questions related to the expression of GAL and its receptors within the CBF in the normal human aged and AD brain.

GALANIN SEQUENCE AND MOLECULAR STRUCTURE

Galanin is a 29 amino acid neuropeptide first isolated from pig intestinal extracts by Mutt and coworkers.[8] Galanin is endogenously synthesized as part of a 123 (124 in humans) amino acid long precursor, which is subsequently cleaved and processed into one signal sequence and two biologically active peptides: GAL and its COOH-terminal flanking peptide, the GAL-message–associated peptide (GMAP).[9,10] The GAL gene has been cloned from several species,[11–13] and the upstream promoter region contains consensus sequences for regulatory factors and hormones such as estrogen.[14–16] Since its initial discovery, GAL has been characterized in a number of species including humans,[8,9,17] and it exerts widespread biologic action throughout the nervous system.[7,18,19] Whereas the first half of the GAL molecule is identical in all species, there are amino acid differences in the COOH-terminal region between species. Also, human GAL (hGAL) contains an additional serine residue and a nonamidated carboxyl terminus (Fig. 1).[9,17] Conformational studies indicate that the GAL structure may conform to a hairpin-like structure with a bend

(1-15 aa) 100 % Homologous

Human, Pig, Rat

H-GLY-TRP-THR-LEU-ASN-SER-ALA-GLY-TYR-LEU-LEU-GLY-PRO-HIS-ALA

(16-30 aa) Human   non-amidated

VAL-GLY-ASN-HIS-ARG-SER-PHE-SER-ASP-LYS-ASN-GLY-LEU-THR-SER-OH

(16-29 aa) Pig

ILE-ASP-ASN-HIS-ARG-SER-PHE-**HIS**-ASP-LYS-**TYR**-GLY-LEU-**ALA**-NH$_2$

(16-29 aa) RAT

ILE-ASP-ASN-HIS-ARG-SER-PHE-SER-ASP-LYS-**HIS**-GLY-LEU-THR-NH$_2$

FIGURE 1. Species differences in the amino acid sequence of endogenous galanin. Differences of amino acids compared with hGAL sequence are indicated in *bold*.

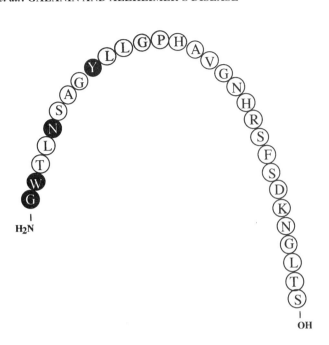

FIGURE 2. Schematic drawing of the molecular structure of galanin, illustrating the putative three-dimensional horseshoe-like structure of the peptide. Note that the two alpha-helical terminals bend around the midportion of the molecule (residues in grey). The underlying pharmacophores of galanin are in *black* and *white* (see text for details).

around amino acids Gly[12]-Pro[13] (FIG. 2).[20,21] Structure-activity relationship studies have demonstrated that the well-conserved NH$_2$-terminal portion of the molecule plays a key role in high-affinity binding of GAL to its receptors.[22] It has been proposed that the NH$_2$-terminal part of GAL is actively involved in binding the GAL receptor (GALR) and that the COOH-terminal fragment functions to protect the NH$_2$-terminal portion from proteolytic attack, resulting in increased bioavailability.[23,24]

SPECIES-DEPENDENT GAL DISTRIBUTION WITHIN THE MAMMALIAN BASAL FOREBRAIN

During the last several years, mounting evidence indicates that the distribution of GAL-like immunoreactivity within the basal forebrain, a region that undergoes severe degeneration in AD,[25] differs among rodents,[26] monkeys,[27] and humans.[5,6,28] In the rat, GAL colocalizes only with cholinergic neurons within the septal diagonal band complex, although to a lesser degree than originally believed.[29,30] Recently, we compared the distribution of galaninergic fibers and perikarya within the basal forebrain of monkeys, lesser (gibbons) and greater (chimpanzee and gorilla) apes as well as humans, using GAL immu-

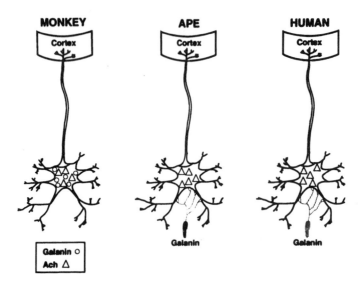

FIGURE 3. Schematic diagram showing the relation between acetylcholine (ACh) and galanin within neurons of the primate cholinergic basal forebrain. Note that in the monkey, all cholinergic basal forebrain neurons colocalize galanin. By contrast, these neurons are galanin negative in apes and humans. In these species, galanin arises from a population of small interneurons (light grey) as well as in an extraforebrain fiber system (not shown) which terminates upon the large cholinergic neurons of the substantia innominata.

nohistochemistry.[28] In the monkey, virtually all CBF neurons (i.e., those within the septal diagonal band complex and nucleus basalis) contain GAL mRNA and GAL-like immunoreactivity,[27,31,32] whereas in apes and humans these neurons lack both the peptide and the gene for GAL (FIG. 3).[6,27,28,32] Interestingly, in apes and humans the basal forebrain contains a small population of noncholinergic galaninergic interneurons. More impressive is a dense galaninergic fiber plexus of unknown origin that innervates the CBF neurons of apes and humans (FIG. 3).[6,28,33] This galaninergic pathway courses through the substantia innominata–nucleus basalis region en route to the hypothalamus, bed nucleus of the stria terminalis, and vertical limb nucleus of the diagonal band. Although the pattern of GAL immunoreactivity within the ape and human basal forebrain was strikingly discordant with that observed in the monkey, the hypothalamus and bed nucleus of the stria terminalis of the these primates displayed similar patterns of cell body and fiber staining, supporting the species-specific pattern seen within the basal forebrain.

GALANIN RECEPTORS

In Vitro Autoradiography of Galanin Receptors in the Human Basal Forebrain

Because GAL acts through its interaction with membrane-bound galanin receptors (GALRs), we undertook studies aimed at assessing the distribution and pharmacologic

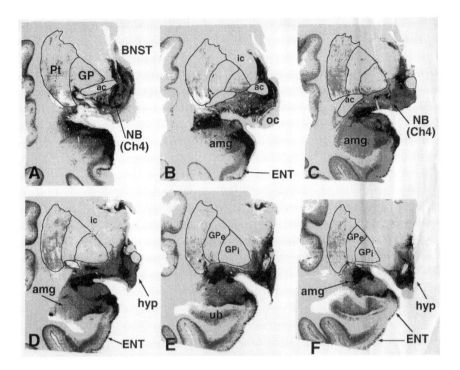

FIGURE 4. Autoradiographic localization of [^{125}I]hGAL binding in human basal forebrain brain (male; 29 years of age). Computer-generated black and white autoradiograms from a series of half-hemisphere coronal sections of the human brain at different anterior to posterior levels through the forebrain. Grey scale indicates intensity of labeling (black = high densities; dark grey = intermediate densities; light grey = low densities). Abbreviations: ac, anterior commissure; amg, amygdala; BNST, bed nucleus of stria terminalis; Ch4, cholinergic basal forebrain subfield; ENT, entorhinal cortex; GP, globus pallidus; GP$_i$, globus pallidus; GP$_e$, globus pallidus; hyp, hypothalamus; ic, internal capsule; NB, nucleus basalis; oc, optic chiasm; Pt, putamen; uh, uncal hippocampus.

characterization of GALRs in the human basal forebrain, using *in vitro* receptor autoradiography and radioligand binding assays.[34,35] Our *in vitro* receptor autoradiography[35] (FIG. 4) and that of others[36] revealed low to high densities of [^{125}I]hGAL binding sites within subfields of the nucleus basalis of the substantia innominata complex, rostrally. At the mid-level of this region, the patchy appearance of [^{125}I]hGAL binding was replaced mainly by a continuous band of high-density labeling that extended into the bed nucleus of the stria terminalis. In addition, medium to high densities of labeling were observed within the anterior hypothalamus, lateral–preoptic area, perifornical region, and amygdaloid complex. In fact, a continuous band of intense GALR labeling was observed between the amygdala and the substantia innominata.[35,36] Moreover, we found a band of intense labeling of the rostral aspect of the entorhinal cortex mainly in layer 2.[35] Additional experiments were done using radioligand binding techniques to characterize the GALRs in the entorhinal cortex. Analysis of the [^{125}I]hGAL saturation experiments depicted a two-site interaction revealing a high and low affinity state of the GALR in entorhinal cortex homogenates.[35] Interestingly, an increase in GALR expression occurs within the entorhinal cortex in AD.[37]

PHARMACOLOGIC CHARACTERIZATION OF GALRs
IN THE HUMAN BASAL FOREBRAIN

Comparative radioligand binding studies were performed on normal human basal forebrain and hypothalamic homogenates (67 ± 15 years) to identify possible biochemical differences between GALRs in these two brain regions.[34] The results of these studies indicate that both [125I]porcine GAL (pGAL) and [125I]galantide (GLT) irreversibly bind with high affinity and act as agonists, based on GppNHp inhibition, at GALRs in the human basal forebrain and hypothalamus. Saturation analysis depicted similar receptor numbers for either radioligand in the basal forebrain, but [125I]pGAL showed higher affinity values for the GALR in this region. By contrast, [125I]pGAL showed lower receptor affinity and labeled 42% more receptors than did [125I]GLT in the hypothalamus (TABLE 1). Saturation analysis revealed that the radioligands in the basal forebrain appear to label the same GALR population with varying affinity, whereas the radioligands labeled two populations of receptors in the hypothalamus. Additional radioligand binding studies were conducted to further characterize possible GALR subtype differences in these two brain regions.[34] Competition studies with GAL and GAL chimeric peptides were performed using either [125I]pGAL or [125I]GLT. On the basis of the results from the saturation experiments, our hypothesis was that inasmuch as both radioligands labeled the same number of GALR in the basal forebrain, rank order affinities of GAL peptide analogs would be the same regardless of the radioligand. Analysis of the data from competition assays revealed different rank order affinities of the GAL peptide analogs within the basal forebrain depending on which radioligand was used. These observations suggest that the radioligands are interacting with different GALRs within the basal forebrain and that two receptor subtypes exist in approximately the same concentration. Hence, on the basis of the saturation and competition studies, there appear to be at least two GALR populations in both the basal forebrain and the hypothalamus. At the time that these studies were conducted, [125I]hGAL was not commercially available. Heterologous radioligands may interact differently with different GALR subtypes.[38] Therefore, saturation experiments were performed using basal forebrain homogenates labeled with [125I]hGAL to determine whether GALR pharmacology varied dependent on species-specific radioligands. Analysis of our preliminary data indicate that the affinity and receptor number values (Deecher and Mufson, unpublished observations) were similar to those values reported for [125I]pGAL (TABLE 1).

GALANIN PLASTICITY WITHIN THE BASAL FOREBRAIN
OF INDIVIDUALS WITH ALZHEIMER'S DISEASE

Recently, we and others have demonstrated that galaninergic fibers hypertrophy and hyperinnervate surviving CBF neurons within the septal diagonal band complex and nucleus basalis of patients with AD (FIG. 5).[5,6] Our group, using confocal laser microscopy, demonstrated that direct appositions are present between GAL-containing fibers and CBF neurons in the normal human brain and that these contacts hypertrophy in AD.[33]

TABLE 1. Saturation of [125I]pGAL or [125I]GLT Binding in Normal Human Basal Forebrain and Hypothalamus[a]

Region	Value	[125I]pGAL	[125I]GLT
Basal forebrain	K_D (pM)	74	221
	B_{max} (fmol/mg protein)	31	32
Hypothalamus	K_D (pM)	264	197
	B_{max} (fmol/mg protein)	125	71

[a]Data are means of triplicate determinations from one experiment that is representative of three other cases. A three-parameter logistic model with parameters B_{max}, K_D, and slope was fitted to evaluate the two-site saturation model. If the slope estimate indicated a one-site model (slope not significantly different from 1), the slope was locked to 1 and the analysis was rerun, giving a linear Rosenthal plot. If a curvilinear plot was generated, then a two-site saturation model was run to determine the binding parameters of each binding site. Saturation models were evaluated using a customized JMP (SAS Institute, Cary, North Carolina) application. The customized JMP applications were developed by Biometrics Research (Wyeth-Ayerst, Princeton, New Jersey).

Although the galaninergic hyperinnervation seen in AD were suggested to be triggered in part by the loss of cholinergic neurons,[5,6] this remains an unresolved issue. We recently questioned this hypothesis in a study of individuals with Down's syndrome, a genetic disorder with many neurodegenerative symptoms resembling AD, including extensive CBF neuron loss.[6] However, despite numerous neuropathologic similarities between the two disorders, Down's syndrome patients failed to display GAL-immunoreactive hypertrophy typically seen in AD.

DISCUSSION

Because galaninergic fibers hyperinnervate remaining CBF neurons in AD,[6,39] it was hypothesized that galaninergic systems play a role in cholinergic cell dysfunction in this disease. In this regard, GAL was shown to inhibit acetylcholine release from the hippocampus[7] and to depress neural circuits underlying working memory in rats.[1,40] Moreover, in humans, GAL is localized mainly to a dense fiber plexus that innervates the GAL-negative cholinergic positive neurons of the basal forebrain. The chemical signature for GAL in humans differs from that in monkeys where all CBF contain GAL and acetylcholine.[28] The change in the chemoanatomic signature of GAL within the basal forebrain through hominoid evolution may reflect an importance for this neuropeptide in the functional regulation of CBF neurons coinciding with the increased evolutionary development in the size of the cortical mantle.[28] The extrinsic innervation of galaninergic fibers upon CBF neurons may allow for greater control over the cellular function of these neurons in the human brain.

In AD, a uniquely human disease, a marked increase occurs in the number of galaninergic fibers upon remaining CBF neurons within the medial septum/diagonal band complex[6] and the more anterior regions of the nucleus basalis.[5,33] We demonstrated by confocal laser microscopy that galaninergic fibers form putative synapses with these neurons in the normal human brain, and that these synaptic contacts hyperinnervate remaining

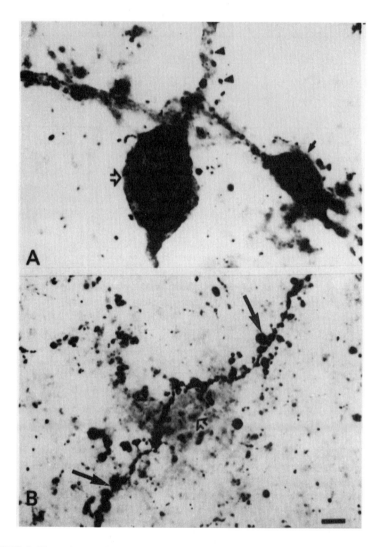

FIGURE 5. Photomicrographs showing the relation between galaninergic profiles and p75^{NTR} immunoreactive neurons in human aged and AD basal forebrain. (**A**) Cholinergic neuron (*open arrow*) within the septal/diagonal band complex containing p75^{NTR} which is decorated by fine galanin-immunoreactive fibers (*arrow heads*) in an aged control case. Note a galanin-immunoreactive neuronal process emanating from a galanin-containing neuron (*small arrow*) which reaches the dendrite of the p75^{NTR} immunopositive neuron. (**B**) Hypertrophied galanin-immunoreactive fibers (*large black arrows*) surrounding a p75^{NTR} positive neuron (*open arrow*) within the septal/diagonal band complex in AD. Bar in B = 15 μm.

CBF neurons in AD.[33] Consistent with this hyperinnervation are the observations that there is an increase in the expression of GAL mRNA in the few small GAL basal forebrain parvicellular neurons[41] and that the GALRs in this region are preserved in patients with AD.[42] Although it is likely that an intrinsic galaninergic fiber system probably provides some of the GALR labeling (i.e., presynaptic receptors) seen within the basal forebrain, an additional extra forebrain component most likely also contributes to this labeling and may arise from the locus coeruleus.[6]

Recently, the first GALR was cloned from Bowes' human melanoma cell line and designated GALR1.[43] The GALR1 receptor is a G-protein–coupled receptor containing seven transmembrane domains and shares common features with other members of this group of receptors.[44] To date, other homologous forms of GALR1 have been found in several human[45] and rat[46] tissue types as well as in cell lines.[47] Following the cloning of GALR1, at least two additional GALR subtypes, GALR2[48–50] and GALR3,[51] have been cloned. Since Miller and colleagues[52] showed that the GALR1 receptor is not coexpressed with cholinergic neurons of the rat basal forebrain, it will be crucial to evaluate the expression of this and other GALRs in the normal versus diseased human brain. Such studies may

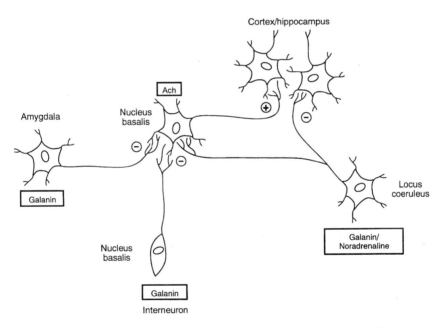

FIGURE 6. Schematic diagram illustrating three putative sources of galaninergic innervation upon the cholinergic neurons of the human basal forebrain. In addition to the intrinsic galaninergic innervation of cholinergic basal neurons, we suggest that additional galanin innervation may arise from the amygdala and the locus coeruleus. However, it remains to be determined whether the inputs from the amygdala and locus coeruleus are also inhibitory as was suggested for the intrinsic galaninergic basal forebrain system. Because each system overexpresses the inhibitory peptide galanin, it is possible that they may either individually or in conjunction downregulate cholinergic basal forebrain cell function in AD.

shed light on which GALR subtype(s) exists within the human basal forebrain and what role these receptors play in the regulation of the basocortical projection system.

Although human CBF neurons do not synthesize GAL, they are innervated by a dense GAL immunoreactive fiber system that courses through this region.[6,28] The source of this GAL fiber system remains to be clearly established. It has been hypothesized that GAL-positive parvicellular neurons are the major source of GAL within the human basal fore-brain.[39] However, it is unlikely that these few GAL immunoreactive cells can account for the rich galaninergic fiber plexus seen within this region.[6,28] One potential source of GAL fiber innervation in the basal forebrain may be the locus coeruleus. In fact, GAL-containing cells within the locus coeruleus also exhibit enhanced GAL expression in AD.[41] Another source of GAL innervation to the forebrain may be the extended amygdaloid complex which contains numerous GAL-containing cell bodies[30] and displays hypertro-phy of galanin-containing fibers in AD (Mufson, unpublished observations). FIGURE 6 summarizes three putative sources of galaninergic input which may play a role in the regu-lation of cholinergic basal forebrain and/or cortical neuronal activity.

THERAPEUTIC POTENTIAL

Current approved drug treatments for AD consist of anticholinesterase agents that act by increasing the availability of synaptic acetylcholine and in the short term improve cog-nitive function.[53,54] Review of the data from functional,[7] biochemical,[55] and behavioral studies[56,57] suggests that GAL acts as an inhibitory modulator of cholinergic function. Anticholinesterase agents increase the available amounts of acetylcholine, resulting in an increased firing rate of remaining cholinergic neurons. It is thought that this increased fir-ing rate increases the release of GAL, which in turn inhibits presynaptic release of acetyl-choline. This negative feedback loop eventually leads to burn-out of the remaining cholinergic neurons. Therefore, it is hypothesized that the increased levels of GAL caused by higher stimulation frequencies of acetylcholine may actually decrease the release of acetylcholine from surviving CBF neurons[58] and effectively diminish benefits from anti-cholinesterase treatment in AD. If the hypothesis of GAL acting as an inhibitory modulator of acetylcholine release is true, then perhaps antagonists towards the GALR could enhance cholinergic transmission by reducing the inhibitory influence of GAL on the firing rate of CBF neurons. The only high-affinity ligands for GAL available today are GAL chimerics which have been proven to exert both agonist and antagonist effects on GALRs.[59-65] How-ever, it is possible that the development of a CNS-specific GAL antagonist used in combi-nation with anticholinesterases, cholinergic agonists, neurotropins and their receptors, or other agents such as anti-inflammatory drugs, apolipoprotein E (apoE) inhibitors, or hor-mones (e.g., estrogen) may provide potential pharmacologic treatment strategies for CBF dysfunction in AD. Indeed, a few scattered clinical studies suggest that patients with AD may be best treated using polypharmacy. For example, an epidemiologic investigation noted an enhanced response to tacrine (a cholinergic inhibitor) in women who had had, or were currently on, estrogen therapy.[66] Although the exact mechanism underlying this effect is unclear, it is worth noting that this hormone influences cholinergic neuron func-tion by altering expression of the genes for choline acetyltransferase and high affinity trkA receptor for the cell survival substance, nerve growth factor.[67] More intriguing are the observations that carriers of the apoE4 allele have severe decreases in forebrain cholinergic function[68–70] and increased GAL within the basal forebrain (Mufson, unpublished observations). Reports indicate that estrogen induces apoE gene expression,[71,72] and studies comparing wild-type versus apoE-knockout mice demonstrated that estradiol increases synaptic sprouting by increased production or uptake of apoE.[73] These findings suggest an apoE-dependent mechanism of estradiol-enhanced synaptic sprouting. Therefore, estrogen deficiency may potentiate the risk of AD associated with the apoE4 genotype. Taken together, we suggest that the hypofunction seen in the cholinergic system in AD may benefit from the combined use of anticholinesterases to increase the levels of available acetylcholine, GAL antagonists to block the inhibitory influence on the rate of cholinergic firing, and estrogenic drugs to preserve/enhance the integrity of the remaining cholinergic neurons.

REFERENCES

1. CRAWLEY, J.N. 1996. Galanin-acetylcholine interactions: Relevance to memory and Alzheimer's disease. Life Sci. **58**: 2185–2199.
2. MESULAM, M.M., E.J. MUFSON, A.I. LEVEY & B.H. WAINER. 1983. Cholinergic innervation of cortex by the basal forebrain: Cytochemistry and cortical connections of the septal area, diagonal band nuclei, nucleus basalis (substantia innominata) and hypothalamus in the rhesus monkey. J. Comp. Neurol. **214**: 170–197.
3. BARTUS, R.T., R.L.D. DEAN, B. BEER & A.S. LIPPA. 1982. The cholinergic hypothesis of geriatric memory dysfunction. Science **217**: 408–414.
4. WILCOCK, G.K., M.M. ESIRI, D.M. BOWEN & C.C. SMITH. 1982. Alzheimer's disease. Correlation of cortical choline acetyltransferase activity with the severity of dementia and histological abnormalities. J. Neurol. Sci. **57**: 407–417.
5. CHAN-PALAY, V. 1988. Galanin hyperinnervates surviving neurons of the human basal nucleus of Meynert in dementias of Alzheimer's and Parkinson's disease: A hypothesis for the role of galanin in accentuating cholinergic dysfunction in dementia. J. Comp. Neurol. **273**: 543–557.
6. MUFSON, E.J., E. COCHRAN, W. BENZING & J.H. KORDOWER. 1993. Galaninergic innervation of the cholinergic vertical limb of the diagonal band (Ch2) and bed nucleus of the stria terminalis in aging, Alzheimer's disease and Down's syndrome. Dementia **4**: 237–250.
7. FISONE, G., C.F. WU, S. CONSOLO, O. NORDSTROM, N. BRYNNE, T. BARTFAI, T. MELANDER & T. HÖKFELT. 1987. Galanin inhibits acetylcholine release in the ventral hippocampus of the rat: Histochemical, autoradiographic, in vivo, and in vitro studies. Proc. Natl. Acad. Sci. USA **84**: 7339–7343.
8. TATEMOTO, K., A. RÖKAEUS, H. JÖRNWALL, T.J. MCDONALD & V. MUTT. 1983. Galanin, a novel biologically active peptide from porcine intestine. FEBS Lett. **164**: 124–128.
9. EVANS, H.F. & J. SHINE. 1991. Human galanin: Molecular cloning reveals a unique structure. Endocrinology **129**: 1682–1684.
10. KAPLAN, L.M., S.C. HOOI, D.R. ABRACZINSKAS, R.M. STRAUSS, M.B. DAVIDSON, D.W. HSU & J.I. KOENIG. 1991 Neuroendocrine regulation of galanin gene expression. *In* Galanin: A Multifunctional Peptide in the Neuro-Endocrine System. T. Hökfelt *et al.*, Eds. :43–65, MacMillan. New York.
11. KAPLAN, L.M., E.R. SPINDEL, K.J. ISSELBACHER & W.W. CHIN. 1988. Tissue-specific expression of rat galanin gene. Proc. Natl. Acad. Sci. USA **85**: 1065–1069.
12. RÖKAEUS, Å. & J.A. WASCHEK. 1994. Primary sequence and functional analysis of the bovine galanin gene promoter in human neuroblastoma cells. DNA Cell Biol. **13**: 845–855.
13. VRONTAKIS, M.E., L.M. PEDEN, M.L. DUCKWORTH & H.G. FRIESEN. 1987. Isolation and characterization of a complementary DNA (galanin) clone from estrogen-induced pituitary tumor messenger RNA. J. Biol. Chem. **262**: 16755–16758.
14. CORNESS, J.D., J.P. BURBACH & T. HOKFELT. 1997. The rat galanin-gene promoter: Response to members of the nuclear hormone receptor family, phorbol ester and forskolin. Brain Res. Molec. Brain Res. **47**: 11–23.

15. HOWARD, G., L.H. PENG & J.F. HYDE. 1997. An estrogen receptor binding site within the human galanin gene. Endocrinology **138:** 4649–4656.
16. VRONTAKIS, M., I. SCHROEDTER, V. LEITE & H.G. FRIESEN. 1993. Estrogen regulation and localization of galanin gene expression in the rat uterus. Biol. Reprod. **49:** 1245–1250.
17. BERSANI, M., A.H. JOHNSEN, P. HØJRUP, B.E. DUNNING, J.J. ANDRESEN & J.J. HOLST. 1991. Human galanin: Primary structure and identification of two molecular forms. FEBS Lett. **283:** 189–194.
18. BARTFAI, T., K. BEDECS, T. LAND, Ü. LANGEL, R. BERTORELLI, P. GIROTTI, S. CONSOLO, X. XU, Z. WIESENFELD-HOLLAND, S. NILSSON, V.A. PIERIBONE & T. HÖKFELT. 1991. M-15: High-affinity chimeric peptide that blocks the neuronal actions of galanin in the hippocampus, locus coeruleus and spinal cord. Proc. Natl. Acad. Sci. USA **88:** 10961–10965.
19. DUTAR, P., Y. LAMOUR & R.A. NICOLL. 1989. Galanin blocks the slow cholinergic EPSP in CA1 pyramidal neurons from ventral hippocampus. Eur. J. Pharmacol. **164:** 355–360.
20. DE LOOF, H., L. NILSSON & R. RIGLER. 1992. Molecular dynamics simulation of galanin in aqueous solution and nonaqueous solution. J. Am. Chem. Soc. **114:** 4028–4035.
21. KULINSKI, T., A.B. WENNERBERG, R. RIGLER, S.W. PROVENCHER, M. POOGA, U. LANGEL & T. BARTFAI. 1997. Conformational analysis of galanin using end to end distance distribution observed by Forster resonance energy transfer. Eur. Biophys. J. **26:** 145–154.
22. FISONE, G., M. BERTHOLD, K. BEDECS, A. UNDEN, T. BARTFAI, R. BERTORELLI, S. CONSOLO, J. CRAWLEY, B. MARTIN & S. NILSSON. 1989. N-terminal galanin-(1-16) fragment is an agonist at the hippocampal galanin receptor. Proc. Natl. Acad. Sci. USA **86:** 9588–9591.
23. BEDECS, K., Ü. LANGEL & T. BARTFAI. 1995. Metabolism of galanin and galanin (1-16) in isolated cerebrospinal fluid and spinal cord membranes. Neuropeptides **29:** 137–143.
24. LAND, T., Ü. LANGEL & T. BARTFAI. 1991. Hypothalamic degradation of galanin(1-29) and galanin(1-16): Identification and characterization of the peptidolytic products. Brain Res. **558:** 245–250.
25. WHITEHOUSE, P.J., D.L. PRICE, R.G. STRUBLE, A.W. CLARK, J.T. COYLE & M.R. DeLONG. 1982. Alzheimer's Disease and senile dementia: loss of neurons in the basal forebrain. Science **215:** 1237–1239.
26. MELANDER, T., W.A. STAINES & A. RÖKAEUS. 1986. Galanin-like immunoreactivity in hippocampal afferents in the rat, with special reference to cholinergic and noradrenergic inputs. Neuroscience **19:** 223–240.
27. KORDOWER, J.H. & E.J. MUFSON. 1990. Galanin-like immunoreactivity within the primate basal forebrain: differential staining patterns between humans and monkeys. J. Comp. Neurol. **294:** 281–292.
28. BENZING, W.C., D.R. BRADY, E.J. MUFSON & D.M. ARMSTRONG. 1993. Evidence that transmitter-containing dystrophic neurites precede those containing paired helical filaments within senile plaques in the entorhinal cortex of nondemented elderly and Alzheimer's disease patients. Brain Res. **619:** 55–68.
29. MELANDER, T., W.A. STAINES, T. HÖKFELT, A. RÖKAEUS, F. ECKENSTEIN, P.M. SALVATERRA & B.H. WAINER. 1985. Galanin-like immunoreactivity in cholinergic neurons of the septum-basal forebrain complex projecting to the hippocampus of the rat. Brain Res. **360:** 130–138.
30. MILLER, M.A., P.E. KOLB, B. PLANAS & M.A. RASKIND. 1998. Few cholinergic neurons in the rat basal forebrain coexpress galanin messenger RNA. J. Comp. Neurol. **391:** 248–258.
31. KORDOWER, J.H., H.K. LE & E.J. MUFSON. 1992. Galanin immunoreactivity in the primate central nervous system. J. Comp. Neurol. **319:** 479–500.
32. WALKER, L.C., N.E. RANCE, D.L. PRICE & W.S. YOUNG. 1991. Galanin mRNA in the nucleus basalis of Meynert complex of baboons and humans. J. Comp. Neurol. **303:** 113–120.
33. BOWSER, R., J.H. KORDOWER & E.J. MUFSON. 1997. A confocal microscopic analysis of galaninergic hyperinnervation of cholinergic basal forebrain neurons in Alzheimer's disease. Brain Pathol. **7:** 723–730.
34. DEECHER, D.C., O.O. ODUSAN & E.J. MUFSON. 1995. Galanin receptors in human basal forebrain differ from receptors in the hypothalamus: Characterization using [^{125}I]galanin (porcine) and [^{125}I]galantide. J. Pharmacol. Exp. Therap. **275:** 720–727.
35. DEECHER, D.C., D.C. MASH, J.K. STALEY & E.J. MUFSON. 1998. Characterization and localization of galanin receptors in human entorhinal cortex. Regul. Pept. **73:** 149–159.

36. KÖHLER, C., A. PERSSON, T. MELANDER, E. THEODORSSON, G. SEDVALL & T. HÖKFELT. 1989. Distribution of galanin-binding sites in the monkey and human telencephalon: Preliminary observations. Exp. Brain Res. **75:** 375–80.
37. RODRIGUEZ-PUERTAS, R., S. NILSSON, J. PASCUAL, A. PAZOS & T. HÖKFELT. 1997. ^{125}I-galanin binding sites in Alzheimer's disease: Increases in hippocampal subfields and a decrease in the caudate nucleus. J. Neurochem. **68:** 1106–1113.
38. DEECHER, D.C. & F.J. LOPEZ. 1996. Porcine and rat galanin label the galanin receptor with different pharmacological properties in rat brain and RINm5F cells. Society Neuroscience, Washington, DC. #694.6.
39. CHAN-PALAY, V. 1988. Neurons with galanin innervate cholinergic cells in the human basal forebrain and galanin and acetylcholine coexist. Brain Res. Bull. 21: 465–472.
40. CRAWLEY, J.N. 1993. Functional interactions of galanin and acetylcholine: Relevance to memory and Alzheimer's disease. Behav. Brain Res. **57:** 133–141.
41. CHAN-PALAY, V., B. JENTSCH, W. LANG, M. HOCHLI & E. ASAN. 1990. Distribution of neuropeptide Y, C-terminal flanking peptide of NPY and galanin and coexistence with catecholamine in the locus coeruleus of normal human Alzheimer's dementia and Parkinson disease brains. Dementia **1:** 18–31.
42. KÖHLER, C. AND V. CHAN-PALAY. 1990. Galanin receptors in the post-mortem human brain. Regional distribution of ^{125}I-galanin binding sites using the method of *in vitro* receptor autoradiography. Neurosci. Lett. **120:** 179–182.
43. HABERT-ORTOLI, E., B. AMIRANOFF, I. LOQUET, M. LABURTHE & J.-F. MAYAUX. 1994. Molecular cloning of a functional human galanin receptor. Proc. Natl. Acad. Sci. USA **91:** 9780–9783.
44. WATSON, S. & S. ARKINSTALL. 1994 The G-protein linked receptor factsbook. :427. Academic Press. San Diego, CA.
45. LORIMER, D.D., K. MATKOWSKJ & R.V. BENYA. 1997. Cloning, chromosomal location, and transcriptional regulation of the human galanin-1 receptor gene (Galn1r). Biochem. Biophys. Res. Commun. **241:** 558–564.
46. BURGEVIN, M.C., I.LOQUET, D. QUATERONET & E. HABERT-ORTOLI. 1995. Cloning, pharmacological characterization, and anatomical distribution of a rat cDNA encoding for a galanin receptor. J. Molec. Neurosci. **6:** 33–41.
47. PARKER, E.M., D.G. IZZARELLI, H.P. NOWAK, C.D. MAHLE, L.G. IBEN, J.C. WANG & M.E. GOLDSTEIN. 1995. Cloning and characterization of the rat GALR1 galanin receptor from Rin14B insulinoma cells. Molec. Brain Res. **34:** 179–189.
48. BLOOMQUIST, B.T., M.R. BEAUCHAMP, L. ZHELNIN, S.E. BROWN, A.R. GOREWILLSE, P. GREGOR & L.J. CORNFIELD. 1998. Cloning and expression of the human galanin receptor Galr2. Biochem. Biophys. Res. Commun. **243:** 474–479.
49. SMITH, K.E., C. FORRAY, M.W. WALKER, K.A. JONES, J.A. TAMM, J. BARD, T.A. BRANCHEK, D.L. LINEMEYER & C. GERALD. 1997. Expression cloning of a rat hypothalamic galanin receptor coupled to phosphoinositide turnover. J. Biol. Chem. **272:** 24612–24616.
50. WANG, S., T. HASHEMI, C.G. HE, C. STRADER & M. BAYNE. 1997. Molecular cloning and pharmacological characterization of a new galanin receptor subtype. Molec. Pharmacol. **52:** 337–343.
51. WANG, S.K., C.G. HE, T. HASHEMI & M. BAYNE. 1997. Cloning and expressional characterization of a novel galanin receptor: Identification of different pharmacophores within galanin for the three galanin receptor subtypes. J. Biol. Chem. **272:** 31949–31952.
52. MILLER, M.A., P.E. KOLB & M.A. RASKIND. 1997. Galr1 galanin receptor Mrna is co-expressed by galanin neurons but not cholinergic neurons in the rat basal forebrain. Molec. Brain Res. **52:** 121–129.
53. DAVIS, K.L., L.J.THAL, E.R. GAMZU, C.S. DAVIS, R.F. WOOLSON, S.I. GRACON, D.A. DRACHMAN, L.S. SCHNEIDER, P.J. WHITEHOUSE, T.M. HOOVER *et al.* 1992. A double-blind, placebo-controlled multicenter study of tacrine for Alzheimer's disease. The Tacrine Collaborative Study Group [see comments]. N. Engl. J. Med. **327:** 1253–1259.
54. FARLOW, M., S.I. GRACON, L.A. HERSHEY, K.W. LEWIS, C.H. SADOWSKY & J. DOLAN-URENO. 1992. A controlled trial of tacrine in Alzheimer's disease. The Tacrine Study Group [see comments]. JAMA **268:** 2523–2529.
55. PALAZZI, E., G. FISONE, T. HOKFELT, T. BARTFAI & S. CONSOLO. 1988. Galanin inhibits the muscarinic stimulation of phosphoinositide turnover in rat ventral hippocampus. Eur. J. Pharmacol. **148:** 479–80.

56. MASTROPAOLO, J., N.S. NADI, N.L. OSTROWSKI & J.N. CRAWLEY. 1988. Galanin antagonizes ace-tylcholine on a memory task in basal forebrain-lesioned rats. Proc. Natl. Acad. Sci. USA **85:** 9841–9845.

57. SUNDSTRÖM, E., T. ARCHER, T. MELANDER & T. HOKFELT. 1988. Galanin impairs acquisition but not retrieval of spatial memory in rats studied in the Morris swim maze. Neurosci. Lett. **88:** 331–335.

58. HÖKFELT, T., D. MILLHORN, K. SEROOGY, Y. TSURUO, S. CECCATELLI, B. LINDH, B. MEISTER, T. MELANDER, M. SCHALLING & T. BARTFAI. 1987. Coexistence of peptides with classical neu-rotransmitters. Experientia **43:** 768–780.

59. DUNNING, B.E., B. AHREN, R.C. VEITH, G. BOTTCHER, F. SUNDLER & G.J. TABORSKY, JR. 1986. Galanin: A novel pancreatic neuropeptide. Am. J. Physiol. E127–E133.

60. GILBEY, S.G., J. STEPHENSON, D.J. O'HALLORAN, J.M. BURRIN & S.R. BLOOM. 1989. High dose porcine galanin infusion and effect on intravenous glucose tolerance in humans. Diabetes **38:** 114–116.

61. GREGERSON, S., S. LINDSKOG, T. LAND, Ü. LANGEL, T. BARTFAI & B. AHRÉN. 1993. Blockade of galanin-induced inhibition of insulin secretion from isolated mouse islets by the non-methion-ine containing antagonist M35. Eur. J. Pharmacol. **232:** 35–39.

62. GU, Z.F., W.J. ROSSOWSKI, D.H. COY, T.K. PRADHAN & R.T. JENSEN. 1993. Chimeric galanin ana-logs that function as antagonists in the CNS are full antagonists in gastrointestinal smooth muscle. J. Pharmacol. Exp. Ther. **266:** 912–918.

63. HOLST, J.J., M. BERSANI, A. HVIDBERG, U. KNIGGE, E. CHRISTIANSEN, S. MADSBAD, H. HARLING & H. KOFOD. 1993. On the effects of human galanin in man. Diabetologia **36:** 653–657.

64. MCDONALD, T.J., E. TU, S. BRENNER, P. ZABEL, M. BEHME, C. PANCHAL, I. HRAMIAK, W.B. BARNETT, D. MILLER & J. DUPRE. 1994. Canine, human, rat plasma insulin responses to galanin administration: Species response differences. Am. J. Physiol. **266:** E612–E617.

65. TAKAHASHI, T., M.G. BELVISI & P.J. BARNES. 1994. Modulation of neurotransmission in guinea-pig airways by galanin and the effect of a new antagonist galantide. Neuropeptides **26:** 245–251.

66. SCHNEIDER, L.S., M.R. FARLOW, V.W. HENDERSON & J.M. POGODA. 1996. Effects of estrogen replacement therapy on response to tacrine in patients with Alzheimer's disease. Neurology **46:** 1580–1584.

67. SOHRABJI, F. & R.C. MIRANDA. 1997. Hormone replacement: Therapeutic strategies in the treat-ment of Alzheimer's disease and ageing-related cognitive disorders [Review]. Expert Opin. Therapeutic Patents **7:** 611–629.

68. ALLEN, S.J., S.H. MACGOWAN, S. TYLER, G.K. WILCOCK, A.G.S. ROBERTSON, P.H. HOLDEN, S.K.F. SMITH & D. DAWBARN. 1997. Reduced cholinergic function in normal and Alzheimer's disease brain is associated with apolipoprotein E4 genotype. Neurosci. Lett. **239:** 33–36.

69. POIRIER, J., M.C. DELISLE, R. QUIRION, I. AUBERT, M. FARLOW, D. LAHIRI, S. HUI, P. BERTRAND, J. NALBANTOGLU, B.M. GILFIX et al. 1995. Apolipoprotein E4 allele as a predictor of cholin-ergic deficits and treatment outcome in Alzheimer disease. Proc. Natl. Acad. Sci. USA **92:** 12260–12264.

70. SOININEN, H., O. KOSUNEN, S. HELISALMI, A. MANNERMAA, L. PALJARVI, S. TALASNIEMI, M. RYYNANEN & P. RIEKKINEN, SR. 1995. A severe loss of choline acetyltransferase in the fron-tal cortex of Alzheimer patients carrying apolipoprotein epsilon 4 allele. Neurosci. Lett. **187:** 79–82.

71. SRIVASTAVA, R.A.K., N. SRIVASTAVA, M. AVERNA, R.C. LIN, K.S. KORACH, D.B. LUBAHN & G. SCHONFELD. 1997. Estrogen up-regulates apolipoprotein E (Apoe) gene expression by increasing ApoE mRNA in the translating pool via the estrogen receptor alpha-mediated path-way. J. Biol. Chem. **272:** 33360–33366.

72. STONE, D.J., I. ROZOVSKY, T.E. MORGAN, C.P. ANDERSON, H. HAJIAN & C.E. FINCH. 1997. Astro-cytes and microglia respond to estrogen with increased apoE mRNA in vivo and in vitro. Exp. Neurol. **143:** 313–318.

73. STONE, D.J., I. ROZOVSKY, T.E. MORGAN, C.P. ANDERSON & C.E. FINCH. 1998. Increased synaptic sprouting in response to estrogen via an apolipoprotein E-dependent mechanism: Implications for Alzheimer's disease. J. Neurosci. **18:** 3180–3185.

Galanin Inhibits Performance on Rodent Memory Tasks

MICHAEL P. McDONALD, THERESA C. GLEASON, JOHN K. ROBINSON,[a] AND JACQUELINE N. CRAWLEY[b]

Section on Behavioral Neuropharmacology, Experimental Therapeutics Branch, National Institute of Mental Health, Bethesda, Maryland 20892-1375, USA

ABSTRACT: Central administration of galanin produces performance deficits on a variety of rodent learning and memory tasks. Galanin impairs acquisition and/or retention of the Morris water task, delayed nonmatching to position, T-maze delayed alternation, starburst radial maze, and passive avoidance in normal rats. A primary site of action is the ventral hippocampus, with an additional modulatory site in the medial septum-diagonal band. The behavioral actions of galanin at rat septohippocampal sites mediating cognitive processes are consistent with previous reports of inhibitory actions of galanin on acetylcholine release and cholinergically activated transduction at the M_1 muscarinic receptor in rat hippocampus. The peptidergic galanin receptor antagonist M40 blocks the inhibitory actions of galanin on memory tasks. Treatment combinations of M40 with an M_1 agonist, TZTP, improves performance on delayed nonmatching to position, in rats with [192]IgG-saporin-induced cholinergic lesions of basal forebrain neurons. Nonpeptide, bioavailable, subtype-selective galanin receptor antagonists may provide tools to test the hypothesis that antagonism of endogenous galanin, which is overexpressed in the basal forebrain in Alzheimer's patients, can contribute to the alleviation of the cognitive deficits associated with Alzheimer's disease.

Galanin is a neuropeptide expressed in brain regions that are thought to mediate learning and memory. Galanin-like immunoreactivity, galanin mRNA, and ^{125}I-galanin binding sites are present in moderate to high levels in the rat and human cerebral cortex, hippocampus, and basal forebrain.[1–12]

Postmortem studies of Alzheimer's disease reveal a striking overexpression of galanin in the basal forebrain.[5, 13–15] Galanin-immunoreactive fibers and terminals are denser and appear to hyperinnervate the remaining cholinergic cell bodies of the nucleus basalis of Meynert, as compared to age-matched controls[5,14,15] (see also Mufson *et al.*, this volume). Galanin overexpression in the region of the basal forebrain neurons that degenerate early in the progression of Alzheimer's disease suggests that galanin may contribute to the memory deficits that characterize Alzheimer's disease.[16–20] To test this hypothesis, our laboratory embarked on a comprehensive investigation of the role of galanin in learning and memory tasks in the normal rat, and in rodent models of Alzheimer's disease.[17–27]

[a]Current address: Dr. John K. Robinson, Biopsychology Area, Department of Psychology, State University of New York at Stony Brook, Stony Brook, NY 11794-2500, USA.

[b]Address for correspondence: Dr. Jacqueline Crawley, Chief, Section on Behavioral Neuropharmacology, Experimental Therapeutics Branch, National Institute of Mental Health, Building 10 Room 4D11, 9000 Rockville Pike, Bethesda, MD 20892-1375. Phone, 301-496-7855; fax, 301-480-1164; e-mail, jncrawle@codon.nih.gov

INHIBITORY ACTIONS OF EXOGENOUSLY ADMINISTERED GALANIN ON LEARNING AND MEMORY TASKS IN RATS

Central administration of galanin results in performance deficits on a wide variety of learning and memory tasks in rodents. Disruptive actions of galanin have been reported on delayed nonmatching to position in rats;[21–25] T-maze delayed alternation in rats;[26,27] starburst radial maze in rats;[28] passive avoidance in mice;[29] and the Morris water task in rats.[30–34] Summarized in TABLE 1, these studies report the inhibitory role of galanin in several distinct aspects of learning or memory and/or in specific anatomical brain sites.

Delayed nonmatching to position is a lever-press operant task that requires a spatial conditional discrimination between right and left levers (position) to obtain a water reward. Water is used as the reinforcer, in water-restricted rats, to avoid the confounding issues of galanin-induced feeding.[35] The rat must choose the lever that is opposite (nonmatching) to the lever that was pressed at the beginning of the trial (sample). The mnemonic component of the task comprises delays ranging from 5–20 seconds interposed between the sample and the choice responses. The primary dependent measure is percent correct on the choice responses. Secondary measures relevant to sensory and motor abilities, attention, and arousal can be analyzed from the DNMTP automated software, to control for nonspecific effects of drugs and lesions.

TABLE 1. Inhibitory Actions of Exogenously Administered Galanin on Learning and Memory Task in Rodents

Task and Route	Effect	Reference
Delayed non-matching to position		
Intraventricular	Delay-independent impairment	Robinson & Crawley,[21] 1993 McDonald & Crawley,[24] 1996
Intrahippocampal	Delay-dependent impairment	Robinson & Crawley,[23] 1994 McDonald & Crawley,[24] 1996
Intraseptal	Potentiates scopolamine-induced impairment	Robinson & Crawley,[22] 1993
T-maze delayed alternation		
Intraventricular	Inhibits acetylcholine-induced improvement in lesioned rats	Mastropaolo et al.,[26] 1988
Intraseptal	Delay-dependent impairment	Givens et al.,[27] 1992
Starburst radial maze		
Intraventricular	Impaired retention	Malin et al.,[28] 1992
Passive avoidance		
Intraventricular	Impaired acquisition	Ukai et al.,[29] 1995
Morris water task		
Intraventricular	Impaired acquisition	Sundstrom et al.,[30] 1988
Intrahippocampal	Impaired acquisition	Ögren et al.,[32] 1996 Schött et al.,[33] 1998
Intraventricular	Impaired acquisition	Gleason & Crawley,[34] 1998

FIGURE 1 shows the impairing actions of intraventricularly administered galanin on DNMTP in normal rats. Doses of galanin, 500 ng – 5 µg (0.16–1.6 nmol), or saline vehicle were administered immediately before the test session. Galanin produced a significant delay-independent impairment in choice accuracy.[22,24] The dose-dependent, delay-inde-

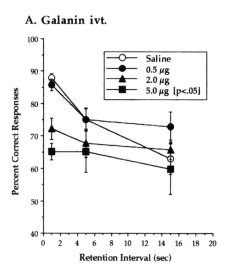

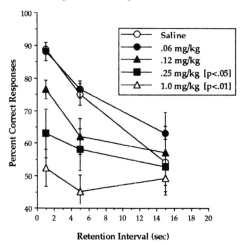

FIGURE 1. Galanin produced a dose-dependent, delay-independent impairment on delayed non-matching to position when administered intraventricularly (ivt) to rats. The impairment profile was analogous to the effects of scopolamine, a muscarinic receptor antagonist, when given intraperitoneally (ip) on this working memory task. Adapted from Robinson and Crawley.[21,22]

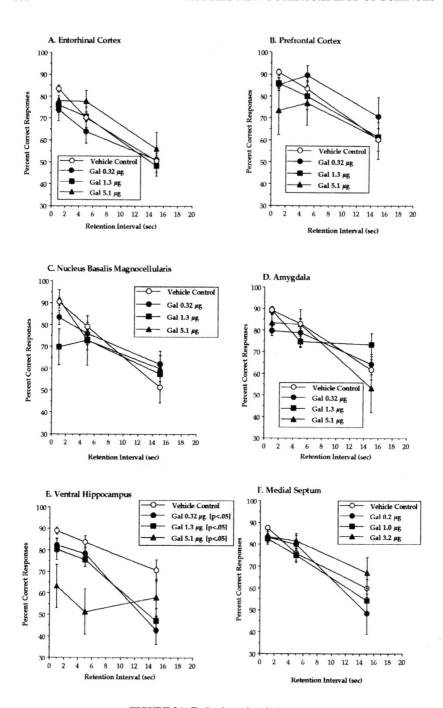

FIGURE 2A–F. *See legend on facing page.*

pendent deficits on DNMTP after galanin treatment are analogous to those produced by the muscarinic receptor antagonist scopolamine, at intraperitoneal doses of 0.25, 0.5, and 1.0 mg/kg.[22]

FIGURE 2 illustrates an anatomical analysis of microinjection sites for galanin administration on DNMTP choice accuracy in normal rats. Doses of 0.1–1.6 nmol had no effect when microinjected into the entorhinal cortex, prefrontal cortex, nucleus basalis magnocellularis, or amygdala.[23] When injected bilaterally into the ventral hippocampus, galanin doses of 0.1 and 0.4 nmol produced a significant delay-dependent impairment in choice accuracy, whereas a larger dose, 1.6 nmol, produced a significant delay-independent impairment in choice accuracy.[23] These results indicate that the ventral hippocampus is a major site for the inhibitory actions of galanin on memory tasks. Furthermore, galanin may produce selective deficits in working memory at the ventral hippocampal site, as opposed to the mnemonic and/or procedural deficits at larger galanin doses and with the intraventricular route of administration. The concentration of ^{125}I-galanin binding sites and the inhibitory effects of galanin on acetylcholine release are greater in the ventral hippocampus than in the dorsal hippocampus.[36] Taken together with our behavioral findings, these three lines of evidence are consistent with the interpretation that galanin has an anatomically specific action in the rat ventral hippocampus.

T-maze delayed alternation is a spatial working memory task. Rats obtain a water reward at one of the two horizontal arms of a T-shaped maze on each trial. The opposite arm is baited (alternation) on successive trials, with a delay of 60 seconds between trials. FIGURE 3 illustrates the dose-dependent reduction in choice accuracy in normal rats treated with galanin either intraventricularly (1 µg, 0.3 nmol[26]) or into the medial septum/diagonal band region (0.2 µg, 0.06 nmol[27]).

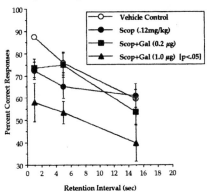

FIGURE 2. Site-specific microinjections of galanin on delayed nonmatching to position in rats. Only the ventral hippocampus site (panel **E**) showed significant galanin-induced impairments on this task. In the ventral hippocampus, smaller doses of galanin (0.32 and 1.3 µg) produced a delay-dependent impairment. A larger dose, 5.1 µg, produced a delay-independent impairment. Although galanin did not produce an impairment in this task when given alone into the medial septum/diagonal band region (panel **F**), galanin produced a synergistic impairment when given in combination with a subthreshold dose of scopolamine, 0.12 mg/kg ip (panel **G**). Adapted from Robinson and Crawley.[21]

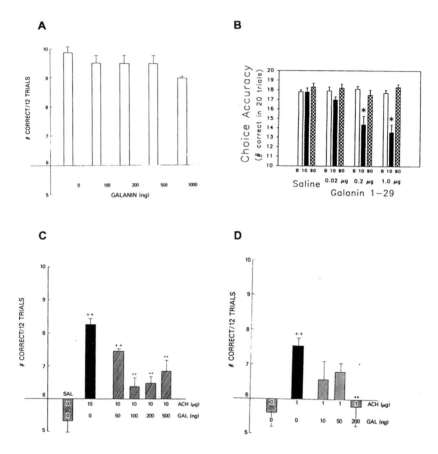

FIGURE 3. (**A**) Galanin produced a dose-dependent impairment in T-maze delayed alternation, significant at the largest dose, 1 µg, administered intraventricularly to control (sham) rats. (**B**) Galanin produced a dose-dependent impairment in T-maze delayed alternation at 10 minutes (10), but not at 90 minutes (90), after administration into the medial septum/diagonal band, as compared to baseline before administration (**B**) and to saline-treated controls. (**C**) Intraventricularly administered galanin attenuated the ability of acetylcholine to improve performance on T-maze delayed alternation in rats with ibotenic acid lesions of the basal forebrain. (**D**) Intrahippocampally administered galanin attenuated the ability of acetylcholine to improve performance on T-maze delayed alternation in rats with ibotenic acid lesions of the basal forebrain. Adapted from Mastropaolo *et al.*[26] and Givens *et al.*[27]

The Morris water maze is an escape task that requires integration of spatial navigation and extramaze cues. Testing occurs in a large, circular pool of water, in which the animals must learn to locate a hidden platform that is submerged below the level of the water. Using visual spatial cues surrounding the pool, rats learn the location of the hidden platform over a series of training trials. In normal animals, latency to reach the platform decreases as the location of the platform is learned over the series of training trials. To assess whether a spatial strategy is used by the animals, a probe trial is given following training. The platform is removed, and the swim path is recorded for 60 seconds. The proportion of swimming activity in the quadrant of the pool that previously contained the platform is the measure of acquisition of the task. Automated videotracking software traces the swim pathway and records the latency to reach the platform as well as time spent in each quadrant of the pool.

FIGURE 4 illustrates the disruptive actions of galanin in the Morris water task in three strains of rats.[34] Sprague-Dawley and Long-Evans rats were first trained for four trials per day over 4 days in the water maze and then given a probe trial. Sprague-Dawley rats treated with galanin, 3 nmol, administered intraventricularly, failed to show a selective search during the probe trial. In contrast, Long-Evans rats did not show any significant effect of galanin treatment in this task. Wistar rats were trained for eight trials per day for 5 days. Rats treated with 1, 3, or 6 nmol galanin, administered intraventricularly, failed to show selective search during the probe trial. The inhibitory actions of galanin on acquisition of the Morris task in our experiments are consistent with previous reports[30,32] and extend the previous findings by indicating genetic differences among strains of rats.

GALANIN-ACETYLCHOLINE INTERACTIONS

Evoked release of acetylcholine in the rat ventral hippocampus is inhibited by galanin.[36–38] *In vitro* assays in rat ventral hippocampal slices report galanin-induced antagonism of the increase in acetylcholine after treatment with concentrations of potassium or electrical stimulation, which induce large increases in acetylcholine release over baseline.[36] *In vivo* microdialysis of the ventral hippocampus in normal rats revealed no effects of galanin alone on the levels of acetylcholine in the extracellular microdialysate, but strong inhibition of scopolamine-induced release of acetylcholine.[36–38] FIGURE 5 illustrates the ability of galanin microinjected intraventricularly at a dose of 1.6 nmol to attenuate the rise in acetylcholine in the ventral hippocampus of awake, behaving rats treated with scopolamine (0.3 mg/kg ip[38]). These findings indicate a presynaptic site of action for galanin-acetylcholine interactions, suggesting that galanin receptors on the terminals of the cholinergic basal forebrain neuron projections act as inhibitory modulators of acetylcholine release.[16]

Because galanin overexpression in Alzheimer's disease appears to surround the cell bodies of the cholinergic basal forebrain, we tested the hypothesis that galanin acts presynaptically on the cell bodies of basal forebrain cholinergic neurons to regulate acetylcholine release. *In vivo* microdialysis in the paradigm just described showed that galanin microinjected into the medial septum/diagonal band region at doses of 0.025–1.6 nmol attenuated scopolamine-induced acetylcholine release in the ventral hippocampus.[38] As shown in FIGURE 5, the potency of galanin at the cell body site was considerably higher than that at the intraventricular microinjection site, suggesting that galanin has specific inhibitory actions at cholinergic cell bodies.

Furthermore, the actions of galanin on cholinergic cell bodies of the basal forebrain were analyzed on T-maze delayed alternation. As shown in FIGURE 3, when microinjected into the medial septum/diagonal band region, the dose of 0.2 μg (0.06 nmol) galanin significantly impaired choice accuracy on T-maze delayed alternation.[27]

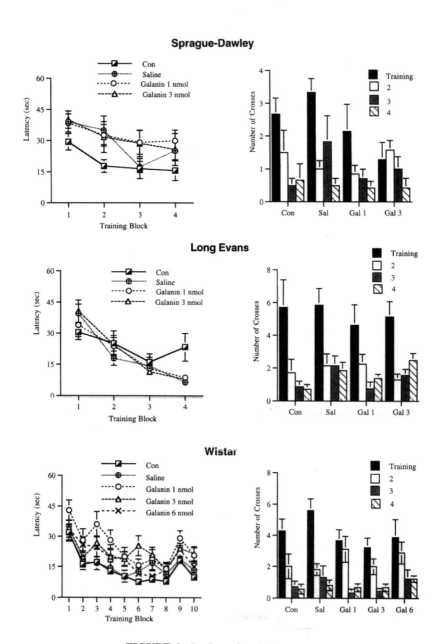

FIGURE 4. *See legend on facing page.*

Rodent paradigms that model the cholinergic loss in Alzheimer's disease typically use cholinergic receptor antagonist drug treatments or lesions of cholinergic basal forebrain neurons. We investigated the actions of galanin in rats with experimentally induced reductions in cholinergic transmission, using three techniques: drug treatment with the muscarinic antagonist scopolamine, ibotenic acid excitotoxin lesions, and [192]IgG saporin immunotoxin lesions. A subthreshold dose of scopolamine (0.12 mg/kg ip) that had no significant effect on DNMTP was combined with doses of galanin (1.0 μg = 0.3 nmol) that had no significant effect on DNMTP when administered alone into the medial septum/diagonal band region.[21] As shown in FIGURE 2, panel G, the combination of scopolamine + galanin produced a large, delay-independent, impairment on DNMTP. This finding demonstrates a synergistic interaction between galanin and a cholinergic antagonist on impairing cognitive processes. The DNMTP results are consistent with the T-maze delayed alternation results shown in FIGURE 3, in which galanin microinjected into the medial septum/diagonal band impaired choice accuracy. These behavioral data are consistent with the microdialysis results shown in FIGURE 5, in which galanin microinjected into the medial septum/diagonal band antagonized evoked acetylcholine release. Taken together, these experiments support an interpretation that galanin overexpression in the region of the cell bodies of the nucleus basalis of Meynert in Alzheimer's disease may contribute to reduced cholinergic transmission.

Lesion studies provide a tool to investigate the behavioral actions of galanin in rats with loss of cholinergic neurons analogous to the characteristic loss of cholinergic neurons of the nucleus basalis of Meynert, medial septum, and diagonal band in Alzheimer's disease.[39,40] Excitotoxin lesions are the method of choice for destroying cell bodies in anatomically selective brain regions. Microinjection of ibotenic acid into the nucleus basalis magnocellularis/medial septum/diagonal band produced an approximately 30% reduction in the cholinergic synthetic enzyme choline acetyltransferase.[26] We found that intraventricularly administered galanin produced no further impairment on T-maze delayed alternation in ibotenic acid lesioned rats, as performance was already close to chance levels.[26] However, when acetylcholine was administered to partially reverse the lesion deficit, galanin treatment blocked the acetylcholine-induced improvement in ibotenic acid-lesioned rats. As shown in FIGURE 3, galanin attenuated the beneficial effects of acetylcholine when the combination treatment was microinjected either intraventricularly or bilaterally into the ventral hippocampus.

Cholinergic immunotoxin lesioning with [192]IgG-saporin[41] is the method of choice for selectively destroying cholinergic cell bodies in the basal forebrain. [192]IgG is an antibody raised against the p75 low affinity nerve growth factor receptor. The antibody is linked to

---

FIGURE 4. Performance on the Morris water task after treatment with galanin or saline vehicle in three strains of rat. Acquisition of this spatial navigation escape task was evaluated by latency to find the hidden platform on successive blocks of training trials (**left panels**) and selective search of the training quadrant when the platform was removed on the probe trial (**right panels**). Untreated controls (Con) and saline-treated controls (Saline) showed significantly more platform crossings in the training quadrant (Training) than in the three untrained quadrants (2,3,4) during the probe trial, reflecting normal acquisition of the Morris task. Galanin-treated Sprague-Dawley and Wistar rats failed to show significantly more platform crossings in the training quadrant (Training) during the probe trial. Galanin did not affect normal probe trial performance in Long-Evans rats at doses that impaired performance in Sprague-Dawley and Wistar rats. Adapted from Gleason and Crawley.[34]

A. Galanin (ivt) + Scopolamine (i.p.)

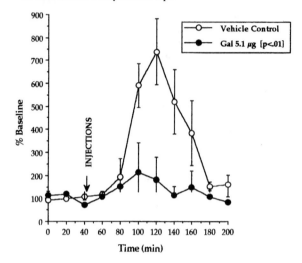

B. Galanin (Medial Septum) + Scopolamine (i.p.)

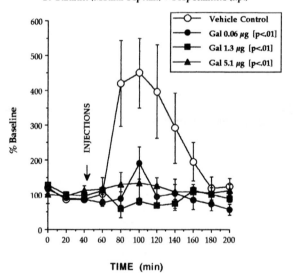

FIGURE 5. Acetylcholine release in the ventral hippocampus of awake, behaving rats as measured by *in vivo* microdialysis. (**A**) Galanin microinjected into the lateral ventricles (ivt) inhibited scopolamine-induced increases in extracellular acetylcholine levels (% baseline). (**B**) Galanin microinjected into the medial septum/diagonal band region (medial septum) inhibited scopolamine-induced increases in extracellular acetylcholine levels (% baseline). Adapted from Robinson *et al.*[38]

saporin, a ribosome-inactivating protein. Because the p75 receptor is localized almost solely on the cell bodies of cholinergic basal forebrain neurons, the antibody binds specifically to the cholinergic cell bodies of the nucleus basalis magnocellularis, medial septum, and diagonal band. The saporin toxin is internalized and kills these neurons only. All of the cholinergic cells of the rat basal forebrain are vulnerable to [192]IgG-saporin, with the exception of the cholinergic basal forebrain neurons that project to the amygdala.[25,42–46] Rats lesioned with [192]IgG-saporin have 50–80% reductions in choline acetyltransferase and show performance deficits on DNMTP[25,45] and several other learning and memory tasks.[42–44,47] As shown in FIGURE 6, immunotoxin-lesioned rats display a severe, lasting impairment in DNMTP choice accuracy. As in the ibotenic acid-lesioned rats on the T-maze task, performance was too close to chance levels to detect any further decrease in performance after galanin treatment. However, a subgroup of [192]IgG-saporin lesioned rats were identified that were unimpaired on DNMTP and had less reduction in choline acetyltransferase in the hippocampus.[25] Partially lesioned, DNMTP-unimpaired rats showed deficits in choice accuracy when treated with galanin, 1.6 nmol intraventricularly. These findings indicate that galanin can exacerbate the deleterious effects of cholinergic lesions on memory processes.

GALANIN RECEPTOR ANTAGONISTS IN MEMORY TASKS

The first galanin receptor antagonists were developed by Bartfai and coworkers[48] (see also Bartfai *et al.*, this volume). These peptidergic compounds were synthesized based on the highly conserved, biologically active NH_2-terminal amino acid sequence of galanin 1-29. Our laboratory has been fortunate to collaborate with Bartfai and coworkers on the characterization of the first generation of galanin receptor antagonists. These high affinity ligands displace ^{125}I-galanin binding and block the inhibitory actions of galanin on evoked acetylcholine release, as described previously[48] (see also Bartfai *et al.*, this volume). In behavioral assays, M40 (galanin 1-12-[Pro-Pro-Pro-Ala-Leu-Ala-Leu-Ala-NH2]) effectively blocked galanin-induced feeding behavior when administered intraventricularly or into the hypothalamus or amygdala of rats.[49–51] This compound was chosen to investigate the role of endogenous galanin in learning and memory tasks in rats.

In normal rats, M40 effectively blocked the inhibitory actions of galanin on DNMTP.[24] As shown in FIGURE 7, M40, 8.0 nmol, administered intraventricularly 5 minutes before intraventricular administration of galanin, 1.6 nmol, completely blocked the galanin-induced delay-independent impairment in choice accuracy on DNMTP. Bilateral microinjection of M40, 2.0 nmol into the ventral hippocampus 5 minutes before bilateral microinjection of galanin, 0.5 nmol, completely blocked the delay-dependent impairment in choice accuracy on DNMTP. Thus, M40 is an effective antagonist of galanin *in vivo* on this cognitive task.

As shown in Figure 8, M40 had no effect alone in sham-treated rats that performed normally on DNMTP, at doses of M40 that blocked the actions of galanin on DNMTP.[25] Furthermore, FIGURE 8 illustrates our findings that M40 had no effect alone on DNMTP in [192]IgG-saporin lesioned rats.[25] This result suggests that antagonism of endogenous galanin cannot increase cholinergic transmission sufficiently to restore DNMTP performance in cholinergically lesioned rats.

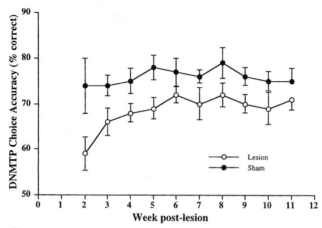

FIGURE 6. [192]IgG-saporin cholinergic immunotoxin treatment produced significant and lasting performance deficits on delayed nonmatching to position in lesioned rats than in sham control rats. Adapted from McDonald *et al.*[25]

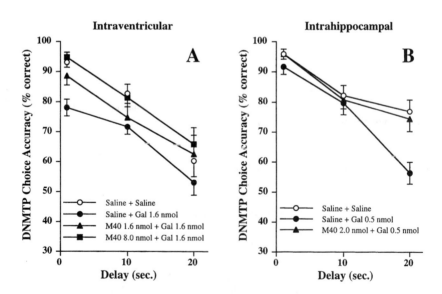

FIGURE 7. M40, a peptidergic galanin receptor ligand, antagonized the delay-independent galanin-induced impairments on delayed nonmatching to position, when both compounds were administered intraventricularly **(left panel)**. Similarly, M40 antagonized the delay-dependent galanin-induced impairments on delayed nonmatching to position when both compounds were administered into the ventral hippocampus **(right panel)**. Adapted from McDonald and Crawley.[24]

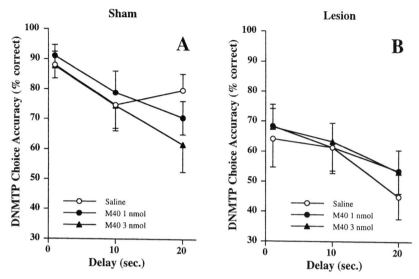

FIGURE 8. M40 had no effect alone on delayed nonmatching to position when administered intraventricularly to sham (**left panel**) or [192]IgG-saporin lesioned (**right panel**) rats. Adapted from McDonald *et al.*[46]

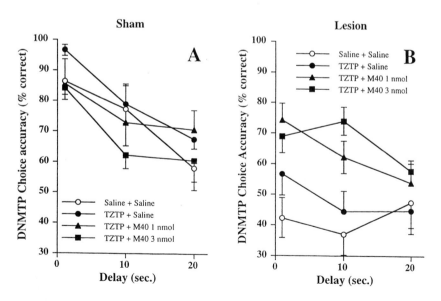

FIGURE 9. The combination of M40 administered intraventricularly, with an M_1 muscarinic agonist, TZTP, administered intraperitoneally, had no effect on delayed nonmatching to position in sham control rats (**left panel**), but significantly improved performance in [192]IgG-saporin lesioned rats (**right panel**). Adapted from McDonald *et al.*[46]

We hypothesized that partial restoration of cholinergic transmission could be facilitated by removal of the putative inhibitory actions of endogenous galanin. Endogenous galanin could exert its putative inhibitory effects at several presynaptic and postsynaptic sites of action. Our first experiments to test this hypothesis were designed to administer M40 intraventricularly in combination with low doses of cholinergic replacement drugs.[46] FIGURE 9 shows the combination of an M_1 agonist TZTP (3-[3-S-n-pentyl-1,2,5-thiadiazol-4-

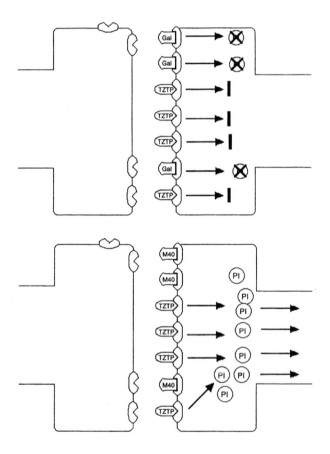

FIGURE 10. Hypothesized mechanism by which M40 improves the efficacy of TZTP on delayed nonmatching to position in cholinergically lesioned rats. Galanin is known to inhibit cholinergically stimulated phosphatidyl inositol hydrolysis, the signal transduction mechanism for postsynaptic M_1 muscarinic receptors.[37,53] As shown in the **top diagram**, endogenous galanin (Gal) may block the stimulatory actions of TZTP on phosphatidyl inositol hydrolysis (PI). As shown in the **bottom diagram**, M40 antagonism of endogenous galanin at postsynaptic galanin receptors could act to prevent the putative inhibitory actions of putative excessive galanin on TZTP-stimulated PI hydrolysis in cholinergically lesioned rats. TZTP acting at postsynaptic M_1 receptors is hypothesized to produce greater stimulation of PI hydrolysis in the presence of M40 than in the absence of M40, resulting in improvement in performance on the memory task in lesioned rats treated with the M40 + TZTP combination.

yl]-1,2,5,6-tetrahydro-1-methylpyridine[52]), 0.1 mg/kg ip, administered 45 minutes before the start of behavioral testing, and M40, 1 or 3 nmol, administered intraventricularly immediately before the start of the behavioral test session. The combination of an M_1 agonist and a galanin antagonist produced a significantly greater improvement in DNMTP choice accuracy in [192]IgG-saporin lesioned rats than did the subthreshold dose of TZTP alone, and as compared to saline vehicle. This drug combination had no significant effect in sham control rats and no significant effects on secondary procedural measures, indicating no complicating side effects of these compounds in the present treatment regimen.

FUTURE DIRECTIONS

Our findings that M40 potentiates the beneficial actions of TZTP on a rodent memory task provide the first evidence for the exciting possibility that a galanin receptor antagonist may potentiate the actions of an M_1 agonist. The clinical relevance of this finding is that a galanin receptor antagonist may be of therapeutic benefit in improving the efficacy of cholinergic drugs for the treatment of the memory loss that is a characteristic symptom of Alzheimer's disease. The hypothesized mechanism underlying this galanin-acetylcholine interaction, based on the postsynaptic inhibitory action of galanin on cholinergically stimulated phosphatidyl inositol hydrolysis,[37,53] is diagrammed in FIGURE 10. Our laboratory plans to pursue other potential sites of galanin-acetylcholine interactions in rodent memory tasks to further investigate the potential therapeutic actions of galanin receptor antagonists on improving the efficacy of other classes of cholinergic drugs.

Three galanin receptor subtype cDNAs have been cloned to date[11,12,54–59] (see also this volume). M40 does not appear to be selective for any one of these three receptor subtypes. Subtype-selective ligands for each of the galanin receptor subtypes will be necessary to determine the receptor mediating the inhibitory actions of galanin on memory tasks. Nonpeptide ligands with good brain bioavailability, long *in vivo* half-life, and receptor subtype selectivity will provide tools to fully test the hypothesis that blocking galanin overexpression in Alzheimer's disease will be of therapeutic benefit.

REFERENCES

1. MELANDER T., T. HÖKFELT & Å. RÖKAEUS. 1986. Distribution of galanin-like immunoreactivity in the rat central nervous system. J. Comp. Neurol. **248:** 475–517.
2. SKOFITSCH, G. & D.M. JACOBOWITZ. 1986. Quantitative distribution of galanin-like immunoreactivity in the rat central nervous system. Peptides **7:** 609–613.
3. SKOFITSCH, G., M.A. SILLS & D.M. JACOBOWITZ. 1986. Autoradiography of ^{125}I-galanin binding sites in the rat central nervous system. Peptides **7:** 1029–1042.
4. MELANDER T., C. KÖHLER, S. NILSSON, T. HÖKFELT, E. BRODIN, E. THEODORSSON & T. BARTFAI. 1988. Autoradiographic quantitation and anatomical mapping of ^{125}I-galanin binding sites in the rat central nervous system. J. Chem. Neuroanat. **1:** 213–233.
5. CHAN-PALAY, V. 1988. Galanin hyperinnervates surviving neurons of the human basal nucleus of Meynert in dementias of Alzheimer's and Parkinson's disease: A hypothesis for the role of galanin in accentuating cholinergic dysfunction in dementia. J. Comp. Neurol. **273:** 543–557.
6. GENTLEMAN, S.M., P. FALKAI, B. BOGERTS, M.T. HERRERO, J.M. POLAK & G.W. ROBERTS. 1989. Distribution of galanin-like immunoreactivity in the human brain. Brain Res. **505:** 311–315.
7. KÖHLER, C. & V. CHAN-PALAY. 1990. Galanin receptors in the post-mortem human brain. Regional distribution of ^{125}I-galanin binding sites using the method of in vitro receptor autoradiography. Neurosci. Lett. **120:** 179–182.

8. BENZING, W.C., J.H. KORDOWER & E.J. MUFSON. 1993. Galanin immunoreactivity within the primate basal forebrain: Evolutionary change between monkeys and apes. J. Comp. Neurol. **336:** 31–39.

9. MERCHENTHALER, I., F.J. LOPEZ & A. NEGRO-VILAR. 1993. Anatomy and physiology of central galanin-containing pathways. Prog. Neurobiol. **40:** 711–769.

10. BURGEVIN, M.C., I. LOQUET, D. QUARTERONET & E. HABERT-ORTOLI. 1995. Cloning, pharmacological characterization, and anatomical distribution of a rat cDNA encoding for a galanin receptor. J. Mol. Neurosci. **6:** 33–41.

11. GUSTAFSON, E.L., K.E. SMITH, M.M. DURKIN, C. GERALD & T.A. BRANCHEK. 1996. Distribution of a rat galanin receptor mRNA in rat brain. NeuroReport **7:** 953–957.

12. FATHI, Z., A.M. CUNNINGHAM, L.G. IBEN, P.B. BATTAGLINO, S.A. WARD, K.A. NICHOL, K.A. PINE, J. WANG, M.E. GOLDSTEIN, T.P. IISMAA & I.A. ZIMANYI. 1997. Cloning, pharmacological characterization and distribution of a novel galanin receptor. Mol. Brain Res. **51:** 49–59.

13. BEAL, M.F., U.M. MACGARVEY & K.J. SWARTZ. 1990. Galanin immunoreactivity is increased in the nucleus basalis of Meynert in Alzheimer's disease. Ann. Neurol. **28:** 157–161.

14. MUFSON, E.J., E. COCHRAN, W. BENZING & J.H. KORDOWER. 1993. Galaninergic innervation of the cholinergic vertical limb of the diagonal band (Ch2) and bed nucleus of the stria terminalis in aging, Alzheimer's disease and Down's syndrome. Dementia **4:** 237–250.

15. BOWSER, R., J.H. KORDOWER & E.J. MUFSON. 1997. A confocal microscopic analysis of galaninergic hyperinnervation of cholinergic basal forebrain neurons in Alzheimer's disease. Brain Pathol. **2:** 723–730.

16. HÖKFELT, T., D. MILLHORN, K. SEROOGY, Y. TSURUO, S. CECATELLI, B. LINDH, B. MEISTER, T. MELANDER, M. SCHALLING, T. BARTFAI & L. TERENIUS. 1987. Coexistence of peptides with classical transmitters. Experientia **43:** 768–780.

17. CRAWLEY, J.N. & G.L. WENK. 1989. Co-existence of galanin and acetylcholine: Is galanin involved in memory processes and dementia? Trends Neurosci. **21:** 278–282.

18. CRAWLEY, J.N., S.M. FISKE, M.C. AUSTIN & B.S. GIVENS. 1991. Behavioral actions of galanin and galanin fragments. *In* Galanin: A New Multifunctional Peptide in the Neuroendocrine System. T. Hökfelt, T. Bartfai, D. Jacobowitz & D. Ottoson, Eds.: 377–392. Macmillan Press. London, UK.

19. CRAWLEY, J.N. 1996. Galanin-acetylcholine interactions: Relevance to memory and Alzheimer's disease. Life Sci. **24:** 2185–2199.

20. MCDONALD, M.P. & J.N. CRAWLEY. 1997. Galanin-acetylcholine interactions in rodent memory tasks and Alzheimer's disease. J. Psychiatry Neurosci. **22:** 303–316.

21. ROBINSON, J.K. & J.N. CRAWLEY. 1993. Intraseptal galanin potentiates scopolamine impairment of delayed nonmatching to sample. J. Neurosci. **13:** 5119–5125.

22. ROBINSON, J.K. & J.N. CRAWLEY. 1993. Intraventricular galanin impairs delayed nonmatching-to-sample performance in rats. Behav. Neurosci. **107:** 458–467.

23. ROBINSON, J.K & J.N. CRAWLEY. 1994. Analysis of anatomical sites at which galanin impairs delayed nonmatching to sample. Behav. Neurosci. **108:** 941–950.

24. MCDONALD, M.P. & J.N. CRAWLEY. 1996. Galanin receptor antagonist M40 blocks galanin-induced choice accuracy deficits on a delayed nonmatching to position task. Behav. Neurosci. **110:** 1025–1032.

25. MCDONALD, M.P., G.L. WENK & J.N. CRAWLEY. 1997. Analysis of galanin and the galanin antagonist M40 on delayed non-matching-to-position performance in rats lesioned with the cholinergic immunotoxin [192]IgG-saporin. Behav. Neurosci. **111:** 552–563.

26. MASTROPAOLO, J., N. NADI, N.L. OSTROWSKI & J.N. CRAWLEY. 1988. Galanin antagonizes acetylcholine on a memory task in basal forebrain-lesioned rats. Proc. Natl. Acad. Sci. USA **85:** 9841–9845.

27. GIVENS, B., D.S. OLTON & J.N. CRAWLEY. 1992. Galanin in the medial septal area impairs working memory. Brain Res. **582:** 71–77.

28. MALIN, D.H., B.J. NOVY, A.E. LETT-BROWN, R.E. PLOTNER, B.T. MAY, S.J. RADULESCU, M.K. CROTHERS, L.D. OSGOOD & J.R. LAKE. 1992. Galanin attenuates retention of one-trial reward learning. Life Sci. **50:** 939–944.

29. UKAI, M., M. MASATAKA, K. TSUTOMU. 1995. Effects of galanin on passive avoidance response, elevated plus-maze learning, and spontaneous alternation performance in mice. Peptides **16:** 1283–1286.

30. Sundström, E., T. Archer, T. Melander & T. Hökfelt. 1988. Galanin impairs acquisition but not retrieval of spatial memory in rats studied in the Morris swim maze. Neurosci. Lett. **88:** 331–335.

31. Ögren, S.O, T. Hökfelt, K. Kask, Ü. Langel & T. Bartfai. 1992. Evidence for a role of the neuropeptide galanin in spatial learning. Neuroscience **51:** 1–5.

32. Ögren, S.O., J. Kehr & P.A. Schött. 1996. Effects of ventral hippocampal galanin on spatial learning and on *in vivo* acetylcholine release in the rat. Neuroscience **75:** 1127–1140.

33. Schött, P.A., B. Bjelke & S.O. Ogren. 1998. Distribution and kinetics of galanin infused into the ventral hippocampus of the rat: Relationship to spatial learning. Neuroscience **83:** 123–126.

34. Gleason, T.C. & J.N. Crawley. 1998. Spatial learning performance following galanin treatment differs across rat strains. Soc. Neurosci. **24:** Abstract 566.15.

35. Crawley, J.N., M.C. Austin, S.M. Fiske, B. Martin, S. Consolo, M. Berthold, Ü. Langel, G. Fisone & T. Bartfai. 1990. Activity of centrally adminstered galanin fragments on stimulation of feeding behavior and on galanin receptor binding in the rat hypothalamus. J. Neurosci. **10:** 3695–3700.

36. Fisone, G., C.F. Wu, S. Consolo, O. Nordstrom, N. Brynne, T. Bartfai, T. Melander & T. Hökfelt. 1987. Galanin inhibits acetylcholine release in the ventral hippocampus of the rat: Histochemical, autoradiographic, in vivo and in vitro studies. Proc. Natl. Acad. Sci. USA **84:** 7339–7343.

37. Consolo, S., R. Bertorelli, P. Girotti, C. La Porta, T. Bartfai & M. Parenti. 1991. Pertussis toxin-sensitive G-protein mediates galanin's inhibition of scopolamine-evoked acetylcholine release in vivo and carbachol-stimulated phosphoinositide turnover in rat ventral hippocampus. Neurosci. Lett. **126:** 29–32.

38. Robinson, J.K., A. Zocchi, A. Pert & J.N. Crawley. 1996. Galanin microinjected into the medial septum inhibits scopolamine-induced acetylcholine overflow in the rat ventral hippocampus. Brain Res. **709:** 81–87.

39. Coyle, J.T., D.L. Price & M.R. DeLong. 1983. Alzheimer's disease: A disorder of cortical cholinergic innervation. Science **219:** 1184–1190.

40. Bierer, L.M., V. Haraoutunian, S. Gabriel, P.J. Knott, L.S. Carlin, D.P. Purohit, D.P. Perl, J. Schmeidler, P. Kanof & K.L. Davis. 1995. Neurochemical correlates of dementia severity in Alzheimer's disease: Relative importance of the cholinergic deficits. J. Neurochem. **64:** 749–760.

41. Book, A.A., R.G. Wiley & J.B. Schweitzer. 1992. Specificity of 192 IgG-saporin for NGF receptor-positive cholinergic basal forebrain neurons in the rat. Brain Res. **590:** 350–355.

42. Heckers, S. & M. Mesulam. 1994. Two types of cholinergic projections to the rat amygdala. Neuroscience **60:** 383–397.

43. Torres, E.M., T.A. Perry, A. Blockland, L.S. Wilkinson, R.G. Wiley, R.G. Lappi & D.A. Dunnett. 1994. Behavioural, histochemical, and biochemical consequences of selective immunolesions in discrete regions of the basal forebrain cholinergic system. Neuroscience **63:** 463–476.

44. Wenk, G.L., J.D. Stoehr, G. Quintana, S. Mobley & R.G. Wiley. 1994. Behavioral, biochemical, histological, and electrophysiological effects of 192 IgG-saporin injections into the basal forebrain of rats. J. Neurosci. **14:** 5986–5995.

45. Robinson, J.K., R.G. Wiley, G.L. Wenk, D.A. Lappi & J.N. Crawley. 1996. [192]IgG-saporin immunotoxin and ibotenic acid lesions of nucleus basalis and medial septum produce comparable deficits on delayed nonmatching-to-sample in rats. Psychobiology **24:** 179–186.

46. McDonald, M.P., L.M. Baker, G.L. Wenk & J.N. Crawley. 1998. Co-administration of galanin antagonist M40 with a muscarinic M1 agonist improves delayed nonmatching to position choice accuracy in rats with cholinergic lesions. J. Neurosci. **18:** 5078–5085.

47. Baxter, M.G., D.J. Bucci, L.K. Gorman, R.G. Wiley & M. Gallagher, 1995. Selective immunotoxin lesions of basal forebrain cholinergic cells: Effects on learning and memory in rats. Behav. Neurosci. **109:** 714–722.

48. Bartfai, T., G. Fisone & Ü. Langel. 1992. Galanin and galanin antagonists: molecular and biochemical properties. Trends Pharmacol. Sci. **13:** 312–317.

49. Crawley J.N., J.K. Robinson, Ü. Langel & T. Bartfai. 1993. Galanin receptor antagonists M40 and C7 block galanin induced feeding. Brain Res. **600:** 268–272.

50. CORWIN, R.L., J.K. ROBINSON & J.N. CRAWLEY. 1993. Galanin antagonists block galanin-induced feeding in the hypothalamus and amygdala of the rat. Eur. J. Neurosci. **5:** 1528–1533.
51. LEIBOWITZ, S.F. & T. KIM. 1992. Impact of a galanin antagonist on exogenous galanin and natural patterns of fat ingestion. Brain Res. **599:** 148–152.
52. SAUERBERG, P., P.H. OLESEN, S. NIELSEN, S. TREPPENDAHL, M.J. SHEARDOWN, T. HONORE, C.H. MITCH, J.S. WARD, A.J. PIKE, F.P. BYMASTER, B.D. SAWYER & H.E. SHANNON. 1992. Novel functional M1 selective muscarinic agonists. Synthesis and structure-activity relationships of 3-(1,2,5-thiadiazolyl)-1,2,5,6-tetrahydro-1-methylpyridines. J. Med. Chem. **35:** 2274–2283.
53. PALAZZI E., G. FISONE, T. HÖKFELT, T. BARTFAI & S. CONSOLO. 1991. Galanin reduces carbachol stimulation of phosphoinositide turnover in rat ventral hippocampus by lowering Ca^{2+} influx through voltage-sensitive Ca^{2+} channels. J. Neurochem. **56:** 739–747.
54. HABERT-ORTOLI, E., B. AMIRANOFF, I. LOQUET, M. LABURTHE & J.F. MAYAUX. 1994. Molecular cloning of a functional human galanin receptor. Proc. Natl. Acad. Sci. USA **91:** 9780–9783.
55. HOWARD, A.D., C. TAN, L.L. SHIAO, O.C. PALYHA, K.K. MCKEE, D.H. WEINBERG, S.D. FEIGHNER, M.A. CASCIERI, R.G. SMITH, L.H.T. VAN DER PLOEG & K.A. SULLIVAN. 1997. Molecular cloning and characterization of new receptor for galanin. FEBS Lett. **405:** 285–290.
56. WANG, S., C. HE, T. HASHEMI & M. BAYNE. 1997. Cloning and expressional characterization of a novel galanin receptor. J. Biol. Chem. **272:** 31949–31952.
57. SMITH, K.E., C. FORRAY, M.W. WALKER, K.A. JONES, J.A. TAMM, J. BARD, T.A. BRANCHEK, D.L. LINEMEYER & C. GERALD. 1997. Expression cloning of a rat hypothalamic galanin receptor coupled to phosphoinositide turnover. J. Biol. Chem. **272:** 24612–24616.
58. BLOOMQUIST, B.T., M.R. BEAUCHAMP, L. ZHELNIN, S.E. BROWN, A.R. GOREWILLSE, P. GREGOR & L.J. CORNFIELD. 1998. Cloning and expression of the human galanin receptor GalR2. Biochem. Biophys. Res. Commun. **243:** 474–479.
59. XU, A.Q.D., T.J. S. SHI & T. HÖKFELT. 1998. Galanin/GMAP- and NPY-like immunoreactivities in locus coeruleus and noradrenergic nerve terminals in the hippocampal formation and cortex with notes on the galanin-R1 and -R2 receptors. J. Comp. Neurol. **392:** 227–251.

Regulation of Galanin in Memory Pathways

MARGARET A. MILLER[a]

*Department of Psychiatry and Behavioral Sciences, University of Washington,
Seattle, Washington 98195, USA*

ABSTRACT: Based on early immunocytochemical findings, galanin (GAL) was postulated to function as an inhibitory cotransmitter in rat cholinergic memory pathways. However, recent studies indicate that in the basal state GAL is not widely expressed by forebrain cholinergic neurons in rats. Inhibition of cholinergic transmission by cosecreted GAL may be enhanced under certain conditions, because GAL gene expression in the cholinergic basal forebrain is significantly increased prior to puberty and following nerve growth factor treatment. Other sources of GAL in rat septohippocampus that could interact with cholinergic pathways include noradrenergic neurons in the locus ceruleus and vasopressinergic neurons in the bed nucleus of the stria terminalis (BST) and medial amygdala (Me). GAL is extensively colocalized within these steroid-sensitive cell groups where its expression is upregulated by gonadal hormones. GAL, acting via the GALR1 receptor subtype, does not appear to directly regulate the activity of cholinergic neurons, but it may regulate the release of vasopressin and GAL into septohippocampus from BST/Me neurons.

The idea that galanin (GAL) functions as an inhibitory cosecreted transmitter in cholinergic memory pathways was first suggested by the observation that GAL immunoreactivity is present in 50–70% of cholinergic neurons in the medial septum-diagonal band complex (MS/DBB) of colchicine-treated rats.[1] Subsequent evidence from *in vitro* and *in vivo* studies led to the hypothesis that GAL, cosecreted with acetylcholine (ACh) into the rat ventral hippocampus, acts at a presynaptic site to inhibit further ACh release and at a postsynaptic site to antagonize the actions of ACh.[2–4] Centrally administered GAL produces behavioral effects in rats that are consistent with the idea that GAL inhibits cholinergic memory processes,[5,6] and treatment with a GAL receptor antagonist facilitates acquisition of the Morris swim maze,[7] indicating that endogenous GAL may tonically inhibit cholinergic transmission.

Identifying the origin of endogenous GAL which interacts with cholinergic memory pathways and the factors that regulate GAL expression within these pathways has become increasingly important for the development of more effective therapeutic strategies to reverse cognitive impairments associated with normal human aging and disease. Hypertrophy of GAL pathways has been postulated to contribute to the cognitive deficits of Alzheimer's disease since GAL immunoreactivity in the cortex[8] and GAL fibers in the basal forebrain[9–11] are increased in patients with this disease. On the basis of immunocytochemical findings, GAL inputs to septohippocampal memory centers originally appeared to differ in rats and humans because GAL immunoreactivity is not extensively colocalized within cholinergic neurons in the human basal forebrain.[9,12] However, our recent finding that few cholinergic neurons in rat forebrain coexpress GAL mRNA provides evidence that as in humans, cholinergic neurons in rats may not be a major source of GAL in the

[a]Address for correspondence: Dr. Margaret Miller, Department of Psychiatry Box 356560, University of Washington, Seattle, Washington 98195. Phone, 206-685-3277; fax, 206-543-9520; e-mail, mam@u.washington.edu

basal state. Here, we summarize a series of experiments directed at elucidating the anatomy and molecular physiology of GAL within three septohippocampal projecting systems in the rat: the cholinergic neurons in the basal forebrain, the noradrenergic (NE) neurons in the locus ceruleus (LC), and the vasopressin (VP) neurons in the bed nucleus of the stria terminalis (BST) and medial amygdala (Me).

GALANIN IN THE CHOLINERGIC BASAL FOREBRAIN

The concept that GAL and ACh are cosecreted into rat ventral hippocampus became a major component of the original model delineating the mechanism by which endogenous GAL regulates cholinergic memory pathways. However, the observation that colchicine treatment, used routinely in immunocytochemistry to enhance detectability of peptidergic neurons in rats, both induces GAL gene expression and inhibits expression of the cholinergic synthetic enzyme choline acetyltransferase (ChAT),[13] suggested to us that the coexistence of GAL and ChAT immunoreactivities observed in the rat following colchicine treatment may have overestimated the actual coexistence of these neurotransmitters in the basal state.

We reevaluated the coexpression of GAL within cholinergic neurons in the basal forebrain of colchicine-untreated male and female Fischer 344 rats using single and double *in situ* hybridization histochemistry.[14] Contrary to previous immunocytochemical findings,[1] we found that relatively few neurons in the cholinergic basal forebrain of adult male rats expressed GAL mRNA (TABLE 1). The greatest number of GAL mRNA expressing cells in the MS/DBB were located within the central aspects of the nucleus of the horizontal diagonal band (HDB), a region that has been shown to project predominantly to dorsal, not ventral, hippocampus.[15] Even in this region, the number of GAL mRNA expressing neurons was considerably lower than that detected in the nearby BST and represented only a

TABLE 1. Neurons in the Cholinergic Basal Forebrain of Adult Male Rats Coexpressing GAL mRNA.[a]

Region	Cell Type	Bregma 1.0 mm	Bregma 0.7 mm	Bregma 0.48 mm	Bregma 0.2 mm	Bregma −0.26 mm	Bregma −0.4 mm
MS	^{35}S-ChAT	27.2 ± 5.2	29.3 ± 3.8	41.5 ± 4.8	44.5 ± 6.5	30.2 ± 9.4	—
	^{35}S-GAL	2.6 ± 0.8	2.7 ± 1.1	1.0 ± 0.6	1.5 ± 0.9	0.5 ± 0.5	—
VDB	^{35}S-ChAT	62.0 ± 14.4	26.0 ± 2.7	40.2 ± 5.2	55.0 ± 7.8	—	—
	^{35}S-GAL	9.3 ± 3.5	2.5 ± 0.6	3.0 ± 0.8	2.8 ± 0.7	—	—
HDB	^{35}S-ChAT	—	43.0 ± 1.6	57.8 ± 2.5	76.7 ± 5.3	57.2 ± 4.5	47.5 ± 4.9
	^{35}S-GAL	—	4.8 ± 0.6	7.2 ± 1.5	9.8 ± 2.6	9.0 ± 3.2	8.2 ± 3.6

[a]Relatively few neurons coexpressed GAL mRNA. The greatest number of GAL mRNA expressing neurons were located in the central aspects of the HDB, but represented a small percentage of ChAT mRNA expressing neurons detected in alternate brain sections. Labeled cells were visualized using transmitted darkfield microscopy in atlas-matched sections. They were counted in the MS, VDB, and counted unilaterally in the HDB. Data are means ± SEM; n = 4. (Reproduced from Miller et al.,[14] with permission.)

small percentage (< 15%) of ChAT mRNA expressing cells. Fewer GAL mRNA expressing neurons were present in the nucleus of the vertical diagonal band (VDB) than the HDB and only occasional neurons labeled for GAL mRNA were detected in the MS, regions that provide the major cholinergic input to the ventral hippocampus. Consistent with previous immunocytochemical findings in the rat, virtually all GAL mRNA expressing neurons in the cholinergic fields of the basal forebrain coexpressed ChAT mRNA. These data suggested to us that in the basal state (1) GAL is not widely cosecreted with ACh into the ventral hippocampus of adult male and female rats, and (2) most GAL fibers in the hippocampus must originate from noncholinergic sources. This interpretation is consistent with the earlier findings of Melander et al.,[16] who reported a large discrepancy in the degree of colocalization of GAL and ChAT immunoreactivities in hippocampal terminals (5–10%) versus forebrain neurons (50–70%) and suggested that the LC may be the origin of many GAL fibers within the rat hippocampus.

REGULATION OF GALANIN GENE EXPRESSION IN THE CHOLINERGIC BASAL FOREBRAIN

Regulation by Gonadal Hormones

In many brain regions as in pituitary,[17–19] GAL immunoreactivity and gene expression are increased by gonadal hormones and enhanced across puberty. Basal forebrain cholinergic neurons express estrogen receptors in rats[20,21] and could therefore respond to gonadal hormone stimulation in both females and males (via aromatization of testosterone to estradiol). Using in situ hybridization histochemistry, we assessed GAL gene expression across the rostrocaudal extent of the HDB in prepubertal (24-day-old) and adult (90-day-old) male rats to determine if GAL expression is also induced in this region with the naturally occurring rise in circulating testosterone.[22] In contrast to another forebrain region in these same animals,[23] we found that the number of GAL mRNA expressing neurons was significantly reduced in the HDB of adult compared to prepubertal animals. Posthoc analysis indicated that this reduction was due to changes in GAL expression within the rostral two thirds of the nucleus, where both the number of labeled neurons and the cellular mRNA content were significantly lower in adult compared to prepubertal males (FIG. 1). In contrast, no significant differences were present in the caudal aspects of the HDB. In this initial study, we did not assess changes in GAL expression within the MS or VDB across puberty but focused instead on the HDB where we had previously detected the largest number of GAL neurons in the cholinergic basal forebrain.

We do not yet understand why GAL mRNA levels are reduced in the rostral HDB, yet increased in other brain regions with puberty. It may be that gonadal hormones exert a region-specific inhibition of GAL gene expression in the HDB. Alternatively, the reduction in GAL expression may be due to age-related changes in some other factor or factors involved in GAL regulation, perhaps a maturation-dependent decline in nerve growth factor (see below). If all GAL mRNA expressing neurons in the HDB of prepubertal males prove to be cholinergic, as we have observed in adult males,[14] these data suggest that the inhibition of cholinergic transmission by cosecreted GAL may be enhanced prior to puberty in neurons located within the rostral and central aspects of the HDB.

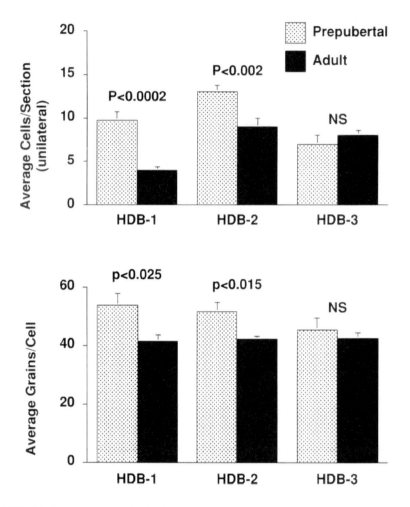

FIGURE 1. GAL gene expression in the cholinergic fields of the HDB declined across puberty in male rats. A lower average number of cells per section was detected in the rostral (HDB-1) and central (HDB-2) subregions of the HDB of adult compared to prepubertal male rats (*top panel*). The average number of grains per cell expressed by GAL neurons in HDB-1 and HDB-2 was also reduced in adult compared to prepubertal males (*bottom panel*). Data are means ± SEM; $n = 7$ per group. (Reproduced from Planas *et al.*,[22] with permission)

In adult female rats, the incidence of GAL coexpression by cholinergic neurons in the HDB is not regulated by chronic estrogen treatment[14] even though most cholinergic neurons in this region contain estrogen receptor-like immunoreactivity.[21] Approximately 16% of ChAT mRNA expressing neurons in the HDB were found to coexpress GAL regardless of estrogen state. We detected a similar incidence of coexpression in the HDB of intact adult male rats assessed in a separate assay. Consistent with the idea that the regulation of this subset of cholinergic neurons by cosecreted GAL is similar in intact adult male and female rats, we also did not find a significant sex difference in the total number of GAL mRNA expressing neurons detected in the cholinergic HDB of intact rats.[24] In agreement with these data, Gibbs[21] did not observe a sex difference in the number of cholinergic neurons in the basal forebrain. Our studies did not assess cellular mRNA content in the HDB or the regulation of GAL gene expression by estrogen within the MS or VDB. As ChAT mRNA expression is upregulated in the MS but not HDB by acute estrogen treatment,[25] it is possible that GAL expression within the MS would also be regulated by estrogen.

Coexpression of VP and GAL in the HDB

As observed originally in the paraventricular and supraoptic nuclei[26] and later in the BST/Me,[27] GAL and VP are also coexpressed in a subset of neurons in the HDB. Using single and double *in situ* hybridization histochemistry, we mapped the distribution of VP mRNA expressing neurons and the colocalization of VP and GAL mRNAs in the HDB.[24] We found that about one third of GAL mRNA expressing neurons in the HDB also contained VP mRNA. Likewise, approximately 50% of cells that were labeled for VP mRNA also contained GAL mRNA. We did not detect sex differences in either the number of neurons labeled for VP mRNA or GAL mRNA or the incidence of VP/GAL coexpression in this region. Follow-up studies confirmed that all VP mRNA expressing neurons in the HDB coexpressed ChAT mRNA (unpublished observations), providing evidence that a subset of cholinergic neurons may synthesize and release a second neuropeptide that has been implicated as a facilitatory modulator of cholinergic transmission.[28–30] Although most cholinergic neurons in the rat basal forebrain do not contain either peptide, these findings suggest that a subset of cholinergic cells in the HDB corelease both peptides, whereas other cholinergic cells corelease either VP or GAL. If VP gene expression in the HDB, like GAL gene expression, is increased prior to puberty, the functional consequences of VP/GAL coexpression within cholinergic neurons may be more readily investigated in younger animals.

Regulation by Nerve Growth Factor

Nerve growth factor (NGF), a target-derived neurotrophic factor for basal forebrain cholinergic neurons, has been proposed as a potential therapeutic agent in the treatment of the cognitive decline associated with Alzheimer's disease. In rats, NGF rescues degenerating cholinergic neurons[31,32] and increases acetylcholine turnover[33] by upregulating ChAT expression.[34] However, NGF upregulates both ChAT[35] and GAL[36] expression in cultured PC12 cells, and an NGF-responsive element has been identified in the promoter region of the GAL gene.[36] These findings suggest that in addition to stimulating ChAT gene expression, *in vivo* NGF treatment may induce the expression of GAL within the cholinergic basal forebrain. Using quantitative *in situ* hybridization histochemistry, we assessed GAL and ChAT gene expression in the cholinergic basal forebrain of young adult male rats following chronic administration (2 weeks, icv) of NGF or the control substance, cytochrome c.[37] Confirming the effectiveness of the NGF treatment, both the number of ChAT mRNA expressing neurons and the intensity of labeling were significantly increased in the MS,

VDB, and HDB. In support of our hypothesis, NGF treatment induced a parallel increase in GAL gene expression measured in alternate brain sections. Both the number of GAL mRNA expressing neurons in the cholinergic basal forebrain and their labeling intensity were significantly enhanced after NGF treatment (FIG. 2). NGF induction of GAL in the cholinergic basal forebrain appeared to be specific, because GAL expression in other forebrain regions including the BST and neurotensin expression in the HDB were unchanged. These data provide the first evidence that *in vivo* administration of NGF specifically induces GAL gene expression in the cholinergic basal forebrain. Although these findings are in complete agreement with the reported upregulation of GAL expression by NGF in cultured PC12 cells, they are in contrast to recent observations that NGF treatment suppresses the injury-induced increase in GAL expression in primary sensory neurons.[38] This discrepancy may be due to differences in the trophic actions of NGF in central versus peripheral neurons or in injured versus uninjured neurons. Our findings may provide a link between the upregulation of endogenous NGF levels recently observed in AD[39] and the hypertrophy of GAL fibers present in this disease.[9-11]

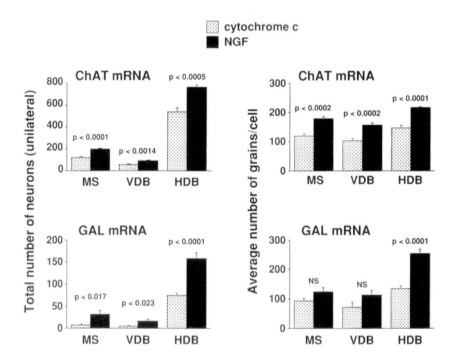

FIGURE 2. Chronic NGF treatment enhanced both ChAT and GAL mRNA levels in the basal forebrain of adult male rats. The number of GAL mRNA expressing neurons was increased in the MS, VDB, and HDB of NGF-infused rats compared with cytochrome c-infused rats. The intensity of labeling was significantly higher in GAL mRNA expressing neurons of the HDB following NGF treatment. Data are means ± SEM; $n = 6$ per group. (Reproduced from Planas *et al.*,[37] with permission.)

Although further work is required to determine if the inhibition by cosecreted GAL is increased, these findings suggest that (1) the trophic effects of NGF on cholinergic function may be blunted by the concurrent induction of GAL and (2) the therapeutic efficacy of NGF in the treatment of human memory disorders may be improved by the concomitant administration of a GAL receptor antagonist. They also raise the possibility that the induction of GAL by NGF may exert beneficial or protective actions within the CNS.[40,41] In addition to colchicine treatment, GAL is upregulated in the basal forebrain by lesion and blockade of neuronal activity.[42,43] Impairment of memory may be a consequence of GAL's role as a neuroprotective agent. The challenge will be to determine whether these two actions can be attributed to different GAL receptor subtypes.

GALANIN IN THE LOCUS CERULEUS

In the rat, NE neurons in the LC project extensively within septohippocampal regions and directly innervate basal forebrain cholinergic neurons.[44] Immunocytochemical evidence indicates that GAL is coexpressed by 80% of NE neurons in the LC,[26,45] and this high level of coexpression can be verified by double *in situ* hybridization histochemistry.[14] In light of the large number of LC neurons and the abundance of GAL gene expression within these neurons, the LC may exhibit the greatest capacity for GAL synthesis of any cell group in the rat brain. Using double immunocytochemistry for GAL and dopamine β-hydroxylase, Xu *et al.*[46] confirmed that the LC is the major source of GAL within the rat cortex[47] and hippocampal formation. However, these researchers also found that a portion of GAL-immunoreactive fibers within the rat ventral hippocampus did not contain dopamine β-hydroxylase immunoreactivity and that these fibers persisted following 6-hydroxydopamine treatment to lesion NE inputs, suggesting that they originated from non-noradrenergic sources.

Regulation of Galanin in the Locus Ceruleus by Estrogen

GAL has been postulated to be an inhibitory modulator of NE transmission because it decreases the activity of LC neurons, inhibits NE release, and antagonizes the postsynaptic actions of NE.[48–50] GAL expression within the LC was previously shown to be upregulated by colchicine treatment, reserpine treatment, social stress, and olfactory bulbectomy.[13,51–53] Inasmuch as GAL is an estrogen-inducible gene and the LC is a target of estrogen's action,[54] we investigated the regulation of GAL expression in the LC following chronic estrogen treatment.[55] Ovariectomized female rats implanted for 2 weeks with a Silastic capsule filled with 17β-estradiol had significantly higher GAL mRNA levels in the central region of the LC than did sham-implanted controls (FIG. 3). By contrast, tyrosine hydroxylase mRNA levels, measured in alternate brain sections, did not differ with estrogen treatment. If GAL inhibits the release and postsynaptic actions of NE as postulated, our findings suggest that estrogen could reduce the noradrenergic tone of the brain by increasing the level of GAL cosecreted with NE from the LC. In addition to modulating NE transmission, GAL released from LC neurons could interact with receptors expressed in postsynaptic target sites including the cholinergic basal forebrain, cortex, and hippocampus.

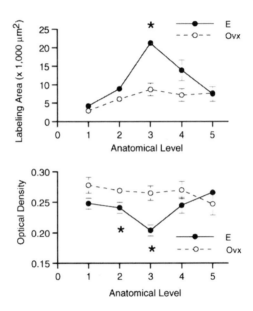

FIGURE 3. GAL gene expression in the LC was significantly greater in ovariectomized female rats treated with estradiol compared to sham-implanted controls. Both the average optical density ($p \leq 0.05$) and the labeling area ($p \leq 0.007$) differed between the groups. Slides were quantified under dark-field microscopy, and therefore reduced optical density indicates enhanced labeling. In contrast, TH gene expression measured in alternate sections did not differ between the groups (data not shown). Data are means ± SEM; $n = 7$ per group. (Reproduced from Tseng et al.,[55] with permission.)

LC neurons in the human also contain GAL immunoreactivity,[56] suggesting that GAL, cosecreted with NE in humans, may modulate those functions in which the LC has been implicated including attention-arousal, stress response, and learning and memory processes. The LC undergoes extensive degeneration in Alzheimer's disease,[57] and remaining LC neurons may be a source of GAL fibers which hyperinnervate the basal forebrain in patients with this disease.[10,11] If estrogen upregulates GAL gene expression in the human LC as in the rat, our findings raise the possibility that the beneficial effects of estrogen replacement therapy for the treatment of cognitive dysfunction may also be enhanced by the concomitant administration of a GAL receptor antagonist.

GALANIN IN THE EXTENDED AMYGDALOID COMPLEX

In addition to the LC, we suggest that another source of GAL innervation to rat ventral hippocampus may be neurons in the extended amygdaloid complex which coexpress VP and GAL.[27] VP/GAL neurons in the BST/Me may be one origin of the dopamine-β hydroxylase negative GAL fibers identified by Xu et al.[46] in rat ventral hippocampus, because these cells are the major source of vasopressinergic innervation to the septohippocampus. VP projections from these neurons have been extensively mapped and include

VDB, lateral septum, lateral habenula, central gray, dorsal raphe, locus ceruleus, and ventral hippocampus.[58,59] The high incidence of VP/GAL coexpression in the BST/Me suggests that these cells must also be a source of GAL innervation to septohippocampus, and the distribution of fibers[61,62] and receptors[63,64] for VP and GAL show a striking similarity within these brain regions. Interestingly, VP was the first peptide identified to have behavioral actions in the rat.[65] In contrast to GAL, VP and the behaviorally active VP fragment 4–9 facilitate performance on a variety of learning and memory tasks,[66] perhaps by activating cholinergic pathways.[28–30] Although the functional consequences of VP/GAL coexpression are not known, GAL, originating in the BST/Me, is anatomically situated to influence memory processes by multiple mechanisms. As originally proposed for GAL colocalized within cholinergic neurons, GAL released from VP/GAL fibers in ventral hippocampus may regulate ACh release or antagonize its postsynaptic actions. Alternatively, GAL may impair central VP release, as it has been shown to inhibit VP release from magnocellular neurons[67] or antagonize the memory-enhancing postsynaptic actions of cosecreted VP.

Coexistence of VP and GAL in the extended amygdaloid complex of the human and non-human primate has not been investigated. VP-immunoreactive neurons are present in the BST and Me of both humans[68] and macaque monkeys.[69] GAL-immunoreactive neurons have been identified in the BST of monkeys but not humans.[56] GAL mRNA expressing neurons are present in the BST and Me of adult macaque monkeys;[70] to our knowledge, the presence of GAL mRNA expressing neurons in the human BST and Me has not been assessed, and the potential role of BST/Me pathways in human memory remains to be clarified.

REGULATION OF GALANIN GENE EXPRESSION IN THE EXTENDED AMYGDALOID COMPLEX

Prior to our observation that VP and GAL are coexpressed in the BST/Me, the regulation of VP in these extrahypothalamic pathways by gonadal hormones had been extensively investigated.[71] VP immunoreactivity and VP gene expression are steroid dependent and sexually dimorphic in these cells. Male rats have more VP-immunoreactive neurons in the BST and a higher density of VP fibers in projection sites than do female rats,[72,73] and this difference results from a sex difference in the level of VP gene expression.[74] VP expression within the BST/Me is extremely dependent on gonadal hormone stimulation,[75] and castration results in a rapid disappearance of VP mRNA expression in the BST with a more gradual but complete disappearance of VP immunoreactive neurons in the BST and fibers in target regions.[61,76] Androgens and estrogens act synergistically to regulate VP expression,[77,78] and estrogen and androgen receptor immunoreactivities are colocalized with VP immunoreactivity in BST/Me neurons.[79,80]

GAL gene expression in the VP/GAL containing neurons of the BST, like VP gene expression, is reduced after castration in adult male rats and restored by testosterone treatment.[81] As expected in a gonadal steroid-responsive system, GAL gene expression in the BST and Me is increased across puberty in both male and female rats.[23,82] However, in contrast to VP expression in these same regions, GAL gene expression does not exhibit sexual dimorphism in either prepubertal or adult rats (FIG. 4). Given the high incidence of VP/GAL coexpression in these regions, this finding suggested to us that the sex difference

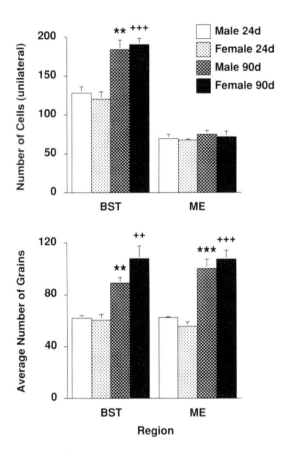

FIGURE 4. GAL gene expression increased across puberty in the BST/Me in both male and female rats. The total number of neurons that express GAL mRNA is increased in the BST (*top panel*) and the average number of grains per labeled cell was increased in both the BST and the Me (*bottom panel*). No sex differences were detected in either the number of GAL mRNA expressing neurons or the number of grains per labeled cell. Data are means ± SEM; $n = 7$ per group. (Reproduced from Planas *et al.*;[82] with permission.)

in the number of VP neurons in the BST resulted from a sex difference in the number of GAL neurons that coexpressed VP. Using double *in situ* hybridization histochemistry to evaluate the distribution and coexpression of VP and GAL mRNAs in the BST in adult rats, we confirmed this hypothesis.[60] We detected a sex difference in the number of GAL neurons that coexpressed VP in the medial but not lateral divisions of the BST. In fact, the reduced incidence of VP/GAL coexpression in the medial division could account for the sex difference in VP cell number within the entire BST. These results suggest that exposure to gonadal hormones during the critical period for sexual differentiation of the brain does not influence the survival and/or proliferation of VP neurons *per se* but regulates instead the capacity of a subset of GAL neurons in the medial BST to coexpress VP.

Although the functional consequences of VP/GAL coexpression are not known, these studies provide evidence that gonadal hormone state may influence the ratio of VP to GAL released into septohippocampus and other target sites. Whereas GAL mRNA levels are markedly reduced following castration, a significant level of gene expression remains at 2 weeks postcastration.[81] By contrast, VP expression in these same neurons virtually disappears immediately following gonadal hormone removal.[76] If our hypothesis that GAL, released from BST/Me neurons, functions as an inhibitory modulator of cholinergic transmission is correct, gonadal hormone deficiency would be predicted to be associated with an impairment of memory processes via activation of GAL receptors which would not be offset by the facilitatory actions of cosecreted VP.

GALANIN RECEPTORS AND EXPRESSION OF GALR1

Regulation of Binding Sites across Puberty

The increase in GAL immunoreactivity and GAL gene expression that occurs across puberty provides indirect evidence that endogenous GAL release increases in multiple brain regions with adulthood. To determine if pubertal activation of GAL pathways resulted in changes in GAL binding site density and/or occupancy of GAL receptors by endogenous ligand, we utilized slice binding and quantitative autoradiography[83] combined with a guanosine 5'-triphosphate (GTP)-dependent desaturation method[84] to induce dissociation of endogenous ligand bound to GAL receptors. As an index of receptor occupancy in specific brain regions, we compared ^{125}I-GAL binding in brain sections of prepubertal (24 day) and adult (90 day) male rats that were preincubated with or without 10^{-5}M GTP. Compared to standard binding conditions, preincubation of sections with GTP significantly increased ^{125}I-GAL binding in several brain regions of both age groups, suggesting that many GAL pathways were tonically active (TABLE 2). However, consistent with the idea that GAL pathways are activated with puberty, more brain regions exhibited enhanced occupancy in adult rats than in prepubertal rats. As shown in TABLE 2, regions that appeared to be specifically activated in adult male rats included the MS, intermediate and ventral parts of the LS (LSI, LSV), VDB, HDB, substantia innominata, the medial and ventral divisions of the BST (BSTM, BSTV), and the septohypothalamic area. These data suggest that the level of GAL inhibition is enhanced in subregions of the cholinergic basal forebrain and the BST in adult animals. Total GAL binding site density was significantly reduced with adulthood in specific regions including the LSV, BSTM, and MePD and increased in the lateral preoptic region.

We have also reported that the density of GAL binding sites in some brain regions, including the MePD, is regulated across puberty in female rats.[85] The density and distribution of ^{125}I-GAL binding sites were similar in adult male and female rats, suggesting that sex differences in GAL receptor number and/or affinity are not a general characteristic of central GAL pathways. However, these data do not rule out the possibility that discrete regional differences in GAL binding, which would not have been detected by our analysis, may contribute to sex differences in particular GAL functions. We did not evaluate age- or sex-related differences in GAL receptor occupancy in this study, and therefore it is unclear whether occupancy of GAL receptors in subregions of the MS/DBB and BST increases across puberty in female rats as we observed previously in males.

TABLE 2. Preincubation of Sections with GTP[a]

Region	Prepubertal		Adult	
	NO GTP	10^{-5}M GTP	NO GTP	10^{-5}M GTP
ICj	0.38 ± 0.04	0.41 ± 0.05	$0.26 \pm 0.02^{*}$	0.29 ± 0.03
LSD	0.18 ± 0.01	0.17 ± 0.01	0.16 ± 0.01	0.18 ± 0.02
LSI	0.18 ± 0.01	0.22 ± 0.03	$0.08 \pm 0.01^{***}$	$0.16 \pm 0.02^{\Diamond\Diamond\Diamond}$
LSV	0.28 ± 0.02	0.33 ± 0.03	$0.09 \pm 0.04^{***}$	$0.22 \pm 0.01^{+,\Diamond\Diamond}$
MS	0.16 ± 0.02	0.21 ± 0.02	$0.09 \pm 0.01^{*}$	$0.21 \pm 0.02^{\Diamond\Diamond}$
SHi	0.88 ± 0.05	0.74 ± 0.05	0.75 ± 0.10	0.84 ± 0.13
SHy	0.37 ± 0.01	0.37 ± 0.03	$0.13 \pm 0.02^{***}$	$0.30 \pm 0.01^{\Diamond\Diamond\Diamond}$
VDB	0.09 ± 0.03	0.19 ± 0.04	0.06 ± 0.01	$0.23 \pm 0.02^{\Diamond\Diamond\Diamond}$
HDB	0.24 ± 0.07	0.30 ± 0.06	0.12 ± 0.02	$0.28 \pm 0.02^{\Diamond\Diamond\Diamond}$
BSTL	0.89 ± 0.07	0.77 ± 0.08	0.88 ± 0.11	0.92 ± 0.09
BSTM	0.54 ± 0.03	0.49 ± 0.03	$0.19 \pm 0.03^{***}$	$0.37 \pm 0.02^{+,\Diamond\Diamond}$
BSTV	0.36 ± 0.03	0.34 ± 0.02	$0.16 \pm 0.03^{**}$	$0.30 \pm 0.02^{\Diamond\Diamond}$
SI	0.32 ± 0.05	0.30 ± 0.01	$0.14 \pm 0.01^{**}$	$0.30 \pm 0.03^{\Diamond\Diamond}$
MePD	0.63 ± 0.10	0.61 ± 0.07	$0.24 \pm 0.02^{**}$	$0.31 \pm 0.04^{++}$
Ce	0.81 ± 0.12	0.86 ± 0.12	0.71 ± 0.10	0.86 ± 0.19
st	0.68 ± 0.05	0.59 ± 0.07	0.61 ± 0.02	$0.80 \pm 0.06^{\Diamond}$
Pe	0.07 ± 0.01	$0.13 \pm 0.02^{\ddagger}$	0.06 ± 0.01	$0.17 \pm 0.02^{\Diamond\Diamond}$
Arc	0.08 ± 0.01	$0.14 \pm 0.01^{\ddagger}$	0.08 ± 0.01	$0.14 \pm 0.02^{\Diamond}$
ME	0.07 ± 0.01	$0.15 \pm 0.01^{\#}$	0.06 ± 0.01	0.11 ± 0.02
MPA	0.08 ± 0.01	$0.19 \pm 0.02^{\#}$	0.05 ± 0.01	$0.26 \pm 0.04^{\Diamond\Diamond}$
LPO	0.09 ± 0.01	$0.19 \pm 0.02^{\#}$	0.08 ± 0.01	$0.30 \pm 0.12^{+,\Diamond\Diamond\Diamond}$
VMH	0.41 ± 0.06	0.46 ± 0.04	$0.25 \pm 0.03^{*}$	$0.38 \pm 0.04^{\Diamond}$
DMH	0.07 ± 0.01	0.12 ± 0.03	0.06 ± 0.01	$0.15 \pm 0.03^{\Diamond}$
LH	0.25 ± 0.04	0.29 ± 0.04	0.16 ± 0.02	$0.28 \pm 0.04^{\Diamond}$
MHb	0.16 ± 0.01	0.17 ± 0.03	$0.11 \pm 0.02^{*}$	0.13 ± 0.03
ZI	0.38 ± 0.06	0.39 ± 0.05	0.28 ± 0.04	0.33 ± 0.06
PV	0.41 ± 0.04	$0.61 \pm 0.03^{\ddagger}$	$0.18 \pm 0.02^{**}$	$0.36 \pm 0.02^{++,\Diamond\Diamond}$
IMD	0.59 ± 0.10	0.79 ± 0.07	$0.14 \pm 0.02^{*}$	$0.30 \pm 0.04^{++,\Diamond}$
CM	0.88 ± 0.08	$1.16 \pm 0.04^{\ddagger}$	1.03 ± 0.06	1.01 ± 0.07
CL	0.80 ± 0.08	$1.07 \pm 0.03^{\ddagger}$	0.93 ± 0.04	0.94 ± 0.06
PC	0.56 ± 0.09	0.72 ± 0.09	0.70 ± 0.05	0.66 ± 0.02
LDDM	0.16 ± 0.01	0.18 ± 0.01	0.15 ± 0.01	0.15 ± 0.03
LDVL	0.14 ± 0.04	0.16 ± 0.03	0.16 ± 0.04	0.15 ± 0.02
Rh	0.53 ± 0.09	0.61 ± 0.09	0.49 ± 0.11	0.52 ± 0.08
Re	0.28 ± 0.01	0.34 ± 0.05	0.28 ± 0.02	0.33 ± 0.06

[a]Specific ^{125}I-GAL binding was increased in several brain regions of both prepubertal (24 days) and adult (90 days) male rats. Consistent with the idea that GAL synthesis and release are increased across puberty, the enhanced binding following GTP pretreatment was greatest in adult males. Regions that were specifically activated in adult male rats included subregions of the cholinergic basal forebrain and BST. Data are means ± SEM, $n = 4$ per group. (Reproduced from Planas et al.,[83] with permission.) (*) prepubertal NO GTP vs adult NO GTP; (+) prepubertal GTP vs adult GTP; (‡) prepubertal NO GTP vs prepubertal GTP; (◊) adult NO GTP vs adult GTP. *, +, ‡, ◊, $p \leq 0.05$; **, ++, ##, ◊◊, $p \leq 0.01$; ***, +++, ###, ◊◊◊, $p \leq 0.001$.

Coexpression of GALR1

Cumulative evidence from behavioral and pharmacologic studies suggests that GAL acts in both the hippocampus and the basal forebrain to inhibit ACh release and impair memory.[2,86] Although GAL binding sites are present in both brain regions,[64,87] the mechanism by which GAL inhibits ACh release is unclear. GAL could directly affect the activity of cholinergic neurons by interacting with receptors located on cholinergic cell bodies and/ or axon terminals. Alternatively, other neurotransmitter systems may mediate the inhibitory actions of GAL on cholinergic transmission.

Using double *in situ* hybridization histochemistry, we tested the hypothesis that GAL, acting via the GALR1 receptor,[88] could directly modulate the activity of basal forebrain cholinergic neurons.[89] We found no evidence for the coexpression of GALR1 and ChAT mRNAs; however, we detected numerous GALR1 mRNA expressing neurons in the immediate vicinity of basal forebrain cholinergic cells (FIG. 5). Although we cannot exclude the possibility that GAL exerts direct actions via a different receptor subtype, these findings do not support the idea that GAL, acting via the GALR1 receptor, directly inhibits ACh release but suggest, instead, that neighboring forebrain neurons play a role in mediating GAL's inhibitory actions on cholinergic transmission. Studies to determine the phenotype of these GALR1 mRNA expressing neurons are underway.

In contrast to the lack of coexpression detected in the cholinergic basal forebrain, GALR1 mRNA is extensively coexpressed with GAL mRNA in VP/GAL neurons of the BST and Me,[89] providing anatomic evidence that GAL could directly modulate the release of VP and/or GAL from these cells into target regions. Neither the location of these receptors (i.e., cell body or axon terminal) nor the origin of endogenous GAL that interacts with these receptors (i.e., the BST/Me neurons themselves or other GAL-containing afferent projections) is known. If VP originating in the BST/Me facilitates acetylcholine release in

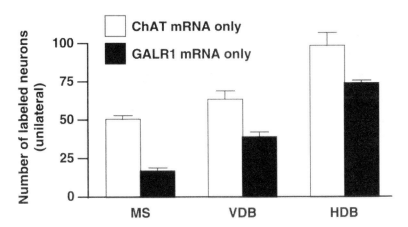

FIGURE 5. Although GALR1 and ChAT mRNAs were not coexpressed, numerous GALR1 mRNA expressing neurons were detected in the immediate vicinity of cholinergic cells in the rat basal forebrain, suggesting that neighboring neurons may mediate the inhibitory actions of GAL on cholinergic transmission. Data are means ± SEM; $n = 5$ per group. (Reproduced from Miller *et al.*,[89] with permission.)

the hippocampus as we have postulated, GAL, acting via GALR1 receptors expressed by VP/GAL neurons, could attenuate these facilitatory actions. Alternatively, GAL, acting via these receptors, may provide a negative feedback mechanism to reduce further GAL release from BST/Me neurons into target sites including the septohippocampus.

SUMMARY

Pharmacologic and behavioral studies provide convincing evidence that GAL impairs memory in rats via inhibition of cholinergic transmission. The anatomy of GAL in memory systems indicates that in the basal state GAL is not widely cosecreted with acetylcholine into rat ventral hippocampus and suggests that GAL, synthesized in the BST/Me and LC, may interact with cholinergic pathways. Despite the low level of expression in the basal state, many forebrain cholinergic neurons have the capacity to synthesize GAL as evidenced by its upregulation following colchicine treatment, lesion, and NGF treatment and prior to puberty. Inasmuch as GAL may also exert beneficial actions in the CNS, the challenge facing researchers interested in human memory disorders will be to determine if these diverse actions can be distinguished on the basis of specific GAL receptor subtypes.

ACKNOWLEDGMENTS

I would like to thank my colleagues and coworkers Dr. Barbara Planas, Pamella Kolb, Janet Tseng, and Dr. Murray Raskind. I am grateful to Dr. Henry G. Friesen, Dr. Maria Vrontakis, Dr. Thomas Sherman, Dr. Eric Parker, and Dr. Richard Palmiter for their gifts of the cDNA clones used in our studies.

REFERENCES

1. MELANDER, T., W.A. STAINES, T. HÖKFELT, Å. RÖKAEUS, F. ECKENSTEIN, P.M. SALVATERRA & B.H. WAINER. 1985. Galanin-like immunoreactivity in cholinergic neurons of the septum-basal forebrain complex projecting to the hippocampus of the rat. Brain Res. **360:** 130–138.
2. FISONE, G., C.F. WU, S. CONSOLO, Ö. NORDSTRÖM, N. BRYNNE, T. BARTFAI, T. MELANDER & T. HÖKFELT. 1987. Galanin inhibits acetylcholine release in ventral hippocampus of the rat. Histochemical, autoradiographic, in vivo, and in vitro studies. Proc. Natl. Acad. Sci. USA **84:** 7339–7343.
3. HÖKFELT, T., D. MILLHORN, K. SEROOGY, Y. TSURUO, S. CECCATELLI, B. LINDH, B. MEISTER, T. MELANDER, M. SCHALLING, T. BARTFAI & L. TERENIUS. 1987. Coexistence of peptides with classical transmitters. Experientia **43:** 768–780.
4. CRAWLEY, J. 1990. Coexistence of neuropeptides and "classical" neurotransmitters. Functional interactions between galanin and acetylcholine. Ann. N.Y. Acad. Sci. **579:** 233–245.
5. SUNDSTRÖM, E., T. ARCHER, T. MELANDER & T. HÖKFELT. 1988. Galanin impairs acquisition but not retrieval of spatial memory in rats studied in the Morris swim maze. Neurosci. Lett. **88:** 331–335.
6. GIVENS, B., D.S. OLTON & J.N. CRAWLEY. 1992. Galanin in the medial septal area impairs working memory. Brain Res. **582:** 71–77.
7. ÖGREN, S.O., T. HÖKFELT, K. KASK, Ü. LANGEL & T. BARTFAI. 1992. Evidence for a role of the neuropeptide galanin in spatial learning. Neuroscience **51:** 1–5.
8. GABRIEL, S.M., L.M. BIERER, M. DAVIDSON, D.P. PUROHIT, D.P. PERL & V. HAROUTUNIAN. 1994. Galanin-like immunoreactivity is increased in the post-mortem cerebral cortex from patients with Alzheimer's disease. J. Neurochem. **62:** 1516–1523.

9. Chan-Palay, V. 1988. Neurons with galanin innervate cholinergic cells in the human basal forebrain and galanin and acetylcholine coexist. Brain Res. Bull. **21:** 465–472.

10. Chan-Palay, V. 1988. Galanin hyperinnervates surviving neurons of the human basal nucleus of Meynert in dementias of Alzheimer's and Parkinson's disease: A hypothesis for the role of galanin in accentuating cholinergic dysfunction in dementia. J. Comp. Neurol. **273:** 543–557.

11. Mufson, E.J., E. Cochran, W. Benzing & J.H. Kordower. 1993. Galaninergic innervation of the cholinergic vertical limb of the diagonal band (Ch2) and bed nucleus of the stria terminalis in aging, Alzheimer's disease and Down's syndrome. Dementia **4:** 237–250.

12. Kordower, J.H. & E.F. Mufson. 1990. Galanin-like immunoreactivity within the primate basal forebrain: Differential staining patterns between humans and monkeys. J. Comp. Neurol. **294:** 281–292.

13. Cortés, R., S. Ceccatelli, M. Schalling & T. Hökfelt. 1990. Differential effects of intracerebroventricular colchicine administration on the expression of mRNAs for neuropeptides and neurotransmitter enzymes, with special emphasis on galanin: An in situ hybridization study. Synapse **6:** 369–391.

14. Miller, M.A., P.E. Kolb, B. Planas & M.A. Raskind. 1998. Few cholinergic neurons in the rat basal forebrain coexpress galanin messenger RNA. J. Comp. Neurol. **391:** 248–258.

15. Gaykema, R.P.A., P.G.M. Luiten, C. Nyakas & J. Traber. 1990. Cortical projection patterns of the medial septum-diagonal band complex. J. Comp. Neurol. **293:** 103–124.

16. Melander, T., W.A. Staines & Å. Rökaeus. 1986. Galanin-like immunoreactivity in hippocampal afferents in the rat, with special reference for cholinergic and noradrenergic inputs. Neuroscience **19:** 223–240.

17. Gabriel, S.M., L.M. Kaplan, J.B. Martin & J.I. Koenig. 1989. Tissue-specific sex differences in galanin-like immunoreactivity and galanin mRNA during development in the rat. Peptides **10:** 369–374.

18. Gabriel S.M., J.I. Koenig & L.M. Kaplan. 1990. Galanin-like immunoreactivity is influenced by estrogen in peripubertal and adult rats. Neuroendocrinology **51:** 168–173.

19. Vrontakis, M.E., T. Yamamoto, I.C. Schroedter, J.I. Nagy & H.G. Friesen. 1989. Estrogen induction of galanin synthesis in the rat anterior pituitary gland demonstrated by *in situ* hybridization and immunocytochemistry. Neurosci. Lett. **100:** 59–64.

20. Toran-Allerand, C.D., R.C. Miranda, W.D.L. Dentham, F. Sohrabji, T.J. Brown, R.B. Hochberg & N.J. MacLusky. 1992. Estrogen receptors colocalize with low-affinity nerve growth factor receptors in cholinergic neurons of the basal forebrain. Proc. Natl. Acad. Sci. USA **89:** 4668–4672.

21. Gibbs, R.B. 1996. Expression of estrogen receptor-like immunoreactivity by different subgroups of basal forebrain cholinergic neurons in gonadectomized male and female rats. Brain Res. **720:** 61–68.

22. Planas, B., P.E. Kolb, M.A. Raskind & M.A. Miller. 1996. Galanin gene expression declines with adulthood in the cholinergic fields of the horizontal diagonal band of male rats. Brain Res. **728:** 57–64.

23. Planas, B., P.E. Kolb, M.A. Raskind & M.A. Miller. 1994. Activation of galanin pathways across puberty in the male rat: Galanin gene expression in the bed nucleus of the stria terminalis and medial amygdala. Neuroscience **63:** 851–858.

24. Planas, B., P.E. Kolb, M.A. Raskind & M.A. Miller. 1995. Vasopressin and galanin mRNAs coexist in the nucleus of the horizontal diagonal band: A novel site of vasopressin gene expression. J. Comp. Neurol. **361:** 48–56.

25. Gibbs, R.B., D. Wu, L.B. Hersh & D.W. Pfaff. 1994. Effects of estrogen replacement on the relative levels of choline acetyltransferase, trkA, and nerve growth factor messenger RNAs in the basal forebrain and hippocampal formation of adult rats. Exp. Neurol. **129:** 70–80.

26. Melander, T., T. Hökfelt, Å. Rökaeus, A.C. Cuello, W.H. Oertel, A. Verhofstad & M. Goldstein. 1986. Coexistence of galanin-like immunoreactivity with catecholamines, 5-hydroxytryptamine, GABA and neuropeptides in the rat CNS. J. Neurosci. **6:** 3640–3654.

27. Miller, M.A., P.E. Kolb & M.A. Raskind. 1993. Extra-hypothalamic vasopressin neurons coexpress galanin messenger RNA as shown by double in situ hybridization histochemistry. J. Comp. Neurol. **329:** 378–384.

28. FAIMAN, C.P., G.A. DE ERAUSQUIN & C.M. BARATTI. 1991. The enhancement of retention induced by vasopressin in mice may be mediated by an activation of central nicotinic cholinergic mechanisms. Behav. Neural. Biol. **56:** 183–199.

29. HORITA, A. & M.A. CARINO. 1991. Centrally administered vasopressin antagonizes pentobarbital-induced narcosis and depresssion of hippocampal cholinergic activity. Peptides **11:** 1021–1025.

30. MAEGAWA, H., N. KATSUBE, T. OKEGAWA, H. AISHITA & A. KAWASAKI. 1992. Arginine-vasopressin fragment 4-9 stimulates acetylcholine release in hippocampus of freely-moving rats. Life Sci. **51:** 285–293.

31. WILLIAMS, L.R., S. VARON, G.M. PETERSON, K. WICTORIN, W. FISCHER, A. BJORKLUND & F.H. GAGE. 1986. Continuous infusion of nerve growth factor prevents basal forebrain neuronal death after fimbria fornix transection. Proc. Natl. Acad. Sci. USA **83:** 9231–9235.

32. FISCHER, W., K. WICTORIN, A. BJORKLUND, L.R. WILLIAMS, S. VARON & F.H. GAGE. 1987. Amelioration of cholinergic neuron atrophy and spatial memory impairment in aged rats by nerve growth factor. Nature **329:** 65–68.

33. RYLETT, R.J., S. GODDARD, B.M. SCHMIDT & L.R. WILLIAMS. 1993. Acetylcholine synthesis and release following continuous intracerebral administration of NGF in adult and aged Fischer 344 rats. J. Neurosci. **13:** 3956–3963.

34. WILLIAMS, L.R. & R.J. RYLETT. 1990. Exogenous nerve growth factor increases the activity of high-affinity choline uptake and choline acetyltransferase in brain of Fisher 344 male rats. J. Neurochem. **55:** 1042–1049.

35. HEUMANN, R., M. SCHWAB, R. MERKL & H. THOENEN. 1984. Nerve growth factor-mediated induction of choline acetyltransferase in PC12 cells: Evaluation of the site of action of nerve growth factor and the involvement of lysosomal degradation products of nerve growth factor. J. Neurosci. **4:** 3039–3050.

36. KAPLAN, L.M., S.C. HOOI, D.R. ABRACZINKAS, R.M. STRAUSS, M.B. DAVIDSON, D.W. HSU & J.I. KOENING. 1991. Neuroendocrine regulation of galanin gene expression. *In* Galanin: A multifunctional peptide in the neuro-endocrine system. T. Hökfelt, Ed.: 43–65. MacMillan. New York, NY.

37. PLANAS, B., P.E. KOLB, M.A. RASKIND & M.A. MILLER. 1997. Nerve growth factor induces galanin gene expression in the rat basal forebrain: Implications for the treatment of cholinergic dysfunction. J. Comp. Neurol. **379:** 563–570.

38. VERGE, V.M., P.M. RICHARDSON, Z. WIESENFELD-HALLIN & T. HOKFELT. 1995. Differential influence of nerve growth factor on neuropeptide expression in vivo: A novel role in peptide suppression in adult sensory neurons. J. Neurosci. **15:** 2081–2096.

39. SCOTT, S.A., E.J. MUFSON, J.A. WEINGARTNER, K.A. SKAU & K.A. CRUTCHER. 1995. Nerve growth factor in Alzheimer's disease: Increased levels throughout the brain coupled with declines in nucleus basalis. J. Neurosci. **15:** 6213–6221.

40. ZINI, S., M.P. ROISIN, C. ARMENGAUD & Y. BEN ARI. 1993. Effect of potassium channel modulators on the release of glutamate induced by ischaemic-like conditions in rat hippocampal slices. Neurosci. Lett. **153:** 202–205.

41. LIU, S., B.G. LYETH & R.J. HAMM. 1994. Protective effect of galanin on behavioral deficits in experimental traumatic brain injury. J. Neurotrauma **11:** 73–82.

42. CORTÉS, R., M.J. VILLAR, A. VERHOFSTAD & T. HÖKFELT. 1990. Effects of central nervous system lesions on the expression of galanin: A comparative in situ hybridization and immunohistochemical study. Proc. Natl. Acad. Sci. USA 87: 7742–7746.

43. AGOSTON, D.V., S. KOMOLY & M. PALKOVITS. 1994. Selective up-regulation of neuropeptide synthesis by blocking the neuronal activity: Galanin expression in septohippocampal neurons. Exp. Neurol. **126:** 247–55.

44. ZABORSKY, L., W.E. CULLINAN & V.N. LUINE. 1993. Catecholaminergic-cholinergic interactions in the basal forebrain. *In* Progress in Brain Research: Cholinergic Function and Dysfunction **98:** 31–49.

45. HOLETS, V.R., T. HÖKFELT, Å. RÖKAEUS, L. TERENIUS & M. GOLDSTEIN. 1988. Locus coeruleus neurons in the rat containing neuropeptide Y, tyrosine hydroxylase or galanin and their efferent projections to the spinal cord, cerebral cortex, and hypothalamus. Neuroscience **24:** 893–906.

46. Xu, Z.D., T.S. Shi & T. Hökfelt. 1998. Galanin/GMAP- and NPY-like immunoreactivities in locus coeruleus and noradrenergic nerve terminals in the hippocampal formation and cortex with notes on the galanin-R1 and -R2 receptors. J. Comp. Neurol. 392: 227–251.

47. Gabriel, S.M., P.J. Knott & V. Haroutunian. 1995. Alterations in cerebral cortical galanin concentrations following neurotransmitter-specific subcortical lesions in the rat. J. Neurosci. 15: 5526–5534.

48. Seutin, V., P. Verbanck, L. Massotte & A. Dresse. 1989. Galanin decreases the activity of locus coeruleus neurons in vitro. Eur. J. Pharmacol. 164: 373–376.

49. Goldstein, M. & A.Y. Deutch. 1989. The inhibitory actions of NPY and galanin on ^{3}H-norepinephrine release in the central nervous system: Relation to a proposed hierarchy of neuronal coexistence. In Neuropeptide Y. Karolinska Institute Nobel Conference Series. V. Mutt, K. Fuxe, T. Hökfelt & J.M. Lundberg, Eds. : 153–162. Raven Press. New York, NY.

50. Nishibori, M., R. Oishi, Y. Itoh & K. Saeki. 1988. Galanin inhibits noradrenaline-induced accumulation of cyclic AMP in the rat cerebral cortex. J. Neurochem. 51: 1953–1988.

51. Austin, M.C., S.L. Cottingham, S.M. Paul & J.N. Crawley. 1990. Tyrosine hydroxylase and galanin mRNA levels in locus coeruleus neurons are increased following reserpine administration. Synapse 6: 351–357.

52. Holmes, P.V., D.C. Blanchard, R.J. Blanchard, L.S. Brady & J.N. Crawley. 1995. Chronic social stress increases levels of preprogalanin mRNA in the rat locus coeruleus. Pharmacol. Biochem. Behav. 50: 655–660.

53. Holmes, P.V. & J.N. Crawley. 1996. Olfactory bulbectomy increases prepro-galanin mRNA levels in the rat locus coeruleus. Mol. Brain Res. 36: 184–188.

54. Sar, M.& W.E. Stumpf. 1981. Central noradrenergic neurones concentrate ^{3}H-oestradiol. Nature 289: 500–502.

55. Tseng, J.Y., P.E. Kolb, M.A. Raskind & M.A. Miller. 1997. Estrogen regulates galanin but not tyrosine hydroxylase gene expression in the rat locus ceruleus. Mol. Brain Res. 50: 100–106.

56. Kordower, J.H., H.K. Le & E.J. Mufson. 1992. Galanin immunoreactivity in the primate central nervous system. J. Comp. Neurol. 319: 479–500.

57. Chan-Palay, V. & E. Asan. 1989. Alterations in catecholamine neurons of the locus coeruleus in senile dementia of the Alzheimer type and in Parkinson's disease with and without dementia and depression. J. Comp. Neurol. 287: 373–92.

58. De Vries, G.J. & R.M. Buijs. 1983. The origin of the vasopressinergic and oxytocinergic innervation of the rat brain with special reference to the lateral septum. Brain Res. 273: 307–317.

59. Caffe, A.R., F.W. Van Leeuwen & P.G.M. Luiten. 1987. Vasopressin cells in the medial amygdala of the rat project to the lateral septum and ventral hippocampus. J. Comp. Neurol. 261: 237–252.

60. Planas, B., P.E. Kolb, M.A. Raskind & M.A. Miller. 1995. Sex difference in coexpression by galanin neurons accounts for sexual dimorphism of vasopressin in the bed nucleus of the stria terminalis. Endocrinology 135: 727–733.

61. De Vries, G.J., R.M. Buijs, F.W. Van Leeuwen, A.R. Caffe & D.F. Swaab. 1985. The vasopressinergic innervation of the brain in normal and castrated rats. J. Comp. Neurol. 233: 236–254.

62. Skofitsch, G. & D.M. Jacobowitz. 1985. Immunohistochemical mapping of galanin-like neurons in the rat central nervous system. Peptides 6: 509–546.

63. Tribollet, E., C. Barberis, S. Jard, M. Dubois-Dauphin & J.J. Dreifuss. 1988. Localization and pharmacological characterization of high affinity binding sites for vasopressin and oxytocin in the rat brain by light microscopic autoradiography. Brain Res. 442: 105–118.

64. Melander, T., C. Kohler, S. Nilsson, T. Hökfelt, E. Brodin, E. Theodorsson & T. Bartfai. 1988. Autoradiographic quantitation and anatomical mapping of ^{125}I-galanin binding sites in the rat central nervous system. J. Chem. Neuroanat. 1: 213–233.

65. De Wied, D. 1965. The influence of the posterior and intermediate lobe of the pituitary and pituitary peptides on the maintenance of a conditioned avoidance response in rats. Int. J. Neuropharmacol. 4: 157–167.63.

66. De Wied, D., M. Diamant & M. Fodor. 1993. Central nervous system effects of the neurohypophyseal hormones and related peptides. Front. Neuroendocrinol. 14: 251–302.

67. Kondo, K., T. Murase, K. Otake, M. Ito, F. Kurimoto & Y. Oiso. 1993. Galanin as a physiological neurotransmitter in hemodynamic control of arginine vasopressin release in rats. Neuroendocrinol. 57: 224–229.

68. FLIERS, E., S.E.F. GULDENAAR, N.V.D. WAL & D.F. SWAAB. 1986. Extrahypothalamic vasopressin and oxytocin in the human brain: Presence of vasopressin cells in the bed nucleus of the stria terminalis. Brain Res. **375**: 363–376.

69. CAFFE, A.R., P.C. VAN RYEN, T.P. VAND DER WOUDE & F.W. VAN LEEUWEN. 1989. Vasopressin and oxytocin systems in the brain and upper spinal cord of Macaca fascicularis. J. Comp. Neurol. **287**: 302–325.

70. EVANS, H.F., G.W. HUNTLEY, J.H. MORRISON & J. SHINE. 1993. Localisation of mRNA encoding the protein precursor of galanin in the monkey hypothalamus and basal forebrain. J. Comp. Neurol. **328**: 203–212.

71. DE VRIES, G.J., H.A. AL-SHAMMA & L. ZHOU. 1994. The sexually dimorphic vasopressin innervation of the brain as a model for steroid modulation of neuropeptide transmission. Ann. N.Y. Acad. Sci. **743**: 95–120.

72. VAN LEEUWEN, F.W., A.R. CAFFE & G.J. DE VRIES. 1985. Vasopressin cells in the bed nucleus of the stria terminalis of the rat: Sex differences and the influence of androgens. Brain Res. **325**: 391–394.

73. DE VRIES, G.J., W. BEST & A.A. SLUITTER. 1983. The influence of androgens on the development of a sex difference in the vasopressinergic innervation of the rat lateral septum. Dev. Brain Res. **8**: 377–380.

74. MILLER, M.A., L. VICIAN, D.K. CLIFTON & D.M. DORSA. 1989. Sex differences in vasopressin neurons in the bed nucleus of the stria terminalis by in situ hybridization. Peptides **10**: 615–619.

75. MILLER, M.A., J.H. URBAN & D.M. DORSA. 1989. Steroid dependency of vasopressin neurons in the bed nucleus of the stria terminalis by in situ hybridization histochemistry. Endocrinology **125**: 2335–2340.

76. MILLER, M.A., G.J. DE VRIES, H. AL-SHAMMA & D.M. DORSA. 1992. Decline of vasopressin mRNA and immunoreactivity in the BNST following castration. J. Neurosci. 12: 2881–2887.

77. DE VRIES, G.J., W. DUETZ, R.M. BUIJS, J. VAN HEERIKHUIZE & J.T.M. VREEBURG. 1986. Effects of androgens and estrogens on the vasopressin and oxytocin innervation of the adult rat brain. Brain Res. **399**: 296–302.

78. DE VRIES, G.J., Z. WANG, N.A. BULLOCK & S. NUMAN. 1994. Sex differences in the effects of testosterone and its metabolites on vasopressin messenger RNA levels in the bed nucleus of the stria terminalis of rats. J. Neurosci. **14**: 1789–1794.

79. AXELSON, J.F. & F.W. VAN LEEUWEN. 1990. Differential localization of estrogen receptors in various vasopressin synthesizing nuclei of the rat brain. J. Neuroendocrinol. **2**: 209–216.

80. ZHOU, L., J.D. BLAUSTEIN & G.J. DE VRIES. 1994. Distribution of androgen receptor immunoreactivity in vasopressin-immunoreactive and oxytocin-immunoreactive neurons in the male rat brain. Endocrinology **134**: 2622–2627.

81. MILLER, M.A., P.E. KOLB & M.A. RASKIND. 1993. Testosterone regulates galanin gene expression in the bed nucleus of the stria terminalis. Brain Res. **611**: 338–341.

82. PLANAS, B., P.E. KOLB, M.A. RASKIND & M.A. MILLER. 1994. Galanin in the bed nucleus of the stria terminalis and medial amygdala of the rat: Lack of sexual dimorphism despite regulation of gene expression across puberty. Endocrinology **143**: 1999–2004.

83. PLANAS, B., P.E. KOLB, M.A. RASKIND & M.A. MILLER. 1994. Activation of galanin pathways across puberty in the male rat: Assessment of galanin binding sites density. Neuroscience **63**: 859–867.

84. LAGNY-POURMIR, I. & J. EPELBAUM. 1992. Regional stimulatory and inhibitory effects of guanine nucleotides on [^{125}I]galanin binding in rat brain: Relationship with the rate of occupancy of galanin receptors by endogenous galanin. Neuroscience **49**: 829–847.

85. PLANAS, B., P.E. KOLB, M.A. RASKIND & M.A. MILLER. 1995. Galanin-binding sites in the female rat brain are regulated across puberty yet similar to the male pattern in adulthood. Neuroendocrinology **61**: 646–654.

86. ROBINSON, J.K., A. ZOCCHI, A. PERT & J.N. CRAWLEY. 1996. Galanin microinjected into the medial septum inhibits scopolamine-induced acetylcholine overflow in the ventral hippocampus. Brain Res. **709**: 81–87.

87. SKOFITSCH, G., M.A. SILLS & D.M. JACOBOWITZ. 1986. Autoradiographic distribution of ^{125}I-galanin binding sites in the rat central nervous system. Peptides **7**: 1029–1042.85.

88. PARKER, E.M., D.G. IZZARELLI, H.P. NOWAK, C.D. MAHLE, L.G. IBEN, J. WANG & M.E. GOLDSTEIN. 1995. Cloning and characterization of the rat GALR1 galanin receptor from Rin14B insulinoma cells. Mol. Brain Res. **34:** 179–189.
89. MILLER, M.A., P.E. KOLB & M.A. RASKIND. 1997. GALR1 galanin receptor mRNA is co-expressed by galanin neurons but not cholinergic neurons in the rat basal forebrain. Mol. Brain Res. **52:** 121–129.

Modulation of Acetylcholine and Serotonin Transmission by Galanin

Relationship to Spatial and Aversive Learning

S.O. ÖGREN,[d] P.A. SCHÖTT, J. KEHR, T. YOSHITAKE,[a] I. MISANE,[b] P. MANNSTRÖM, AND J. SANDIN[c]

Department of Neuroscience, Karolinska Institute, S-171 77 Stockholm, Sweden

[a]*Chemical Biotesting Center, Chemical Inspection & Testing Institute, Hita, Oita 877, Japan*

[b]*Laboratory of Pharmacology, Latvian Institute of Organic Synthesis, Riga, Latvia*

[c]*Department of Clinical Neuroscience, Karolinska Institute, S-171 76 Stockholm, Sweden*

ABSTRACT: This paper presents evidence that galanin is a potent *in vivo* modulator of basal acetylcholine release in the rat brain with qualitatively and quantitatively differential effects in the dorsal and ventral hippocampus. Galanin perfused through the microdialysis probe decreased basal acetylcholine release in the ventral hippocampus, while it enhanced acetylcholine release in the dorsal hippocampus. Galanin (3 nmol/rat) infused into the ventral hippocampus impaired spatial learning acquisition, while it tended to facilitate acquisition when injected into the dorsal hippocampus. These effects appear to be related to activation of GAL-R1 (ventral hippocampus) and GAL-R2 (dorsal hippocampus) receptors, respectively. However, the effects of galanin on acetylcholine release and on spatial learning appear not to be directly related to cholinergic mechanisms, but they may also involve interactions with noradrenaline and/or glutamate transmission. Galanin administered into the lateral ventricle failed to affect acetylcholine release, while this route of administration produced a long-lasting reduction in 5-HT release in the ventral hippocampus, indicating that galanin is a potent inhibitor of mesencephalic 5-HT neurotransmission *in vivo*. Subsequent studies supported this hypothesis, showing that the effects on 5-HT release *in vivo* are most likely mediated by a galanin receptor in the dorsal raphe. The implications of these findings are discussed in relation to the role of acetylcholine in cognitive functions in the forebrain and the role of the raphe 5-HT neurons in affective disorders.

Both animal and human studies in the last decade suggest that the neuropeptide galanin (GAL)[1,2] may participate in the spectrum of events related to learning and memory, particularly during pathologic conditions.[3–5] Cognitive impairments in the elderly or in senile dementia of the Alzheimer type are related to dysfunction of cholinergic cell groups in the basal forebrain,[6–8] resulting in both cortical and hippocampal cholinergic neuronal loss.[9] GAL may contribute to the cognitive impairment in patients with Alzheimer's disease by hyperinnervating the degenerating cholinergic basal forebrain neurons[10–12] and/or by overexpressing hippocampal GAL binding sites.[13]

[d]Address for correspondence: Professor Sven Ove Ögren, Department of Neuroscience, Karolinska Institute, S-171 77 Stockholm, Sweden. Phone, +46-8-728 7074; fax, + 46-8-30 28 75; e-mail: Sven.Ove.Ogren@neuro.ki.se

Since the late 1980s, GAL-like immunoreactivity (GAL-like ir) has been known to coexist with several "classic" neurotransmitters in the brain[14] known to play a role in cognition. From these findings studies were initiated on its role in cognition in rodents. Of particular importance was the demonstration (in colchicine-treated rats) that GAL is colocalized with acetylcholine (ACh) in a population of ACh neurons in the septal nucleus and diagonal band of Broca area (MS/dBBA) projecting to the hippocampal formation.[15,16] On the other hand, cholinergic neurons in the nucleus basalis of Meynert (nBM), which innervate cortical areas, do not contain GAL-like ir in the rat. In the brain stem of the rat, GAL-like ir was found in noradrenergic (NA) neurons of the locus coeruleus[17,18] and in the serotonin (5-HT) neurons of the dorsal and medial raphe nuclei,[19] projecting inter alia to the hippo-campus and cortex. In view of this anatomy, the physiologic effects of GAL might involve multiple interactions at both pre- and postjunctional levels, producing both changes in neurotransmitter release and actions at various G-protein–coupled receptors.[20] Studies in the rat have also shown that central administration of GAL can affect (mostly impair) learning and memory in a variety of tasks.[21] The effects of GAL on cognition have been related mainly to inhibitory effects on ACh transmission.[4] However, the neuronal mechanisms behind the behavioral effects of GAL are far from clear, because limited information exists as to the effects of exogenously administrated GAL on neurotransmitter function *in vivo*. The recent development of HPLC methodology with increased sensitivity has made it feasible for the first time to measure the very low levels of ACh and 5-HT in the awake rat in the hippocampus,[22,23] making it possible to examine the effects of GAL on both basal and evoked ACh release in anatomically relevant areas, such as the hippocampus, and to relate these changes to the behavioral effects of the infused peptide.

This paper reviews this development and presents evidence for exogenous GAL as a potent *in vivo* modulator of both brain ACh and 5-HT transmission. The consequences of the GAL-mediated modulation of basal ACh and 5-HT transmission for learning and memory in two different types of tasks, such as the spatial swim maze task and the aversive paradigm, the passive avoidance task, are presented and discussed.

EFFECTS OF GALANIN INFUSIONS INTO THE VENTRAL HIPPOCAMPUS ON SPATIAL LEARNING

Previous studies in the rat indicated that GAL acts as an inhibitor of brain cholinergic transmission in the basal forebrain, acting by decreasing the evoked ACh release. Thus, GAL administered through the lateral ventricle (icv) blocked scopolamine-induced ACh release *in vitro* and *in vivo* in the ventral but not in the dorsal part of the hippocampus.[24,25] Moreover, GAL given icv also reduced potassium-evoked ACh release in awake rats.[26] These findings support the general notion that GAL affects learning via inhibitory modulation of ACh release in the basal forebrain, such as the ventral hippocampus.[3,4] Therefore, analysis of the function of the cholinergic systems in the basal forebrain is required to understand the role of GAL in cognition.

Both cortical and hippocampal cholinergic systems have been implicated in the neuronal and molecular mechanisms underlying learning and memory in humans and in the rat.[27–29] The projection from the medial septum (e.g., the septohippocampal projection) gives rise to an extensive cholinergic innervation of the entire hippocampal formation.[30] Damage to the medial septum (MS) mimics many of the effects on cognition observed after extensive damage to the hippocampus. For example, electrolytic or excitotoxic lesions of the MS result in severe disturbances of both acquisition and retention in various spatial learning memory tasks,[29,31,32] giving evidence for an important role for this pathway in spatial memory.[29,32] However, later lesioning studies of the MS/dBBA with more selective excitotoxins, such as AMPA, failed to find a direct correlation between impairment of spatial performance and loss of ACh neurons.[6,28,33] This suggests that the effects of electrolytic lesioning on learning may at least partly reflect concomitant damages to GABAergic cells in the MS.[28,34] Interpretation of the role of the cholinergic neurons in the hippocampus was further complicated by studies using intracerebral microinjections of the neuronal immunotoxin 192IgG-saporin which causes an extensive and selective loss of cholinergic cells in the MS/dBBA.[6,35] The results with 192IgG-saporin are complex but generally indicate that the selective lesioning of hippocampal ACh neurons produces only marginal effects on spatial learning and memory.[6] Thus, microinjections of 192IgG-saporin into either the nBM or MS/dBBA produced unimpaired or marginal effects on swim maze acquisition.[36,37] By contrast, systemic administration of nonselective muscarinic antagonists such as scopolamine produced profound impairment in spatial learning.[28] These discrepancies suggest differential roles for cholinergic pathways within the septo-hippocampal projection. Alternatively, multiple neurotransmitter dysfunctions might be required for a behavioral deficit. Therefore, it seems likely that the roles of GAL may differ depending on the type of GAL/neurotransmitter coexistence within the hippocampus. It is notable that in the rat most GAL-ACh–containing neurons derived from the cholinergic cells in MS/dBBA and projecting to the hippocampus innervate mainly the ventral and, to a lesser extent, the dorsal hippocampus.[15,18]

These considerations led us to use site-specific injections of GAL into the ventral part of the hippocampus which contains the majority of ACh/GAL coexisting neurons and many GAL binding sites.[38] The effects of ventral hippocampal GAL were examined in the Morris swim maze task, which is a test for visuospatial learning.[39] Performance in this task depends on the integrity of the hippocampal formation.[40] Rats are required to localize a hidden platform that is submerged below the surface of a pool filled with water.[41] Spatial cues surrounding the water tank (extra-maze cues) are unchanged from trial to trial, and they are used to locate the platform. Importantly, this reference-memory task must clearly be distinguished from spatial working-memory tasks in which the rat has to remember the information from the previous trial.

Daily bilateral microinjections of porcine GAL were performed with coordinates aimed at the medial part of the ventral hippocampus.[41] This area of the ventral hippocampus has been implicated in spatial learning since discrete kainic-acid lesions of the CA3 hippocampal subregion were shown to produce marked deficits in spatial learning and memory.[42] In several studies, injections of GAL (3 nmol/rat, 1.5 nmol/side for 5 days via chronic cannulas placed in the ventral hippocampus, ivh) using these coordinates have consistently been shown to produce a small, but significant impairment of acquisition of the spatial swim task (FIG. 1). This deficit was evidenced by increased escape latencies to find the submerged platform and longer swim-paths compared with control rats.[41,43,44] The acquisition impairment was not dose-related because the 1-nmol dose of GAL facilitated acquisition,[41] whereas GAL given at a higher dose (6 nmol/rat) failed to affect performance (FIG. 1). This suggests that GAL behaves in a biphasic manner typical for many neuropeptides seen in different learning tasks. The acquisition deficit appeared not to be due to nonlearning impairments involving motor dysfunction or motivational factors since

swim speed was unaffected by intrahippocampal GAL.[41,44] In contrast systemic administration of antimuscarinic agents such as scopolamine consistently increases swim speed.[41]
It remains unclear how this motor dysfunction is related to the marked cognitive deficits
seen after systemic scopolamine.

The acquisition deficit after intrahippocampal GAL (3 nmol/rat) was small compared
to the marked impairments following subcutaneous systemic administration (sc) of scopolamine (0.1–0.3 mg/kg sc).[41] This difference probably reflects the fact that systemic scopolamine blocks many muscarinic receptors in both the cortex and the hippocampus,
whereas local administration of GAL affects a relatively limited area of the ventral hippocampus. Most of the GAL infusion sites were localized in the vicinity of the CA3 area
in the ventral hippocampus (FIG. 2).[44] The recent observation that GAL given icv failed to
produce any significant short-term impairment of swim maze acquisition (to be published)
supports the view of a site-specific action of GAL with respect to spatial learning. To test
this hypothesis, scopolamine was injected into the ventral hippocampus using the same
coordinates as for GAL. Scopolamine (10 µg/rat) infused ivh caused a marked acquisition
deficit much greater than that of GAL (3 nmol; FIG. 3).[45] This finding clearly shows that
cholinergic muscarinic blockade in the ventral hippocampus results in cognitive impairment. Furthermore, since swim speed was only slightly affected by intrahippocampal scopolamine (FIG. 3), similar to GAL, the scopolamine-induced impairment appears not to be

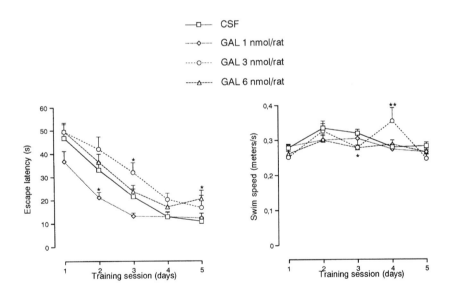

FIGURE 1. Dose-dependent effects of galanin (GAL) on the acquisition of a spatial learning task.
Three different doses of porcine GAL were injected via permanent cannulas placed in the ventral hippocampus (1 nmol, $n = 8$; 3 nmol, $n = 8$; 6 nmol/rat/µl, $n = 16$ or CSF, $n = 16$). The latency to find the
hidden platform as well as swim speed is shown. GAL-treated groups were compared with the CSF
control group using a repeated measure of variance (ANOVA). Fisher's PLSD test was used to compare the different treatments vs control (*$p < 0.05$, **$p < 0.01$). GAL, galanin in all figures. Data
taken from Ögren *et al.*[41] with permission from Elsevier Science.

due to changes in nonlearning factors.[45] Therefore, these data are not in agreement with the reports that selective lesions of hippocampal ACh do not result in behavioral deficits in the Morris swim maze.[36] The results are incompatible with the view that only widespread cortical cholinergic denervation involving both the cortical and the hippocampal projection is a prerequisite for spatial learning deficits in the rat.[46] The discrepancies between pharmacologic blockade of muscarinic cholinergic transmission and disruptive effects of 192IgG-saporin within the hippocampus indicate that different populations of cholinergic neurons may subserve different functional roles in spatial learning. Alternatively, removal of cholinergic neurons by the neurotoxin may result in compensatory changes at efferent targets which result in functional compensation.

However, the behavioral effects of scopolamine clearly are mainly due to blocking action of postsynaptic muscarinic receptors. GAL is also a modulator of muscarinic transmission *in vitro* because it inhibits the muscarinic M_1-receptor–mediated actions on phospholipase C.[47] However, when GAL (3 nmol/rat ivh) was coinfused with scopolamine (10 μg/rat), GAL did not produce any synergistic effect on the inhibitory effect on spatial learning induced by the muscarinic antagonist (FIG. 3).[45] This confirms previous data in which GAL (3 nmol/rat ivh) was given in combination with scopolamine (0.1 mg/kg sc).[41] Besides spatial learning, icv GAL has been reported to impair passive avoidance retention in the rat.[48] Since nucleus basalis-amygdala cholinergic systems are crucially involved in passive avoidance,[49] it is possible that interactions between GAL and ACh occur in limbic

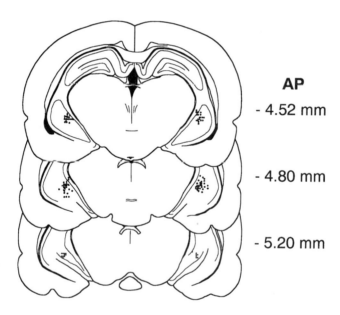

FIGURE 2. Histologic examination (using thionon-stained slides) of the animal receiving porcine GAL or CSF. Each point represents an injection site (*left and right side*) and represents results from 100 animals. Some injection sites are the same for different animals. Brain plates from the Paxinos and Watsons atlas showing, from top, AP −4.52 mm, AP −4.80 mm, and AP −5.20 mm. Data taken from Ögren *et al.*[41] and Schött *et al.*,[44] with permission from Elsevier Science.

areas such as the amygdala. However, in our studies, GAL (0.3–3 nmol/rat, icv) did not alter passive avoidance retention. Furthermore, GAL (3 nmol icv) did not alter the effects of a threshold dose of scopolamine (30 μg/rat icv) (FIG. 4). These findings suggest that cooperative mechanisms of GAL and postsynaptic muscarinic receptors do not contribute to the spatial learning deficit induced by GAL or to interactions with ACh in an aversive learning   task.[41]

Consistent with the effects on acquisition, scopolamine given sc or ivh caused a marked decline in retention examined in a probe trial (without the platform present) 24 hours after the last training trial.[45] By contrast, animals trained under the influence of the 3-nmol dose of GAL were not affected in the spatial retention test when examined 24 hours after the last training session.[44] However, a clear trend for impairment of long-term memory (examined 7 days after the last training session) was observed after the 3-nmol dose of GAL, whereas the 1-nmol dose facilitated retention performance.[41] This suggests a potential effect of GAL on the temporal decay of memory. These data are generally consistent with the view that the GAL-mediated deficit in spatial learning is mainly due to the effects on acquisition mechanisms.[41] However, this conclusion may require revision because recent studies indicate that subtypes of GAL receptors, located heterogeneously in hippocampal subsystems, may subserve different aspects of cognition (see below).

Because the hippocampal formation is considered to operate as a temporary memory buffer,[50] it is critical to investigate the *in vivo* tissue distribution and kinetics of GAL infused ivh with the temporal effect of GAL on spatial learning in the rat. If learning is related to changes in cholinergic transmission, coexisting peptides such as GAL could intervene at various stages in the temporal processing of the information. The importance of *in vivo* kinetics was confirmed when GAL (1.5 nmol/side for 5 days) was infused in the ventral hippocampus at various times before acquisition.[44] An acquisition deficit was seen when GAL (3 nmol/rat) was infused 20 minutes but not 5 minutes before the daily training session. A trend for impairment was observed only when GAL was infused 60 minutes before training.[44] Interestingly, this time-dependent effect on acquisition did not exactly coincide with the peak distribution of the infused peptide (FIG. 5). With an antibody raised against porcine GAL, GAL-like ir was found within the ventral hippocampus with a peak effect 5 minutes after GAL infusion.[44] However, GAL-like ir was rapidly cleared from the extracellular space between 5 and 20 minutes after injection. Thus, five minutes after GAL infusion, immunoreactive nerve cells appeared in the ventral hippocampus both within and outside the zone of extracellularly located GAL (FIG. 6). Morphologically these cells appear to be middle-sized neurons with a similar position as cells showing neuropeptide Y-like immunoreactivity. At 20 and 60 minutes after infusion of GAL, no nerve cells with detectable levels of GAL-like ir could be seen. It seems likely that infused GAL can be internalized as in the case of β-endorphin[51] and rapidly degraded by intracellular peptidases. It is not excluded that metabolically stable short GAL fragments may contribute to some aspects of the effects of GAL on cognition.[52] Together, these results support the view that infused GAL exerts its effects not only via membrane-bound GAL receptors (see below), but also via long-term actions on intracellular events following endocytotic uptake. The rapid clearance of infused GAL indicates that its main action initially is related to actions on the "working memory" components of the spatial learning tasks, whereas at later stages its actions may also affect subsequent processing of reference memory.

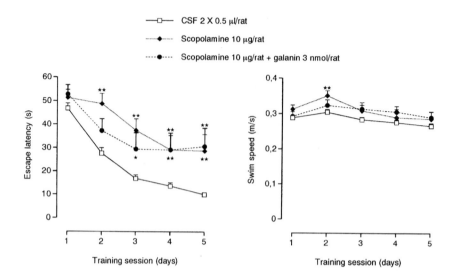

FIGURE 3. Effects of intrahippocampal injections of the muscarinic antagonist scopolamine on swim maze acquisition. Bilateral injection of scopolamine (10 μg/rat/μl) with or without GAL (3 nmol/rat/μl) via permanent cannulas placed in the ventral hippocampus using the same coordinates as in FIGURE 1. Animals ($n = 8$/group) were operated on 7 days prior to the start of the first training session. For further details, see legend of FIGURE 1.

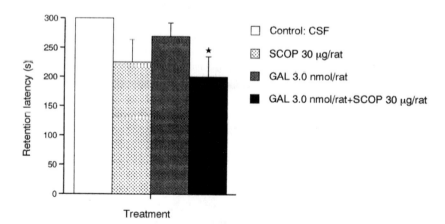

FIGURE 4. Combined effects of GAL and centrally administered scopolamine on passive avoidance (PA) retention in the rat. Rats were injected with scopolamine (30 μg/rat icv bilaterally) and/or GAL (3.0 nmol/rat icv bilaterally) 20 minutes before the training session (exposure to inescapable foot-shock). The CSF (icv bilaterally, 2 μl/side) control group was run concurrently with the scopolamine-and/or GAL-treated group. The retention test was performed 24 hours later. *Vertical bars* represent means (± SEM) of retention latencies in groups of eight to nine ($n = 8$–9) animals. Maximal time of latency was set at 300 seconds (cut-off time). Statistical analysis was performed by two-way ANOVA followed by Fisher's PLSD test. *$p < 0.05$ vs CSF control group. GAL, galanin; SCOP, scopolamine.

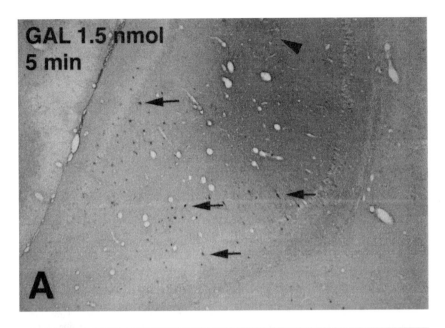

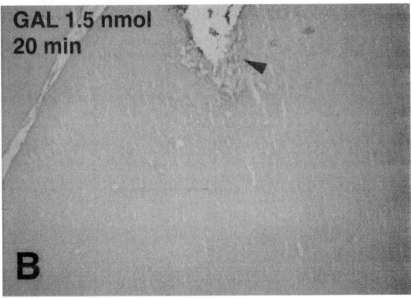

FIGURE 5. *See legend on next page.*

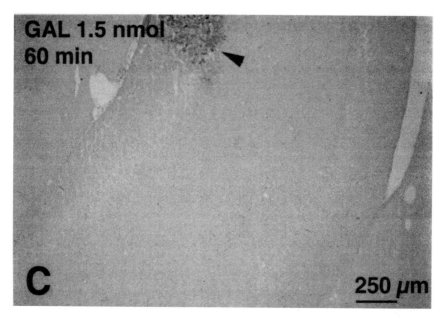

FIGURE 5. Distribution of infused porcine GAL in the ventral hippocampus visualized immunohistochemically using an antibody to porcine GAL. Coronal 14-μm thick cryostat sections showing GAL-like ir in the ventral part of hippocampus. In the upper part of each figure (A-C), the site of infusion tips of the cannula tract is indicated (*arrowhead*). In panel A, 5 minutes after GAL infusion an intense zone of GAL-like ir was observed in the neuropil around the site of infusion, almost covering the entire ventral hippocampus. Numerous cells within the ventral hippocampus also show a GAL-like ir (indicated by *arrows*). At 20 minutes after GAL infusion, panel B, almost no GAL-like ir was observed in the neuropil and no GAL-like ir cells were seen. In panel C, 60 minutes after GAL infusion, no exogenous GAL-like ir was observed in the neuropil. (At the site of infusion a small amount of bleeding was observed). Bars indicate 250 μm. Data taken from Schött *et al.*,[44] with permission from Elsevier Science.

INVOLVEMENT OF DIFFERENT GALANIN
RECEPTORS IN SPATIAL LEARNING

The recent development of chimeric GAL ligands has resulted in GAL antagonists that provide the means to explore the involvement of GAL receptor subtypes in behavior and the role of endogenous GAL in the brain. The role of GAL receptors in spatial learning was analyzed by the use of the high-affinity GAL receptor antagonist M35 which is a chimeric peptide [galanin(1-13)-bradykinin(2-9)-amide].[1] M35 at higher doses caused a reduction of extracellular ACh when perfused through the striatum and in the hippocampus (like GAL), suggesting a partial agonistic profile.[53] Therefore, a lower dose (1 nmol/rat) of M35 was employed in the *in vivo* studies. This dose blocked the GAL-induced reduction in basal ACh extracellular concentrations without influencing the basal levels of ACh.[53]

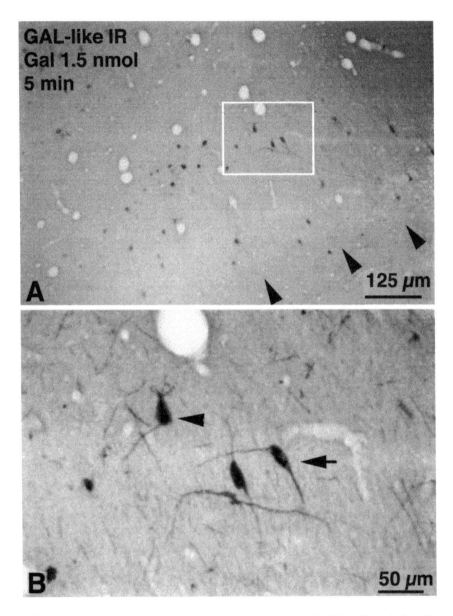

FIGURE 6. GAL-like ir cells in the ventral hippocampus 5 minutes after GAL infusion in the region (**A**). Cells in the framed area are shown at higher magnification in **B**. The ventral part of CA1 is outlined by *arrowheads* in **A**. The GAL-like ir cells (**B**) are from a morphologic point of view medium-sized neurons showing intense immunoreactivity. The location of the GAL-like ir cells in **A**, indicated by *arrows* and *arrowheads* in **B**, are in the vicinity of the CA3 region in the ventral hippocampus. Bars indicate 125 or 50 μm. Data taken from Schött *et al.*,[44] with permission from Elsevier Science.

The acquisition impairment induced by GAL (3 nmol/rat ivh) was completely blocked by M35 (1 nmol/rat ivh), suggesting that GAL at least partly exerts its action at the level of the ventral hippocampus via membrane-bound high-affinity GAL receptors.[45] Importantly, M35 (1 nmol/rat) injected into the ventral hippocampus did not by itself affect acquisition.[45] This suggests that GAL has a permissive role in spatial learning. Alternatively, multiple GAL receptor subtypes at several anatomic locations have to be affected to influence acquisition. However, the recent discovery of at least two GAL receptors with different anatomic locations in the brain has complicated the interpretation of the in vivo effects of infused GAL. The GAL-R1-receptor mRNA expression is high in the ventral hippocampus and correlates roughly with the pattern of [^{125}I]GAL binding.[54–56] The recently discovered GAL-R2 receptor[57] was found to be expressed mainly in the dorsal hippocampus, particularly the granular cell layer in the dentate gyrus.[58] That M35 has about equal affinity for the two receptors[58] implies that the inhibitory effect on spatial learning induced by exogenous GAL in the ventral hippocampus is mainly mediated via the GAL-R1 subtype.

The lack of effect on cognition after intrahippocampal M35 contrasts with earlier findings of a potential involvement of endogenous GAL in spatial learning. Thus, icv administration of M35 (6 but not 3 nmol/rat) significantly facilitated acquisition in the Morris swim maze without significantly altering swim speed.[5] M35 (6 nmol) also tended to facilitate retention when tested 7 days after training. The receptor autoradiographic analysis revealed that when given icv [^{125}I]M35 bound preferentially in the periventricular regions including the hippocampus, especially its ventral part, suggesting that the antagonist could influence ACh transmission in this region. However, M3,[5] (icv) failed to affect basal ACh release in the ventral hippocampus (unpublished data). On the other hand, icv M35 influenced evoked ACh release in this region, because it fully counteracted the inhibitory effects of GAL (icv) on scopolamine-induced increase in ACh release in the ventral hippocampus.[25] Together, given the distribution of icv M35, GAL receptors located in the locus coeruleus and dorsal raphe and to some extent the cerebral cortex will be occupied by M3.[5] This suggests that cognitive effects of GAL involve multiple neurotransmitter systems besides that of ACh.

EFFECTS OF GALANIN ON ACETYLCHOLINE RELEASE IN THE VENTRAL HIPPOCAMPUS: RELATIONSHIP TO SPATIAL LEARNING

Evidence for the existence of antagonistic GAL/ACh interactions in the hippocampus was first obtained in studies on potassium-evoked release of [^{3}H]-ACh. GAL induced inhibition of evoked [^{3}H]-ACh release in slices from rats or monkeys, however, could only be demonstrated in the ventral but not the dorsal hippocampus.[24,26] GAL given icv also inhibited ACh release induced by scopolamine in the forebrain.[24] The first direct evidence for an inhibitory effect of GAL on basal and scopolamine-evoked release of ACh in the ventral hippocampus in vivo was provided by microdialysis studies.[41] GAL was perfused through the ventral hippocampus in freely moving rats to avoid the profound effects of anesthesia on the action of GAL.

Perfusion (100 min) with GAL (0.1 nmol or 0.3 nmol/1.25 µl/min) through the ventral hippocampal probe (using the same coordinates as in the studies on spatial learning) resulted in a dose-dependent reduction of basal ACh release (FIG. 7). The inhibiting effect of GAL was reversible within 20–30 minutes after cessation of perfusion through the

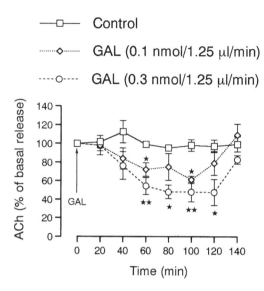

FIGURE 7. Effects of GAL on basal ACh release in the ventral hippocampus in freely moving rats. GAL was infused (0.1 or 0.3 nmol/1.25 μl/min, by adding to the perfusion liquid) for 100 minutes locally into the ventral hippocampus. *Arrow* indicates the start of GAL infusion. Each value represents the average ACh concentration (mean ± SEM) in 20-minute samples from three different groups of rats (n = 4/group). *p < 0.05, **p < 0.01 versus all corresponding time points for the concurrent control values (Fisher's PLSD test). Data taken from Ögren *et al.*[41] with permission from Elsevier Science.

probe, confirming earlier findings that GAL is rapidly cleared from the site of perfusion or injection.[44] The inhibitory effects of GAL on basal ACh release appeared to be mediated by GAL receptors, because it was blocked by M35.[53] These findings indicate that GAL in the ventral hippocampus modulates basal ACh transmission mainly by stimulating GAL-R1 receptors. On the other hand, GAL (3 nmol/10 μl icv or through the probe [0.3 nmol/1.25 μl/min]) attenuated the increase in scopolamine (0.1 mg/kg sc; 0.001 nmol/1.25 μl/min through the probe)-evoked ACh release. GAL (3 nmol/10 μl icv) failed to affect basal ACh release in this region,[41] which is consistent with earlier data.[24] These results point to the similarity in mechanism(s) underlying GAL-mediated inhibition of scopolamine induced and basal ACh release.[41]

GAL infused into the ventral hippocampus can inhibit spatial learning and also reduce ACh release *in vivo* by stimulating GAL receptors which probably are of the GAL-R1 type. However, the causal relation between these two events is not clear. Thus, the inhibitory effect of exogenous GAL on spatial learning cannot strictly be related to changes in *in vivo* cholinergic transmission in the ventral hippocampus. The effect of exogenous GAL on cognition is not dose-related, unlike the effect on ACh release which suggests partial involvement of noncholinergic neurons, such as glutamate and/or NA. Future studies should attempt to directly relate the temporary reduction in ACh release after injected GAL to cognitive performance. This point is especially relevant, because recent double-labeling studies have shown that most immunohistochemically detectable GAL in the hippocampus is found in NA neurons.[59] Because GAL inhibits NA release from hypothalamic slices *in vitro* mediated partly via α_2-adrenergic receptors,[60] a role for NA in the cognitive actions of GAL can be envisioned. Although it is generally believed that GAL receptors located presynaptically regulate ACh release in the septohippocampal projection,[21,24] there appears to be no coexpression of GAL-R1 mRNA within cholinergic neurons in the MS/ dBBA of the rat.[61] By contrast, extensive coexpression of GAL-R1 mRNA was detected within neurons of the bed nucleus of the stria terminals and medial amygdala which coexpress vasopressin and GAL.[61] These neurons project to both the hippocampus and the septum. Therefore, our data suggests that the inhibiting action of GAL on both cognition and basal ACh release could partly be due to noncholinergic mechanisms[41] that indirectly influence ACh release.

EVIDENCE FOR A DIFFERENTIAL ROLE OF GALANIN ON SPATIAL LEARNING AND BASAL ACETYLCHOLINE RELEASE IN DORSAL VERSUS VENTRAL HIPPOCAMPUS

Unlike the ventral hippocampus, the dorsal hippocampus contains a low density of high affinity [^{125}I]-GAL binding sites with many GAL fragment (1-15) binding sites.[62,63] Previous studies have also shown marked differences in the innervation of GAL in these two parts of the rat hippocampus.[64,65] In a recent immunohistochemical study using double-labeling technique all GAL-containing neurons in the dorsal hippocampus were localized within NA neurons derived from the locus coeruleus.[59] Furthermore, GAL did not affect evoked [^{3}H]-ACh in slices prepared from the dorsal region.[24] It was therefore assumed that GAL infused through this region would not modulate basal ACh release. Contrary to this expectation, perfusion of GAL through the probe evoked a marked dose-related increase in basal ACh release in the awake rat (FIG. 8).[45] A significant elevation of basal ACh release was observed when GAL was perfused through the dialysis probe at a concentration of 0.3 nmol/1.25 µl/min, whereas no effect was noted at 0.1 nmol/1.25 µl/min, which is the same concentration range as that found earlier for the inhibitory effect of GAL on ACh release in the ventral hippocampus.[41] This increase in basal ACh release was related to the time of perfusion of the peptide, because the level of ACh returned to baseline within 20 minutes after cessation of perfusion.[41,53] This finding further underlines the importance of the kinetics of GAL for its *in vivo* action also in the dorsal hippocampus.[44] The stimulatory effect of GAL on ACh in the dorsal hippocampus was fully blocked by coperfusion with M35 (0.1 nmol/1.25 µl/min), indicating possible mediation via GAL-R2 receptors.[59] Because there is no evidence for GAL receptors on septohippocampal cholinergic terminals[61] and in view of the GAL-NA coexistence in this region,[59] the increase in basal ACh release might be mediated via NA transmission. GAL-mediated stimulation of GAL-R2 receptors located at the prejunctional level may alter the action of hippocampal NA neurons, resulting in subsequent changes in ACh release. An alternative interpretation is that the GAL-mediated stimulatory effect on ACh involves action on GAL fragment receptors, which are numerous in this region.[52]

In view of the facilitatory effects on ACh release, one would predict changes in spatial learning. In these studies GAL was injected in the dorsal CA1 subregion of the hippocampus which, based on excitotoxic kainic acid lesioning, has been implicated in spatial learning.[42] Interestingly, GAL was reported to inhibit long-term potentiation at Schaffer collateral-CA1 synapses in guinea pig hippocampal slices,[66] whereas local injections of

GAL into this area failed to affect short-term memory in the rat (operant delayed non-matching to sample task).[67] However, local injection of GAL at the 1-nmol dose clearly facilitated the acquisition of the spatial task during the first 3 days of training without any change in swim speed (FIG. 9). Consistent with the results in the ventral hippocampus, this facilitatory effect was not dose-dependent because the 3-nmol dose produced only a trend for a facilitation (FIG. 9). Thus, unlike the ventral hippocampus, dorsal hippocampal injections of GAL do not result in cognitive impairment.

Taken together, GAL in the dorsal hippocampus might modulate ACh transmission and facilitate spatial learning by mechanisms that involve stimulation of GAL receptors, possibly the GAL-R2 receptor. These results support our early notion that the mechanisms underlying the GAL-mediated effects on ACh release and on cognition are not directly related.[41] Furthermore, these findings are also consistent with the view that subareas of the hippocampus may play differential roles in information processing.[68] Inasmuch as dorsal and ventral hippocampus have different afferent and efferent connections,[69] the exciting possibility exists that GAL-mediated dissociative actions on divisions of the hippocampus may, depending on the configuration of the afferent cholinergic input, result in functional compensation or severe dysfunction.

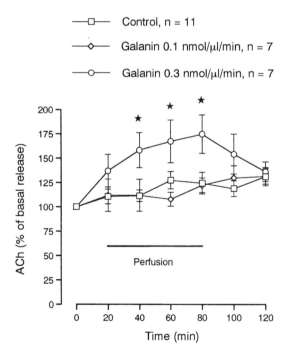

FIGURE 8. Effects of GAL on basal ACh release in the dorsal hippocampus in freely moving rats. GAL was infused (0.1 or 0.3 nmol/1.25 μl/minute, by adding to the perfusion liquid) for 80 minutes locally into the dorsal hippocampus. Each value represents the average ACh concentration (mean ± SEM) in 20-minute samples from three different groups of rats (*n* = 4/group). *p < 0.05, **P < 0.01 vs all the corresponding time points for the concurrent control values (Fisher's PLSD test). Data taken from Schött *et al.*,[44] submitted manuscript.

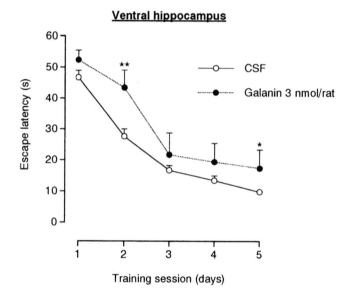

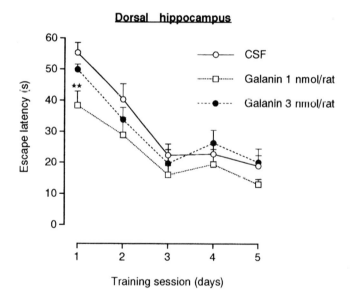

FIGURE 9. Effects of GAL infusion in the dorsal hippocampus on swim maze acquisition. Two different doses of GAL were injected via permanent cannulas in the dorsal hippocampus (1 nmol, $n = 8$; 3 nmol/rat/µl, $n = 8$ or CSF, $n = 8$). Latency to find the hidden platform is shown. For further details, see legend of FIGURE 1. Data taken from Schött et al.,[44] submitted manuscript.

INTRAVENTRICULAR GALANIN AS A POTENT MODULATOR OF 5-HT RELEASE IN THE FOREBRAIN: RELATION TO PASSIVE AVOIDANCE

In vitro and *in vivo* studies have emphasized the importance of interactions between GAL and central 5-HT_{1A} receptors at the pre- and postjunctional level.[52] For instance, GAL was found to attenuate the deficit of passive avoidance retention induced by the 5-HT_{1A} agonist 8-OH-DPAT in the rat.[70] This deficit induced by 8-OH-DPAT is mainly due to stimulation of postsynaptic 5-HT_{1A} receptors.[71] Based on the *in vivo* distribution of injected GAL, these results indicate that GAL can exert a short-term modification of postsynaptic 5-HT_{1A}-mediated transmission *in vivo* in discrete cell populations in forebrain regions such as the dorsal and ventral hippocampus.[70] There is also evidence that galaninergic mechanisms related to 5-HT neurons in the dorsal raphe nucleus of the rat can regulate 5-HT neuronal activity at the level of the cell body.[52,72]

In a recent study the effects of icv administered GAL on 5-HT release in the ventral hippocampus were measured by *in vivo* microdialysis.[23] A newly developed, highly sensitive method for detecting concentrations as low as 80 attomol 5-HT in the microdialysis samples[73] allowed determination of basal extracellular 5-HT without the need for citalopram (or another 5-HT reuptake blocker) in the perfusion medium. GAL (0.5 and 1.5 nmol icv) caused a dose-related and long-lasting (more than 3 hours) suppression of basal 5-HT levels in the rat ventral hippocampus (FIG. 10). This reduction was almost completely blocked by icv injection of the antagonist M35 at a dose of 1.5 nmol 120 minutes before GAL administration.[23] However, at higher doses, M35 itself reduced basal extracellular 5-HT in the rat hippocampus, indicating a partial agonistic mode of action also in 5-HT neurons.

The mechanism of the long-lasting effect of GAL on hippocampal 5-HT release *in vivo* is currently under investigation. In view of the results with M35, icv GAL may exert its action by blocking GAL receptors in the dorsal raphe. This conclusion is supported by our recent finding that perfusion of GAL via probes in the ventral hippocampus failed to affect 5-HT release.[23] Electron microscopic immunohistochemical studies provide clear evidence for the existence of at least three types of synaptic contacts in the dorsal raphe:[72] (a) GAL-positive axons making synaptic contacts on non-GAL dendrites, (b) axon terminals contacting dendrites that contain both GAL and 5-HT, and (c) GAL-positive, 5-HT–negative axon terminals making contacts with 5-HT immunoreactive dendrites. The accompanying measurements of GAL-R1 receptor expression by *in situ* hybridization did not prove the existence of the GAL-R1 receptor in the raphe nuclei,[72] indicating that GAL-R2 or a third type of GAL receptor may be expressed by 5-HT-ergic raphe neurons. However, a recent report using an autoradiographic receptor binding technique indicated moderate GAL-R1 and GAL-R2 receptor binding in the raphe nucleus with equal occupancy of the respective receptors.[74]

The long-lasting effect of icv GAL on basal 5-HT release is intriguing, because the half-life of the injected peptide in brain tissue appears to be short.[44] However, other data also indicate that the physiologic effects of GAL in the ventricular space may be long-lasting. GAL induced intense c-Fos expression in the nucleus of the solitary tract and reticular nuclei 6 hours after its intracisternal injection.[75] Also, the effects of GAL on ingestive behavior indicate long-lasting inhibitory effects of icv GAL, manifested by suppression of food and water intake for at least 8 hours following the initial stimulation of eating.[76] Studies are in progress to identify whether internalization in target cells by cell

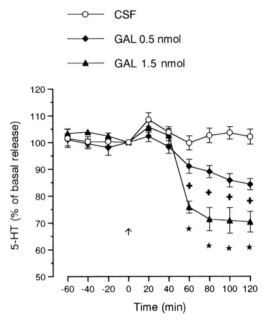

FIGURE 10. Reduction of GAL administered icv on basal 5-HT release in the ventral hippocampus. GAL (0.5 or 1.5 nmol/rat) or artificial CSF was infused via a unilateral cannula in the lateral ventricle. The microdialysis probe was placed in the ventral part of the hippocampus using the coordinates in FIGURE 1. *Arrow* indicates the time for GAL or CSF injection. Each value represents the average 5-HT concentration (mean ± SEM) in 20-minute samples from three different groups of rats (n = 4/ group). For further details, see legend of FIGURE 7. Data taken from Kehr *et al.*,[23] submitted manuscript.

surface receptors and/or formation of GAL fragments contributes to this prolonged action of the neuropeptide.[52,70]

The observation that GAL (3 nmol/rat) given icv inhibits 5-HT release but fails to affect ACh release in the ventral hippocampus[41] is interesting and points to differential effects on aspects of cognitive performance. This difference is not simply due to differential brain kinetics, because after icv injection of GAL, GAL-like ir appeared in nerve cells in both the dorsal and the ventral hippocampus[70] and at the level of the dorsal raphe nucleus. Despite the marked reduction in hippocampal 5-HT release, GAL (3 nmol/rat) given icv failed to impair swim maze acquisition (to be published) and also passive avoidance retention.[70] The passive avoidance task was highly sensitive to 5-HT$_{1A}$ receptor-mediated transmission in the limbic forebrain.[71] The observation that injected GAL attenuated the impairment induced by the 5-HT$_{1A}$ agonist 8-OH-DPAT in this task suggests that the functional interaction between GAL and 5-HT occurs at the postjunctional level. It is also likely that changes in 5-HT release in the forebrain will functionally affect certain aspects of muscarinic receptor-mediated transmission. Furthermore, a recent study showed a powerful interaction between 5-HT$_{1A}$ and muscarinic receptors in the control of passive avoidance retention.[77]

CONCLUSION

These findings show that GAL is a potent *in vivo* modulator of basal ACh release in the rat brain with a differential action in the dorsal and ventral hippocampus. Although the mechanism behind these differential effects is not clear, the effects of GAL seem to involve noncholinergic mechanisms that indirectly modify presynaptic ACh transmission. GAL also exerts differential effects on spatial learning in the dorsal and ventral hippocampus which probably partly reflects noncholinergic mechanisms, such as glutamate and/or NA transmission. These results therefore indicate that depending on the cholinergic pathways involved, GAL can dissociate between different aspects of hippocampal information transfer. Since the dorsal and ventral hippocampus have a different input/output relationship, the possibility of severe cognitive deficits could follow if the cholinergic dysregulation is combined with galaninergic upregulation in the entire hippocampal formation. This seems to be the case in Alzheimer's disease in which GAL receptors are upregulated in the hippocampal formation including the subiculum.[13] This gives potential for integrative effects of GAL on hippocampal transmission at both the afferent and efferent side (output). The failure of increases in ACh transmission via cholinesterase inhibition to restore hippocampally mediated function may be due to a failure to effectively overcome imbalances at the input-output level controlled mainly by glutamate and GABA. In this context an effective GAL antagonist may be of value to "normalize" synaptic input in the hippocampal subsystems.

The hyperpolarizing action of GAL on dorsal raphe neurons *in vitro*[72] and the potent and long-lasting inhibition of 5-HT release *in vivo* indicate that centrally administered GAL is a potent inhibitor of mesencephalic 5-HT neurotransmission. From the current data it seems likely that the *in vivo* actions on 5-HT release are mediated by a GAL receptor in the dorsal raphe, whereas the role for the somatodendritic 5-HT$_{1A}$ receptor has not been clarified as yet. In addition, centrally administrated GAL has potent modulatory effects on 5-HT$_{1A}$-mediated responses in the forebrain.[70] These *in vivo* actions occur at surprisingly low doses (3 nmol/rat icv) suggesting that GAL or possibly GAL fragments released in the ventricular space can exert long-term physiologic effects. In conclusion, the potential role of GAL–5-HT interactions in a variety of 5-HT–related CNS pathologic conditions warrant further exploration.

REFERENCES

1. BARTFAI, T., G. FISONE & Ü. LANGEL. 1992. Galanin and galanin antagonists: Molecular and biochemical perspectives. Trends Pharmacol. Sci. **13:** 312–317.
2. TATEMOTO, K., Å. RÖKAEUS, H. JÖRNVALL, T.J. MCDONALD & V. MUTT. 1983. Galanin: A novel biologically active peptide from porcine intestine. FEBS Lett. **164:** 124–128.
3. CRAWLEY, J.N. & G.L. WENK. 1989. Co-existence of galanin and acetylcholine: Is galanin involved in memory processes and dementia? Trends Neurosci. **12:** 278–282.
4. CRAWLEY, J.N. 1993. Functional interactions of galanin and acetylcholine: Relevance to memory and Alzheimer's disease. Behav. Brain Res. **57:** 133–141.
5. ÖGREN, S.O., T. HÖKFELT, K. KASK, Ü. LANGEL & T. BARTFAI. 1992. Evidence for a role of the neuropeptide galanin in spatial learning. Neuroscience **51:** 1–5.
6. GALLAGHER, M. & P.J. COLOMBO. 1995. Ageing: The cholinergic hypothesis of cognitive decline. Curr. Opin. Neurobiol. **5:** 161–168.

7. COYLE, J.T., D.L. PRICE & M.R. DELONG. 1983. Alzheimer's disease: A disorder of cortical cholinergic innervation. Science **219:** 1184–1190.

8. BARTUS, R.T., R.L.D. DEAN, B. BEER & A.S. LIPPA. 1982. The cholinergic hypothesis of geriatric memory dysfunction. Science **217:** 408–414.

9. TERRY, R.D. & P. DAVIES. 1980. Dementia of the Alzheimer type. Annu. Rev. Neurosci. **3:** 77–95.

10. BEAL, M.F., U. MACGARVEY & K.J. SWARTZ. 1990. Galanin immunoreactivity is increased in the nucleus basalis of Meynert in Alzheimer's disease. Ann. Neurol. **28:** 157–161.

11. CHAN-PALAY, V. 1988. Neurons with galanin innervate cholinergic cells in the human basal forebrain and galanin and acetylcholine coexist. Brain Res. Bull. **21:** 465–472.

12. MUFSON, E.J., E. COCHRAN, W. BENZING & J.H. KORDOWER. 1993. Galaninergic innervation of the cholinergic vertical limb of the diagonal band (Ch2) and bed nucleus of the stria terminalis in aging, Alzheimer's disease and Down's syndrome. Dementia **4:** 237–250.

13. RODRIGUEZ-PUERTAS, R., S. NILSSON, J. PASCUAL, A. PAZOS & T. HÖKFELT. 1997. ^{125}I-galanin binding sites in Alzheimer's disease: Increases in hippocampal subfields and a decrease in the caudate nucleus. J. Neurochem. **68:** 1106–1113.

14. HÖKFELT, T., D. MILLHOR, K. SEROOGY, Y. TSURUO, S. CECCATELLI, B. LINDH, B. MEISTER, T. MELANDER, M. SCHALLING, T. BARTFAI & L. TERENIUS. 1987. Coexistence of peptides with classical neurotransmitters. Experimentia **43:** 768–780.

15. SENUT, M.C., D. MENETREY & Y. LAMOUR. 1989. Cholinergic and peptidergic projections from the medial septum and the nucleus of the diagonal band of Broca to dorsal hippocampus, cingulate cortex and olfactory bulb: A combined wheatgerm agglutinin-apohorseradish peroxidase-gold immunohistochemical study. Neuroscience **30:** 385–403.

16. MELANDER, T., W.A. STAINES, T. HÖKFELT, Å. RÖKAEUS, F. ECKENSTEIN, P.M. SALVATERRA & B.H. WAINER. 1985. Galanin-like immunoreactivity in cholinergic neurons of the septum-basal forebrain complex projecting to the hippocampus of the rat. Brain Res. **360:** 130–138.

17. HOLETS, V.R., T. HÖKFELT, Å. RÖKAEUS, L. TERENIUS & M. GOLDSTEIN. 1988. Locus coeruleus neurons in the rat containing neuropeptide Y, tyrosine hydroxylase or galanin and their efferent projections to the spinal cord, cerebral cortex and hypothalamus. Neuroscience **24:** 893–906.

18. MELANDER, T., T. HÖKFELT & Å. RÖKAEUS. 1986. Distribution of galanin-like immunoreactivity in the rat central nervous system. J. Comp. Neurol. **248:** 475–517.

19. MELANDER, T., T. HÖKFELT, Å. RÖKAEUS, A.C. CUELLO, W.H. OERTEL, A. VERHOFSTAD & M. GOLDSTEIN. 1986. Co-existence of galanin-like immunoreactivity with catecholamines, 5-hydroxytryptamine, GABA and neuropeptides in the rat CNS. J. Neurosci. **6:** 3640–3654.

20. KARELSON, E. & Ü. LANGEL. 1998. Galaninergic signalling and adenylate cyclase. Neuropeptides **32:** 197–210.

21. CRAWLEY, J.N. 1996. Minireview: Galanin-acetylcholine interactions: Relevance to memory and Alzheimer's disease. Life Sci. **58:** 2186–2199.

22. KEHR, J., P. DECHENT & S.O. ÖGREN. 1998. Simultaneous determination of acetylcholine, choline and physostigmine in microdialysis samples from rat hippocampus by microbore liquid chromatography/electrochemistry on peroxidase redox polymer coated electrodes. J. Neurosci. Methods **83:** 143–150.

23. KEHR, J., T. YOSHITAKE, F.-H. WANG, L. GIMENEZ-LLORT, J. ISHIDA, M. YAMAMGUCHI & S.O. ÖGREN. 1998. Galanin is a potent modulator of mesencephalic serotonergic neurotransmission. Eur. J. Neurosci. Submitted.

24. FISONE, G., C.F. WU, S. CONSOLO, Ö. NORDSTRÖM, N. BRYNNE, T. BARTFAI, T. MELANDER & T. HÖKFELT. 1987. Galanin inhibits acetylcholine release in the ventral hippocampus of the rat: Histochemical, autoradiographic, *in vivo*, and *in vitro* studies. Proc. Natl. Acad. Sci. USA **84:** 7339–7343.

25. CONSOLO, S., R. BERTORELLI, P. GIROTTI, P.C. LA, T. BARTFAI, M. PARENTI & M. ZAMBELLI. 1991. Pertussis toxin-sensitive G-protein mediates galanin's inhibition of scopolamine-evoked acetylcholine release *in vivo* and carbachol-stimulated phosphoinositide turnover in rat ventral hippocampus. Neurosci. Lett. **126:** 29–32.

26. FISONE, G., T. BARTFAI, S. NILSSON & T. HÖKFELT. 1991. Galanin inhibits the potassium-evoked release of acetylcholine and the muscarinic receptor-mediated stimulation of phosphoinositide turnover in slices of monkey hippocampus. Brain Res. **568:** 279–284.

27. BARTUS, R.T., R.L. DEAN, M.J. PONTECORVO & C. FLICKER. 1985. The cholinergic hypothesis: A historical overview, current perspective, and future directions. Ann. N.Y. Acad. Sci. **444**: 332–358.

28. FIBIGER, H.C. 1991. Cholinergic mechanisms in learning, memory and dementia: A review of recent evidence. Trends Neurosci. **14**: 220–223.

29. OLTON, D.S., B.S. GIVENS, A.M. MARKOWSKA, M. SHAPIRO & S. GOLSKI. 1992. Mnemonic functions of the cholinergic septohippocampal system. *In* Memory: Organization and Locus of Change. L.R. Squire, N.M. Weinberger, G. Lynch & J.L. McGaugh, Eds. :250–269. Oxford University Press. New York.

30. KOLIATSOS, V.E., L.J. MARTIN & D.L. PRICE. 1990. Efferent organization of the mammalian basal forebrain. *In* Brain Cholinergic Systems. M. Steriade & D. Biesold, Eds. :120–152. Oxford University Press. New York.

31. HAGAN, J.J. & R.G.M. MORRIS. 1988. The cholinergic hypothesis of memory: A review of animal experiments. *In* Handbook of Psychopharmacology. L.L. Iversen, S.D. Iversen & S.H. Snyder, Eds. :237–323. Plenum Press. London.

32. HAGAN, J.J., J.D. SALAMONE, J. SIMPSON, S.D. IVERSEN & R.G. MORRIS. 1988. Place navigation in rats is impaired by lesions of medial septum and diagonal band but not nucleus basalis magnocellularis. Behav. Brain Res. **27**: 9–20.

33. DUNNETT, S.B., B.J. EVERITT & T.W. ROBBINS. 1991. The basal forebrain-cortical cholinergic system: Interpreting the functional consequences of excitotoxic lesions. Trends Neurosci **14**: 494–501.

34. SHEN, R., L.M. TILLEKERATNE, J.R. KIRCHHOFF & R.A. HUDSON. 1996. 6-Hydroxycatecholine, a choline-mimicking analogue of the selective neurotoxin, 6-hydroxydopamine. Biochem. Biophys. Res. Commun. **228**: 187–192.

35. BOOK, A.A., R.G. WILEY & J.B. SCHWEITZER. 1992. Specificity of 192 IgG-saporin for NGF receptor-positive cholinergic basal forebrain neurons in the rat. Brain Res. **590**: 350–355.

36. BAXTER, M.G., D.J. BUCCI, L.K. GORMAN, R.G. WILEY & M. GALLAGHER. 1995. Selective immunotoxic lesions of basal forebrain cholinergic cells: Effects on learning and memory in rats. Behav. Neurosci. **109**: 714–722.

37. BERGER-SWEENEY, J., S. HECKERS, M.-M. MESULAM, R. WILEY, D.A. LAPPI & M. SHARMA. 1994. Differential effects on spatial navigation of immunotoxin-induced cholinergic lesions of the medial septal area and nucleus basalis magnocellularis. J. Neurosci. **14**: 4507–4519.

38. MELANDER, T., C. KÖHLER, S. NILSSON, T. HÖKFELT, E. BRODIN, E. THEODORSSON & T. BARTFAI. 1988. Autoradiographic quantitation and anatomical mapping of ^{125}I-galanin binding sites in the rat central nervous system. J. Chem. Neuroanat. **1**: 213–233.

39. MORRIS, R.G.M. 1981. Spatial localization does not require the presence of local cues. Learn. Motiv. **12**: 239–260.

40. MORRIS, R.G., P. GARRUD, J.N. RAWLINS & J. O'KEEFE. 1982. Place navigation impaired in rats with hippocampal lesions. Nature **297**: 681–683.

41. ÖGREN, S.O., J. KEHR & P.A. SCHÖTT. 1996. Effects of ventral hippocampal galanin on spatial learning and on *in vivo* acetylcholine release in the rat. Neuroscience **75**: 1127–1140.

42. STUBLEY-WEATHERLY, L., J.W. HARDING & J.W. WRIGHT. 1996. Effects of discrete kainic acid-induced hippocampal lesions on spatial and contextual learning and memory in rats. Brain Res. **716**: 29–38.

43. ÖGREN, S.O. & A. PRAMANIK. 1991. Galanin: Regulation of cholinergic function and behaviour. *In* Cholinergic Basis for Alzheimer Therapy. R. Becker & E. Giacobini, Eds. :193–199. Birkhäuser. Boston.

44. SCHÖTT, P.A., B. BJELKE & S.O. ÖGREN. 1998. Distribution and kinetics of galanin infused into the ventral hippocampus of the rat: Relationship to spatial learning. Neuroscience **83**: 123–136.

45. SCHÖTT, P.A., J. KEHR, J. SANDIN & S.O. ÖGREN. 1998. Galanin differentially modulates spatial learning and *in vivo* acetylcholine release in ventral and dorsal hippocampus of the rat. Neuroscience. Submitted.

46. LEANZA, G., J. MUIR, O.G. NILSSON, R.G. WILEY, S.B. DUNNETT & A. BJÖRKLUND. 1996. Selective immunolesioning of the basal forebrain cholinergic system disrupts short-term memory in rats. Eur. J. Neurosci. **8**: 1535–1544.

47. PALAZZI, E., S. FELINSKA, M. ZAMBELLI, G. FISONE, T. BARTFAI & S. CONSOLO. 1991. Galanin reduces carbachol stimulation of phosphoinositide turnover in rat ventral hippocampus by lowering Ca^{2+} influx through voltage- sensitive Ca^{2+} channels. J. Neurochem. **56:** 739–747.
48. HIRAMATSU, M., H. MORI, H. MURASAWA & T. KAMEYAMA. 1996. Improvement by dynorphin A (1-13) of galanin-induced impairment of memory accompanied by blockade of reductions in acetylcholine release in rats. Br. J. Pharmacol. **118:** 255–260.
49. RIEKKINEN, P., JR., M. RIEKKINEN & J. SIRVIO. 1993. Cholinergic drugs regulate passive avoidance performance via the amygdala. J. Pharmacol. Exp. Ther. **267:** 1484–1492.
50. EICHENBAUM, H., T. OTTO & N.J. COHEN. 1992. The hippocampus--what does it do? Behav. Neural. Biol. **57:** 2–36.
51. FUXE, K., X.-M. LI, B. BJELKE, P.B. HEDLUND, G. BIAGINI & L.F. AGNATI. 1994. Possible mechanisms for the powerful actions of neuropeptides. *In* Models of Neuropeptide Action. F.L. Strand, B. Beckwith, B. Chronwall & C.A. Sandman, Eds. :42–59. Ann. N.Y. Acad. Sci. New York.
52. FUXE, K., A. JANSSON, Z. DIAZ-CABIALE, A. ANDERSSON, B. TINNER, U.-B. FINNMAN, I. MISANE, H. RAZANI, F.-H. WANG, L.F. AGNATI & S.O. ÖGREN. 1998. Galanin modulates 5-hydroxy-tryptamine functions. Focus on galanin and galanin fragment/5-hydroxytryptamine1A receptor interactions in the brain. Ann. N.Y. Acad. Sci. This volume.
53. ANTONIOU, K., J. KEHR, K. SNITT & S.O. ÖGREN. 1997. Differential effects of the neuropeptide galanin on striatal acetylcholine release in anaesthetized and awake rats. Br. J. Pharmacol. **121:** 1180–1186.
54. PARKER, E.M., D.G. IZZARELLI, H.P. NOWAK, C.D. MAHLE, L.G. IBEN, J. WANG & M.E. GOLDSTEIN. 1995. Cloning and characterization of the rat GALR1 galanin receptor from Rin14B insulinoma cells. Mol. Brain Res. **34:** 179–189.
55. BURGEVIN, M.C., I. LOQUET, D. QUARTERONET & E. HABERT-ORTOLI. 1995. Cloning, pharmacological characterization, and anatomical distribution of a rat cDNA encoding for a galanin receptor. J. Mol. Neurosci. **6:** 33–41.
56. HABERT-ORTOLI, E., B. AMIRANOFF, I. LOQUET, M. LABURTHE & J.F. MAYAUX. 1994. Molecular cloning of a functional human galanin receptor. Proc. Natl. Acad. Sci. USA **91:** 9780–9783.
57. HOWARD, A.D., C. TAN, L.L. SHIAO, O.C. PALYHA, K.K. MCKEE, D.H. WEINBERG, S.C. GEGHNER, M.A. CASCIERI, R.G. SMITH, L.H.T. VAN DER PLOEG & K.A. SULLIVAN. 1997. Molecular cloning and characterization of a new receptor for galanin. FEBS Lett. **405:** 285–290.
58. FATHI, Z., A.M. CUNNINGHAM, L.G. IBEN, P.B. BATTAGLINO, S.A. WARD, K.A. NICHOL, K.A. PINE, J. WANG, M.E. GOLDSTEIN, T.P. IISMAA & I.A. ZIMANYI. 1997. Cloning, pharmacological characterization and distribution of a novel galanin receptor. Mol. Brain Res. **51:** 49–59.
59. XU, Z.-Q.D., T.-J.S. SHI & T. HÖKFELT. 1998. Galanin/GMAP- and NPY-like immunoreactivities in locus coeruleus and noradrenergic nerve terminals in the hippocampal formation and cortex with notes on the galanin-R1 and -R2 receptors. J. Comp. Neurol. **392:** 227–251.
60. TSUDA, K., H. YOKOO & M. GOLDSTEIN. 1989. Neuropeptide Y and galanin in norepinephrine release in hypothalamic slices. Hypertension **14:** 81–86.
61. MILLER, M.A., P.E. KOLB & M.A. RASKIND. 1997. GALR1 galanin receptor mRNA is co-expressed by galanin neurons but not cholinergic neurons in the rat basal forebrain. Mol. Brain Res. **52:** 121–129.
62. MELANDER, T., T. HÖKFELT, S. NILSSON & E. BRODIN. 1986. Visualization of galanin binding sites in the rat central nervous system. Eur. J. Pharmacol. **124:** 381–382.
63. HEDLUND, P.B., N. YANAIHARA & K. FUXE. 1992. Evidence for specific N-terminal fragment binding sites in the rat brain. Eur. J. Pharmacol. **224:** 203–205.
64. MELANDER, T. & W.A. STAINES. 1986. A galanin-like peptide coexists in putative cholinergic somata of the septum-basal forebrain complex and in acetylcholinesterase-containing fibers and varicosities within the hippocampus in the owl monkey (*Aotus trivirgatus*). Neurosci. Lett. **68:** 17–22.
65. GABRIEL, S.M., P.J. KNOTT & V. HAROUTUNIAN. 1995. Alterations in cerebral cortical galanin concentrations following neurotransmitter-specific subcortical lesions in the rat. J. Neurosci. **15:** 5526–5534.
66. SAKURAI, E., T. MAEDA, S. KANEKO, A. AKAIKE & M. SATOH. 1996. Galanin inhibits long-term potentiation at Schaffer collateral-CA1 synapses in guinea-pig hippocampal slices. Neurosci. Lett. **212:** 21–24.

67. ROBINSON, J.K. & J.N. CRAWLEY. 1994. Analysis of anatomical sites at which galanin impairs delayed nonmatching to sample in rats. Behav. Neurosci. **108:** 941–950.
68. ROBINSON, J.K. & J.B. MAO. 1997. Differential effects on delayed non-matching-to-position in rats of microinjections of muscarinic receptor antagonist scopolamine or NMDA receptor antagonist MK-801 into the dorsal or ventral extent of the hippocampus. Brain Res. 765: 51–60.
69. JONES, E.G. & T.P.S. POWELL. 1970. An anatomical study of converging pathways within *the cerebral* cortex of monkey. Brain **93:** 793–820.
70. MISANE, I., H. RAZANI, F.-H. WANG, A. JANSSON, K. FUXE & S.O. ÖGREN. 1998. Intraventricular galanin modulates a $5-HT_{1A}$ receptor-mediated behavioural response in the rat. Eur. J. Neurosci. **10:** 1230–1240.
71. MISANE, I. C. JOHANSSON & S.O. ÖGREN. 1998. Analysis of the $5-HT_{1A}$ receptor involvement in passive avoidance in the rat. Br. J. Pharmacol. **125:** 499–509.
72. XU, Z.-Q.D., X. ZHANG, V.A. PIERIBONE, S. GRILLNER & T. HÖKFELT. 1998. Galanin-5-hydroxytryptamine interactions: Electrophysiological, immunohistochemical and *in situ* hybridization studies on rat dorsal raphe neurons with a note on galanin R1 and R2 receptors. Neuroscience **87:** 79–94.
73. ISHIDA, J., T. YOSHITAKE, K. FUJINO, K. KAWANO, J. KEHR & M. YAMAGUCHI. 1998. Serotonin monitoring in microdialysate from rat brain by microbore-HPLC with fluorescence detection. Anal. Chim. Acta **365:** 227–232.
74. BRANCHEK, T.A., E.L. GUSTAFSON, M.W. WALKER, C. FORRAY, K.E. SMITH, C. GERALD & M.M. DURKIN. 1997. Autoradiographic localization of the GALR2 receptor subtype in the rat CNS [abstr.]. Soc. Neurosci. Abstr. **23:** 965.
75. DIAZ, Z., P. MARCOS, M.P. CORDON, R. COVENAS, J.A. AGUIRRE, P.B. HEDLUND & K. FUXE. 1997. C-fos expression induced by galanin in brainstem nuclei of the rat [abstr.]. Soc. Neurosci. Abstr. **23:** 966.
76. ERVIN, G.N., A.P. DUNN, C.A. TALBOT, S.A. BRAMER, A. SCHOFIELD, T.A. BRANCHEK, S.A. NOBLE & W.E. HEYDORN. 1997. Unique features of feeding induced by intraventricular galanin 1–29 (GAL) in the rat [abstr.]. Soc. Neurosci. Abstr. **23:** 1074.
77. MISANE, I., F.-H. WANG, A. FISHER & S.O. ÖGREN. 1998. Interactions between central muscarinic and $5-HT_{1A}$ receptors in passive avoidance in the rat. Eur. J. Neurosci. Submitted.

Galanin: A Significant Role in Depression?

JAY M. WEISS,[a] ROBERT W. BONSALL, MELISSA K. DEMETRIKOPOULOS,
MILBURN S. EMERY, AND CHARLES H.K. WEST

*Emory University School of Medicine, Department of Psychiatry and Behavioral Sciences,
1256 Briarcliff Road, Atlanta, Georgia 30306, USA*

ABSTRACT: This paper describes a hypothesis that attempts to account for how changes in noradrenergic systems in the brain can affect depression-related behaviors and symptoms. It is hypothesized that increased activity of the locus coeruleus (LC) neurons, the principal norepinephrine (NE)-containing cells in the brain, causes release of galanin (GAL) in the ventral tegmentum (VTA) from LC axon terminals in which GAL is colocalized with NE. It is proposed that GAL release in VTA inhibits the activity of dopaminergic cell bodies in this region whose axons project to forebrain, thereby resulting in two of the principal symptoms seen in depression, decreased motor activation and decreased appreciation of pleasurable stimuli (anhedonia). The genesis of this hypothesis, which derives from studies using an animal model of depression, is described as well as recent data consistent with the hypothesis. The formulation proposed suggests that GAL antagonists may be of therapeutic benefit in the treatment of depression.

The research described here addresses the question of how noradrenergic neurons can affect symptoms seen in depression. Although it has been evident for more than 30 years that noradrenergic neurons can play a significant role in ameliorating depression, how this occurs has not been evident. The major difficulty in formulating such an explanation is that basic research provides little evidence of a link between noradrenergic activity in the brain and depression-related behavior. The hypothesis explored here is that the major noradrenergic neuronal system in the brain, the locus coeruleus (LC) dorsal bundle noradrenergic system, influences depressive symptoms by affecting the activity of dopaminergic neurons in the ventral tegmental region of the brain. In regard to the focus of this volume, it is suggested that this significant influence of LC neurons is exerted via release of galanin from terminals on LC axons.

AN ANIMAL MODEL FOR STUDY OF DEPRESSION

We have studied depression for more than two decades using a rodent model. In this model, laboratory rats are exposed to electric shocks that they cannot control, after which they show numerous behavioral changes seen in depression (see summary in Weiss[1]). Insofar as human clinical depression is preceded by stressful events, this model bears etiologic similarity to depression. With respect to the symptoms seen in the model, after exposure to the uncontrollable stressor, rats show decreased motor activity, decreased food/water consumption accompanied by weight loss, decreased grooming, and decreased competitive behavior. The animals also show sleep disturbance characterized by "early morning awakening," increased errors in discrimination tasks, and decreased responding for "rewarding brain stimulation." These symptoms closely correspond to those listed for the

[a]Author for correspondence. Phone, 404/894-5948; fax, 404/894-5901; e-mail, jweis01@emory.edu

diagnosis of depression in recent editions of the "Diagnostic and Statistical Manual of the American Psychiatric Association."[2,3] In addition to resembling depression in terms of symptoms, several effective treatments for relieving depression, such as electroconvulsive shock and drug therapy, have been shown to counteract the stress-induced behavioral deficits enumerated above or to prevent their occurrence. In summary, the model resembles clinical depression with respect to aspects of etiology, symptoms, and responsiveness to treatment. It approximates human depression in at least as many respects as does any other animal model currently in use.[4–6]

Much effort has focused on analyzing physiologic changes responsible for the depression-like symptoms in the aforedescribed model, the rationale being that uncovering these physiologic changes is likely to reveal processes that are relevant to the pathophysiology of depression in view of the similarity of the model to human clinical depression. Beginning in the late 1960s, various studies showed a relationship between the depression-like behavioral changes seen in this model and disturbance of norepinephrine (NE) in the brain (see summary in Weiss *et al.*[7]). In the early 1980s, investigators began to localize the NE disturbance, reporting that NE depletion of large magnitude in the LC region of the brain was particularly closely associated with the behavioral changes seen in the model.[8–11] This led to a hypothesis describing the functional significance of this change.[12] It was hypothesized that large-magnitude depletion of NE in the LC region resulted in decreased release of NE that normally stimulates inhibitory α_2-receptors on LC neurons. Thus, depression-related symptoms in the model were hypothesized to result from a stress-induced "functional blockade" of inhibitory somatodendritic α_2-receptors on LC neurons. Various pharmacologic manipulations of α_2-receptors in the LC region, both blockade and stimulation of these receptors, produced changes in depression-like behavior that were consistent with this formulation.[13–15] Electrophysiologic single-unit recordings of LC activity also yielded results consistent with this formulation. Functional blockade of inhibitory α_2-receptors in the LC region would be expected to produce hyperresponsivity of LC neurons, particularly an increase in "burst firing" of LC neurons that occurs in response to excitatory stimuli.[16] Electrophysiologic recording of LC neurons indicated that animals manifesting depression-like behavioral changes showed increased LC activity and LC hyperresponsivity, and that the degree of behavioral depression observed in individual animals was related to the degree of LC hyperresponsivity shown by these animals.[17]

By tracing depression-like behavior to elevated activity of LC neurons, the research just reviewed confronts us with the question of how increased activity of LC neurons might cause depression-like behavior. Increased activity of LC neurons would be expected to cause an increase in the amount of NE released from LC terminals throughout the forebrain. However, this simply raises once again a major issue for the neurobiology of depression, which is how a formulation that points to a change in brain NE (and this includes explanations of drug action, such as tricyclic antidepressants) can explain changes in depression-related behavior. This issue is based on many years of research that has failed to reveal how altering brain NE influences behavior related to depression. Experimentally produced changes in brain NE have been reported to affect motor activity,[18] investigatory behavior,[19] and sleep,[20] but the effects seen are small and subtle and point in no clear way to how altering this neurotransmitter directly affects depression-related symptoms (e.g., see refs. 21–24). (Actually, the same issue applies to serotonin in the brain, so that the mechanism by which drugs that alter 5HT in the brain affect depression-related behavior is also unclear.) But in contrast to NE, research related to dopamine (DA) in the brain has revealed that this monoamine exerts a strong influence on behavioral responses and processes highly relevant to depression. Manipulation of forebrain DA profoundly affects motor activity (e.g., see refs. 25–27) and processes related to reward (hedonic value of stimuli) (e.g., see refs. 28–30). Thus, at least two of the major symptoms of depression, decreased motor activity and decreased appreciation of pleasure, represent responses that are importantly influenced by brain DA. Decreases in normal DA release and/or DA postsynaptic receptor stimulation in the forebrain would be expected to produce these symptoms. One possibility, then, by which NE might influence depression would be for NE to modulate activity of brain DA systems and thereby affect depression-related symptoms.

A POTENTIALLY IMPORTANT NEW FINDING

One suggestion for how this might occur, and a possibility that we feel is potentially important for this entire area of research, developed from an article published by Grenhoff *et al.* in 1993.[31] In their paper, the latest of a series that examined electrophysiologic links between NE and DA neurons,[32–34] the investigators demonstrated that NE released from terminals on axons that originate in the LC and project to the ventral tegmentum (VTA) potentiates firing of dopaminergic cell bodies in the VTA whose axons then project to the limbic forebrain (nucleus accumbens [NACC], prefrontal cortex [PFC]). This was done by stimulating the LC region with a single electrical pulse and observing augmented firing of VTA cells projecting to dopaminergic regions in the forebrain. The excitatory influence of NE was mediated, as might be expected, through an α_1 receptor, which was demonstrated by blocking this effect with prazosin but not with idazoxan or timolol. Unfortunately, defining an excitatory influence of LC activity on VTA-DA cells offered nothing new for explaining depression-related symptoms. Not only would excitation of VTA-DA neurons be expected to produce the opposite of behavioral depression, but also the indication that LC-NE activity could potentiate DA cell activity in VTA had first been reported almost 20 years earlier.[35,36]

However, Grenhoff *et al.* then conducted an important additional manipulation; they repeatedly stimulated the LC region to try to reproduce the burst firing pattern of LC neurons that occurs *in vivo* in response to excitatory input. Instead of finding an even larger potentiation of VTA-DA electrophysiologic cell activity than that which occurred with single-pulse LC stimulation, these investigators found that simulation of burst firing produced a marked suppression of DA cell activity. FIGURE 1 shows the contrast between what occurs when a single electrical pulse or 20 pulses are delivered to the LC prior to electrophysiologic recording from a DA cell in the VTA. Whereas a single pulse causes excitation of the DA cell, multiple pulses delivered to the LC result in profound inhibition of the VTA-DA cell. In relation to the pathophysiology of depression as described previously in this paper, Grenhoff *et al.* appeared to have discovered a circumstance in which heightened LC activity will inhibit DA cell depolarization, thus potentially providing the link between the NE and DA systems that is needed to explain the pathophysiology of depression-like behavioral changes. Moreover, their finding specifically linked the LC-derived inhibition of VTA-DA cells to burst firing of LC neurons, which the electrophysiologic studies cited above[17] had shown to be the particular parameter of LC activity that was most affected in the animal model of depression described here. This pointed to a hypothesis that will now be described.

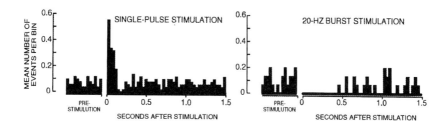

FIGURE 1. Electrophysiologic activity of a dopaminergic cell in the ventral tegmentum (VTA) following electrical stimulation of the locus coeruleus (LC). At top is shown the number of depolarizations recorded from a VTA dopamine (DA) cell body after the LC was stimulated with a single 0.5-ms electrical stimulus delivered to the LC region. At the bottom is shown the number of depolarizations recorded after delivery of a train of 20 such electrical pulses to the LC with 49.5 ms intervening between each pulse. Data for this figure were constructed from computer scanning of Figures 1 and 3 of Grenhoff *et al.* (1993). These data show that VTA DA cell depolarizations were increased over the baseline (i.e., prestimulation) firing rate after a single electrical pulse to the LC but were markedly inhibited after a train of 20 pulses.

LINKING BRAIN NOREPINEPHRINE TO DEPRESSION-RELATED RESPONSES VIA DOPAMINE AND GALANIN

Findings by Grenhoff *et al.* suggest that heightened burst firing of LC neurons will inhibit the electrophysiologic activity of DA neurons in the VTA, which would result in reduced DA release in the forebrain and thus produce depression-related behavioral changes such as reduced motor activity and lack of responsivity to rewarding stimuli. This formulation can link activity of NE-containing neurons to depression-like behavior. But how does one explain how LC activity inhibits DA cell firing when NE release in the VTA potentiates DA cell activity through an α_1 receptor? Grenhoff *et al.* rejected the notion that NE itself might inhibit VTA neuronal activity (as had been suggested by microiontophoretic studies using very high doses of NE) because (1) pharmacologic treatment to block adrenoreceptors did not affect the inhibition, and (2) reserpine-treated rats, which failed to show VTA activation by single-pulse LC stimulation, did show VTA inhibition in response to burst-type stimulation of the LC. Such results suggest a non-noradrenergic mechanism for the inhibition. One possibility discussed by Grenhoff *et al.*, which is central to the hypothesis described here, is that the inhibition of DA neurons in the VTA is accomplished through the release of the peptide galanin from LC terminals.

Galanin (GAL) is colocalized with NE in most LC neurons (80–100%)[37–40] and therefore will be released from NE-containing terminals on LC axons (e.g., ref. 41). The VTA contains GAL-immunoreactive fibers[38,39] and ^{125}I-GAL binding sites[42,43] that are presumed to represent the GAL receptor. Also of importance for the present discussion is the evidence that suggests that the release of GAL and NE from the terminals in which they are colocalized is not well correlated; instead, when NE neurons depolarize at slow, regular rates, little or no GAL is released, but when the terminal membrane depolarizes rapidly, as in burst firing, release of GAL then increases. For example, Consolo *et al.*,[44] using microdialysis, reported that high-frequency stimulation (50 Hz) of the ventral limb of the

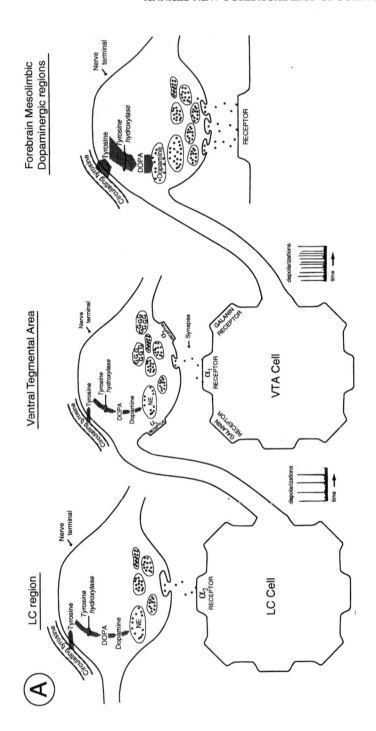

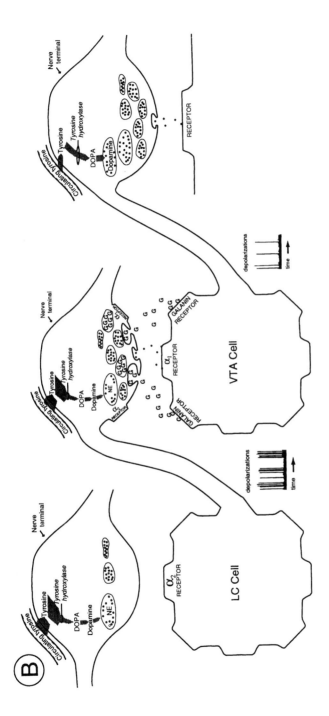

FIGURE 2. Hypothesized neural events that mediate stress-induced behavioral depression. (**A**) The functioning of these neural connections in normal (nonstress) conditions where normal inhibition of LC firing is exerted via NE stimulation of α_2 receptors on LC cell bodies, resulting in moderate depolarization and release of NE onto α_1 receptors in the VTA, thereby promoting release of DA in mesolimbic forebrain regions. (**B**) Hypothesized sequence in stress-induced behavioral depression. In this instance, large-magnitude NE depletion in terminals in the LC region reduces stimulation of inhibitory α_2 receptors on LC cells (i.e., causes "functional blockade" of α_2 receptors), thereby producing increased "burst" firing of these neurons, which leads to release of GAL in the VTA, which, in turn, inhibits firing of the VTA DA neurons and thereby decreases release of DA in the forebrain.

diagonal band caused release of GAL in the ventral hippocampus, whereas lower frequency (10 Hz) stimulation was largely ineffective in producing GAL release. Extrapolating this to the projection regions of the LC, base-rate firing of an LC neuron would be
expected to cause little or no GAL to be released from LC terminals, whereas burst firing
of LC cells, and especially augmented burst firing, would result in release of significant
amounts of GAL. Finally, and of considerable relevance for the hypothesis being
described here, GAL is known to hyperpolarize neurons, including monoaminergic neurons,[45] and to have inhibitory effects on dopaminergic neurons,[46–49] so this peptide would
be expected to inhibit depolarization of VTA DA cells.

The hypothesis is presented in FIGURE 2. Under normal conditions, shown at the top of
the figure (Part A), LC neurons depolarize mostly in a regular manner, and consequently
terminals on LC axons release NE but little GAL in the VTA; this stimulates DA cells in
the VTA by NE released onto excitatory α_1 receptors. By contrast, what is proposed to
occur when stress produces behavioral depression is shown in the lower portion of the figure (Part B). Severe stress produces NE depletion in the LC region which results in functionally blocked α_2 receptors, leading to augmented burst firing of LC neurons. As a
consequence, GAL is released in large amounts from LC terminals in the VTA so that the
excitatory effect of NE on DA cells via α_1 receptors is overwhelmed by the hyperpolarizing influence of GAL on these cells, and DA cell firing in the VTA is inhibited. The result
of this is decreased DA release in the forebrain regions to which these neurons project,
causing certain behavioral symptoms observed in stress-induced depression, such as
decreased motor activity and anhedonia.

EFFECTS OF STRESSFUL CONDITIONS ON DOPAMINE

How does the hypothesis that a highly stressful condition (exposure to an uncontrollable stressor) will produce depression-like behavioral changes by decreasing DA release in
VTA-DA projection regions fit with previous studies of how stress affects DA release? It
surely does not escape notice that many studies found that the DA systems are activated by
stress. DA metabolite ratios (i.e., DOPAC/DA and HVA/DA ratios), indicative of increased
DA activity, were elevated by acute stressors such as restraint, foot shock, or tail pinch in
NACC, PFC, and striatum (e.g., refs. 50–55). Microdialysis studies confirmed the activating effects of acute stress with respect to DA and its metabolites in these regions (e.g., refs.
56–58). These data offer no support for the hypothesis described above. However, several
recent studies employing stressful conditions similar to those used to generate behavioral
depression in the model described above have reported that such conditions decrease
dopaminergic activity. These include studies using forced swimming,[59] prolonged immo-
bilization,[60] and repeated application of restraint.[61] Also, similar findings were reported in
studies using uncontrollable foot shock[62] and uncontrollable versus controllable foot
shock in which uncontrollable shock showed evidence of decreased release.[63]

A recent study provides the most direct indication to date of whether DA release in
VTA projection regions, particularly in NACC, is decreased in the animal model of
depression just described. As reported by Scott et al.,[64] we estimated turnover by measuring DA and its metabolite DOPAC in NACC and striatum (STR) after the 3.0 hour uncontrollable shock session used to induce behavioral depression; also measured were changes
observed after a much milder stressor–30-minute exposure to a grid-floor compartment in

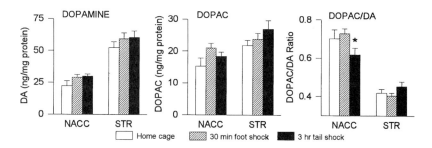

FIGURE 3. Concentration of DA, DOPAC, and DOPAC/DA ratio in the nucleus accumbens (NACC) and striatum (STR) in animals simply removed from their home cage and sacrificed (home cage), animals given a 30-minute footshock session in which they received 7 relatively mild foot shocks (30-minute foot shock), and animals given the standard 3-hour tail-shock session used to produce behavioral depression (3-hour tail shock). Means and standard errors are shown. * Differs significantly (at least $p < 0.05$) from other two conditions.

which the animals received a small number of grid shocks (7 shocks in 30 minutes, each shock 0.4 mA, 2-second duration). Two different selectively bred types of animals were used in this study, but this is not of consequence here as both types of animal responded to these stressors with similar acute changes in DA and DOPAC in NACC and STR. The results (combined across both animal types) are shown below in FIGURE 3. The level of DA rose slightly and equally in both brain regions in response to either stressor condition (30-minute grid shock or 3.0-hour tail shock). However, the concentration of DOPAC in NACC was lower after the 3-hour tail shock than after the 30-minute grid shock, and the DOPAC/DA ratio (right side of figure) was significantly lower in animals that had undergone the 3-hour uncontrollable shock session than it was in animals given no shock (home cage) or the 30-minute stress session. These results indicate that DA activity in NACC was reduced in animals that had been exposed to the uncontrollable shock procedure used in the animal model of depression. Interestingly, DA activity in the STR was not affected in this manner; the DOPAC/DA ratio rose with exposure to the 3-hour stressor condition. These data suggest that the uncontrollable shock procedure used to induce behavioral depression in the model described above results in decreased DA turnover in NACC.

IS THERE GALANIN IN THE VTA REGION THAT IS IN THE LC-NE TERMINALS?

Immunohistochemical studies have demonstrated that GAL is colocalized with NE in most cells of the LC and that GAL is also present in VTA; however, we found no study that specifically addressed the issue of whether any of the GAL in VTA derives from the LC, which is required by the hypothesis shown in FIGURE 2. To address this issue, we made lesions (via 6-hydroxydopamine [6-OHDA]) aimed at the NE dorsal bundle (DB), the main axonal outflow pathway from the LC, and subsequently measured GAL in projection regions of the LC (and also NE and metabolites). Evidence that there is GAL in terminal regions of the LC, including the VTA, that derives from terminals on LC axons would be obtained if GAL found in these terminal regions decreased as a result of the DB lesion. Additionally, as Moore and Gustafson[65] suggested that GAL is transported in axons of the NE ventral bundle (and consequently would appear to be colocalized in NE cells of the caudal brain stem that give rise to the NE ventral bundle), lesions of the ventral bundle (VB) were made as well.

The details of this experiment are as follows: lesions were made by infusion of 6-OHDA aimed at DB using the coordinates of Mason and Iversen.[66] These coordinates were (nosepiece 10 mm below level for flat skull): A-P = −0.6 mm (from lambda), lat = 1.2 mm (from midline), and depth = −6.0 mm (from dura). For lesioning VB the coordinates were (flat skull; cannula angled 10 degrees towards midline): A-P = −4.4 mm (from lambda), lat = 4.3 mm (from midline), and depth = −8.0 mm. In the case of the VB, it is important to emphasize that we therefore lesioned the central tegmental tract posterior to the LC so that any potential innervation of the LC by VB would be interrupted by placement of the lesion here. By comparison, the coordinates for the LC (used for cannula implantations, lesions, or electrophysiologic recording) were (nosepiece 10 mm below flat skull level): A-P = −3.6 mm (from lambda), lat = 1.2 mm (from midline), and depth = −6.0 mm (below dura). Lesions were produced (in halothane-anesthetized animals) by infusion of freshly dissolved 6-OHDA (4 μg/μl; 4μl infused bilaterally; 2-minute infusion time) into the sites just indicated. Following surgery, animals were returned to their home cages where they remained for 2 months (to allow for complete degeneration of NE terminals), at which time animals were sacrificed and brains dissected; subsequently, we measured NE and metabolites DHPG and MHPG, DA and metabolites HVA and DOPAC, serotonin (5-HT) and 5-HIAA, and the peptide GAL in several brain regions. The monoamines and their respective metabolites were assayed by standard HPLC techniques with electrochemical detection (sensitivities ranged from 0.1 to 0.5 pg), whereas GAL was measured by radioimmunoassay using antiserum generously provided by Dr. Steven Gabriel (sensitivity <0.5 pg). (The study described here was also repeated with animals sacrificed 21 days after being lesioned, but for the sake of brevity only the initial study is presented here [i.e., sac. at 60 days postlesion] as the findings of the second study were highly similar.)

The focus of the study was to determine if there would be a relation between NE and GAL in LC terminal regions and if GAL concentration would fall in these regions in lesioned animals. FIGURE 4 shows, in six brain regions, the concentration of NE in relation to the concentration of GAL measured in unoperated control animals (n = 10), animals with 6-OHDA DB lesions (n = 10), and animals with 6-OHDA VB lesions (n = 5). Destruction of DB indeed affected GAL in projection regions of the LC. The most dramatic example was the parietal cortex, where the relation between NE and GAL indicates that all of the GAL in this brain region is colocalized with NE (i.e., total destruction of NE terminals results in total loss of GAL). The relation between NE and GAL in the hippocampus was almost as strong, suggesting that nearly all of the GAL in the hippocampus is colocalized in NE terminals. Most important for the focus of the present study were changes in the ventral tegmental region (VTA). DB lesions resulted in a highly significant decrease in GAL content in the VTA (t = 3.3, $p < 0.005$). The mean GAL content in the VTA of DB-lesioned animals was 39% lower than the mean level in nonlesioned animals; if only those DB-lesioned rats are considered whose NE in the VTA was less than 50% of the mean NE for nonlesioned animals so that only highly effective lesions are included, the GAL level in these animals was 45% lower than that in nonlesioned subjects.

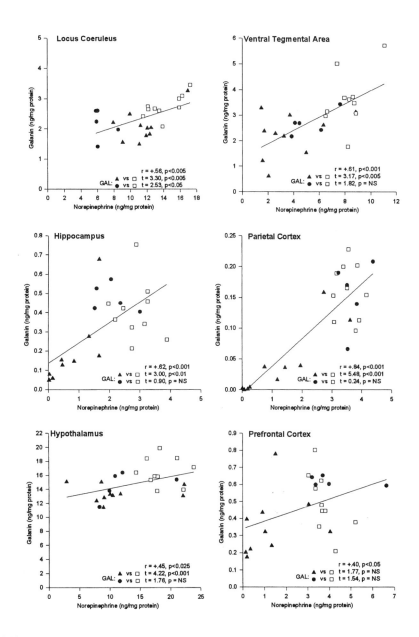

FIGURE 4. Relation between GAL and NE in various brain regions of normal nonlesioned animals (*open squares* □) and animals having had 6-OHDA lesions aimed at either the NE dorsal bundle (DB; *solid triangles* ▲) or NE ventral bundle (VB; *solid circles* ●). At bottom of each graph is the correlation between GAL and NE and the *t* tests comparing GAL concentrations of lesioned and nonlesioned rats.

The findings in FIGURE 4 also make it clear that, as expected, much of the GAL in certain forebrain regions (i.e., hypothalamus, VTA, and prefrontal cortex) is not colocalized with NE. The prime example of this is the hypothalamus. In this case, DB lesions caused a statistically significant reduction in GAL content compared to that in nonlesioned animals, but the magnitude of the decrease was not large (mean change 19%). Lesioning of VB, which significantly reduced NE in the hypothalamus (even including one lesioned animal whose NE in the hypothalamus was not diminished, indicating a "missed" or ineffective lesion in this case), also produced only a small (and nonsignificant) decrease in GAL (mean change 12% [excluding the animal with the "missed" lesion]). Thus, NE terminals in the hypothalamus do not seem to contribute more than about 30% of GAL in the hypothalamus. With respect to the VTA, the findings described here similarly indicate that an appreciable amount of GAL in the VTA is not in NE terminals, although the amount attributable to NE terminals is larger than that in for the hypothalamus (i.e., combining the loss from DB and VB lesions adds up to a decrease in VTA GAL of approximately 60%). It should be kept in mind that for LC neurons to influence VTA-DA cells via GAL does not require all GAL in VTA to derive from LC, only that there is GAL in the VTA which is in LC-NE terminals. The results in FIGURE 5 are consistent with the hypothesis that LC-derived terminals in the VTA contribute GAL to the VTA.

Regarding the contribution of VB NE terminals to GAL in the VTA, the decreases in GAL after lesioning of VB that are shown in FIGURE 4 did not reach statistical significance; however, the decrease in VTA GAL after lesioning of VB was highly significant in the next study in which animals were sacrificed 21 days after lesioning, thus indicating that this pathway indeed contributes GAL to the VTA.

DOES GALANIN MICROINJECTED INTO THE VTA ELICIT DEPRESSION-LIKE RESPONSES?

A major test of the hypothesis that GAL released from NE terminals in the VTA mediates behavioral depression in the model described here is to microinject GAL into the VTA region of animals that have not been exposed to stressful conditions that depress active behavior to determine if GAL acting in the VTA of "nonstressed" animals will cause depression-like behavior. This study is analogous to one we carried out soon after it was hypothesized that stress-induced behavioral depression resulted from "functional blockade" of somatodendritic α_2 receptors in the LC region[13]; in that study, drugs microinjected into normal nonstressed animals to block α_2 receptors in the LC caused decreases in motor activity similar to those seen in stressed animals. Microinjection of GAL into the VTA is a similar next step for the hypothesis described here. Several experiments have now been carried out to examine this.

In all of these studies, bilateral cannulas for microinjection were implanted into the VTA or other brain regions (except for one group given microinjection into the lateral ventricle, for which a single cannula was implanted). Following surgery, animals recovered in their home cages and then were tested 7–10 days later. For testing, animals were removed to a quiet room, cannulas were opened, an infusion device was attached to each cannula, and vehicle (artificial cerebrospinal fluid [CSF]) or GAL (in artificial CSF) was injected. In all studies described here, 3 μl of solution was introduced slowly over a period of 6–7 minutes into awake, ambulatory animals. Following injection, cannulas were closed, and the animal was placed in the appropriate testing apparatus. After the behavioral test, animals were sacrificed, their brains examined for accuracy of cannula placement, and in some cases brain regions were retained for neurochemical analysis.

Effects on Spontaneous Ambulation

In the first experiment, ambulatory activity was measured in a moderate-sized compartment (15×15-inch floor area) that was novel to the animal; photobeam sensors recorded activity during a 40-minute exposure to this compartment. FIGURE 5 shows the effects of microinjecting GAL and control substances (vehicle or heat-treated GAL solution) into the VTA and other brain regions. The microinjection of GAL into the VTA significantly reduced motor activity (both ambulatory and rearing) in this environment. Most noteworthy was that following the first 8 minutes of exploratory activity in this novel environment, ambulation of animals that received GAL into the VTA virtually ceased. When GAL was injected into the lateral ventricle, only rearing behavior but not ambulation decreased; however, injection of GAL into the hypothalamus also decreased ambulation and rearing, thus indicating that GAL acting in other brain regions might also produce an effect on activity in these testing conditions similar to that produced by GAL in the VTA. The hypothesis articulated here does not predict that GAL can only affect motor activity when acting in the VTA. On the other hand, subsequent findings using the swim test (see next two paragraphs) indicated that the activity-reducing effects of GAL, at least in that test situation, were specific to the VTA (see section "C" of FIGURE 6).

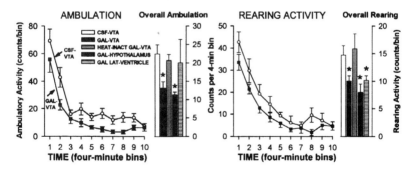

FIGURE 5. Effect of bilateral infusion of GAL (3.0 µg on each side of brain) or control substances (artificial CSF, heat-inactivated GAL) into the VTA on spontaneous ambulatory and rearing activity in a novel environment. Same dose of GAL was also infused bilaterally into the lateral hypothalamus (HYPOTHALAMUS) and into the lateral ventricle via a single cannula (LAT VENTRICLE). Ambulation and rearing in 4-minute periods over the 40 minutes of the activity measurement session is shown as well as the average activity (expressed as counts per 4-minute period) shown by all groups in the entire session. Means and standard errors are shown. To quantify ambulation, repetitive interruptions of the same light beam are ignored so that counts are registered only when the animal moves from one place to another. To quantify rearing, a gross number of interruptions of the upper set of beams was recorded. Statistical significance: *Differs from CSF-infused group at $p < 0.05$ or less.

Effects on Swim-Test Activity

The test we most often employed to quantify reduced motor activity in the model of depression described herein is a modification of the swim test developed by Porsolt to screen for antidepressant medications.[67] In this modification, the tank is larger so that the animal cannot remain immobile by standing on the bottom of the tank, and the animal also wears "water wings" to prevent any sinking that might occur when the animal ceases activity and begins to float. The test therefore quantifies active behavior in a mildly threatening situation whose characteristics tend to evoke active responding. Two responses in the swim test are measured (i.e., duration of behavior is timed): "struggling," defined as all four of the rat's limbs being in motion with the front feet breaking through the surface of the water, and "floating," defined as all four limbs being motionless in the water. Animals whose ambulatory activity is shown in FIGURE 5 were placed into this swim test after ambulatory activity was measured. These particular animals had been bred for higher-than-normal "struggling" activity in the swim test. Among animals that had never been exposed to the swim test previously, VTA GAL versus vehicle had no effect on activity in the swim test. But among those animals ($n = 12$) that had been given a single swim test approximately 1 month earlier so that their tendency to be active in the test was somewhat reduced, GAL microinjection into the VTA significantly ($p < 0.03$) decreased struggling behavior relative to vehicle-injected animals. However, activity in the swim test had not been the primary focus in this study, which is why the measure was not taken until after ambulatory activity was quantified. Swim test activity was the focus of four subsequent experiments, whose results *are shown below.* In these studies, (1) the effects of microinjection into the VTA were tested in normal, nonselected Sprague-Dawley rats, and (2) the test in the water tank was conducted immediately after the microinjections were completed.

In each experiment shown below, floating behavior (i.e., time spent without any limb movement in the water; what Porsolt calls "immobility") was significantly affected by the drug conditions, as we reported previously with drug manipulations of the LC.[14,15] In the first experiment (FIG. 6A), microinjection of GAL into the VTA significantly increased floating in comparison with the artificial CSF vehicle. The next study (B) showed that the ability of VTA GAL to increase floating was dose related and that a statistically significant effect (relative to CSF vehicle control) was found with a thousand-fold dilution of the original 3.0-µg dose (i.e., .003 µg). The next experiment (C) showed that GAL (0.3 µg) injected into other brain regions around the VTA (i.e., 2.0 mm anterior to the VTA [hypothalamus, or HYPO] or 3.0 mm dorsal to the VTA [midbrain reticular formation, or MID]) or into the lateral ventricle did not increase floating as did GAL in the VTA. Finally, an experiment was undertaken to determine if the effect of VTA GAL seen in FIGURE 6A, B, and C could be blocked by a GAL antagonist. In this study, galantide (GTD), an antagonist of GAL,[68] or vehicle was loaded into the microinjection tubing, so that it would be injected just prior to either GAL or its vehicle (CSF). For both GAL and galantide, the dose used was 0.3 µg. The results (FIG. 6D) show that animals given only GAL (i.e., vehicle followed by GAL, or VEH-GAL) showed more floating than did animals given no drug (VEH-CSF). When galantide was given before GAL (GTD-GAL), the increase in floating normally produced by GAL was completely blocked. Finally, and of much interest, galantide alone (GTD-CSF) significantly reduced floating behavior below the level of animals given only vehicle (VEH-CSF).

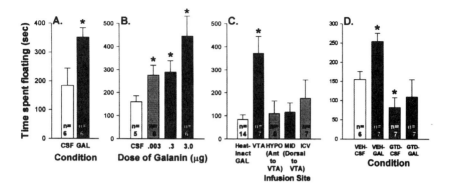

FIGURE 6. Swim test activity (time spent floating) of animals given bilateral microinjections of GAL into the VTA. (**A**) Effect of 3.0 μg GAL versus CSF vehicle. (Doses stated are amount given into each side of brain; icv dose was total given bilaterally.) (**B**) Effect of increasing doses of GAL compared to CSF. (**C**) Effect of microinjecting GAL (3.0 μg) into the VTA, anterior to the VTA (hypothalamus [HYPO]), dorsal to VTA (MID), or into lateral ventricle (ICV). Control was heat-inactivated GAL. Also, female rats were used in this study. (**D**) Effect of infusing GAL antagonist galantide (0.3 μg, GTD) or vehicle (VEH) just before microinjection of GAL (0.3 μg) or CSF. Means and standard errors are shown. *Significantly different (at least $p < 0.05$) from vehicle-injected animals (CSF or VEH-CSF).

Summarizing the results shown in FIGURE 6, GAL in the VTA also reduces motor activity in the swim test and can do so at rather low doses of GAL. The "immobility-producing" effect of GAL in the VTA is not produced by GAL injections nearby or into the lateral ventricle. Also, this effect of GAL in the VTA can be blocked by prior infusion of the GAL antagonist galantide. We observed that microinjection of galantide alone resulted in more motor activity in the swim test than that in animals given no drug (i.e., treated only with vehicles). An explanation for this last result that is consistent with the foregoing, is as follows: the microinjection procedure itself is moderately stressful in that the animal is removed from its home cage and handled, tubes are affixed to its head, and the injection process then occurs in a novel environment over several minutes. These moderately stressful conditions cause endogenous GAL to be released into the VTA, thereby causing some reduction in motor activity even in nondrug (vehicle-treated) animals, and galantide blocks this effect. In summary, data just reported support the view that GAL released in the VTA reduces motor activity.

CONCLUSION

In concluding this presentation, several of ancillary points can be made.

1. Recent findings in humans also suggest that LC neurons are hyperactive in depression. Ordway and colleagues[69] reported that tyrosine hydroxylase is elevated in the LC of persons who have committed suicide, indicating that LC activity was elevated for a considerable period of time prior to death because this enzyme is induced by a high firing rate.

However, higher-than-normal activity of LC neurons can be produced in a variety of ways. For example, some depressed individuals may have a low endogenous concentration of LC somatodendritic α_2 receptors on the LC (for review, see ref. 70) and therefore might show high activity of LC neurons because of a diminished inhibitory influence on LC activity. Although the particular animal model just described manifests increased LC activity because of one specific mechanism (i.e., hypostimulation of inhibitory somatodendritic α_2 receptors on LC neurons), it is important to note that the critical pathogenic factor to which the model directs attention is LC hyperactivity, and human depression could be characterized by LC hyperactivity as a result of different mechanisms only one of which is hypostimulation of somatodendritic α_2 receptors.

2. One issue that informed readers might raise is how the hypothesis presented here can be integrated with the predominant action of certain antidepressants, which is to block NE reuptake and therefore increase the level of NE in the synapse. In this regard, we would point out that an important result of blocking NE reuptake is to profoundly stimulate the inhibitory α_2 somatodendritic receptors on LC neurons and thereby inhibit the firing of LC neurons. Thus, the proposed hypothesis would point to the inhibition of LC neuronal activity and the resultant decrease in GAL release in the VTA as being the potential basis of antidepressant action of such drugs rather than the elevation of NE in synapses throughout much of the brain. In this regard, a significant study by Nestler and colleagues[71] reported that a number of antidepressant drugs administered chronically (which is the therapeutic regimen for such drugs) decreased the concentration of tyrosine hydroxylase in the LC. Whereas a decrease in tyrosine hydroxylase in LC neurons may prove to be an important aspect of the antidepressant action of these drugs, the hypothesis proposed here suggests that another peptide colocalized in LC neurons, GAL, which also is likely to be decreased by a drug-produced decrease in LC activity, may be an even more important part of the therapeutic schema than is the decrease in tyrosine hydroxylase. Decreased GAL synthesis in the LC, resulting from a drug-induced decrease in LC activity, would be proposed to eventually result in decreased GAL release in the VTA with resultant decreased inhibition of VTA-DA neurons, thereby producing an antidepressant effect.

ACKNOWLEDGMENT

The authors wish to express their sincere appreciation to Lorna Clarke for her invaluable assistance in the preparation of this manuscript.

REFERENCES

1. WEISS, J.M. 1991. Stress-induced depression: Critical neurochemical and electrophysiological changes. *In* Neurobiology of Learning, Emotion and Affect. J. Madden, IV, Ed.: 123–154. Raven Press. New York, NY.
2. American Psychiatric Association Diagnostic and Statistical Manual of Mental Disorders. 1980. American Psychiatric Association. Washington, DC.
3. American Psychiatric Association Diagnostic and Statistical Manual of Mental Disorders. 1994. American Psychiatric Association. Washington, DC.
4. WEISS, J.M. & C.D. KILTS. 1998. Animal models of depression and schizophrenia. *In* American Psychiatric Press Textbook of Psychopharmacology, 2nd Ed. C.B. Nemeroff & A.F. Schatzberg, Eds.: 89–131. American Psychiatric Press. Washington, DC.
5. WILLNER, P. 1991. Animal models as simulations of depression. Trends Pharmacol. Sci. **12:** 131–136.

6. MATTHYSSE, S. 1986. Animal models in psychiatric research. Prog. Brain Res. **65:** 259–270.
7. WEISS, J.M., M.K. DEMETRIKOPOULOS, C.H.K. WEST & R.W. BONSALL. 1996. Hypothesis linking the noradrenergic and dopaminergic systems in depression. Depression **3:** 225–245.
8. WEISS, J.M., W.H. BAILEY, L.A. POHORECKY, D. KORZENIOWSKI & G. GRILLIONE. 1980. Stress-induced depression of motor activity correlates with regional changes in brain norepinephrine but not dopamine. Neurochem. Res. **5:** 9–22.
9. WEISS, J.M., P.A. GOODMAN, B.G. LOSITO, S. CORRIGAN, J.M. CHARRY & W.H. BAILEY. 1981. Behavioral depression produced by an uncontrollable stressor: relationship to norepinephrine, dopamine, and serotonin levels in various regions of the rat brain. Brain Res. Rev. **3:** 167–205.
10. HUGHES, C.W., T.A. KENT, J. CAMPBELL, A. OKE, H. CROSKELL & S.H. PRESKORN. 1984. Cerebral blood flow and cerebrovascular permeability in an inescapable shock (learned helplessness) animal model of depression. Pharmacol. Biochem. Behav. **21:** 891–894.
11. LEHNERT, H., D.K. REINSTEIN, B.W. STROWBRIDGE & R.J. WURTMAN. 1984. Neurochemical and behavioral consequences of acute, uncontrollable stress: effects of dietary tyrosine. Brain Res. **303:** 215–223.
12. WEISS, J.M., W.H. BAILEY, P.E. GOODMAN, L.J. HOFFMAN, M.J. AMBROSE, S. SALMAN & J.M. CHARRY. 1982. A model for neurochemical study of depression. *In* Behavioral Models and the Analysis of Drug Action. M.Y. Spiegelstein & A. Levy, Eds.: 195–223. Elsevier. Amsterdam.
13. WEISS, J.M., P.G. SIMSON, L.J. HOFFMAN, M.J. AMBROSE, S. COOPER & A. WEBSTER. 1986. Infusion of noradrenergic receptor agonists and antagonists into the locus coeruleus and ventricular system of the brain. Effects on swim-motivated and spontaneous locomotor activity. Neuropharmacology **25:** 367–384.
14. SIMSON, P.G., J.M. WEISS, M.J. AMBROSE & A. WEBSTER. 1986. Infusion of a monoamine oxidase inhibitor into the locus coeruleus can prevent stress-induced behavioral depression. Biol. Psychiatry **21:** 724–734.
15. SIMSON, P.G., J.M. WEISS, L.J. HOFFMAN & M.J. AMBROSE. 1986. Reversal of behavioral depression by infusion of alpha-2 adrenergic agonist into the locus coeruleus. Neuropharmacology **25:** 385–389.
16. SIMSON, P.E. & J.M. WEISS. 1987. Alpha-2 receptor blockade increases responsiveness of locus coeruleus neurons to excitatory stimulation. J. Neurosci. **7:** 1732–1740.
17. SIMSON, P.E. & J.M. WEISS. 1988. Altered activity of the locus coeruleus in an animal model of depression. Neuropsychopharmacology **1:** 287–295.
18. CAREY, R.J. 1976. Effects of selective forebrain depletions of norepinephrine and serotonin on the activity and food intake effects of amphetamine and fenfluramine. Pharmacol. Biochem. Behav. **5:** 519–523.
19. DELINI-STULA, A., E. MOGILNICKA, C. HUNN & D.J. DOOLEY. 1984. Novelty-oriented behavior in the rat after selective damage of locus coeruleus projections by DSP-4, a new noradrenergic neurotoxin. Pharmacol. Biochem. Behav. **20:** 613–618.
20. KAITIN, K.I., D.L. BLIWISE, C. GLEASON, G. NINO-MURCIA, W.C. DEMENT & B. LIBET. 1986. Sleep disturbance produced by electrical stimulation of the locus coeruleus in a human subject. Biol. Psychiatry **21:** 710–716.
21. AMARAL, D.G. & H.M. SINNAMON. 1977. The locus coeruleus: Neurobiology of a central noradrenergic nucleus. Prog. Neurobiol. **9:** 147–196.
22. CARLI, M., T.W. ROBBINS, J.L. EVENDEN & B.J. EVERITT. 1983. Effects of lesions to ascending noradrenergic neurons on performance of a 5-choice serial reaction task in rats; implication for theories of dorsal noradrenergic bundle function based on selective attention and arousal. Behav. Brain Res. **9:** 361–380.
23. CROW, T.J., J.F.W. DEAKIN, S.E. FILE, A. LONGDEN & S. WENDLANDT. 1978. The locus coeruleus noradrenergic system: Evidence against a role in attention, habituation, anxiety and motor activity. Brain Res. **155:** 249–261.
24. MASON, S.T. 1981. Noradrenaline in the brain: Progress in theories of behavioural function. Prog. Neurobiol. **16:** 263–303.
25. MOGENSON, G.J. & M. NIELSEN. 1984. A study of the contribution of hippocampal-accumbens-subpallidal projections to locomotor activity. Behav. Neural Biol. **42:** 38–51.
26. PIJNENBURG, A.J.J. & J.M. VAN ROSSUM. 1973. Stimulation of locomotor activity following injection of dopamine into the nucleus accumbens. J. Pharm. Pharmacol. **25:** 1003–1005.

27. Museo, E. & R.A. Wise. 1990. Microinjections of a nicotinic agonist into dopamine terminal fields: Effects on locomotion. Pharmacol. Biochem. Behav. **37:** 113–116.
28. Smith, G.P. 1995 Dopamine and food reward. *In* Progress in Psychobiology and Physiological Psychology. A. Morrison & S. Fluharty, Eds. Academic Press. New York, NY.
29. Stellar, J.R. & E. Stellar. 1985. The Neurobiology of Motivation and Reward. Springer-Verlag. New York, NY.
30. Wise, R.A., M. Fotuhi & L.M. Cole. 1989. Facilitation of feeding by nucleus accumbens amphetamine injections: Latency and speed measures. Pharmacol. Biochem. Behav. **32:** 769–772.
31. Grenhoff, J., M. Nisell, S. Ferre, G. Aston-Jones & T.H. Svensson. 1993. Noradrenergic modulation of midbrain dopamine cell firing elicited by stimulation of the locus coeruleus in the rat. J. Neural Transm. Gen. Sect. **93:** 11–25.
32. Grenhoff, J. & T.H. Svensson. 1988. Clonidine regularizes substantia nigra dopamine cell firing. Life Sci. **42:** 2003–2009.
33. Grenhoff, J. & T.H. Svensson. 1989. Clonidine modulates dopamine cell firing in rat ventral tegmental area. Eur. J. Pharmacol. **165:** 11–18.
34. Grenhoff, J. & T.H. Svensson. 1993. Prazosin modulates the firing pattern of dopamine neurons in rat ventral tegmental area. Eur. J. Pharmacol. **233:** 79–84.
35. Anden, N.-E. & M. Grabowska. 1976. Pharmacological evidence for a stimulation of dopamine neurons by noradrenaline in the brain. Eur. J. Pharmacol. **39:** 275–282.
36. Donaldson, I.M., A. Dolphin, P. Jenner, C.D. Marsden & C. Pycock. 1976. The roles of noradrenaline and dopamine in contraversive circling behavior seen after electrolytic lesions of the locus coeruleus. Eur. J. Pharmacol. **39:** 179–191.
37. Holets, V.R., T. Hökfelt, A. Rökaeus, L. Terenius & M. Goldstein. 1988. Locus coeruleus neurons in the rat containing neuropeptide Y, tyrosine hydroxylase or galanin and their efferent projections to the spinal cord, cerebral cortex and hypothalamus. Neurosciences **24:** 893–906.
38. Melander, T., T. Hökfelt & A. Rökaeus. 1986. Distribution of galaninlike immunoreactivity in the rat central nervous system. J. Comp. Neurol. **248:** 475–517.
39. Skofitsch, G. & D.M. Jacobowitz. 1985. Immunohistochemical mapping of galanin-like neurons in the rat central nervous system. Peptides **6:** 509–546.
40. Sutin, E.L. & D.M. Jacobowitz. 1991. Neurochemicals in the dorsal pontine tegmentum. Prog. Brain Res. **88:** 3–14.
41. Bartfai, T., K. Iverfeldt & G. Fisone. 1988. Regulation of the release of coexisting neurotransmitters. Ann. Rev. Pharmacol. Toxicol. **28:** 285–310.
42. Melander, T., C. Kohler, S. Nilsson, T. Hokfelt, E. Brodin, E. Theodorsson & T. Bartfai. 1988. Autoradiographic quantitation and anatomical mapping of ^{125}I-galanin binding sites in the rat central nervous system. J. Chem. Neuroanat. **1:** 213–233.
43. Skofitsch, G., M.A. Sills & D.M. Jacobowitz. 1986. Autoradiographic distribution of ^{125}I-galanin binding sites in the rat central nervous system. Peptides **7:** 1029–1042.
44. Consolo, S., G. Baldi, G. Russi, G. Civenni, T. Bartfai & A. Vezzani. 1994. Impulse flow dependency of galanin release in vivo in the rat ventral hippocampus. Proc. Natl. Acad. Sci. USA **91:** 8047–8051.
45. Seutin, V., P. Verbanck, L. Massotte & A. Dresse. 1989. Galanin decreases the activity of locus coeruleus neurons in vitro. Eur. J. Pharmacol. **164:** 373–376.
46. Gopalan, C., Y. Tian, K.E. Moore & K.J. Lookingland. 1993. Neurochemical evidence that the inhibitory effect of galanin on tuberoinfundibular dopamine neurons is activity dependent. Neuroendocrinology **58:** 287–293.
47. de Weille, J.R., M. Fosset, H. Schmid-Antomarchi & M. Lazdunski. 1989. Galanin inhibits dopamine secretion and activates a potassium channel in pheochromocytoma cells. Brain Res. **485:** 199–203.
48. Jansson, A., K. Kuxe, P. Eneroth & L.F. Agnati. 1989. Centrally administered galanin reduces dopamine utilization in the median eminence and increases dopamine utilization in the medial neostriatum of the male rat. Acta Physiol. Scand. **135:** 199–200.
49. Nordstrom, O., T. Melander, T. Hökfelt, T. Bartfai & M. Goldstein. 1987. Evidence for an inhibitory effect of the peptide galanin on dopamine release from the rat median eminence. Neurosci. Lett. **73:** 21–26.

50. DUNN, A.J. & S.E. FILE. 1983. Cold restraint alters dopamine metabolism in frontal cortex, nucleus accumbens and neostriatum. Physiol. Behav. **31:** 511–513.

51. FADDA, F., A. ARGIOLAS, M.R. MELIS, A.H. TISSARI, P.L. ONALI & G.L. GESSA. 1978. Stress-induced increase in 3,4-dihydroxyphenylacetic acid (DOPAC) levels in the cerebral cortex and in n. accumbens: reversal by diazepam. Life Sci. **23:** 2219–2224.

52. HERMAN, J.P., D. GUILLONNEAU, R. DANTZER, B. SCATTON, L. SEMERDJIAN-ROUQUIER & M. LE MOAL. 1982. Differential effects of inescapable footshocks and of stimuli previously paired with inescapable footshocks on dopamine turnover in cortical and limbic areas of the rat. Life Sci. **30:** 2207–2214.

53. LAVIELLE, S., J.P. TASSIN, A.M. THIERRY, G. BLANC, D. HERVE, C. BARTHELEMY & J. GLOWINSKI. 1979. Blockade by benzodiazepines of the selective high increase in dopamine turnover induced by stress in mesocortical dopaminergic neurons of the rat. Brain Res. **168:** 585–594.

54. THIERRY, A.M., J.P. TASSIN, G. BLANC & J. GLOWINSKI. 1976. Selective activation of the mesocortical DA system by stress. Nature **263:** 242–244.

55. KALIVAS, P.W. & P. DUFFY. 1989. Similar effects of daily cocaine and stress on mesocorticolimbic dopamine neurotransmission in the rat. Biol. Psychiatry **25:** 913–928.

56. KALIVAS, P.W. & P. DUFFY. 1995. Selective activation of dopamine transmission in the shell of the nucleus accumbens by stress. Brain Res. **675:** 325–328.

57. BOUTELLE, M.G., T. ZETTERSTROM, Q. PEI, L. SVENSSON & M. FILLENZ. 1990. In vivo neurochemical effects of tail pinch. J. Neurosci. Methods **34:** 151–157.

58. FINLAY, J.M., M.J. ZIGMOND & E.D. ABERCROMBIE. 1995. Increased dopamine and norepinephrine release in medial prefrontal cortex induced by acute and chronic stress: effects of diazepam. Neuroscience **64:** 619–628.

59. ROSSETTI, Z.L., M. LAI, Y. HMAIDAN & G.L. GESSA. 1993. Depletion of mesolimbic dopamine during behavioral despair: partial reversal by chronic imipramine. Eur. J. Pharmacol. **242:** 313–315.

60. PUGLISI-ALLEGRA, S., A. IMPERATO, L. ANGELUCCI & S. CABIB. 1991. Acute stress induces time-dependent responses in dopamine mesolimbic system. Brain Res. **554:** 217–222.

61. IMPERATO, A., S. CABIB & S. PUGLISI-ALLEGRA. 1993. Repeated stressful experiences differently affect the time-dependent responses of the mesolimbic dopamine system to the stressor. Brain Res. **601:** 333–336.

62. FRIEDHOFF, A.J., K.D. CARR, S. UYSAL & J. SCHWEITZER. 1995. Repeated inescapable stress produces a neuroleptic effect on the conditioned avoidance response. Neuropsychopharmacology **13:** 129–138.

63. CABIB, S. & S. PUGLISI-ALLEGRA. 1994. Opposite responses of mesolimbic dopamine system to controllable and uncontrollable aversive experiences. J. Neurosci. **14:** 3333–3340.

64. SCOTT, P.A., M.A. CIERPIAL, C.D. KILTS & J.M. WEISS. 1996. Susceptibility and resistance of rats to stress-induced decreases in swim-test activity: a selective breeding study. Brain Res. **725:** 217–230.

65. MOORE, R.Y. & E.L. GUSTAFSON. 1989. The distribution of dopamine-β-hydroxylase, neuropeptide Y and galanin in locus coeruleus neurons. J. Chem. Neuroanat. **2:** 95–106.

66. MASON, S.T. & S.D. IVERSEN. 1977. An investigation of the role of cortical and cerebellar noradrenaline in associative motor learning in the rat. Brain Res. **134:** 513–527.

67. PORSOLT, R.D., M. LE PICHON & M. JALFRE. 1977. Depression: A new animal model sensitive to antidepressant procedures. Nature **226:** 730–732.

68. BARTFAI, T., K. BEDECS, T. LAND, U. LANGEL, R. BERTORELLI, P. GIROTTI, S. CONSOLO, X. XU, Z. WIESENFELD-HALLIN, S. NILSSON, V.A. PIERIBONE & T. HÖKFELT. 1991. M-15: High-affinity chimeric peptide that blocks the neuronal actions of galanin in the hippocampus, locus coeruleus, and spinal cord. Proc. Natl. Acad. Sci. USA **88:** 10961–10965.

69. ORDWAY, G.A., K.S. SMITH & J.W. HAYCOCK. 1994. Elevated tyrosine hydroxylase in the locus coeruleus of suicide victims. J. Neurochem. **62:** 680–685.

70. MANJI, H.K., M.E. SCHMIDT, F. GROSSMAN, K. DAWKINS & W.Z. POTTER. 1997. α_2 Adrenergic receptors in the pathophysiology and treatment of depression. *In* α_2-Adrenergic receptors: Structure, Function and Therapeutic Implications. S.M. Lanier & L.E. Limbird, Eds.: 149–160. Harwood Academic Publishers. Amsterdam.

71. NESTLER, E.J., A. MCMAHON, E.L. SABBAN, J.F. TALLMAN & R.S. DUMAN. 1990. Chronic antidepressant administration decreases the expression of tyrosine hydroxylase in the rat locus coeruleus. Proc. Natl. Acad. Sci. USA **87:** 7522–7526.

Galanin in Somatosensory Function[a]

ZSUZSANNA WIESENFELD-HALLIN[b] AND XIAO-JUN XU

Department of Medical Laboratory Sciences and Technology,
Division of Clinical Neurophysiology, Karolinska Institute,
Huddinge University Hospital, Huddinge, Sweden

ABSTRACT: Galanin-like immunoreactivity and galanin receptors are found in dorsal root ganglion (DRG) cells and in dorsal horn interneurons, suggesting that this neuropeptide may have a role in sensory transmission and modulation at the spinal level. Expression of galanin or galanin receptors in the DRG and spinal cord are altered, sometimes in a dramatic fashion, by peripheral nerve injury or inflammation. Under normal conditions, galanin occurs in a small population of primary sensory neurons as well as in spinal interneurons. However, following peripheral nerve injury or inflammation, expression of galanin in primary afferents and spinal cord is upregulated. We examined the role of galanin in spinal processing of nociceptive information under normal and pathologic conditions in a large series of electrophysiologic and behavioral studies. Results suggest that under normal conditions galanin exerts tonic inhibition of nociceptive input to the central nervous system. After peripheral nerve injury the inhibitory control exerted by endogenous galanin, probably released from DRG neurons, is increased. During inflammation, galanin presumably released from dorsal horn interneurons also exerts an inhibitory function. Thus, stable galanin agonists may be useful in the treatment of inflammatory and neuropathic pain.

DISTRIBUTION OF GALANIN AND ITS RECEPTORS IN DORSAL ROOT GANGLIA AND SPINAL CORD UNDER NORMAL AND PATHOLOGIC CONDITIONS

Galanin mRNA and galanin-like immunoreactivity in normal rats and monkeys occur in a small population of small-diameter dorsal root ganglion (DRG) neurons.[1–4] Peripheral nerve injury induces a rapid and extensive upregulation of galanin synthesis in both species, resulting in the detection of galanin-like immunoreactivity in about 50% of DRG neurons of all sizes.[4–6] The increased expression of both galanin-like immunoreactivity and mRNA is seen already 24 hours after nerve injury, reaches maximum within a week, and is maintained if nerve regeneration does not take place. After axotomy, galanin coexists with vasoactive intestinal peptide (VIP), which is also upregulated following axotomy.[7] Galanin receptors of both R1 and R2 types[8,9] are expressed in normal DRG neurons.[10,11] Following axotomy, galanin receptors are downregulated in DRG.[10,11]

In the spinal cord dorsal horn, galanin-like immunoreactivity has been localized in small neurons, mainly in lamina II, where it coexists with GABA, enkephalin, and neuropeptide Y.[12,13] Another population of galanin-like immunoreactive neurons is found in

[a]This work was supported by the Swedish Medical Research Council (project 07913), the Biomed II programme of the European Commission (project BMH4-CT95-0172), and Astra Pain Control AB.

[b]Address for correspondence: Professor Zsuzsanna Wiesenfeld-Hallin, Division of Clinical Neurophysiology, Huddinge University Hospital, SE-141 86 Huddinge, Sweden. Phone, +46-8-585 87085; fax, +46-8-585 87050; e-mail, zsuzsanna.wiesenfeld-hallin@neurophys.hs.sll.se

areas around the central canal. A dense network of galanin-like immunoreactive fibers is visualized in the superficial dorsal horn. Because dorsal rhizotomy or neonatal capsaicin treatment significantly reduces this immunoreactivity, it may be concluded that many of these fibers and terminals originate from primary afferents.[1,2] This finding has been supported by studies on the ultrastructural level where coexistence of galanin-like immunoreactivity and calcitonin gene-related peptide (CGRP)-like immunoreactivity in afferent terminals and vericosities has been observed.[13,14] Following peripheral nerve injury there is an increase in the distribution of galanin-like immunoreactivity in the dorsal horn, presumably derived from primary afferents.[4,15] The number of dorsal horn interneurons expressing galanin-like immunoreactivity is unchanged after nerve injury, but some ultrastructural changes are observed.[15] Very high density galanin binding sites are located in spinal cord laminae I, II, and X of the normal rat and monkey.[16,17] These binding sites are not affected by dorsal rhizotomy or neonatal capsaicin treatment, indicating that they are derived primarily from postsynaptic neurons.

Peripheral inflammation also induces complex changes in messengers in sensory neurons and in the spinal cord, and many of these changes are different from those occurring after peripheral nerve injury.[18,19] By contrast to the extensive upregulation of galanin-like immunoreactivity in DRG cells following peripheral nerve injury, a decrease in the number of neurons expressing galanin-like immunoreactivity was seen 3 days after carrageenan-induced inflammation.[20,21] The mRNA coding for the galanin R1 receptor found in normal DRG cells in rat was transiently downregulated during inflammation,[10] whereas the R2 galanin receptor was upregulated.[11] By contrast to DRG, the number of dorsal horn neurons that express galanin mRNA was increased in the superficial dorsal horn at this time.[20,21] Inflammation also alters the release of galanin. Joint inflammation increased basal release of galanin in the dorsal horn, and stimulation of the inflamed joints suppressed such release.[22]

FUNCTION OF GALANIN IN NORMAL SOMATOSENSORY TRANSMISSION

Because of the extensive presence of galanin-like immunoreactivity and galanin receptor mRNAs in DRG cells and in dorsal horn interneurons, galanin has been suggested to be a possible transmitter or modulator in spinal nociception (see ref. 23 for review). Most functional studies in normal animals have shown that intrathecal galanin reduced spinal nociception/transmission,[7,24–29] although hyperalgesia has also been reported.[30] An antinociceptive effect of galanin is further supported by the finding that intrathecal galanin significantly potentiated the spinal analgesic effect of the opiate morphine in behavioral and electrophysiologic studies.[23,31] Interestingly, spinal administration of galanin receptor antagonist (see below) blocked the antinociceptive effect of morphine, suggesting that the spinal effect of morphine is mediated in part by the inhibitory action of galanin.[29]

Strong evidence supporting an antinociceptive role for galanin has been obtained in electrophysiologic studies. Galanin hyperpolarizes dorsal horn neurons in the rat[32] and depresses C-afferent mediated ventral root potentials elicited by capsaicin or electrical stimulation.[24,33] Galanin inhibited the flexor reflex and reduced spinal cord hyperexcitability following repetitive activation of C-afferents. Such repetitive conditioning stimulation of C-fibers leads to a gradual increase in the excitability of dorsal horn interneurons (wind-up) followed by a period of spinal hyperexcitability, which may be a model of hyperalgesia.[7,26,34]

Although application of exogenous galanin has revealed an antinociceptive function of this peptide, receptor antagonists are needed to study the role of the endogenous peptide under normal and pathologic conditions. A series of chimeric peptides have been developed that act as highly potent galanin receptor antagonists *in vivo*.[35] These drugs have been shown to antagonize the effect of galanin in the spinal cord. Intrathecal injection of one of these antagonists, M-35 [galanin (1-13)-bradykinin-(2-9)], significantly potentiated the facilitation of the flexor reflex induced by C-fiber conditioning stimulation under normal conditions, indicating that galanin exerts a tonic inhibitory control on spinal cord excitability.[36]

EFFECT OF PERIPHERAL NERVE INJURY ON THE ROLE OF GALANIN

Galanin expression is strongly upregulated in DRG neurons after peripheral nerve injury, and we have shown that following axotomy galanin may be tonically active in inhibiting nociceptive input from injured peripheral nerves. In electrophysiologic studies, intrathecal galanin was more effective in depressing the baseline flexor reflex in axotomized than in normal animals.[27] Galanin also blocked the facilitation of the flexor reflex induced by repetitive stimulation of C-fibers in axotomized rats.[7] Interestingly, the potentiation by M-35 of the facilitation of the flexor reflex induced by repetitive C-fiber stimulation was greatly increased in axotomized rats than in normals, indicating that the inhibitory role of endogenous galanin on spinal cord hyperexcitability following activation of axotomized C-afferents was enhanced. Thus, upregulation of galanin following nerve injury may reduce neuropathic pain.[36] In supporting this hypothesis, we and others have shown in behavioral studies that chronic infusion of the antagonist M-35 or galanin antisense oligonucleotides enhanced autotomy behavior, a sign of neuropathic pain, following peripheral nerve injury.[37,38] Also in agreement with a putative increased tonic inhibition by galanin following nerve injury, enhanced release of galanin was detected in the dorsal horn after ipsilateral peripheral nerve axotomy.[39]

We recently developed a rat model of partial sciatic nerve injury of ischemic origin in which rats exhibited behavioral signs of allodynia or hyperalgesia to mechanical or cold stimulation.[40,41] Intrathecal galanin reversed mechanical allodynia and reduced cold hyperalgesia in these rats without causing noticeable side effects (Hao *et al.*, submitted). Intrathecal M-35, on the other hand, did not significantly enhance the pain-like behaviors in these rat, unlike in the axotomized rats. This may be due to a much less profound upregulation of galanin synthesis in the DRG in this model of partial sciatic nerve injury compared to axotomy. Thus, involvement of endogenous galanin in depressing nociceptive input after nerve injury may be model-dependent.

The site of action of galanin is of interest in understanding its mechanism of action in axotomized rats. Galanin receptors of both R1 and R2 types have been expressed in DRG neurons.[10,11] However, a presynaptic mechanism for the antinociceptive effect of galanin is unlikely because peripheral nerve injury is associated with downregulation of galanin receptors in DRG,[10,11] whereas an enhanced effect for galanin is observed after nerve injury. Thus, our data suggest that galanin inhibits spinal nociception primarily through postsynaptic mechanisms. This substantiates the finding that galanin reduced the excitatory effect of exogenously applied substance P.[7]

EFFECT OF INFLAMMATION ON THE ROLE OF GALANIN

In a recent electrophysiologic study,[42] the effects of endogenous and exogenous galanin on spinal flexor reflex excitability were evaluated after the induction of inflammation by subcutaneous injection of carrageenan in the rat hindpaw. The results are in sharp contrast to those in normal animals, where repetitive activation of C-afferents causes wind-up and sensitization of the spinal cord. At the peak of inflammation, the magnitude and duration of the reflex were significantly increased over those of normal animals; however, wind-up and reflex hyperexcitability were significantly reduced. In fact, reduced reflex excitability during repetitive C-fiber activation (wind-down), which is not seen in normal or axotomized animals, was sometimes observed. This effect was often followed by reflex depression.

As already mentioned, an increase in spinal excitability following repetitive C-fiber activation is reduced by galanin in normal and axotomized animals. Intrathecal galanin also reduced spinal hyperexcitability during inflammation, but it was less potent than in normal or axotomized animals. However, the antagonist M-35 strongly enhanced wind-up and reflex hyperexcitability, much more than in normals. These results indicate that endogenous galanin has a potent inhibitory effect during inflammation.

Why does exogenous galanin become less effective in blocking the facilitation of the flexor reflex induced by repetitive C-fiber activation during inflammation? It is possible that this is partially due to a reduction of galanin receptors in DRG,[10] but not in the dorsal horn,[21] during inflammation. The fact that M-35 exerted a strong potentiating effect on wind-up and spinal hyperexcitability indicates that endogenous galanin was still effective in its antinociceptive role. This may indicate that active receptors were still present in the terminals of afferents in the dorsal horn at a time when receptor protein was reduced in the cell bodies in the DRG. Furthermore, it is possible that a strong inhibitory control exerted by endogenous galanin reduced the effect of exogenous galanin. Unlike in normal animals, where galanin antagonist only moderately enhances wind-up and central sensitization, during inflammation M-35 strongly enhances these effects, indicating a strong, tonic galaninergic control during inflammation. Increased basal release of galanin in the dorsal horn has been reported after joint inflammation.[22]

The source of endogenous galanin is probably spinal cord interneurons, because upregulation of galanin mRNA in dorsal horn neurons has been observed during inflammation.[21] These results suggest complex functional plasticity in the role of endogenous galanin in mediating spinal excitability during inflammation. Galanin appears to exert an enhanced endogenous inhibitory control on C-afferent input during the peak of inflammation, which may explain the relative ineffectiveness of exogenous galanin.

CONCLUSIONS

Studies on the somatosensory effect of galanin are largely consistent, suggesting that this peptide exerts an inhibitory function. The results further indicate that endogenous galanin has an enhanced antinociceptive role in chronic pain of neuropathic or inflammatory origin. After nerve injury, the source of galanin is probably DRG neurons. During inflammation, galanin released from spinal cord interneurons may be increased. Stable galanin agonists, alone or in combination with other analgesics, such as opiates, may be useful in relieving chronic pain conditions.

REFERENCES

1. CH'NG, J.L.C., N.D. CHRISTOFIDES, P. ANAND, S.J. GIBSON, Y.S. ALLEN, H.C. SU, K. TATEMOTO, J.F.B. MORRISON, J.M. POLAK & S.R. BLOOM. 1985. Distribution of galanin immunoreactivity in the central nervous system and responses of galanin-containing neuronal pathways to injury. Neuroscience **16:** 343–354.
2. SKOFITSCH, G. & D. JACOBOWITZ. 1985. Galanin-like immunoreactivity in capsaicin sensitive sensory neurons and ganglia. Brain Res. Bull. **15:** 191–195.
3. MELANDER, T., T. HÖKFELT & Å. RÖKAEUS. 1986. Distribution of galanin-like immunoreactivity in the rat central nervous system. J. Comp. Neurol. **248:** 475–517.
4. ZHANG, X., G. JU, R. ELDE & T. HÖKFELT. 1993. Effect of peripheral nerve cut on neuropeptides in dorsal root ganglia and the spinal cord of monkey with special reference to galanin. J. Neurocytol. **22:** 342–381.
5. HÖKFELT, T., Z. WIESENFELD-HALLIN, M. VILLAR & T. MELANDER. 1987. Increase of galanin-like immunoreactivity in rat dorsal root ganglion cells after peripheral axotomy. Neurosci. Lett. **83:** 217–220.
6. VILLAR, M.J., R. CORTÉS, E. THEODORSSON, Z. WIESENFELD-HALLIN, M. SCHALLING, J. FAHRENKRUG, P.C. EMSON & T. HÖKFELT. 1989. Neuropeptide expression in rat dorsal root ganglion cells and spinal cord after peripheral nerve injury with special reference to galanin. Neuroscience **33:** 587–604
7. XU. X.-J., Z. WIESENFELD-HALLIN, M.J. VILLAR, J. FAHRENKRUG & T. HÖKFELT. 1990. On the role of galanin, substance P and other neuropeptides in primary sensory neurons of the rat: Studies on spinal reflex excitability and peripheral axotomy. Eur. J. Neurosci. **2:** 733–743.
8. PARKER, E.M., D.G. IZZARELLI, H.P. NOWAK, C.D. MAHLE, J. WANG & M.E. GOLDSTEIN. 1995. Cloning and characterization of the rat GAL R1 galanin receptor from Rin14B insulinoma cells. Mol. Brain Res. **34:** 179–189.
9. GUSTAFSSON, E.L., K.E. SMITH, M.M. DURKIN, C. GERALD & T.A. BRANCHEK. 1996. Distribution of a rat galanin receptor mRNA in rat brain. NeuroReport **7:** 953–957.
10. XU, Z.-Q., T.-J. SHI, M. LANDRY & T. HÖKFELT. 1996. Evidence for galanin receptors in primary sensory neurones and effect of axotomy and inflammation. NeuroReport **8:** 237–242.
11. SHI, T.J.S., X. ZHANG, K. HOLMBERG, Z.Q.D. XU & T. HÖKFELT. 1997. Expression and regulation of galanin-R2 receptors in rat primary sensory neurons. Effect of axotomy and inflammation. Neurosci. Lett. **237:** 57–60.
12. SIMMONS, D.R., R.C. SPIKE & A.J. TODD. 1995. Galanin is contained in GABAergic neurons in the rat spinal dorsal horn. Neurosci. Lett. **187:** 119–122.
13. ZHANG, X., A.P. NICHOLAS & T. HÖKFELT. 1995. Ultrastructural studies on peptides in the dorsal horn of the rat spinal cord. I. Coexistence of galanin with other peptides in local neurons. Neuroscience **64:** 875–891.
14. TUSCHERER, M.M. & V.S. SEYBOLD. 1989. A quantitative study of the coexistence of peptides in varicosities within the superficial laminae of the doral horn of the rat spinal cord. J. Neurosci. **9:** 195–205.
15. ZHANG X., A.J. BEAN, Z. WIESENFELD-HALLIN, X.-J.XU & T. HÖKFELT. 1995. Ultrastructural studies on peptides in the dorsal horn of the rat spinal cord III. Effects of peripheral axotomy with special reference to galanin. Neuroscience 64: 893–915.
16. KAR, S. & R. QUIRION. 1994. Galanin receptor binding sites in adult rat spinal cord respond differentially to neonatal capsaicin, dorsal rhizotomy and peripheral axotomy. Eur. J. Neurosci. **6:** 1917–1921.
17. ZHANG, X., R.R. JI, S. NILSSON, M. VILLAR, R. UBINK, G. JU, Z. WIESENFELD-HALLIN & T. HÖKFELT. 1995. Neuropeptide Y and galanin binding sites in rat and monkey lumbar dorsal root ganglia and spinal cord and effect of peripheral axotomy. Eur. J. Neurosci. **7:** 367–380.
18. HÖKFELT, T., X. ZHANG & Z. WIESENFELD-HALLIN. 1994. Messenger plasticity in primary sensory neurons following axotomy and its functional implications. Trends Neurosci. **17:** 22–30.
19. HÖKFELT, T., X. ZHANG, Z.-Q. XU, R.-R. JI, T. SHI, J. CORNESS, N. KEREKES, M. LANDRY, M. RYDH-RINDER, C. BROBERGER, Z. WIESENFELD-HALLIN, T. BARTFAI, R. ELDE & G. JU. 1997. Transition of pain from acute to chronic: cellular and synaptic mechanisms. *In* Proceedings of the 8th World Congress on Pain. Prog. Pain Res. Manag. Vol. 8. T.S. Jensen, J.A. Turner & Z. Wiesenfeld-Hallin, Eds. :133–154. IASP Press.

20. Togunaga A, E. Senba, Y. Manabe, T. Shida, Y. Ueda & M. Tohyama. 1992. Orofacial pain increase mRNA level for galanin in the trigeminal nucleus caudalis of the rat. Peptides **13:** 1067–1072.

21. Ji, R.R., X. Zhang, Q. Zhang, A. Dagerlind, S. Nilsson, Z. Wiesenfeld-Hallin & T. Hökfelt. 1995. Central and peripheral expression of galanin in response to inflammation. Neuroscience **68:** 563–576.

22. Hope, P.J., C.W. Lang, B.D. Grubb & A.W. Duggan. 1994. Release of immunoreactive galanin in the spinal cord of rats with ankle inflammation: studies with antibody microprobes. Neuroscience **60:** 801–807.

23. Wiesenfeld-Hallin, Z., T. Bartfai & T. Hökfelt. 1992. Galanin in sensory neurons in the spinal cord. Frontiers Neuroendocrinol. **13:** 319–343.

24. Yanagisawa, M., N. Yagi, M. Otsuka, C. Yanaihara & N. Yanaihara. 1986. Inhibitory effects of galanin on the isolated spinal cord of the newborn rat. Neurosci. Lett. **70:** 278–282.

25. Post, C., L. Alari & T. Hökfelt. 198. Intrathecal galanin increases the latency in the tail flick and hot plate tests in mouse. Acta Physiol. Scand. **132:** 583–584.

26. Wiesenfeld-Hallin, Z., M.J. Villar & T. Hökfelt. 1989. The effect of intrathecal galanin and C-fiber stimulation on the flexor reflex in the rat. Brain Res. **486:** 205–213.

27. Wiesenfeld-Hallin, Z., X-J. Xu, M.J. Villar & T. Hökfelt. 1989. The effect of intrathecal galanin on the flexor reflex in rat: Increased depression after sciatic nerve section. Neurosci. Lett. **105:** 149–154.

28. Wiesenfeld-Hallin, Z., X.J. Xu, J.X. Hao & T. Hökfelt. 1993. The behavioural effects of intrathecal galanin on tests of thermal and mechanical nociception in the rat. Acta Physiol. Scand. **147:** 457–458.

29. Reimann, W., W. Englberger, E. Friderichs, N. Selve & B. Wilffert. 1994. Spinal antinociception by morphine is antagonised by galanin receptor antagonists. Naunyn-Schmiedeberg's Arch. Pharmacol. **350:** 380–386.

30. Kuraishi Y., M. Kawamura, H. Yamaguchi, T. Houtani, S. Kawabata, S. Futaki, N. Fujii & M. Satoh. 1991. Intrathecal injections of galanin and its antiserum effect nociceptive response of rat to mechanical, but not thermal, stimuli. Pain **44:** 321–324.

31. Wiesenfeld-Hallin, Z., X.-J. Xu, M.J. Villar & T. Hökfelt. 1990. Intrathecal galanin potentiates the spinal analgesic effect of morphine: Electrophysiological and behavioural studies. Neurosci. Lett. **109:** 217–221.

32. Randic, M., G. Gerber, P.D. Ryu & I. Kangrga. 1987. Inhibitory actions of galanin and somatostatin 28 on rat spinal dorsal horn neurons. Abstr. Soc. Neurosci. **17:** 1308.

33. Nussbaumer, J.-C., M. Yanagisawa & M. Otsuka. 1989. Pharmacological properties of a C-fibre response evoked by saphenous nerve stimulation in an isolated spinal cord-nerve preparation of the newborn rat. Br. J. Pharmacol. **98:** 373–382.

34. Xu, X.-J., Z. Wiesenfeld-Hallin & T. Hökfelt. 1991. Intrathecal galanin blocks the prolonged increase in spinal cord flexor reflex induced by conditioning stimulation of unmyelinated muscle afferents in the rat. Brain Res. **541:** 350–353.

35. Bartfai T., K. Bedecs, T. Land, Ü. Langel, R. Bertorelli, P. Girotti, S. Consolo, X.-J. Xu, Z. Wiesenfeld-Hallin, S. Nilsson, V.A. Pieribone & T. Hökfelt. 1991. M-15: High-affinity chimeric peptide that blocks the neuronal actions of galanin in the hippocampus, locus coeruleus, and spinal cord. Proc. Natl. Acad. Sci. USA **88:** 10961–10965.

36. Wiesenfeld-Hallin, Z., X.-J. Xu, Ü. Langel, K. Bedecs, T. Hökfelt & T. Bartfai. 1992. Galanin-mediated control of pain: Enhanced role after nerve injury. Proc. Natl. Acad. Sci. USA **89:** 3334–3337.

37. Verge, V.M., X.J. Xu, Ü. Langel, T. Hökfelt, Z. Wiesenfeld-Hallin & T. Bartfai. 1993. Evidence for endogenous inhibition of autotomy by galanin in the rat after sciatic nerve section: Demonstrated by chronic intrathecal infusion of a high affinity galanin receptor antagonist. Neurosci. Lett. **149:** 193–197

38. Ji, R.R., Q. Zhang, K. Bedecs, J. Arvidsson, X. Zhang, X.J. Xu, Z. Wiesenfeld-Hallin, T. Bartfai & T. Hökfelt. 1994. Galanin antisense oligonucleotides reduce galanin levels in dorsal root ganglia and induce autotomy in rats after axotomy. Proc. Natl. Acad. Sci. USA **91:** 12540–12543.

39. Colvin, L.A., M.A. Mark & A.W. Duggan. 1997. The effect of a peripheral mononeuropathy on immunoreactive (ir)-galanin release in the spinal cord of the rat. Brain Res. **766:** 259–261.

40. GAZELIUS, B., J.-G. CUI, M. SVENSSON, B. MEYERSON & B. LINDEROTH. 1996. Photochemically induced ischaemic lesion of the rat sciatic nerve. A novel method providing high incidence of mononeuropathy. NeuroReport **7:** 2619–2623.

41. KUPERS, R.C., Y. WEI, J.K.E. PERSSON, X.-J. XU & Z. WIESENFELD-HALLIN. 1998. Photochemically-induced ischemia of the rat sciatic nerve produces a dose-dependent and highly reproducible mechanical, heat and cold allodynia, and signs of spontaneous pain. Pain. In press.

42. XU, I.S., S. GRASS, X.-J. XU & Z. WIESENFELD-HALLIN. 1998. On the role of galanin in mediating spinal flexor reflex excitability in inflammation. Neuroscience **85:** 827–835.

Galanin Expression in Neuropathic Pain: Friend or Foe?[a]

MATTHEW S. RAMER,[b,d] WEIYA MA,[b] PATRICIA G. MURPHY,[c]
PETER M. RICHARDSON,[c] AND MARK A. BISBY[b]

[b]Department of Physiology, Queen's University, Kingston, Ontario, Canada K7L 3N6

[c]Division of Neurosurgery, Montreal General Hospital and McGill University,
Montreal, Province Quebec, Canada H3G 1A4

ABSTRACT: We investigated a possible link between galanin expression and evoked pain accompanying painful partial sciatic nerve lesions. Increased galanin immunoreactivity (IR) in the dorsal horn, in gracile nucleus, and in sensory neurons following chronic constriction injury (CCI) compared to complete sciatic transection suggested a facilitatory role in thermal and mechanical hypersensitivity (allodynia). We therefore investigated the effects of endogenous interleukin-6 (IL-6) and nerve growth factor (NGF) on allodynia and neuropeptide expression. IL-6 knockout mice showed decreased allodynia and galanin-IR compared to wild-type mice, but also decreased substance P (SP)-IR in the dorsal horn. Anti-NGF–treated rats with CCI also showed decreased allodynia and SP-IR, but increased galanin-IR in the dorsal horn. These results suggest that evoked pain is more tightly linked to SP than to galanin expression. If galanin's effects are inhibitory as the bulk of the literature suggests, its effects are subordinate to those of SP and to other changes following CCI.

NEUROPATHIC PAIN

Trauma to peripheral nerves can lead to debilitating and intractable pain for which treatments are few and of limited value. This inadequacy is due to a lack of understanding of mechanisms underlying this common clinical condition. Often the most severe peripheral neuropathic pain in humans results from partially injuring or compressing nerves (e.g., colles fractures, carpal tunnel syndrome, and sciatica). Three commonly employed rodent models of neuropathic pain involve partial lesions to the sciatic nerve: chronic constriction injury (CCI),[1] induced by loosely tying the sciatic nerve with chromic gut ligatures, results in the slow edematous axotomy of predominantly large-diameter myelinated axons;[2] partial sciatic nerve lesion (PSNL)[3] results in the nonselective axotomy of one third to one half the sciatic nerve's axons; segmental spinal nerve ligation (SNL)[4] causes the degeneration of all L5 and/or L6 spinal nerve-derived fibers. The result of these injuries is that a sciatic nerve connection to the periphery is spared and the uninjured axons reside for a time in a peripheral nerve environment in which Wallerian degeneration is occurring and in which factors affecting neuropeptide synthesis, such as nerve growth factor (NGF)[5] and leukemia inhibitory factor (LIF),[6] are upregulated.

[a]This work supported by Canadian MRC grants to M.A.B. and P.M.R. M.S.R. receives a Canadian MRC studentship. WM holds a Rick Hansen Man in Motion Legacy Foundation Fellowship.

[d]Current address: Guy's, King's, and St. Thomas' School of Biomedical Sciences, King's College London, Division of Physiology, Sherrington Bldg, St. Thomas' Campus, Lambeth Palace Rd, London SE1 7EH. Phone, +44 0171 928 9292; fax, +44 0171 928 0724; e-mail, m.ramer@umds.ac.uk

GALANIN EXPRESSION AFTER NERVE INJURY

While in normal dorsal root ganglia (DRG) galanin and its mRNA are nearly undetectable, nerve injury induces its expression, mainly in small DRG neurons,[7] suggesting a role in sensory function following axotomy. Galanin plays a predominantly inhibitory role in spinal nociception: application of galanin to the spinal cord suppresses the spinal nociceptive flexor reflex, and this effect is enhanced following axotomy.[8,9] Additionally, autotomy following sciatic nerve injury (a self-mutilating behavior thought to be reflective of painful paresthesia) is exacerbated with the application of galanin antagonists.[10] However, it is important to keep in mind that these results have all been obtained using complete nerve lesions, and it is of great interest to investigate the pattern of galanin expression following partial nerve injury: if galanin has an antinociceptive role, partial nerve injury (which evokes greater behavioral manifestations of neuropathic pain than complete transection) might cause a lower degree of galanin expression than complete sciatic nerve injury.

CCI is the most widely used rodent neuropathic pain model and is characterized by a reproducible thermal and mechanical allodynia (e.g., FIG. 5) as well as consistent neuropathology involving the axotomy of mostly large-diameter axons. Given that galanin upregulation following complete nerve injury occurs mainly in small neurons, we expected that its expression would be diminished following CCI than after complete sciatic nerve transection (CSNT).[11]

Lumbar spinal cord, brainstem, and DRG from rats with CSNT and CCI were processed with galanin immunocytochemistry. As expected, the superficial layers of the ipsilateral dorsal horn of CSNT-treated rats contained many more galanin-immunoreactive (IR) terminals and fibers than did the contralateral side (FIG. 1A and B). Surprisingly, increased galanin-IR was present in the ipsilateral superficial dorsal horn of CCI-treated rats than of rats receiving CSNT, and the fibers and terminals extended well into the deeper laminae (III–IV) (FIG. 1C). A similar pattern of galanin-IR was observed in the gracile nucleus, with a modest increase in CSNT rats compared to the dense network of axons and terminals in the gracile nucleus of CCI rats (FIG. 1D and E).

The galanin-IR in the deep layers of the dorsal horn and in the gracile nucleus following CCI suggested the upregulation of galanin in large-diameter neurons in greater numbers than following CSNT. Size-intensity distribution analysis of galanin-IR DRG neurons confirmed this, showing that a substantial number of large-diameter cells from CCI rats were intensely stained, whereas only a moderate number of large cells from CSNT rats were galanin-IR (FIG. 2A and B). Overall, a significantly greater number of DRG neurons were galanin-IR following CCI than following CSNT. This finding suggested that signals other than axotomy itself may be sufficient to bring about galanin induction in sensory neurons and that intact as well as axotomized cells were synthesizing galanin.

The PSNT model (which also generates thermal and mechanical hypersensitivity,[3] and which showed an identical pattern of galanin expression to CCI in all regions examined) was used to determine which DRG neurons were upregulating galanin (axotomized and/or intact): rhodamine injected at the lesion labeled axotomized DRG neurons, while fluorogold injected distal to the lesion labeled spared DRG neurons. Quantitative analysis revealed that the majority of galanin-positive, dye-labeled cells were axotomized (rhodamine-filled) and 30% were spared (fluorogold-filled) (FIG. 2C). Interestingly, of the fluorogold-labeled cells (spared), 34% were galanin-IR, and this was significantly increased over the number of galanin-IR cells in uninjured ganglia (10%, FIG. 2C).

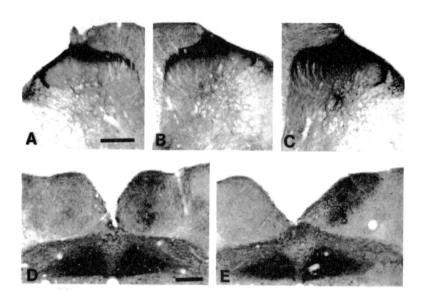

FIGURE 1. Galanin-IR in the dorsal horn (**A,B,C**) and gracile nucleus (**D,E**) from rats that had received complete sciatic nerve transection (CSNT) (**A,B,D**) or a chronic constriction injury (CCI) (**C,E**) 2 weeks earlier. In the dorsal horn, galanin-IR was greatest in animals receiving a CCI (**C**), with intense staining in both the superficial and deeper laminae. CSNT-induced galanin expression was much less dramatic (**B**) than that of the uninjured dorsal horn (**A**). Similarly, in the gracile nucleus, galanin expression after CCI (**E**) was greater than that after CSNT (**D**).

These results refute the hypothesis that galanin expression is inversely related to peripherally evoked pain. The simplest interpretation is that galanin and evoked pain are unrelated. Alternately, these results may suggest a nociceptive role for galanin; its increased expression may in fact mediate the thermal and mechanical allodynia observed following CCI. Low doses of intrathecally applied galanin generate hyperalgesia in rats,[12] and the spontaneous release of galanin in the superficial dorsal horn following CCI has been suggested to be associated with ectopic activity within sensory neurons and hence with the CCI-induced pain.[13] An alternative interpretation, based on galanin's previously demonstrated inhibitory nature, is that the increased levels after CCI represent an insufficient compensatory measure for other changes leading to pain. For example, CCI causes an increase in the nociceptive neuropeptide substance P (SP) in undamaged lumbar DRG neurons, leading to insignificant changes in SP-IR in the dorsal horn compared to pronounced decreases following CSNT.[14]

The differential regulation of galanin expression following partial and complete nerve injury may be due to spared axon access to the Wallerian-degenerating distal nerve stump and/or the partially denervated target which contains supernormal amounts of trophic substances,[5,15] many of which have been implicated in abnormal nociception following nerve injury. Following CCI, Aδ and C fibers are spared to the greatest extent, and have the capacity to retrograde transport trophic molecules such as NGF,[16] LIF,[17] and ciliary neu-

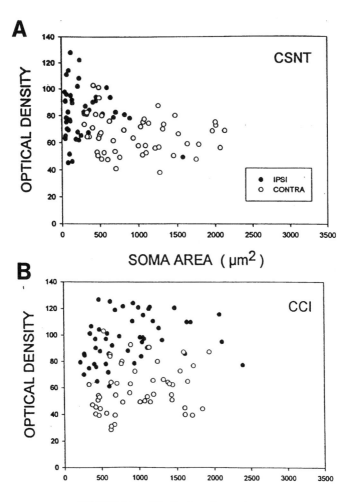

FIGURE 2A and B. *See legend on next page.*

rotrophic factor[18] to the DRG where they may influence galanin expression in small DRG neurons. Puzzling, however, is the apparently greater number of large galanin-IR DRG neurons following CCI than after CSNT despite the fact that large-diameter axons are damaged in either case. Following CCI, this may be a result of either the maintained connection of severed large axons to the trophic distal stump or the release of stump/target-derived substances (or secondary factors) from peripherally connected small neurons within the DRG which can regulate galanin expression in the large DRG neurons. One such factor may be the pleiotropic cytokine Interleukin-6 (IL-6), as discussed in the next section.

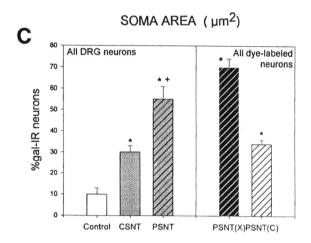

FIGURE 2. Size-optical density scattergrams of galanin-positive DRG neurons 2 weeks following complete sciatic nerve transection (CSNT) (**A**) or chronic constriction injury (CCI) (**B**). There were many more strongly labeled large-diameter DRG neurons following CCI than following CSNT. DRG from rats with partial sciatic nerve transection (PSNT) contained significantly more galanin-IR neurons than did DRG from CSNT rats (**C**). Most of the galanin-IR neurons following PSNT were rhodamine-labeled and hence axotomized (PSNT(X)). Of the fluorogold-labeled (spared) DRG neurons from ipsilateral ganglia following CCI (PSNT[C]), 34% were galanin-IR compared to 10% in contralateral ganglia (**C**). *Asterisks*: significant difference from uninjured ganglia (ANOVA); Plus sign (+): significant difference from CSNT rats (*t* test).

IL-6 AS MEDIATOR OF NEUROPEPTIDE EXPRESSION AND NEUROPATHIC PAIN

Peripheral nerve injury induces the production of IL-6 by Schwann cells[19] and DRG neurons,[20] and both sympathetic and sensory neurons express the IL-6 receptor subunit gp80.[21] IL-6 has trophic actions on sensory neurons[22] and, when applied intrathecally, can induce allodynia and hyperalgesia in rats.[23] The gp130 IL-6 receptor component transduces signals not only from IL-6, but also from CNTF and LIF,[24] the latter of which has been shown to regulate galanin expression.[25,26] We sought to determine whether galanin expression and neuropathic pain were related to endogenous IL-6.

The availability of IL-6 knockout mice[27] allowed for the determination of the role of endogenous IL-6, not only in galanin and SP expression, but also in the development of CCI-induced pain. Behavior was assessed in CCI-treated animals using standard tests for decreases in pain threshold (i.e., allodynia) to mechanical and thermal stimulation (von Frey filaments; radiant heat). No contralateral threshold decreases were observed, so data were plotted as difference scores (contralateral minus ipsilateral responses). As anticipated, by 2 weeks following CCI, normal mice were allodynic to both classes of stimuli[1] (FIG. 3A and B). The CCI-treated IL-6 knockout mice did not develop the thermal and mechanical hypersensitivity (FIG. 3A and B). These results suggested that endogenous IL-6 can mediate neuropathic pain, and further experiments focused on possible neuropeptidergic intermediates. Intrathecal IL-6 infusion in rats induced the upregulation of both

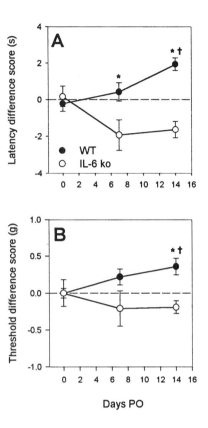

FIGURE 3. Neuropathic pain behavior in wild-type (WT) and IL-6 knockout (IL-6 KO) mice following a chronic constriction injury (CCI). Data represent difference scores (uninjured minus injured hindpaws). Unlike wild-type mice, IL-6 knockout mice do not develop thermal (**A**) or mechanical (**B**) allodynia following CCI. *Asterisks*: significant difference between genotypes (*t* test); *dagger*: significant difference from preoperative score (ANOVA).

galanin and substance P (SP) mRNA in rat DRG neurons (not shown). Galanin and immunocytochemistry were performed on lumber spinal cord and brainstem, and it was found that galanin upregulation following CCI in wild-type mice was similar to that occurring in rats,[11] but it was significantly less robust in IL-6 knockout mice in both the dorsal horn and gracile nucleus (FIG. 4A and B). In addition, the basal (contralateral) SP-IR was decreased in the dorsal horn of IL-6 knockout than of wild-type mice (FIG. 4C and D). Furthermore, while SP-IR in the ipsilateral dorsal horn of wild-type mice following CCI was relatively unchanged (similar to the negligible change in SP-IR in the dorsal horn of CCI-treated rats[14]), there was a marked ipsilateral decrease in SP-IR in the dorsal horn of IL-6 knockout mice after CCI (FIG. 4D). These results suggest that IL-6 is involved in the regulation of the injury-induced upregulation of galanin following CCI, the level of basal SP expression in the dorsal horn, and the lack of downregulation of SP in the central projec-

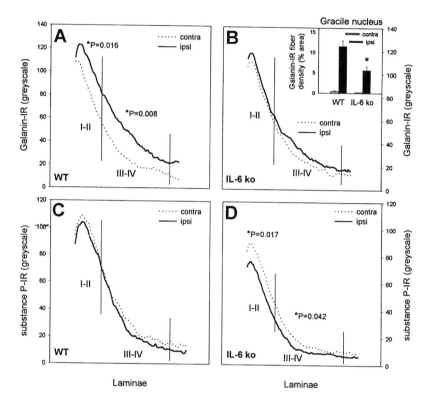

FIGURE 4. Galanin (**A,B**) and substance P (**C,D**) expression in the dorsal horn and gracile nucleus (**B,** inset) 2 weeks following CCI. In wild-type (WT) mice, galanin expression was significantly increased in superficial and deep laminae of the ipsilateral dorsal horn (*solid line*) (**A**) and in the ipsilateral gracile nucleus (**B,** inset). In IL-6 knockout (IL-6 KO) mice, the apparent increase in galanin-IR in the ipsilateral dorsal horn was not significant (**B**), and the galanin-IR fiber density in the gracile nucleus of IL-6 KO mice was significantly reduced compared to that of WT mice (**B,** *inset*). In WT mice, there was no difference in substance P expression between the ipsilateral and contralateral (*dotted line*) dorsal horn 2 weeks post-CCI (**C**). In IL-6 KO mice, the basal level of substance P was reduced significantly compared to that of WT mice (*dotted line*), and substance P-IR decreased dramatically ipsilaterally (*solid line*) following CCI in knockout mice unlike in WT mice (**D**). Significant differences of average immunoreactivity in superficial (I-II) and deep (III-IV) laminae are indicated by *asterisks* (paired *t* test).

tions of DRG neurons following CCI. Thus, in the IL-6 knockout mice, a reduced galanin response to CCI was associated with absence of neuropathic pain. However, difficulty with ascribing a role for galanin in neuropathic pain at this stage lies in the fact that wherever allodynia and galanin-IR are reduced, SP-IR is also reduced. If galanin and SP expression can be modulated in opposite directions following CCI, analysis of the pain behavior will indicate to which peptide pain is more tightly linked. We have achieved this through treatment with NGF antiserum, as described below.

NGF AS A MEDIATOR OF NEUROPEPTIDE EXPRESSION
AND NEUROPATHIC PAIN

The effects of NGF on neuropeptide expression in intact nerves and after complete axotomy are well known and can be demonstrated by application of exogenous NGF to the distal stump of a severed nerve, which rescues SP and calcitonin gene-related peptide (CGRP) expression, and suppresses axotomy-induced galanin and neuropeptide tyrosine (NPY) upregulation.[28] NGF also plays an important role in the development of inflammatory pain.[29] NGF's contribution to partial nerve injury-induced neuropathic pain is not as well understood, given the contradictory results of studies using NGF or its antiserum.[30,31] We have previously hypothesized that the situation of intact small-diameter C and Aδ fibers in the degenerating distal stump and their connection to partially denervated targets result in the retrograde transport of upregulated molecules such as NGF to the DRG where

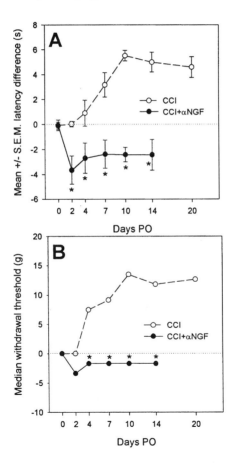

FIGURE 5. Effect of anti-NGF treatment on CCI-induced thermal (**A**) and mechanical (**B**) allodynia. Daily systemic anti-NGF treatment abolished both thermal and mechanical allodynia in rats with a CCI. *Asterisks* indicate significant difference from untreated rats (*t* test).

they may affect neuropeptide expression in the spared neurons themselves or in their axotomized neighbors.

We found that the effect of daily systemic anti-NGF[32,33] on behavior was dramatic, completely preventing the development of either thermal or mechanical allodynia that occurred in normal serum-treated rats after CCI (FIG. 5). These results confirm earlier reports on the alleviating effects of NGF antiserum applied directly to the lesion.[30] In normal serum-treated rats, galanin-IR was increased in superficial (I-II) and deeper (III-IV) laminae of the spinal cord and in the gracile nucleus (FIG. 6A), as described previously.[11]

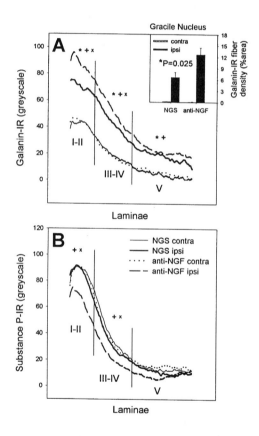

FIGURE 6. Galanin (**A**) and substance P (**B**) immunoreactivity in the dorsal horn and gracile nucleus (**A,** inset) 2 weeks following CCI and the effect of anti-NGF. In untreated rats, galanin-IR was significantly increased in the ipsilateral dorsal horn (*thick unbroken line*) compared to the contralateral side (*thin unbroken line*) after CCI. Anti-NGF induced a further increase in galanin-IR ipsilaterally (*dashed line*) but had no contralateral effect (*dotted line*). Substance P expression in the ipsilateral dorsal horn of untreated animals was unaffected by CCI (compare thick and thin unbroken lines), but was significantly reduced by anti-NGF treatment (*dashed line*). Anti-NGF had no contralateral effect in CCI-treated animals (*dotted line*). Asterisks: significant difference between ipsilateral and contralateral side in untreated rats (paired *t* test); plus sign (+): significant difference between ipsilateral and contralateral sides in anti-NGF–treated rats (paired *t* test); ×: significant difference between ipsilateral sides of treated and untreated rats (*t* test).

Also as anticipated,[14] SP-IR in the dorsal horn was unchanged in the ipsilateral dorsal horn following CCI (FIG. 6B). Treatment with NGF antiserum resulted in a significant further increase in galanin-IR in both the superficial and deeper laminae of the dorsal horn as well as in the gracile nucleus (FIG. 6A), and a reduction in SP-IR in the dorsal horn which was characteristic of the decrease that accompanies CSNT (FIG. 6B).[14] No differences in contralateral galanin- or SP-IR were observed between normal serum and anti-NGF–treated rats, implying that injury-induced changes in neuropeptide expression are more sensitive to NGF depletion than is SP and galanin expression in intact rats. These results are also intriguing since anti-NGF increases galanin-IR in the terminal regions of large-diameter DRG neurons, which do not express the NGF-specific receptor trkA,[34] suggesting that NGF normally suppresses the action of another factor (IL-6? LIF?) to which large diameter sensory neurons are responsive. These results demonstrated that increased upregulation of galanin following CCI was actually associated with decreased neuropathic pain, suggesting a dissociation between the two.

CONCLUSION

From these data it can be concluded that endogenous galanin most likely does not have a simple excitatory role in thermal and mechanical hypersensitivity as we suggested following detection of its increased expression after CCI.[11] We are left with three possible interpretations. The first is that galanin does not have any role to play in evoked pain; it is more likely that CCI-induced allodynia is linked to SP expression, because in addition to its well known role in spinal nociception,[35] SP expression paralleled hypersensitivity in all of the experiments described here. The second is that evokable pain results from a change in the balance of neuropeptides in the spinal cord, with SP weighing more heavily than galanin: when excess SP expression is combined with excess galanin expression (as after CCI), SP is the dominant factor and allodynia develops. On the other hand, when a reduction in SP is combined with an increase in galanin expression (as after CCI in anti-NGF–treated animals), the balance is shifted towards the inhibitory influence of galanin. The final possibility is that separate behavioral abnormalities (spontaneous autotomy versus evoked allodynia) are modulated by separate neuropeptides (galanin versus SP). If any behavioral modulation can be linked to galanin expression, it is suppression of autotomy; complete nerve injuries that result in the highest degree of autotomy also result in lower levels of galanin expression. Conversely, partial nerve injury results not only in a high level of galanin expression, but also in a greatly reduced degree of autotomy (ref. 3 and our unpublished observations). These possibilities highlight the need for further investigations into the interaction of neuropeptides in the spinal cord and on the relationship between sensory-modulating peptides and different behavioral manifestations of nerve injury.

ACKNOWLEDGMENTS

We thank Dr. Jack Diamond for the generous donation of NGF-antiserum, Kevan McRae and Serap Erdebil for excellent technical assistance, and Patty Pauls for assistance with the figures.

REFERENCES

1. BENNETT, G.J. & Y.K. XIE. 1988. A peripheral mononeuropathy in rat that produces disorders of pain sensation like those seen in man. Pain **33:** 87–107.
2. BASBAUM, A.I., M. GAUTRON, F. JAZAT, M. MAYES & G. GUILBAUD. 1991. The spectrum of fiber loss in a model of neuropathic pain in the rat: An electron microscopic study. Pain **47:** 359–367.
3. SELTZER, Z., R. DUBNER & Y. SHIR. 1990. A novel behavioral model of neuropathic pain disorders produced in rats by partial sciatic nerve injury. Pain **43:** 205–218.
4. KIM, S.H. & J.M. CHUNG. 1992. An experimental model for peripheral neuropathy produced by segmental spinal nerve ligation in the rat. Pain **50:** 355–363.
5. HEUMANN, R., S. KORSCHING, C. BANDTLOW & H. THOENEN. 1987. Changes of nerve growth factor synthesis in non-neuronal cells in response to sciatic nerve transection. J. Cell. Biol. **104:** 1623–1631.
6. BANNER, L.R. & P.H. PATTERSON. 1994. Major changes in the expression of the mRNAs for cholinergic differentiation factor/leukemia inhibitory factor and its receptor after injury to adult peripheral nerves and ganglia. Proc. Natl. Acad. Sci. USA **91:** 7109–7113.
7. HÖKFELT, T., Z. WIESENFELD-HALLIN, M. VILLAR & T. MELANDER. 1987. Increase of galanin-like immunoreactivity in rat dorsal root ganglion cells after peripheral axotomy. Neurosci. Lett. **83:** 217–220.
8. WIESENFELD-HALLIN, Z., X.-J. XU, U. LANGEL, K. BEDECS, T. HÖKFELT & T. BARTFAI. 1992. Galanin-mediated control of pain: Enhanced role after nerve injury. Proc. Natl. Acad. Sci. USA **89:** 3334–3337.
9. WIESENFELD-HALLIN, Z., X.-J. XU, M. VILLAR & T. HÖKFELT. 1989. The effect of galanin on the flexor reflex in rat: increased depression after sciatic nerve section. Neurosci. Lett. **105:** 149–154.
10. VERGE, V.M.K., X.J. XU, U. LANGEL, T. HÖKFELT, Z. WIESENFELD-HALLIN & T. BARTFAI. 1993. Evidence for endogenous inhibition of autotomy by galanin in the rat after sciatic nerve section, demonstrated by chronic intrathecal infusion of a high affinity galanin receptor antagonist. Neurosci. Lett. **149:** 193–197.
11. MA, W. & M.A. BISBY. 1997. Differential expression of galanin immunoreactivities in the primary sensory neurons following partial and complete sciatic nerve injuries. Neuroscience **79:** 1183–1195.
12. WIESENFELD HALLIN, Z., M.J. VILLAR & T. HÖKFELT. 1988. Intrathecal galanin at low doses increases spinal reflex excitability in rats more to thermal than mechanical stimuli. Exp. Brain. Res. **71:** 663–666.
13. COLVIN, L.A., M.A. MARK & A.W. DUGGAN. 1997. The effect of a peripheral mononeuropathy on immunoreactive (ir)-galanin release in the spinal cord of the rat. Brain Res. **766:** 259–261.
14. MA, W. & M.A. BISBY. 1998. Increase of preprotachykinin mRNA and substance P immunoreactivity in spared primary sensory neurons following partial sciatic nerve injuries. Eur. J. Neurosci. In press.
15. MEAROW, K.M., Y. KRIL & J. DIAMOND. 1993. Increased NGF messenger RNA expression in denervated rat skin. Neuroreport **4:** 351–354.
16. RICHARDSON, P.M., & R.J. RIOPELLE. 1984. Uptake of nerve growth factor along peripheral and spinal axons of primary sensory neurons. J. Neurosci. **4:** 1683–1689.
17. CURTIS, R., S.S. SCHERER, R. SOMOGYI, K.M. ADRYAN, N.Y. IP, Y. ZHU, R.M. LINDSAY & P.S. DISTEFANO. 1994. Retrograde axonal transport of LIF is increased by peripheral nerve injury: Correlation with increased LIF expression in distal Nerve. Neuron **12:** 191–204.
18. CURTIS, R., K.M. ADRYAN, Y. ZHU, P.J. HARKNESS, R.M. LINDSAY & P.S. DISTEFANO. 1993. Retrograde axonal transport of ciliary neurotrophic factor is increased by peripheral nerve injury. Nature **365:** 253–255.
19. BOLIN, L.M., A.N. VERITY, J.E. SILVER, E.M. SHOOTER & J.S. ABRAMS. 1995. Interleukin-6 production by Schwann cells and induction in sciatic nerve injury. J. Neurochem. **64:** 850–858.
20. MURPHY, P.G., J. GRONDIN, M. ALTARES & P.M. RICHARDSON. 1995. Induction of interleukin-6 in axotomized sensory neurons. J. Neurosci. **15:** 5130–5138.
21. GADIENT, R.A. & U. OTTEN. 1996. Postnatal expression of interleukin-6 (IL-6) and IL-6 receptor mRNAs in rat sympathetic and sensory ganglia. Brain Res. **724:** 41–46.

22. MURPHY, P.G., M. ALTARES, J. GAULDIE & P.M. RICHARDSON. 1997. Interleukin-6 promotes the survival of sensory neurons. Soc. Neurosci. Abstr. **23:** 890.

23. DELEO, J.A., R.W. COLBURN, M. NICHOLS & A. MALHOTRA. 1996. Interleukin-6-mediated hyperalgesia/allodynia and increased spinal IL-6 expression in a rat mononeuropathy model. J. Int. Cytokine Res. **16:** 695–700.

24. IP, N.Y., S.H. NYE, T.G. BOULTON, S. DAVIS, T. TAGA, Y.P. LI, S.J. BIRREN, K. YASUKAWA, T. KISHIMOTO, D.J. ANDERSON, N. STAHL & G.D. YANCOPOULOS. 1992. CNTF and LIF act on neuronal cells via shared signaling pathways that involve the IL-6 signal transducing receptor component gp130. Cell. **69:** 1121–1132.

25. CORNESS, J., T.J. SHI, Z.Q. XU, P. BRULET & T. HÖKFELT. 1996. Influence of leukemia inhibitory factor on galanin/GMAP and neuropeptide Y expression in mouse primary sensory neurons after axotomy. Exp. Brain Res. **112:** 79–88.

26. KURAISHI, Y., M. KAWAMURA, T. YAMAGUCHI, T. HOUTANI, S. KAWABATA, S. FUTAKI, N. FIJII & M. SATOH. 1991. Intrathecal injections of galanin and its antiserum affect nociceptive response of rat to mechanical, but not thermal, stimuli. Pain **44:** 321–324.

27. KOPF, M., H. BAUMANN, G. FREER, M. FREUDENBERG, M. LAMERS, T. KISHIMOTO & R. ZINKERNAGEL. 1994. Impaired immune and acute-phase responses in interleukin-6-deficient mice. Nature **368:** 339–342.

28. VERGE, V.M.K., P.M. RICHARDSON, Z. WIESENFELD-HALLIN & T. HÖKFELT. 1995. Differential influence of nerve growth factor on neuropeptide expression in vivo: A novel role in peptide suppression in adult sensory neurons. J. Neurosci. **15:** 2081–2096.

29. WOOLF, C.J., B. SAFIEHGARABEDIAN, Q.P. MA, P. CRILLY & J. WINTER. 1994. Nerve growth factor contributes to the generation of inflammatory sensory hypersensitivity. Neuroscience **62:** 327–331.

30. HERZBEUG, U., E. ELIAV, J.M. DORSEY, R.H. GRACELY & I.J. KOPIN. 1997. NGF involvement in pain induced by chronic constriction injury of the rat sciatic nerve. Neuroreport **8:** 1613–1618.

31. REN, K., D.A. THOMAS & R. DUBNER. 1995. Nerve growth factor alleviates a painful peripheral neuropathy in rats. Brain Res. **699:** 286–292.

32. DIAMOND, J., A. FOERSTER, M. HOLMES & M. COUGHLIN. 1992. Sensory nerves in adult rats regenerate and restore sensory function to the skin independently of endogenous NGF. J. Neurosci. **12:** 1467–1476.

33. GLOSTER, A. & J. DIAMOND. 1992. Sympathetic nerves in adult rats regenerate normally and restore pilomotor function during an anti-NGF treatment that prevents their collateral sprouting. J. Comp. Neurol. **326:** 363–374.

34. VERGE, V.M.K., J.P. MERLIO, J. GRONDIN, P. ERNFORS, H. PERSSON, R.J. RIOPELLE, T. HÖKFELT & P.M. RICHARDSON. 1992. Colocalization of NGF binding sites, trk messenger RNA, and low-affinity NGF receptor messenger RNA in primary sensory neurons: Responses to injury and infusion of NGF. J. Neurosci. **12:** 4011–4022.

35. TRAUB, R.J. 1996. The spinal contribution of substance P to the generation and maintenance of inflammatory hyperalgesia in the rat. Pain **67:** 151–161.

Regulation of Expression of Galanin and Galanin Receptors in Dorsal Root Ganglia and Spinal Cord after Axotomy and Inflammation[a]

XU ZHANG,[b,c] ZHI-QING XU,[b] TIE-JUN SHI,[b] MARC LANDRY,[b]
KRISTINA HOLMBERG,[b] GONG JU,[c] YONG-GUANG TONG,[c] LAN BAO,[c]
XI-PING CHENG,[c] ZSUZSANNA WIESENFELD-HALLIN,[d] ANDRES LOZANO,[e]
JONATHAN DOSTROVSKY,[f] AND TOMAS HÖKFELT[b,g]

[b]Department of Neuroscience, S-171 77, Karolinska Institute, Stockholm, Sweden

[c]Institute of Neuroscience, Fourth Military Medical University, Xi'an, P.R. China

[d]Department of Clinical Physiology, Section of Clinical Neurophysiology,
Huddinge University, Karolinska Institute, Huddinge, Sweden

Departments of [e]Neurosurgery and [f]Physiology, University of Toronto, Toronto, Canada

ABSTRACT: Galanin can normally be detected only in a few dorsal root ganglion (DRG) neurons, but it is dramatically upregulated after peripheral nerve injury in both rat and monkey. Galanin is stored in large dense core vesicles, which after axotomy are often found close to the membrane of afferent nerve endings in the dorsal horn. In the monkey there is an increase in galanin in many nerve terminals in the superficial dorsal horn after axotomy, but such an increase is more difficult to detect in the rat. Galanin is also present in local dorsal horn neurons, where it is upregulated by peripheral inflammation. Both galanin-R1 and galanin-R2 receptor mRNAs are expressed in rat DRGs, mainly in, respectively, large and small DRG neurons. Galanin-R1 receptor mRNA is downregulated in DRG neurons after axotomy, and a small decrease in galanin-R2 receptor mRNA levels can also be seen. After peripheral tissue inflammation galanin-R1 receptor mRNA levels decrease and galanin-R2 receptor mRNA levels increase. The present results show that galanin and galanin receptors are present in sensory and local dorsal horn neurons and are regulated by nerve injury and inflammation. Galanin may therefore be involved in processing of pain information, primarily exerting analgesic effects. Whereas local dorsal horn neurons represent a defense system against inflammatory pain, we have proposed that a second defense system, against neuropathic pain, is intrinsic to DRG neurons.

G alanin is a 29 amino acid residue peptide originally isolated from pig intestine.[1] It has a wide distribution in the nervous system and in some endocrine glands and may be involved in numerous functions (see Proceedings of the First Galanin Meeting[2]). For example, evidence indicates that galanin is involved in processing of sensory information.[3] Under normal circumstances galanin is present in low numbers of small dorsal root ganglion (DRG) neurons and in neurons in the superficial dorsal horn of the spinal cord.[4–7] Peripheral inflammation and axotomy are two animal pain models, whereby the latter is used to study some aspects of neuropathic pain (nerve injury-induced pain). It was early

[a]These studies were supported by grants from the Swedish Medical Research Council (04X-2887), Marianne and Marcus Wallenbergs Stiftelse, the European Commission (BMH4-CT95-0172), Astra Pain Control AB, and the Nature Science Foundation of China (39525010 and 39500045).

[g]To whom correspondence should be addressed. Phone, 46 8-7287070; fax, 46 8-331692; e-mail, Tomas.Hökfelt@neuro.ki.se

observed that peripheral nerve injury induces marked upregulation of galanin synthesis in DRG neurons of the rat.[8,9] Subsequently, numerous studies on gene expression, cell biologic mechanisms, and functional significance of the regulation of galanin in primary sensory neurons have been carried out in both neuropathic and inflammatory animal pain models. Recently, three subtypes of galanin receptors were cloned,[10–16] which further expands our means to understand the possible functional significance of galanin in pain processing.

GALANIN IN DORSAL ROOT GANGLIA AND SPINAL CORD OF RAT AND MONKEY

Under normal circumstances, only low levels of galanin are expressed in about 5% of all neurons in rat lumbar (L) 4 and L5 DRGs[9] and in 17% of all neurons in monkey L4 and L5 DRGs.[17] They are mainly small neurons and also contain substance P (SP) and calcitonin gene-related peptide (CGRP). In the cell bodies of these DRG neurons, galanin is packed into large dense-core vesicles (LDCVs) in the Golgi complex.[18] The LDCVs containing neuropeptides are transported to the central terminals in laminae I and II of the spinal cord,[6] where galanin-positive afferent terminals often form glomeruli in lamina II. Under normal conditions about 50% of the CGRP-positive primary afferent terminals in the lamina II of rat spinal cord contain galanin-like immunoreactivity.[6] This is higher than expected, because only a small percentage of the DRG neurons are galanin positive, whereas almost 50% are CGRP immunoreactive, suggesting that electron microscopic analysis has a high sensitivity. In fact, Klein *et al.*,[19] also using the electron microscope, reported that around 50% of all axons in dorsal roots are galanin positive. In terminals positive for both galanin and CGRP, that is, presumably primary afferents, galanin-like immunoreactivity could be detected in about 20% of the LDCVs, whereas CGRP was found in 65%.[6] Galanin was co-stored with substance P and/or CGRP in the same LDCVs in primary afferent terminals, suggesting that galanin even under normal circumstances can be released together with substance P and/or CGRP. These findings in the dorsal horn are in good agreement with the quantitative analysis of Tuchscherer and Seybold,[20] demonstrating a high degree of coexistence of galanin and substance P in those fibers that disappear after rhizotomy.

Several dorsal horn neurons express galanin in lamina II of rat spinal cord.[7] They are of the islet cell type. Galanin-like immunoreactivity is colocalized with enkephalin-, neuropeptide Y-, or substance P-like immunoreactivity in the cell bodies and terminals of these neurons. However, in laminae I and II of monkey spinal cord, galanin-positive local neurons could not be detected. This, however, might be due to low peptide levels.

In the dorsal horn of normal rats, basal release of galanin was demonstrated,[21,22] which may originate from primary afferent terminals, intrinsic neurons, and perhaps even supraspinally derived fibers.

EXPERIMENTALLY INDUCED CHANGES IN GALANIN EXPRESSION

A marked increase in the number of galanin-immunoreactive neurons was observed in rat DRGs after sciatic nerve transection.[8,9,23,24] About 50% of the neurons express galanin in rat DRGs. Galanin is not the only neuropeptide that is increased in rat DRGs after peripheral axotomy. For example, vasoactive intestinal polypeptide[25] and neuropeptide Y[26] are also upregulated after axotomy, and this occurs in certain subpopulations of DRG neurons. Vasoactive intestinal polypeptide is almost exclusively observed in small neurons,[25] neuropeptide Y mainly in large DRG neurons,[26] and galanin-positive neurons are mainly small in size, but medium-sized and large DRG neurons are also observed. Vasoactive intestinal polypeptide is mostly present in the small galanin neurons,[27,28] and about 60% of all galanin-positive DRG neurons contain neuropeptide Y (Landry et al., in preparation). Galanin is also colocalized with c-JUN transcription factor in DRG neurons after axotomy.[29] In the dorsal horn, around 65% of all CGRP-positive primary afferent terminals in lamina II contain detectable galanin-like immunoreactivity after axotomy.[30]

Newly synthesized galanin is packed into the LDCVs and is transported to the terminals in the dorsal horn of the spinal cord, which results in a moderate increase in the number of galanin-positive primary afferent terminals in laminae I and II but a fairly limited expansion of galanin-like immunoreactivity into lamina III of rat spinal cord. This expansion is somewhat larger if the axotomy is made closer to the DRG.[30] However, the intensity of galanin-like immunoreactivity in these nerve fibers is not markedly increased.[30] No significant change is noted in the total number of LDCVs containing galanin-like immunoreactivity per terminal. However, the number of LDCVs containing galanin alone is almost doubled, whereas the number of CGRP/substance P-positive, galanin-negative vesicles is markedly reduced, suggesting that galanin to a considerable extent has "replaced" CGRP and substance P in these vesicles.[30] Interestingly, in another pain model based on chronic nerve constriction, a more pronounced expansion into the deeper layers of the dorsal horn was reported[24] (see Ramer et al., this volume).

In lamina II of the spinal cord three types of galanin-containing afferent terminals can be identified at the ultrastructural level in axotomized rats. The first type of terminal undergoes degeneration, and the second type is involved in labyrinth formation. The third and most common type contains many galanin-immunoreactive LDCVs (FIG. 1) and is strongly positive for galanin as judged from the number of gold particles overlying these vesicles.[30] Some LDCVs can be found close to the plasmalemma of the terminals, and exocytosis sites can be seen, indicating an increased release of galanin from the terminals. In fact, Colvin et al.,[22] using the microprobe technique,[31] showed a spontaneous, increased release of galanin in lamina II of the spinal cord after nerve injury. Interestingly, release of galanin in the dorsal horn of the spinal cord was also demonstrated in rats with ankle inflammation.[21] Thus, an enhanced release may explain why no marked increase in the intensity of galanin-like immunoreactivity can be detected in laminae I and II of rat spinal cord despite the dramatic increase in galanin synthesis and centrifugal transport.[23]

So far galanin is the only neuropeptide that is markedly upregulated in monkey DRG neurons after peripheral axotomy.[17] Only a small increase in the number of neuropeptide Y-positive neurons and no upregulation of vascoactive intestinal polypeptide are seen in monkey DRGs. After axotomy about 70% of the neurons express galanin and they are small neurons. An increase in galanin-like immunoreactivity is observed in many nerve fibers and terminals in laminae I and II of monkey spinal cord (FIG. 2a and b). This increase is especially strong in the inner lamina II, where galanin-immunoreactive nerve fibers form distinct patches of densely packed nerve fibers. Although galanin-immunoreactive nerve fibers occupy a larger area in the dorsal horn of the spinal cord on the lesion side, most galanin-positive nerve fibers are very fine fibers and contain low levels of gala-

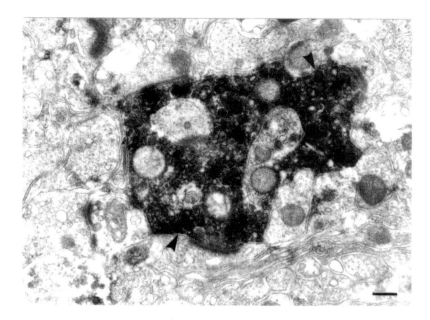

FIGURE 1. Pre-embedding immunoperoxidase electron microscopy shows a galanin-immunoreactive primary afferent terminal containing many large dense-core vesicles in lamina II of the spinal cord of a rat 14 days after sciatic nerve cut. Some galanin-positive large dense-core vesicles are close to the plasmalemma (*arrowheads*). Bar indicates 250 nm.

nin-like immunoreactivity. Immunoelectron microscopic studies show that galanin-like immunoreactivity is present in some large terminals containing many galanin-positive LDCVs and in some terminals with signs of degeneration. Many fine nerve fibers appear galanin-positive in lamina II of the dorsal horn on the lesion side, especially in the inner lamina II. These galanin-positive nerve fibers contain many microtubules and a few large dense-core vesicles, and often form small bundles.

Upregulation of expression of galanin in primary sensory neurons occurs not only after peripheral axotomy, but also in other situations when the peripheral nerve is injured, such as nerve crush,[9] chronic constriction injury,[24,32] nerve ligation,[33] local application of vinblastine,[34] herpes simplex infection,[35,36] and systemic administration of resiniferatoxin.[37] In fact, high levels of galanin mRNA were demonstrated in many small neurons in herpes simplex-infected human DRGs (FIG. 3).

In the superficial dorsal horn of the spinal cord of the rat and monkey, a change in galanin expression in the local neurons has not been detected after peripheral nerve injury. However, upregulation of expression of galanin in the local neurons is seen in lamina II of rat spinal cord following peripheral tissue inflammation induced by injection of 4% carrageenan into the hind paw.[38] In this pain model, the expression of galanin in DRG neurons is slightly downregulated.[38]

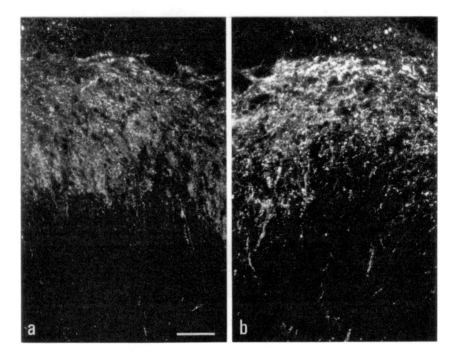

FIGURE 2. Immunofluorescence micrographs of the ipsilateral (**a**) and contralateral (**b**) dorsal horn of monkey spinal cord 14 days after unilateral sciatic nerve cut. (**a**) After peripheral axotomy, expansion of the area covered by galanin-immunoreactive nerve fibers is seen in lamina II, especially in the inner lamina II. (**b**) In the contralateral dorsal horn, a galanin-positive nerve fiber plexus is observed in laminae I and II with fewer nerve fibers in the inner lamina II. Bar indicates 100 μm.

GALANIN RECEPTORS IN DRG AND SPINAL CORD OF RAT AND MONKEY

Receptor autoradiography[39] shows a high density of galanin binding sites in laminae I and II of the spinal cord of rat and monkey,[40,41] with less labeling in laminae III and IV. Galanin binding sites can be seen in monkey lumbar DRGs, but could not be detected in rat lumbar DRGs. Recently, the cDNAs of three subtypes of galanin receptors, namely, the GAL-R1, GAL-R2, and GAL-R3 receptors, were cloned.[10–16] Under normal circumstances, GAL-R1 can be observed in about 20% of all neuron profiles in L4 and L5 DRGs of the rat, mainly constituting large and medium-sized neurons (FIG. 4a).[42] Almost all of these neurons express CGRP. About 25% of all DRG neuron profiles are GAL-R2 receptor mRNA-positive, and the majority are of the small type with some medium-sized neurons (FIG. 4b).[43] Eighty percent of GAL-R2 receptor mRNA-positive neurons colocalize with CGRP mRNA and about 20% with GAL-R1 receptor mRNA. However, in our electrophysiologic studies application of galanin to acutely extirpated DRGs from normal rats did not affect the membrane potential of DRG neurons,[44] suggesting that neither GAL-R1 nor GAL-R2 receptors are somatic receptors. Instead, they may be transported to terminals

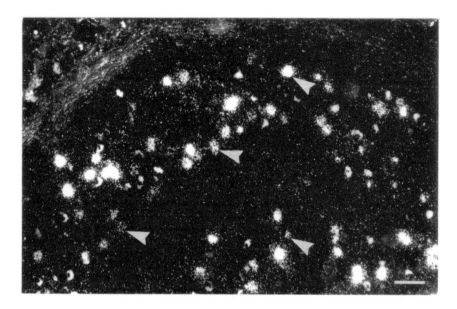

FIGURE 3. Dark-field micrograph of a herpes simplex–infected human dorsal root ganglion after hybridization with probes complementary to mRNA for galanin. Galanin mRNA is found in many small neurons (*arrowheads*). Bar indicates 200 μm.

acting as presynaptic or prejunctional receptors. Alternatively they may mediate metabolic or trophic effects on primary sensory neurons.

Many intrinsic neurons express the GAL-R1 receptor in laminae I and II (FIG. 5 and b), and some GAL-R1 mRNA-positive neurons can be found in laminae III-V of rat spinal cord (FIG. 5a). Only a few neurons express GAL-R2 receptor mRNA in the dorsal horn of rat spinal cord. Taken together, these results suggest that galanin binding sites in the superficial dorsal horn reflect both primary afferents and local neurons in the spinal dorsal horn and that galanin can act on both pre- and postjunctional receptors at the spinal level.

EXPERIMENTALLY INDUCED CHANGES IN EXPRESSION OF GALANIN RECEPTORS

After sciatic nerve cut Kar and Quirion[41] reported a decrease in galanin binding sites in the dorsal horn. In our studies no marked changes in intensity and distribution of galanin binding sites could be detected in rat and monkey DRGs and spinal cord.[40] Moreover, *in situ* hybridization shows that the number of GAL-R1 receptor mRNA-positive neurons is reduced in rat DRGs after axotomy,[42] perhaps reflecting the decreased binding shown by Kar and Quirion.[41] Expression of GAL-R2 receptor mRNA levels is only slightly down-regulated in rat DRGs 2 weeks after axotomy with a somewhat more pronounced reduction 3 weeks after axotomy, when about 10% of all DRG neuron profiles contain GAL-R2

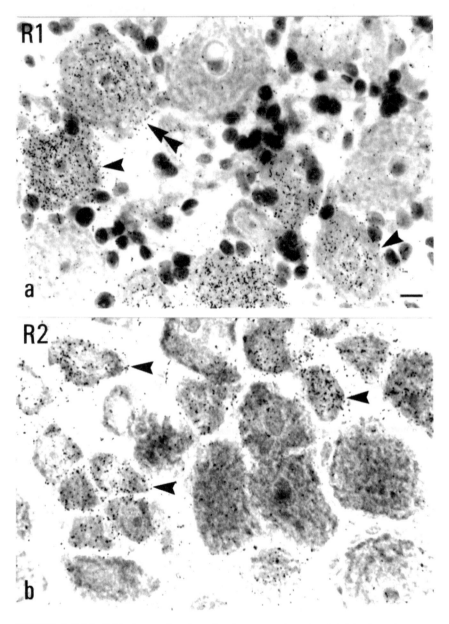

FIGURE 4. Bright-field micrographs of rat dorsal root ganglion after hybridization with probes complementary to mRNA for GAL-R1 (**a**) and GAL-R2 receptor (**b**). (**a**) GAL-R1 mRNA is mainly localized in many large neurons (*double arrowhead*) and some medium-sized neurons (*arrowheads*). (**b**) GAL-R2 mRNA is seen in many small neurons (*arrowheads*). Bar indicates 10 μm.

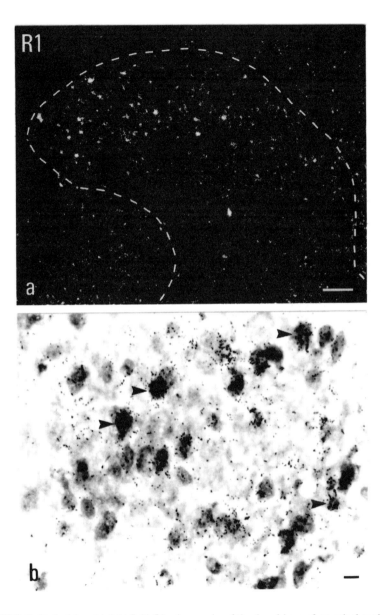

FIGURE 5. Dark- (**a**) and bright-field (**b**) micrographs of the dorsal horn of rat spinal cord after hybridization with probes complementary to mRNA for GAL-R1 receptor. (**a**) Many intrinsic neurons in laminae I and II and some neurons in laminae III and IV are GAL-R1 mRNA-positive. (**b**) Intense labeling for GAL-R1 receptor mRNA is observed in many neurons (*arrowheads*) in lamina II of rat spinal cord. Bars indicate 250 μm in **a** and 10 μm in **b**.

receptor mRNA versus 25% in controls.[43] These data indicate that DRG neurons become less "sensitive" to galanin after peripheral axotomy. However, in contrast to the situation in normal ganglion cell bodies, galanin causes depolarization in both small and large DRG neurons when DRGs are removed 7 days after sciatic nerve cut.[44] It is thus possible that DRG neurons after peripheral axotomy express a further subtype of galanin receptor, which is responsible for the galanin-induced depolarization and which perhaps is related to regenerative processes. No marked change in the expression of GAL-R1 and GAL-R2 receptors in the dorsal horn of the spinal cord has been seen after peripheral axotomy.

Taken together, changes in the subtypes of galanin receptor may represent one type of adaptation of DRG neurons in response to peripheral nerve injury. The GAL-R1 receptor in dorsal horn neurons appears to be the major postjunctional receptor for galanin released from primary afferent fibers after peripheral nerve injury.

Peripheral tissue inflammation causes downregulation of the GAL-R1 receptor mRNA levels in rat DRGs and a strong, transient increase in the number and intensity of GAL-R2 receptor mRNA-positive neurons.[43,44] In the dorsal horn, galanin mRNA is upregulated. If GAL-R2 receptors are presynaptic on primary afferents, then the increased amounts of galanin released from the dorsal horn after inflammation should exert a more pronounced effect on sensory inputs to the dorsal horn, presumably exerting an analgesic effect, as do opiate agonists.

CONCLUSION

Under normal circumstances galanin can only be detected in a few small DRG neurons, but it is probably expressed at low levels in almost half of all DRG neurons. It is colocalized with substance P and/or CGRP. Galanin-immunoreactive intrinsic neurons and primary afferent terminals are located in laminae I and II of the spinal cord. GAL-R1 receptors are expressed in many large DRG neurons and some medium-sized and small neurons, and GAL-R2 receptors mainly in small neurons. They colocalize to a large extent with CGRP, whereby GAL-R1 is mainly in large and GAL-R2 mainly in small CGRP neurons. A similar subdivision has been observed for neuropeptide Y1 and Y2 receptors which are expressed in small and large CGRP neurons, respectively.[45,46] GAL-R1 and GAL-R2 receptors colocalize in some DRG neurons of the rat. Dense galanin binding sites are present in the superficial dorsal horn of the spinal cord of the rat and monkey and in several neurons in monkey DRGs. Peripheral axotomy induces upregulation of galanin in many DRG neurons of the rat and monkey and downregulation of GAL-R1 and GAL-R2 receptors in DRG neurons of the rat. Electrophysiologic analysis suggests that in addition to GAL-R1 and GAL-R2 receptors, a further subtype of galanin receptor may be expressed in DRG neurons after peripheral axotomy, which mediates galanin-induced depolarization. However, no marked changes in the intensity and distribution of the abundant galanin binding sites could be seen in the spinal dorsal horn after peripheral axotomy. It is thus likely that galanin binding in the dorsal horn mainly represents binding to the GAL-R1 receptor on local neurons. Currently, it can only be speculated on the functional role of these two receptors. Analysis of the nociceptive reflex has revealed a biphasic effect of galanin, whereby the facilitation seen at low doses is attenuated after peripheral axotomy leading to increased inhibition.[47,48] It is possible that the inhibitory effects reported in electrophysiologic studies[49,50] are related to the postsynaptic GAL-R1 receptor, which does not appear to change after axotomy.

Peripheral tissue inflammation induces downregulation of galanin in DRG neurons and strong upregulation of galanin in local neurons in lamina II of the spinal cord. Galanin in such dorsal horn neurons, like enkephalin and dynorphin, presumably causes inhibition in the dorsal horn as does enkephalin and dynorphin, perhaps resulting in a decrease in inflammatory pain. The reciprocal change of galanin (down) versus substance P and CGRP (up) in inflammation is similar to the reciprocal changes seen after nerve injury, although in the reversed direction (galanin up, substance P and CGRP down) (see above). Expression of the GAL-R1 receptor was decreased and that of the GAL-R2 receptor increased in DRG neurons after inflammation.[43] It is possible that the GAL-R1–positive local dorsal horn neurons represent the main inhibitory galanin elements in the spinal cord, whereby they are activated by galanin release from primary afferents in neuropathic pain and by galanin released from local dorsal horn neurons in inflammatory pain.

The present findings suggest the existence of two pain defense systems at the spinal level. The first is related to neurons in the superficial dorsal horn of the spinal cord and responds to acute inflammatory pain, which induces marked changes in the expression of inhibitory dorsal horn peptides such as dynorphin, enkephalin, neuropeptide Y, and galanin. The second one is represented by DRG neurons and is activated by chronic neuropathic pain, changing the expression of neuropeptides, neuropeptide receptors, and other messenger molecules. Galanin and its receptors are regulated in both these pain defense systems, strongly suggesting that galanin might play a role in both types of pain.

REFERENCES

1. TATEMOTO, K., Å. RÖKAEUS, H. JÖRNVALL, T.J. McDONALD & V. MUTT. 1983. Galanin: A novel biologically active peptide from porcine intestine. FEBS. Lett. **164:** 124–128.
2. HÖKFELT, T., T. BARTFAI, D. JACOBWITZ & D. OTTOSON, Eds. 1991. Galanin: A New Multifunctional Peptide in the Neuro-Endocrine System. Wenner-Gren Center International Symposium Series, Vol. 58. MacMillan. London.
3. WIESENFELD-HALLIN, Z., T. BARTFAI & T. HÖKFELT. 1992. Galanin in sensory neurons in the spinal cord. Front. Neuroendocrinol. **13:** 319–343.
4. CH'NG, J.L.C., N.D. CHRISTOFIDES, P. ANAND, S.J. GIBSON, Y.S. ALLEN, H.C. SU, K. TATEMOTO, J.F.B. MORRISON, J.M. POLAK & S.R. BLOOM. 1985. Distribution of galanin immunoreactivity in the central nervous system and responses of galanin-containing neuronal pathways to injury. Neuroscience **16:** 343–354.
5. SKOFITSCH, G. & D.M. JACOBOWITZ. 1985. Galanin-like immunoreactivity in capsaicin sensitive sensory neurons and ganglia. Brain Res. Bull. **15:** 191–195.
6. ZHANG, X., A.P. NICHOLAS & T. HÖKFELT. 1993. Ultrastructural studies on peptides in the dorsal horn of the spinal cord. I. Co-existence of galanin with other peptides in primary afferents in normal rats. Neuroscience **7:** 365–384.
7. ZHANG, X., A.P. NICHOLAS & T. HÖKFELT. 1995. Ultrastructural studies on peptides in the dorsal horn of the spinal cord-II. Coexistence of galanin with other peptides in local neurons. Neuroscience **64:** 875–891.
8. HÖKFELT, T., Z. WIESENFELD-HALLIN, M.J. VILLAR & T. MELANDER. 1987. Increase of galanin-like immunoreactivity in rat dorsal root ganglion cells after peripheral axotomy. Neurosci. Lett. **83:** 217–220.
9. VILLAR, M.J., R. CORTÉS, E. THEODORSSON, Z. WIESENFELD-HALLIN, M. SCHALLING, J. FAHRENKRUG, P.C. EMSON & T. HÖKFELT. 1989. Neuropeptide expression in rat dorsal root ganglion cells and spinal cord after peripheral nerve injury with special reference to galanin. Neuroscience **3:** 587–604.
10. BURGEVIN, M.-C., I. LOQUET, D. QUARTERONE & E. HABERT-ORTOLI. 1995. Cloning, pharmacological characterization, and anatomical distribution of a rat cDNA encoding for a galanin receptor. J. Mol. Neurosci. **6:** 33–41.

11. Habert-Ortholi, E., B. Amiranoff, I. Loquet, M. Laburthe & J.F. Mayaux. 1994. Molecular cloning of a functonal human galanin receptor. Proc. Natl. Acad. Sci. USA **91:** 9780–9783.
12. Parker, E.M., D.G. Izzarelli, H.P. Nowak, C.D. Mahle, L.G. Iben, J. Wang & M.E. Goldstein. 1995. Cloning and characterization of the rat GALR1 galanin receptor from Rin 14B insulinoma cells. Mol. Brain Res. **34:** 179–189.
13. Ahmad, S., S.H. Shen, P. Walker & C. Wahlestedt. 1996. Molecular cloning of a novel widely distributed galanin receptor subtype (GALR2). 8th World Congress on Pain, **81:** 134 (abstr.). IASP Press. Seattle, WA.
14. Howard, A.D., C. Tan, L.-L. Shiao, O.C. Palyha, K.K. McKee, D.H. Weinberg, S.C. Geighner, M.A. Cascieri, R.G. Smith, L.H.T. Van der Ploeg & K.A. Sullivan. 1997. Molecular cloning and characterization of a new receptor for galanin. FEBS Lett. **405:** 285–290.
15. Wang, S., C. He, T. Hashemi & M. Bayne. 1997. Cloning and expressional characterization of a novel galanin receptor. J. Biol. Chem. **272:** 31949–31952.
16. Wang, S., T. Hashemi, C. He, C. Strader & M. Bayne. 1997. Molecular cloning and pharmacological characterization of a new galanin receptor subtype. Mol. Pharmacol. **52:** 337–343.
17. Zhang, X., G. Ju, R. Elde & T. Hökfelt. 1993. Effect of peripheral nerve cut on neuropeptides in dorsal root ganglia and the spinal cord of monkey with special reference to galanin. J. Neurocytol. **22:** 342–381.
18. Zhang, X., K. Åman & T. Hökfelt. 1995. Secretory pathways of neuropeptides in rat lumbar dorsal root ganglion neurons and effects of peripheral axotomy. J. Comp. Neurol. **352:** 481–500.
19. Klein, C.M., K.N. Westlund & R.E. Coggeshall. 1990. Percentages of dorsal root axons immunoreactive for galanin are higher than those immunoreactive for calcitonin gene-related peptide in the rat. Brain Res. **519:** 97–101.
20. Tuchscherer, M.M. & S. Seybold. 1989. A quantitative study of the coexistence of peptides in varicosities within the superficial laminae of the dorsal horn of the rat spinal cord. J. Neurosci. **9:** 195–205.
21. Hope, P.J., C.W. Lang, B.D. Grubb & A.W. Duggan. 1994. Release of immunoreactive galanin in the spinal cord of rats with ankle inflammation: Studies with antibody microprobes. Neuroscience **60:** 801–807.
22. Colvin, L.A., M.A. Mark & A.W. Duggan. 1997. The effect of a peripheral mononeuropathy on immunoreactive (ir)-galanin release in the spinal cord of the rat. Brain Res. **766:** 259–261.
23. Villar, M.J., Z. Wiesenfeld-Hallin, X.-J. Xu, E. Theodorsson, P.C. Emson & T. Hökfelt. 1991. Further studies on galanin-, substance P-, and CGRP-like immunoreactivities in primary sensory neurons and spinal cord: Effects of dorsal rhizotomies and sciatic nerve lesions. Exp. Neurol. **112:** 29–39.
24. Ma, W. & M. Bisby. 1997. Differential expression of galanin immunoreactivities in the primary sensory neurons following partial and complete sciatic nerve injuries. Neuroscience **79:** 1183–1195.
25. Shehab, S.A. & M.E. Atkinson. 1986. Vasoactive intestinal polypeptide (VIP) increases in the spinal cord after peripheral axotomy of the sciatic nerve originate from primary afferent neurons. Brain Res. **372:** 37–44.
26. Wakisaka, S., K.C. Kajander & G.J. Bennett. 1991. Increased neuropeptide (NPY)-like immunoreactivity in rat sensory neurons following peripheral axotomy. Neurosci. Lett. **124:** 200–203.
27. Xu, X.-J., Z. Wiesenfeld-Hallin, M.J. Villar, J. Fahrenkrug & T. Hökfelt. 1990. On the role of galanin, substance P and other neuropeptides in primary sensory neurons of the rat: Studies on spinal reflex excitability and peripheral axotomy. Eur. J. Neurosci. **2:** 733–743.
28. Kashiba, H., E. Senba, Y. Ueda & M. Tohyama. 1992. Co-localized but target-unrelated expression of vasoactive intestinal polypeptide and galanin in rat dorsal root ganglion neurons after peripheral nerve crush injury. Brain Res. **582:** 47–57.
29. Herdegen, T., C.E. Fiallos-Estrada, R. Bravo & M. Zimmermann. 1993. Colocalisation and covariation of c-JUN transcription factor with galanin in primary afferent neurons and with CGRP in spinal motoneurons following transection of rat sciatic nerve. Mol. Brain Res. **17:** 147–154.
30. Zhang, X., A.J. Bean, Z. Wiesenfeld-Hallin, X.-J. Xu & T. Hökfelt. 1995. Ultrastructural studies on peptides in the dorsal horn of the spinal cord. III. Effects of peripheral axotomy with special reference to galanin. Neuroscience **64:** 893–915.

31. DUGGAN, A.W., I.A. HENDRY, J.L. GREEN, C.R. MORTON & W.D. HUTCHINSON. 1988. The preparation and use of antibody microprobes. J. Neurosci. Meth. **23:** 241–248.
32. NAHIN, R.L., K. REN, M. DE LEÓN & M. RUDA. 1994. Primary sensory neurons exhibit altered gene expression in a rat model of neuropathic pain. Pain **58:** 95–108.
33. CARLTON, S.M. & R.E. COGGESHALL. 1996. Stereological analysis of galanin and CGRP synapses in the dorsal horn of neuropathic primates. Brain Res. **711:** 16–25.
34. KASHIBA, H., E. SENBA, Y. KAWAI, Y. UEDA & M. TOHYAMA. 1992. Axonal blockade induces the expression of vasoactive intestinal polypeptide and galanin in rat dorsal root ganglion neurons. Brain Res. **577:** 19–28.
35. HENKEN, D.B. & J.R. MARTIN. 1992. The proportion of galanin-immunoreactive neurons in mouse trigeminal ganglia is transiently increased following corneal inoculation of herpes simplex virus type-l. Neurosci. Lett. **140:** 177–180.
36. HENKEN, D.B. & J.R. MARTIN. 1992. Herpes simplex virus infection induces a selective increase in the proportion of galanin-positive neurons in mouse sensory ganglia. Exp. Neurol. **118:** 195–203.
37. FARKAS-SZALLASI, T., J.M. LUNDBERG, Z. WIESENFELD-HALLIN, T. HÖKFELT & A. SZALLASI. 1995. Increased levels of GMAP, VIP and nitric oxide synthase, and their mRNAs, in lumbar dorsal root ganglia of the rat following systemic resiniferatoxin treatment. NeuroReport **6:** 2230–2234.
38. JI, R.-R., X. ZHANG, Q. ZHANG, Å. DAGERLIND, S. NILSSON, Z. WIESENFELD-HALLIN & T. HÖKFELT. 1995. Central and peripheral expression of galanin in response to inflammation. Neuroscience **48:** 563–576.
39. YOUNG, W.S. & M.J. KUHAR. 1979. A new method for receptor autoradiography. ^{3}H-opioid receptor labeling in mounted tissue sections. Brain Res. **179:** 255–270.
40. ZHANG, X., R.-R. JI, S. NILSSON, M. VILLAR, R. UBINK, G. JU, Z. WIESENFELD-HALLIN & T. HÖKFELT. 1995. Neuropeptide Y and galanin binding sites in rat and monkey lumbar dorsal root ganglia and spinal cord and effect of peripheral axotomy. Eur. J. Neurosci. **7:** 367–380.
41. KAR, S. & R. QUIRION. 1994. Galanin receptor binding sites in adult rat spinal cord respond differentially to neonatal capsaicin, dorsal rhizotomy and peripheral axotomy. Eur. J. Neuorsci. **6:** 1917–1921.
42. XU, Z.-Q., T.-J. SHI, M. LANDRY & T. HÖKFELT. 1996. Evidence for galanin receptors in primary sensory neurones and effect of axotomy and inflammation. NeuroReport **8:** 237–242.
43. SHI, T.-J.S., X. ZHANG, K. HOLMBERG, Z.-Q.D. XU & T. HÖKFELT. 1997. Expression and regulation of galanin-R2 receptors in rat primary sensory neurons: effect of axotomy and inflammation. Neurosci. Lett. **237:** 57–60.
44. XU, Z.-Q.D., X. ZHANG, S. GRILLNER & T. HÖKFELT. 1997. Electrophysiological studies on rat dorsal root ganglion neurons after peripheral axotomy: Changes in responses to neuropeptides. Proc. Natl. Acad. Sci. USA **94:** 13262–13266.
45. ZHANG, X., L. BAO, Z.-Q XU, J. KOPP, U. ARVIDSSON, R. ELDE & T. HÖKFELT. 1994. Localization of neuropeptide Y Y1 receptors in the rat nervous system with special reference to somatic receptors on small dorsal root ganglion neurons. Proc. Natl. Acad. Sci. USA **91:** 11738–11742.
46. ZHANG, X., T.-J. SHI, K. HOLMBERG, M. LANDRY, W. HUAN, H. XIAO, G. JU & T. HÖKFELT. 1997. Expression and regulation of the neuropeptide Y Y2 receptor in sensory and autonomic ganglia. Proc. Natl. Acad. Sci. USA **4:** 729–734.
47. WIESENFELD-HALLIN, Z., X.-J. XU, M.J. VILLAR & T. HÖKFELT. 1989. The effect of intrathecal galanin on the flexor reflex in rat: increased depression after sciatic nerve section. Neurosci. Lett. **105:** 149–154.
48. WIESENFELD-HALLIN, Z., X.-J. XU, Ü. LANGEL, K. BEDECS, T. HÖKFELT & T. BARTFAI. 1992. Galanin-mediated control of pain: enhanced role after nerve injury. Proc. Natl. Acad. Sci. USA **89:** 3334–3337.
49. YANAGISAWA, M., N. YAGI, M. OTSUKA, C. YANAIHARA & N. YANAIHARA. 1986. Inhibitory effects of galanin on the isolated spinal cord of the newborn rat. Neurosci. Lett. **70:** 278–282.
50. RANDIC, M., G. GERBER, P.D. RYU & I. KANGRGA. 1987. Inhibitory actions of galanin and somatostatin 28 on rat spinal dorsal horn neurons. Soc. Neurosci. **13:** 1308.

Syntheses of Galanins, Their Fragments, and Analogs[a]

L. BALASPIRI,[b,g] T. JANAKY,[b] M. MAK,[f] G. BLAZSO,[c] R. JOZSA,[g] T. TAKACS,[g] AND P. KASA[e]

[b]Departments of Medical Chemistry,[c] Pharmacodynamics,[d] First Department of Medicine and [e]Alzheimer's Disease Research Centre, A. Szent-Gyorgyi Medical University, Szeged, Hungary

[f]Central Research Institute for Chemistry of the Hungarian Academy of Sciences, Budapest, Hungary

[g]Department of Anatomy, Medical University, Pecs, Hungary

The galanins (GALs) are linear peptides containing 29 or 30 (in man) amino acid residues derived from preproGAL precursor proteins (123 or 124 amino acids). Since the discovery of pig GAL 16 years ago, close to 1,000 papers and reviews have been published on different GALs. To date the structures of 15 GALs from different species, including pig, rat, sheep, cow, dog, dogfish, tuna, and chicken are known. Three excellent reviews[1-3] have surveyed the outstanding chemical, physiologic, and other results in this field.

MATERIALS AND METHODS

In the last 5 years, we have been dealing with the synthesis of GAL mainly from porcine, rat, human, and chicken. During this period, the full sequences of these species, 26 fragments and 10 analogs with amide ends or containing uncoded amino acids, have been synthesized and published in part.[4-6] Synthesis involved SPS technology manually and with synthesizers (ACT model 80 or Applied Biosystems 430A). The peptides were elongated on 1% Merrifield (0.5 mmol/g), on p-methylbenzhydrylamine (0.35 mmol/g), on TentaGel S PHB (0.24 mmol/g), and on TentaGel S RAM (0.24 mmol/g) resins using Boc and Fmoc techniques. Amino acid derivatives in all cases were successfully coupled with DCC-HOBt in three- to fourfold excess in DCM, DMF, or DCM/DMF. During manual synthesis, the qualitative nynhidrine test was systematically applied. α-protecting groups were removed in the usual way with 50% trifluoroacetic acid (TFA)/DCM or 20% piperidine. The crude peptides were removed from the resins with HF or different TFA/DCM mixtures. The peptides were dissolved in different concentrations of AcOH and lyophilized or after TFA evaporation in vacuum were precipitated with cold ether.

RESULTS AND DISCUSSION

The crude peptides were purified by RP-HPLC on a Lichrosorb 10 C18 column (16 × 250 mm) with a 0.1% TFA/acetonitrile solvent system gradient and lyophilized. Purity and

[a]This work was supported by Grants OTKA T 016565, T 016563, T 022683, T 026624, T 17235, and T 016356 from the National Research Fund.

identification were controlled by RP-HPLC, FAB- or ES-MS, HPCE (in 2 systems),[7] amino acid analysis, and regular sequencing or after enzymatic hydrolysis with FAB-MS.[8] The pure peptides were used for further chemical and physiological studies.

For more information on their conformations, human and chicken GALs and their NH_2- and COOH-terminal fragments were subjected to CD spectroscopy in trifluoroethanol (TFE) in water and in 50% TFE/water, and to 1H nuclear magnetic resonance studies using DQF-COSY, TOCSY, and ROESY methods (Bruker 400-mHz wide-bore spectrometer). In water, neither GAL has a fixed conformation, but in TFE, both adopt a predominantly helical structure. This conformational flexibility may be significant for the physiologic roles; the helical structure may be adopted on binding to their receptors/subreceptors.

For human Gal 1-30 and 1-19 and chicken GAL 1-29, 1-16, and 17-29, polyclonal antibodies were raised in rabbits and used by our collaborators for immunohistochemical localization of GAL-immunoreactive neurons in different human organs, chicken brain, pigeon, and earthworm. Human GAL 1-30 and 1-19 can be found in different parts of the brain, spinal cord, gastrointestinal tract (stomach, small and large intestine), pancreas, urinary tract, and muscle, but not in the skin as earlier reported.[3] All three chicken antisera revealed widespread localization of cell bodies and fibers throughout the chicken brain (hypothalamus and brain stem). Almost the same results were found with the antisera in pigeon (probably great similarity in structure with chicken GAL.)

Single sequence determination methods were also developed for the GALs, where enzymatic hydrolysis is followed by FAB-MS determination.[8] All of our synthetic GALs, fragments, and analogs were compared with standard rat and pig GALs (gifts from Peninsula) as regards the contractile action of substance P on the smooth muscle in rat, pig, and dog ileum.[4–5] In the periphery, the effects of GALs and fragments on pancreatic secretion in anesthetized and conscious rats with or without CCK-OP stimulation were studied.[9] Human GAL and its fragment were studied as concerns the coexistence in the hypothalamus with oxytocin (OT), arginine-vasopressin (AVP), desmopressin (dDAVP), with and without two specific OT and AVP antagonists (gifts from Prof. M. Manning, USA). Studies with endogenous human GALs and fragments on feeding and behavior have started. The coexistence of GALs with neurotransmitters, especially acetylcholine, were investigated.[10] Another presentation in this series deals with some of these results (Kasa *et al.*).

There are at least two or three "active centers" in human GAL 1-30. This agrees with the minimum of 2–3 receptors/subreceptors theory of human GAL. GAL opens the ATP-sensitive K^+ channels and closes the Ca^{2+} channels. GAL is a regulatory peptide; they are neurotransmitters/neuromodulators.

REFERENCES

1. BARTFAI, T., G. FISONE & U. LANGEL. 1992. TIPS Rev. **13:** 312–317.
2. BARTFAI, T., T. HÖKFELT & U. LANGEL. 1993. Crit. Rev. Neurobiol. **7:** 229–274.
3. ROKAEUS, A. 1994. *In* Gut Peptides: Biochemistry and Physiology J.H. Wals & G.J. Docray, Eds. :525–552. Raven Press, Ltd. New York.
4. BALASPIRI, L., G. BLAZSO, T. JANAKY, P. KASA, M. MAK, A. RILL & L. OTVOS. 1995. Peptides 1994, Proceedings of the 22nd European Peptide Symposium, 595–596. ESCOM. Leiden.
5. BALASPIRI, L., F. SIROKMAN, B. VARGA, L. KOVACS & A.F. LASZLO. 1994. Innovation and Perspectives in Solid Phase Synthesis. R. Epton, Ed. :207–211, Intercept Limited, Andover.

6. BALASPIRI, L., T. JANAKY, C.S. SOMLAI, M. MAK, T. TAKACS, G. JANCSO, G. BLAZSO & P. KASA. 1996. Proceedings of the Innovation and Perspectives in Solid Phase Synthesis. :227–232. R. Epton, Ed. Mayflower Scientific Limited.
7. JANAKY, T., E. SZABO, L. BALASPIRI, B. ADY & B. PENKE. 1996. J. Chromatogr. B. **676:** 7–12.
8. MAK, M., & J. TAMAS. 1992. J.Org.Mass Spectrom. **28:** 542–545.
9. TAKACS, T., L. BALASPIRI & J. LONOVICS. 1997. Biomed. Res. In press.
10. KASA, P., Z. FARKAS, L. BALASPIRI & J.R. WOLF. 1996. Neuroscience **72:** 709–723.

Galanin Upregulation in Glial Cells after Colchicine Injection Is Dependent on Thyroid Hormone[a]

L. CALZÀ,[b,c,f] L. GIARDINO,[d] AND T. HÖKFELT[e]

[b]Pathophysiology Center for the Nervous System, Hesperia Hospital, Modena, Italy

[c]Department of Biochemistry and Human Physiology, University of Cagliari, Cagliari, Italy

[d]Institute of ORL 2, University of Milan, Milan, Italy

[e]Department of Neuroscience, Karolinska Institute, Stockholm, Sweden

The *in vivo* synthesis of galanin and galanin message associated peptide (GMAP) is strongly influenced by the endocrine status. Estrogens are potent inducers of galanin synthesis in the pituitary,[1] and thyroid hormone depletion suppresses galanin synthesis in selected hypothalamic areas and in the pituitary gland.[2–4] Recently, a binding site for thyroid hormone was identified between –41 and –132 bp upstream of the transcription start site in the promoter of the rat galanin gene.[5] Galanin expression is also modulated by brain and nerve, one example being a strong upregulation of galanin synthesis in neurons and in glial cells after intracerebroventricular (icv) colchicine injection.[6,7] To further investigate the *in vivo* regulation of galanin/GMAP synthesis, we challenged adult hypothyroid rats with colchicine. We demonstrated that the upregulation of galanin/GMAP synthesis induced by colchicine in glial cells was strongly suppressed in hypothyroid rats.

Postpuberal male rats, made hypothyroid by thyroidectomy, were icv injected with colchicine (120 µg/10 µl/ animal) or saline 60 days after thyroidectomy. The animals were then killed 24 or 48 hours after injection. Sections were processed for *in situ* hybridization using ^{35}S-dATP 3′-end–labeled oligoprobes with sequences complementary to mRNA encoding prepro-galanin (pp-GAL) (nucleotides 152-199 and 230-277) according to our standard procedure.[8] Briefly, sections were covered with a hybridization buffer containing 50% formamide, 4xSSC (1xSSC: 0.15 M NaCl, 0.015 M sodium citrate), 1 x Denhardt's solution (0.02% polyvinyl-pyrrolidone, 0.02% bovine serum albumin and 0.02% Ficoll), 1% sarcosyl, 0.02 M phosphate buffer (pH 7.0), 10% dextran sulfate, 500 µg/ml heat-denatured salmon sperm DNA, and 200 mM DTT and 40 ng/µl of the labeled probes, placed in a humid chamber and incubated for 15–20 hours at 50°C. Afterwards, sections were rinsed in 1xSSC at 55°C for 1 hour with six changes and washed in the same buffer for 1 hour at room temperature. Slides were rinsed in distilled water and 60% and 95% ethanol (2 minutes each) and air dried. Sections were then dipped in nuclear track emulsion and developed 3 weeks later.

Some animals were also perfused with buffered 4% paraformaldehyde, and 14-µm thick brain sections were processed for galanin visualization by the indirect immunofluorescence method (anti-galanin antibody was purchased from Peninsula).

[a]This work was supported by CNR (94.02574.CT04LC) and by MURST (LC ex60% Cagliari University).

[f]Phone, (39) 59 449176; fax, (39) 59 394840; e-mail, cefisnmo@tin.it

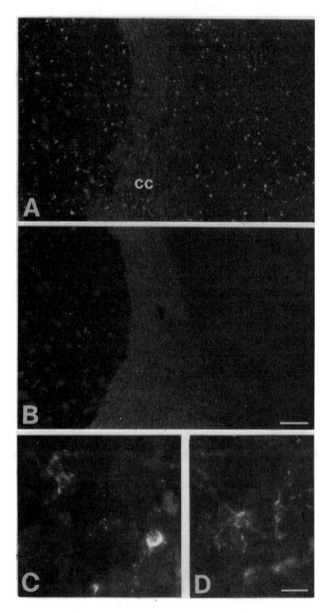

FIGURE 1. Dark-field micrograph of galanin message associated peptide (GMAP) mRNA express-ing cells in the dorsal caudate putamen and in the cerebral cortex in euthyroid animals 48 hours after colchicine injection (**A**). This regulation is not present in hypothyroid rats (**B**). cc, corpus callosum. Galanin-positive cells in the same area in the caudate putamen (**C,D**). Bars: (**B**) 100 μm; (**D**) 50 μm.

Colchicine injection in euthyroid rats induced a dramatic upregulation of pp-GAL mRNA levels, apparently also in cells normally devoid of this peptide. In particular, many small cells were found in a wide area around the colchicine injection site, extending from the basal ganglia to the posterior hypothalamus, distributed in the grey as well as in the white matter (FIG. 1A). The caudate putamen, cerebral cortex, septal nuclei, hippocampus, thalamus, hypothalamus, and amydgaloid complex contained many such pp-GAL mRNA expressing cells. Also, the peptide was present in the same areas (FIG. 1C and D). Immunocytochemical staining revealed that the galanin-positive cells were small, with multiple short processes (FIG. 1C and D). The effect was time-dependent, being stronger 48 than 24 hours after colchicine.

In hypothyroid rats, almost no pp-GAL mRNA positive glial cells with a corresponding distribution could be seen after colchicine injection (FIG. 1B). Only very few elements close to the lateral ventricle were found at both time intervals studied.

The present results suggest that thyroid hormone is an important factor for colchicine-induced upregulation of galanin/GMAP synthesis in glial cells. Thyroid hormone could act through its nuclear receptor regulating galanin-gene transcription, or this effect could be related to more general metabolic and structural alterations due to prolonged hypothyroidism. Glial cells express different isoforms of thyroid hormone receptors, and the enzymes needed for conversion of the inactive to the active form of thyroid hormone are also present in these cells. Moreover, thyroid hormone affects synthesis and assembly of different structural proteins in glial cells, including tubulin, actin, integrin, and glial fibrillary acid protein.[9] In particular, in mouse and chicken brain cultures, colchicine binding to tubulin is increased by triiodothyronine in glial cells.[10] High-affinity binding to the β-subunit of tubulin is considered the mechanism by which colchicine severely affects axonal transport and, more generally, the intracellular traffic of different substances.[11] This could also affect the regulation of galanin/GMAP gene transcription.

The difference in glial reaction to a "toxic" substance that we observed in hypothyroid versus euthyroid rats could also partially account for the peculiar responsiveness to brain injuries observed during hypothyroidism. Thus, hypothyroidism is known to protect from ischemic injury,[12] probably because of an attenuated formation of free radicals as a consequence of a reduced metabolic rate,[13] but also because of a decrease in glutamate release.[14] Glial cells, in fact, participate in many aspects of brain injury reaction, including (1) scavenging cellular debris, (2) regulating extracellular neurotransmitter and ion concentrations, and (3) secreting reactive oxygen species such as nitric oxide as well as glutamate.

REFERENCES

1. VRONTAKIS, M.E., L.M. PEDEN, M.L. DUCKWORTH & H.G. FRIESEN. 1987. Isolation and characterization of a complementary DNA (galanin) clone from estrogen-induced pituitary tumor messenger RNA. J. Biol. Chem. **262:** 16755–16758
2. HOOI, S.C., J.I. KOENIG, S.M. GABRIEL, D. MAITER & J.B. MARTIN. 1990. Influence of thyroid hormone on the concentration of galanin in the rat brain and pituitary. Neuroendocrinology **51:** 351–356.
3. GIARDINO, L., A. VELARDO, A. GALLINELLI & L. CALZÀ. 1992. Deficit of galanin-like immunostaining in the median eminence of adult hypothyroid rats. Neuroendocrinology **55:** 237–247.
4. CECCATELLI, S., L. GIARDINO & L. CALZÀ. 1992. Response of hypothalamic peptide mRNAs to thyroidectomy. Neuroendocrinology **56:** 694–703.

5. Hooi, S.C., J.I. Koenig, D.R. Abraczinskas & L.M. Kaplan. 1997. Regulation of anterior pituitary galanin gene expression by thyroid hormone. Mol. Brain Res. **51:** 15–22.
6. Cortes, R., S. Ceccatelli, M. Shalling & T. Hökfelt. 1990. Differential effects of intracerebroventricular colchicine administration on the expression of mRNAs for neuropeptides and neurotransmitter enzymes, with special emphasis on galanin: An *in situ* hybridization study. Synapse **6:** 369–391.
7. Xu, Z., R. Cortes, M. Villar, P. Molino, M.N. Castel & T. Hökfelt. 1992. Evidence for upregulation of galanin synthesis in rat glial cells in vivo after colchicine. Neurosci. Lett. **145:** 185–188.
8. Dagerlind, A.-J., K. Friberg, A. Bean & T. Hökfelt. 1992. Sensitive mRNA detection using unfixed tissue: Combined radioactive and non-radioactive in situ hybridization histochemistry. Histochemistry **98:** 39–49.
9. Garcia-Segura, L.M., J.A. Chowen & F. Naftolin. 1996. Endocrine glia: Roles of glial cells in the brain actions of steroid and thyroid hormones and in the regulation of hormone secretion. Front. Neuroendocrinol. **17:** 180–211.
10. Sherline, P., J.T. Leung & D.M. Kipnis. 1975. Binding of colchicine to purified microtubule protein. J. Biol. Chem. **250:** 5481–5486.
11. De, A., S. Chaudhury & P.K. Sarkar. 1991. Thyroidal stimulation of tubulin and actin in primary cultures of neuronal and glial cells of the rat brain. Int. J. Dev. Neurosci. **9:** 381–390.
12. Shuaib, A., S. Ijaz, R. Mazagri, J. Kalra, S. Hemmings, A. Senthilsvlvan & N. Crosby. 1994. Hypothyroidism protects the brain during transient forebrain ischemia in gerbils. Exp. Neurol. **127:** 119–125.
13. Calzà, L., L. Giardino & L. Aloe. 1997. Thyroid hormone-induced plasticity in the adult rat brain. Brain Res. Bull. **44:** 549–557.
14. Shuaib, A., S. Ijaz, S. Hemmings, P. Galazka, R. Ishaqzay, L. Liu, J. Ravindran & H. Miyashita. 1994. Decreased glutamate release during hypothyroidism may contribute to protection in cerebral ischemia. Exp. Neurol. **128:** 260–265.

Galanin and NH$_2$-Terminal Galanin Fragments in Central Cardiovascular Regulation[a]

Z. DÍAZ-CABIALE,[b–d] J.A. NARVÁEZ,[b] P. MARCOS,[b] M.P. CORDÓN,[b] R. COVEÑAS,[b] K. FUXE,[c] AND S. GONZÁLEZ-BARON[b]

[b]Department of Physiology, University of Malaga, Malaga, Spain

[c] Department of Neuroscience, Karolinska Institute, Stockholm, Sweden

Galanin is a peptide involved in different autonomic functions, including central cardiovascular regulation (CVR). Intracisternal injections of galanin elicit hypotension and tachycardia,[1–3] and in spontaneously hypertensive rats the presence of galanin within the nucleus tractus solitarius is increased.[4] By contrast, central administration of the NH$_2$-terminal galanin fragment (1-15) [gal-(1-15)] elicits hypertension and tachycardia and counteracts the cardiovascular actions of the parent molecule [gal-(1-29)].[3] Furthermore, gal-(1-15) decreases baroreceptor reflex sensitivity, whereas gal-(1-29) has no effect[5] and the galanin antagonist M40 blocks the cardiovascular responses of gal-(1-15) without affecting those elicited by gal(1-29).[6] These results strongly support the existence of a specific galanin fragment receptor distinct from the galanin receptor in central cardiovascular regulation. Since several galanin fragments have been shown to exert biologic activity at different levels,[7] the aim of this work was to investigate the probable participation of other galanin fragments on CVR as well as the possible mechanism of action of NH$_2$-terminal galanin fragments.

MATERIAL AND METHODS

Groups of urethane-anesthetized rats (1.1 g/kg bw) were injected intracisternally with porcine gal-(1-29), gal-(1-15), the NH$_2$-terminal galanin fragment (1-16) [gal-(1-16)], or the COOH-terminal galanin fragment (10-29) [gal-(10-29)]. The dose administered in all cases was 3.0 nmol/rat, which is the effective dose for the cardiovascular effects of gal-(1-29) and gal-(1-15).[3] Control rats received artificial cerebrospinal fluid alone. Mean arterial pressure (MAP) and heart rate (HR) were recorded from the femoral artery during 60 minutes after injections. To study the possible mechanism of action of NH$_2$-terminal galanin fragments, a group of urethane-anesthetized rats pre-treated with atropine (125 µg/kg bw, iv) received 10 minutes later intracisternal injections of gal-(1-15) (3 nmol/rat) or gal-(1-29) (3.0 nmol/rat). Another group was pre-treated with propranolol (1 mg/kg bw, iv) and received 10 minutes later intracisternal injections of gal-(1-15) or gal-(1-29) at the same doses. MAP and HR were recorded from the femoral artery during 30 minutes after intracisternal injections. Data were analyzed by a two-way ANOVA followed by the Fisher post-hoc test.

[a]This work was supported by the Spanish DIDGICYT (PB93-0992 and PB96-1467).

[d]Address for correspondence: Zaida Díaz-Cabiale, Department of Neuroscience, Karolinska Institute, S-171 77 Stockholm, Sweden. Phone, + 46-8-728 7081; fax, +46-8-33 79 41; e-mail, Zaida.Diaz@neuro.ki.se

RESULTS

Intracisternal injections of gal-(1-15) and gal-(1-16) produced a vasopressor response significantly different from that induced by gal-(1-29) and from the control group ($p < 0.01$) (FIG. 1), whereas the response induced by gal-(10-29) was not different from the control or the gal-(1-29) response. Both gal-(1-15) and gal-(1-16) induced tachycardic responses of similar intensity to that found with gal-(1-29), and all treatments gave significantly different responses from those of the control group ($p < 0.01$, and $p < 0.05$, respectively). However, the effect of gal-(10-29) on HR was no different from that of the control group.

The hypertension elicited by gal-(1-15) was not observed in propranolol pre-treated rats, but pre-treatment with atropine did not significantly modify this response (FIG. 2). This was true also for its tachycardic action. However, the cardiovascular actions of gal-(1-29) were unchanged during propranolol pre-treatment, but in atropine-treated rats gal-(1-29) elicited hypertension and tachycardia.

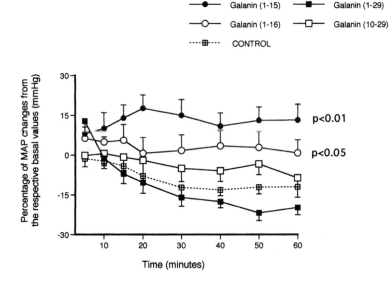

FIGURE 1. Effects of intracisternal injections of porcine galanin (1-29) (■), the NH$_2$-terminal galanin fragment (1-15) (●), the NH$_2$-terminal galanin fragment (1-16) (○), or the COOH-terminal galanin fragment (10-29) (□) (3.0 nmol/rat in all cases) on mean arterial blood pressure over a 60-minute recording period. Means ± SEM are shown as percentages of changes from the respective basal values. $n = 6$–8 rats per group. Basal values were: control group 86 ± 6 mm Hg; galanin-(l-15) group 85 ± 3 mm Hg; galanin-(1-16) group 98 ± 10 mm Hg; galanin-(1-29) group 90 ± 3 mmHg; galanin-(10-29) group 88 ± 10 mm Hg. $p < 0.01$ and $p < 0.05$ are the significance levels of the gal-(1-15) and gal-(1-16) groups versus the control group (Fisher post-hoc test), when considering the entire observation period.

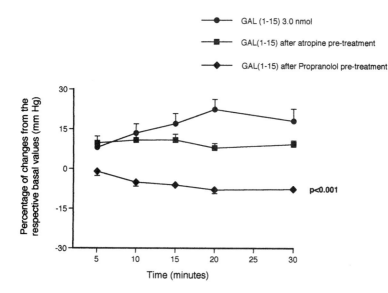

FIGURE 2. Effects of intracisternal injections of 3.0 nmol galanin-(1-15) (●) or 3.0 nmol galanin-(1-15) after atropine pre-treatment (■) or 3.0 nmol galanin-(1-15) after propranolol pre-treatment (◆) on mean arterial blood pressure over a 30-minute recording period. Means ± SEM are shown as percentages of changes from the respective basal values. n = 6–8 rats per group. Basal values were: galanin-(1-15) group 85 ± 3mm Hg; galanin-(1-15)-propranolol group 91 ± 7 mm Hg; galanin-(1-15)-atropine group 87 ± 6 mm Hg. $p < 0.001$ is the significance level of the gal-(1-15)-propranolol group versus gal-(1-15) group (Fisher post-hoc test) when considering the entire observation period.

DISCUSSION

The two NH$_2$-terminal galanin fragments showed similar cardiovascular effects, but opposite to those elicited by gal-(1-29), whereas the COOH-terminal galanin fragment (10-29) did not appear to play any role in central cardiovascular regulation. These results give further functional indications to support the existence of a unique galanin fragment receptor recognizing NH$_2$-terminal fragments, but not COOH-terminal fragments.

Furthermore, unlike atropine, the beta-adrenergic antagonist propranolol blocked the cardiovascular actions of gal-(1-15), suggesting that these actions of the NH$_2$-terminal fragments may be mediated through changes in sympathetic outflow. The absence of modulation of the cardiovascular effects of gal-(1-29) under propranolol treatment and the modification of its responses in atropine pre-treated rats suggests that for its actions the galanin receptor depends on cholinergic systems, possibly at a central level.

In conclusion, it is proposed that NH$_2$-terminal galanin fragments centrally through activation of a galanin fragment receptor distinct from galanin receptors induce hypertension and tachycardia through increases in central sympathetic outflow.

REFERENCES

1. Härfstrand, A., K. Fuxe, T. Melander, T. Hökfelt & L.F. Agnati. 1987. Evidence for a cardiovascular role of central galanin neurons: Focus on interactions with α2-adrenergic and neuropeptide Y mechanisms. J. Cardiovasc. Pharmacol. **10:** 199–204.
2. Hedlund, P., J.A. Aguirre, J.A. Narvaez & K. Fuxe. 1991. Intracisternally coinjected galanin and a 5-HT$_{1A}$ receptor agonist act synergistically to produce vasodrepessor responses in the α-chloralose anaesthetized male rat. Eur. J. Pharmacol. **204:** 87–95.
3. Narvaez, J.A., Z. Diaz, J.A. Aguirre, S. Gonzalez-Baron, N. Yanaihara, K. Fuxe & P.B. Hedlund. 1994. Intracisternally injected galanin-(1-15) modulates the cardiovascular responses of galanin-(1-29) and the 5-HT$_{1A}$ receptor agonist 8-OH-DPAT. Eur. J. Pharmacol. **257:** 257–265.
4. Kunkler, P.E., G.-M. Wang & B.H. Hwang. 1994. Galanin-containing neurons in the solitary nucleus and locus coeruleus of spontaneously hypertensive rats are associated with genetic hypertension. Brain Res. **651:** 349–352.
5. Diaz, Z., J.A. Narvaez, P.B. Hedlund, J.A. Aguirre, S. Gonzalez-Baron & K. Fuxe. 1996. Centrally infused galanin-(1-15) but not galanin-(1-29) reduces the baroreceptor reflex sensitivity in the rat. Brain Res. **741:** 32–37.
6. Narvaez, J.A., Z. Diaz, P.B. Hedlund, J.A. Aguirre, R. Covenas, S. Gonzalez-Baron & K. Fuxe. Galanin antagonist M40 blocks the cardiovascular effects elicited by the galanin N-terminal fragment (1-15) but not by galanin (1-29). Eur. J. Pharmacol. Submitted.
7. Crawley, J.N., M.C. Austin, S.M. Fiske, B. Martin, S. Consolo, M. Berthold, U. Langel, G. Fisone & T. Bartfai. 1990. Activity of centrally administered galanin fragments on stimulation of feeding behaviour and on galanin receptor binding in the rat hypothalamus. J. Neurosci. **10:** 3695–3700.

Expression of Galanin and the GALR1 Galanin Receptor Subtype in the Colon of Children with Paradoxical Fecal Incontinence

A. ENGELIS,[a] DZ. MOZGIS,[a] K.A. PINE,[b] J. SHINE,[b] T.P. IISMAA,[b] AND M. PILMANE[c,d]

[a]*Latvian Medical Academy, State Children's Hospital, Vienibas Gatve 45, LV 1004, Riga, Latvia*

[b]*The Garvan Institute of Medical Research, 384 Victoria Street, Sydney, NSW 2010, Australia*

[c]*Latvian Postgraduate and Continuing Medical Education Institute, Skolas Street 1a, Riga, LV 1010, Latvia*

Galanin is a 29-30 amino acid peptide originally isolated from porcine upper small intestine and subsequently from a number of vertebrate species.[1] Galanin is expressed in the neurons and nerve fibers of the gastrointestinal tract of mammals,[2,3] and regulates ion absorption in ileal tissue[4] and the contractile activity of digestive smooth muscle.[5-7] Three galanin receptor subtypes have been cloned to date.[1] The GALR1 subtype is expressed in the normal human gastrointestinal tract,[8] but its expression in diseased gastrointestinal tissue is not known. In this study, we examined the distribution of galaninergic fibers and expression of GALR1 in mucosal epithelial cells in the colon of children with evacuation disorders of the bowel.

MATERIALS AND METHODS

Patients. Colon biopsies were obtained from nine children aged 1–15 years with paradoxical fecal incontinence and from one (control) child during polipoextirpation, from each of the regions of the linea pectinea and the colon 10 cm from the anus, according to the method of Scharli.[9]

Immunohistochemistry. Tissue samples were fixed in 10% formalin for 24 hours, embedded in paraffin, and then sectioned at a thickness of 5 μm. Galanin-containing nerve fibers were detected with rabbit anti-galanin antiserum[10] (working dilution 1:800), using biotin/avidin immunohistochemistry as described by the manufacturer (Vector, Burlingame, California, USA). Immunoreactivity with synaptophysin (mouse, Sigma, St. Louis, Missouri, USA; working dilution 1:300) and protein gene peptide 9.5 (PGP 9.5, rabbit, Ultraclone, Cambridge, UK; working dilution 1:1600) was detected using indirect immunofluorescence.[11] Light microscopy sections stained with hematoxylin and eosin were prepared for each biopsy.

[d]Address for correspondence: Mara Pilmane, Latvian Postgraduate and Continuing Medical Education Institute, Skolas Street 1a, Riga, LV 1010, Latvia. Phone, 371 7 240 368; fax, 371 7 288 734; e-mail, pilmane@com.latnet.lv

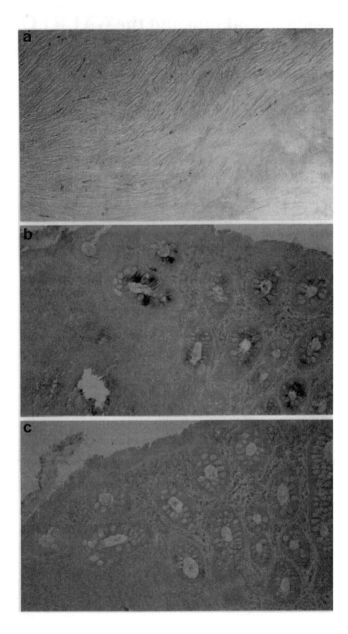

FIGURE 1. Light micrographs of human colon in patients with paradoxical fecal incontinence. (a) Galanin immunoreactive nerve fibers in the connective tissue of submucous layer (biotin and avidin histochemistry; ×200). (b and c) GALR1 mRNA *in situ* hybridization in mucosal epithelial cells: antisense riboprobe (b), ×200; sense riboprobe (c), ×200.

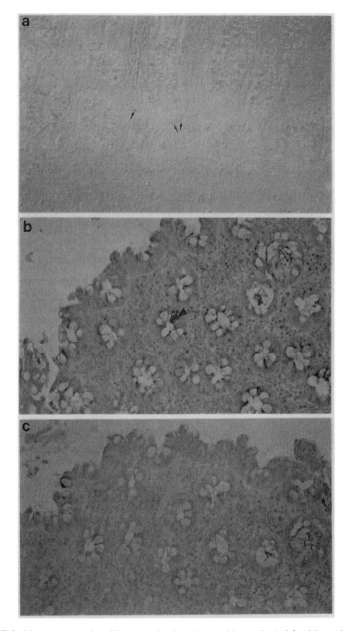

FIGURE 2. Light micrographs of human colon in patients with paradoxical fecal incontinence. (a) galanin-containing nerve fibers around the crypts in the mucous layer of the colon (biotin and avidin histochemistry; ×200). (b and c) GALR1 mRNA *in situ* hybridization in epitheliocytes: antisense riboprobe (b), ×200; sense riboprobe (c), ×200.

In situ Hybridization. Digoxygenin-labeled sense and antisense riboprobes were synthesized from a construct of a 376-bp fragment, corresponding to the segment extending from the third intracellular loop to the COOH-terminus of human GALR1,[12] according to directions of the manufacturer (Dla RNA Labelling kit [SP6/T7]; Boehringer-Mannheim). *In situ* hybridization was performed on 5-μm sections of biopsy material, as described previously.[13]

RESULTS AND DISCUSSION

All biopsies possessed a mucous and a submucous layer of colon and showed infiltration by white blood cells. The general neuronal markers PGP 9.5 and synaptophysin stained fine nerve fibers around crypts, epitheliocytes, and some nerve trunks in the submucous layer. Two types of distribution of galanin-containing nerve fibers were observed in tissue of both the region of the linea pectinea and the colon 10 cm from the anus. In seven of nine biopsies of diseased tissue, many fine galanin-immunoreactive nerve fibers occurred around the crypts, beneath the surface epithelium, and in the submucous connective tissue (FIG. 1a). Occasional galanin-containing nerve fibers were seen in these locations in two biopsies and in control tissue (FIG. 2a). Positive signal for GALR1 was detected in many epitheliocytes in tissue densely innervated with galanin-containing nerve fibers (FIGS. 1b and c), whereas biopsy and control tissues that contained occasional galanin-immunoreactive nerve fibers contained few epitheliocytes expressing GALR1 mRNA (FIGS. 2b and c). This study suggests that a correlation may exist between expression of GALR1 mRNA in epitheliocytes and the relative abundance of galanin-containing nerve fibers in mucosal and submucosal layers. The significance of this finding in the functioning of the diseased bowel and its relevance to inflammation in gut tissue remain to be determined.

REFERENCES

1. FATHI, Z., W.B. CHURCH & T.P. IISMAA. 1998. Galanin receptors: Recent developments and potential use as therapeutic targets. Ann. Rep. Med. Chem. In press.
2. BAUER, F.E., T.E. ADRIAN, N.D. CHRISTOFIDES, G.L. FERRI, N.Y. YANAIHARA, J.M. POLAK & S.R. BLOOM. 1986. Distribution and molecular heterogeneity of galanin in human, pig, guinea pig and rat gastrointestinal tract. Gastroenterology **91:** 877–883.
3. BISHOP, A., J. POLACK, F.E. BAUER, N.D. CHRISTOFIDES, F. CARBI & S.R. BLOOM. 1986. Occurrence and distribution of a newly discovered peptide, galanin, in the mammalian enteric nervous system. Gut **27:** 849–857.
4. HOMAIDAN, F.R., S.H. TANG, M. DONOWITZ & G.W. SCHARP. 1994. Peptides 15: 1431–1436.
5. FOX, J.E.T., T.J. MCDONALD, S. CIPRIS, Z. WOSKOWSKA & E.E. DANIEL. 1991. Galanin inhibition of vasoactive intestinal polypeptide release and circular muscle motility in the isolated perfused canine ileum. Gastroenterology **101:** 1471–1476.
6. KUWAHARA, A., T. OZAKI & N. YANAIHARA. 1990. Structural requirements for galanin action in the guinea-pig ileum. Regul. Pept. **29:** 23–29.
7. KATSOULIS, S., A. CLEMENTS, C. MORYS-WORTMANN, H. SCHWÖRER, H. SCHAUBE, H.J. KLOMP, H.J. FÖLSCH & W.E. SCHMIDT. 1996. Human galanin modulates human colonic motility in vitro. Characterization of structural requirements. Scand. J. Gastroenterol. **31:** 446–451.
8. LORIMER, D.D. & R.V. BENYA. 1996. Cloning and quantification of galanin-1 receptor expression by mucosal cells lining the human gastrointestinal tract. Chem. Biophy. Res. Commun. **222:** 379–385.

9. Scharli, A.F. 1992. Neuronal intestinal dysplasia. Pediatr. Surg. Int. **7:** 2–7.

10. Carey, D.G., T.P. Iismaa, K.Y. Ho, I.A. Rajkovic, J. Kelly, E.W. Kraegen, J. Ferguson, A.S. Inglis, J. Shine & D.J. Chisholm. 1993. Potent effects of human galanin in man: Growth hormone secretion and vagal blockade. J. Clin. Endocrinol. Metab. **77:** 90–93.

11. Coons, A.D., R.E.H. Leduc & J.M. Connoly. 1955. Studies of antibody production. A method for the histochemical demonstration of specific antibody and its application to a study of the hyperimmune rabbit. J. Exp. Med. **102:** 49–60.

12. Jacoby, A.S., A.C. Webb, M.L. Liu, B. Kofler, Y.T. Hort, Z. Fathi, C.D.K. Bottema & J. Shine. 1997. Structural organization of the mouse and human GALR1 galanin receptor genes (*galnr* and *GALNR*) and chromosomal localization of the mouse gene. Genomics **45:** 446–508.

13. Fathi, Z., A.M. Cunningham, L.G. Iben, P.B. Battaglino, S.A. Ward, K.A. Nichol, K.A. Pine, J. Wang, M.E. Goldstein, T.P. Iismaa & I. Antal Zimanyi. 1997. Cloning, pharmacological characterization and distribution of a novel galanin receptor. Mol. Brain Res. **51:** 49–53.

Effects of Antimetabolites to Glucose and Fatty Acids on Galanin-1 Receptor mRNA Levels in the Hypothalamic Paraventricular and Supraoptic Nuclei[a]

O. GORBATYUK AND T. HÖKFELT[b]

Department of Neuroscience, Karolinska Institutet, S-171 77 Stockholm, Sweden

Galanin-R1 receptor (GAL-R1) mRNA has a wide distribution in the rat brain, including the hypothalamic paraventricular (PVN) and supraoptic (SON) nuclei.[1–4] It was previously shown that galanin is involved in the central regulation of food intake. Thus, galanin injected into the hypothalamus of satiated rats activates food intake.[5,6] The hypothalamic PVN and, to some extent, the SON are known to play an important role[7,8] in addition to their involvement in general control of autonomic functions.[9,10]

To determine the possible involvement of the GAL-R1 in the PVN and SON in the control of food intake, we induced pharmacologic blockade of glucose utilization by 2-deoxy-D-glucose (2-DG) and of fatty acid oxidation by mercaptoacetate (MA). In our experimental model repeated injections of DG and MA (four times for DG and two injections for MA during 8 hours) were given, and GAL-R1 mRNA levels were monitored in the PVN and SON.

Male Sprague-Dawley rats (body weight 200–220 g, B&K Universal, Stockholm, Sweden) were used. All animals had free access to laboratory chow. Some rats were used in preliminary experiments to define appropriate doses. As a result, rats were subjected to intraperitoneal administration of repeated doses of DG or MA (four injections of DG, 500 mg/kg, with 2-hour intervals, or two injections of MA 57 mg/kg with 4-hour intervals) over a period of 8 hours.

Cryostat sections (14 μm) of unfixed brain tissue were processed for *in situ* hybridization histochemistry, as described earlier.[11] Sequences were complementary to nucleotides 4-51, 506-553, 784-831, and 975-1022 of the cDNA encoding the rat GAL-R1.

After hybridization, sections were covered with Amersham-β-max X-ray film (Amersham) for 3 weeks, developed, and processed for quantitative analysis. The average isotope concentration of control tissue sections was set to 100%, and changes during experimental conditions were expressed in percentage of control ± SEM. Statistical analysis was carried out using analysis of variance (ANOVA) followed by Dunett's test.

In situ hybridization histochemistry revealed that the GAL-R1 mRNA levels significantly increased in both the PVN and SON after prolonged stimulation by 2-DG as well as by MA. Compared to control levels the increase in GAL-R1 mRNA expression was $60 \pm 5.8\%$ ($p < 0.01$) in the PVN and $93 \pm 10.1\%$ ($p < 0.01$) in the SON for 2-DG–treated

[a]This study was supported by the Swedish MRC (04X-2887), Marianne och Marcus Wallenbergs Stiftelse, and a Fellowship to Oleg Gorbatyuk from the Swedish Royal Academy of Sciences.

[b]Author to whom correspondence should be addressed. Phone, 46 8-7287070; fax, 46 8-331692; e-mail, Tomas.Hokfelt@neuro.ki.se

rats. Repeated injections of MA also resulted in a highly significant GAL-R1 mRNA transcript elevation in the PVN ($88 \pm 6.5\%$) and SON ($77 \pm 7.4\%$).

These findings suggest that both glucoprivation and lipoprivation enhance the sensitivity of PVN and SON neurons to galanin and that this enhancement may contribute to the subsequent compensatory increase in food intake.

REFERENCES

1. BURGEVIN, M.-C., I. LOQUET, D. QUARTERONET & E. HABERT-ORTOLI. 1995. Cloning, pharmacological characterization, and anatomical distribution of a rat cDNA encoding for a galanin receptor. J. Mol. Neurosci. **6:** 33–41.
2. PARKER, E.M., D.G. IZZARELLI, H.P. NOWAK, C.D. MAHLE, L.G. IBEN, J. WANG & M.E. GOLDSTEIN. 1995. Cloning and characterization of the rat GALR1 galanin receptor from Rin14B insulinoma cells. Mol. Brain Res. **34:** 179–189.
3. GUSTAFSON, E.L., K.E. SMITH, M.M. DURKIN, C. GERALD & T.A. BRANCHEK. 1996. Distribution of a rat galanin receptor mRNA in rat brain. NeuroReport **7:** 953–957.
4. MITCHELL, V., E. HABERT-ORTOLI, J. EPELBAUM, J.-P. AUBERT & J.-C. BEAUVILLAIN. 1997. Semiquantitative distribution of galanin-receptor (GAL-R1)mRNA-containing cells in the male rat hypothalamus. Neuroendocrinology, **66:** 160–172.
5. KYRKOULI, S.E., B.G. STANLEY & S.F. LEIBOWITZ. 1986. Galanin: Stimulation of feeding induced by medial hypothalamic injection of this novel peptide. Eur. J. Pharmacol. **122:** 159–160.
6. CRAWLEY, J., M.C. AUSTIN, S.M. FISKE, B. MARTIN, S. CONSOLO, M. BERTHOLD, Ü. LANGEL, G. FISONE & T. BARTFAI. 1990. Activity of centrally administered galanin fragments on stimulation of feeding behaviour and on galanin receptor binding in the rat hypothalamus. J. Neurosci. **10:** 3695.
7. LEIBOWITZ, S.F. 1995. Brain peptides and obesity: Pharmacological treatment. Obes. Res. **3:** 573S–589S.
8. KALRA, S.P. 1997. Appetite and body weight regulation: Is it all in the brain? Neuron **19:** 227–230.
9. SWANSON L.W. & P.E. SAWCHENKO. 1983. Hypothalamic integrations: Organization of the paraventricular and supraoptic nuclei. Annu. Rev. Neurosci. **6:** 269–324.
10. LUITEN P.G., G.J. TER HORST & A.B. STEFFENS. 1987. The hypothalamic, intrinsic connections and outflow pathways to the endocrine system in relation to the control of feeding and metabolism. Prog. Neurobiol. **28:** 1–54.
11. DAGERLIND, Å., K. FRIBERG, A. BEAN & T. HÖKFELT. 1992. Sensitive mRNA detection using unfixed tissue: combined radioactive and non-radioactive *in situ* hybridization histochemistry. Histochemistry **98:** 39–49.

Hypothalamic Galanin Is Upregulated during Hyperphagia[a]

P.S. KALRA,[b,d] S. PU,[c] T. EDWARDS,[b] AND M.G. DUBE[b]

Departments of [b]Physiology and [c]Neuroscience, University of Florida College of Medicine, Gainesville, Florida 32610, USA

Impairment of neural signaling in the ventromedial hypothalamus (VMH) by electrolytic lesions induces persistent hyperphagia and excessive body weight gain. Hyperphagia may also be induced by microinjection of colchicine (COL), a neurotoxin that blocks neuronal axoplasmic flow, into the ventromedial nucleus (VMN) of the hypothalamus. COL-induced hyperphagia is rapid in onset and temporary. It is characterized by a loss of regulated feeding, with rats consuming equal amounts of food during the dark and light phases for 4 days postinjection.[1] The neural signaling mechanisms accountable for this phenomenon are not known; however, the current view is that altered signaling in the orexigenic and anorexigenic networks may underlie the disturbed appetitive behavior. For the last few years we have systematically analyzed the pattern of orexigenic signaling during this transient hyperphagia in an attempt to identify the neurochemical substrate of obesity. We recently reported that in VMN-COL–microinjected rats, the levels and gene expression of neuropeptide Y (NPY), the most potent and abundant orexigenic peptide in the hypothalamus, were markedly reduced concurrent with increases in NPY Y_1 receptor mRNA levels.[1] These results suggested that increased expression of NPY Y_1 receptors in hypothalamic sites involved in ingestive behavior may account for increased food intake despite the low levels of endogenous NPY in these rats.[2]

The role of galanin (GAL) in feeding has been extensively studied since the demonstration that central administration of GAL stimulated feeding, with rats displaying a preference for a high fat diet. (For a review see refs. 3 and 4.) Because continuous infusion of GAL failed to produce sustained hyperphagia and body weight gain,[5] the physiologic relevance of GAL in the regulation of daily food intake and in the development of obesity is unclear. To determine the role of GAL in the experimental model of transient hyperphagia induced by COL microinjection into the VMN, we analyzed hypothalamic GAL levels and gene expression and examined appetitive behavior in response to intracerebroventricular administration of GAL in these rats.

GALANIN GENE EXPRESSION IN THE HYPOTHALAMUS

GAL gene expression, as analyzed by the ribonuclease protection assay in the whole hypothalamus, was rapidly upregulated. Within 24 hours of COL injection, GAL mRNA

[a]This work was supported by Grant NS32727 from the National Institutes of Health.

[d]Address for correspondence: Pushpa S. Kalra, PhD, University of Florida College of Medicine, Department of Physiology, Box 100274, Gainesville, FL 32610-0274. Phone, 352-392-4169; fax, 352-846-0270; e-mail, pkalra@phys.med.ufl.edu

levels were more than twofold higher than these in control rats similarly injected with saline solution in the VMN. These high levels were maintained throughout the period of avid hyperphagia until day 4. Inasmuch as GAL is known to elicit multiple neuroendocrine effects and is produced in a number of sites in the hypothalamus, it was important to determine if this COL-induced upregulation occurred in hypothalamic sites implicated in the regulation of appetite. Regional analysis of GAL gene expression on day 4 after COL injection was conducted by *in situ* hybridization. Interestingly, maximal increases were detected in the arcuate and dorsal-medial nuclei of the hypothalamus; significant increases were also seen in the parvocellular regions of the paraventricular nucleus and in the supraoptic nuclei.

GALANIN CONCENTRATION IN THE HYPOTHALAMUS

To determine if this increase in GAL gene expression is translated to increased levels of the peptide, immunoreactive GAL was quantitated in microdissected hypothalamic nuclei of rats after COL microinjection. Progressive increases in GAL concentration were seen in hypothalamic sites known to be relevant for appetite regulation. In the dorsal-medial nuclei and paraventricular nuclei of COL-injected rats, GAL levels were three- to fourfold higher than those in saline-injected control rats. Significant increases were also seen in the median eminence-arcuate, VMN, lateral preoptic area, and perifornicle and lateral hypothalamic areas. The implication that these increases, especially those in the paraventricular nucleus, lateral hypothalamus, and VMN, induce hyperphagia is supported by the finding that microinjection of GAL into these sites stimulated feeding.[6]

RESPONSE TO GALANIN ADMINISTRATION

We extended these studies to determine if COL-injected rats were hyperresponsive to the appetite-stimulating effects of GAL. One-hour food intake in response to GAL (2 nmol icv) was significantly and consistently higher in COL-injected rats than in control rats on days 2–10 post-COL injection (6.1 ± 0.38 g vs 3.4 ± 0.3g; $p < 0.001$); latency to initiate feeding was significantly decreased during this period.

SUMMARY

In summary, a multifaceted approach was employed to assess the role of GAL in hyperphagia and obesity. The results showed that unlike NPY, GAL synthesis (gene expression and peptide levels) increased in various hypothalamic sites known to be important for central regulation of appetite. Also, hyperphagic rats were hyperresponsive to GAL administration. These observations are the first demonstration of a tight temporal correlation between hypothalamic GAL signaling and hyperphagia leading to excessive body weight gain.

REFERENCES

1. KALRA, P.S., M.G. DUBE, B. XU, & S.P. KALRA. 1997. Increased receptor sensitivity to neuropeptide Y in the hypothalamus may underlie transient hyperphagia and body weight gain. Regul. Pept. **72:** 121–130.
2. KALRA, P.S., M.G. DUBE, B. XU, W.G. FARMERIE & S.P. KALRA. 1998. Neuropeptide Y (NPY) Y$_1$ receptor mRNA is upregulated in association with transient hyperphagia and body weight gain: Evidence for concurrent development of leptin resistance. J. Neuroendocrinol. **10:** 43–49.
3. LEIBOWITZ, S.F. 1995. Brain peptides and obesity: Pharmacologic treatment. Obesity Res. **3:** 573S–589S.
4. KALRA, S.P., B. XU, M.G. DUBE, S. PU & P.S. KALRA. 1999. Interactive appetite regulating pathways in the hypothalamic regulation of body weight. Endocrine Rev. In press.
5. SMITH, B.K., D.A. YORK & G.A. BRAY. 1994. Chronic cerebroventricular galanin does not induce sustained hyperphagia or obesity. Peptides **15:** 1267–1272.
6. KRYKOULI, S.E., B.G. STANLEY, R.D. SEIRAL & S.F. LEIBOWITZ. 1990. Stimulation of feeding by galanin: Anatomical localization and behavioral specificity of the peptide's effects in the brain. Peptides **11:** 995–1100.

Effects of Different Galanins on the Release of Acetylcholine in the Various Areas of Rat Brain[a]

PETER KASA, ZOLTAN FARKAS, MONIKA FORGON, HENRIETTA PAPP, AND LAJOS BALASPIRI[b]

Alzheimer's Disease Research Centre and [b]Department of Medical Chemistry, A. Szent-Gyorgyi Medical University, H-6720 Szeged, Hungary

The various areas of the central nervous system (CNS) are innervated differentially by galaninergic nerve fibers. Neurochemical, histochemical, and immunohistochemical observations reveal that the elements of the cholinergic system are reduced, whereas the number of galanin (GAL)-positive nerve fibers is significantly increased in Alzheimer's disease. It was suggested earlier that GAL has a crucial role in the regulation of cholinergic function and may be involved in the cognitive dysfunctions associated with Alzheimer's disease. In neuropharmacologic experiments pGAL1-29 inhibits K^+-evoked acetylcholine (ACh) release from the hippocampus, whereas it stimulates the basal release of ACh from the striatum of the rat.[1] In the CNS, pGAL1-29 reduces the evoked release of ACh from the ventral hippocampus and initiates inhibitory modulation of several central neurotransmitters at both pre- and postsynaptic levels. Because the number of excitatory cholinergic neurons in the basal forebrain is reduced and the number of inhibitory GAL-containing nerve fibers is increased in Alzheimer's disease, it is suggested that GAL may be involved in the etiology of the disease. GAL actions are mediated by different types of GAL receptors, and the receptor antagonist may have therapeutic potential in the treatment of Alzheimer's disease.[3] In this study we compared the effects of hGAL1-30 and its NH_2-terminal (hGAL1-19) and COOH-terminal parts (hGAL17-30, hGAL21-30, and hGAL26-30) with those of pGAL1-29 on the basal release of ACh and evoked by K^+ or electrical stimulation in different areas of the CNS of the rat.

NEUROPHARMACOLOGY

The basal forebrain, striatum, and main olfactory bulb of Sprague-Dawley male rats was dissected and sliced to a thickness of 0.35 mm. The tissue slices were incubated for 60 minutes at 37°C in Krebs-Ringer buffer solutions (KRS) containing 2 µCi/ml [^{3}H]choline (82 Ci/mmol; 37 MBq/ml; Amersham). Slices were then processed for ACh release as described.[2]

EFFECT OF DIFFERENT GALANINS

In neuropharmacologic experiments, direct stimulatory effects of 200 nM hGAL1-30, hGAL21-30, hGAL26-30, and pGAL1-29 on ACh release could be demonstrated in the

[a]This work was supported by Grants MKM-36, OTKA-T022683, T016565, and ETT-584/1996.

basal forebrain of the rat. pGAL1-29 increased the basal release of ACh in a dose-dependent manner, and this effect was antagonized by 1 μM M15. The 50 mM K$^+$-evoked ACh release was not modulated by 200 nM hGAL1-30, whereas the amount of ACh released was inhibited by 500 nM pGAL1-29. Electrically evoked [^{3}H]ACh release was reduced by 200 nM hGAL1-30, but not by 200 nM hGAL1-19. The COOH-terminal fragment hGAL21-30 had a similar inhibitory effect on ACh release as could be demonstrated with hGAL1-30. The evoked release process was Ca^{2+}-dependent. The GAL receptor antagonist M15 (1 mM) did not prevent the inhibitory effects of hGAL1-30 and hGAL21-30 on the electrically evoked ACh release. The results clearly demonstrate the modulatory effects of galanins on cholinergic neuronal transmission (FIG. 1). We concluded that the COOH-terminal fragments (hGAL21-30 and hGAL26-30) can effectively modulate ACh release mechanism in the basal forebrain.

In the striatum, results show that 500 nM hGAL1-30, hGAL1-19, and hGAL17-30 and 1 μM galantide (M15) had no effect, whereas 200 nM pGAL1-29 stimulated the basal release of ACh. Also, 500 nM hGAL1-30, hGAL17-30, and hGAL26-30 diminished both the K$^+$ and electrically evoked release, but 500 nM hGAL1-19 had no inhibitory effect on the K$^+$-evoked ACh release. The inhibitory effect of hGAL1-30 and hGAL26-30 on K$^+$-evoked ACh release was antagonized by 1 μM M15; no such effect of M15 was observed during electrical stimulation.The combination of nifedipine with hGAL1-30 dramatically reduced electrically induced ACh release, but nifedipine had no such effect on K$^+$-evoked ACh release. The most interesting finding is the inhibitory effect of the COOH-terminal fragments of the peptide (hGAL17-30 and hGAL26-30) on K$^+$-induced [^{3}H]ACh release

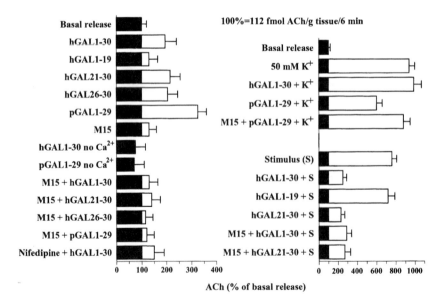

FIGURE 1. Effects of different substances on the release of acetylcholine from the basal forebrain of the rat.

in the striatum. Such a modulatory effect of the NH_2-terminal fragment (hGAL1-19) on the transmitter release could not be demonstrated.

The effects of GAL on basal release and on 50 mM K^+-stimulated [^{3}H]ACh release were investigated on main olfactory bulb tissue slices too. It was demonstrated that 200 nM hGAL1-30 had no effect, whereas 200 nM pGAL1-29 administered to the tissue samples exerted a significant stimulatory effect on the basal release of ACh. This excitatory effect was prevented by 400 nM M15. The effect of 50 mM K^+ on ACh release was not reduced by either 200 nM pGAL1-29 or hGAL1-30. The stimulatory effect of 200 nM pGAL1-29, however, was Ca^{2+}-dependent, because it was blocked by 1 mM EDTA.

CONCLUSION

hGAL and pGAL can modulate the *in vitro* release of ACh, but the effects of the peptides in various regions of the CNS of the rat may differ.

REFERENCES

1. PRAMANIK, A. & S.O. OGREN. 1992. Brain Res. **574:** 317–319.
2. KASA, P., Z. FARKAS, L. BALASPIRI & J. R. WOLFF. 1996. Neuroscience **72:** 709–723.
3. HÖKFELT, T., D. MILLHORN, Y. TSURUO, S. CECCATELLI, B. LINDH, B. MEISTER, T. MELANDER, M. SCHALLING, T. BARTFAI & L. TERENIUS. 1987. Experientia **43:** 768–780.

Galanin and Galanin Receptor Expression in Neuroblastoma[a]

C. TUECHLER,[b] R. HAMETNER,[c] N. JONES,[b] R. JONES,[b] T.P. IISMAA,[d] W. SPERL,[b] AND B. KOFLER[b,e]

[b]Children's Hospital and [c]Department of Dermatology, General Hospital Salzburg, Salzburg, Austria

[d]Garvan Institute of Medical Research, Sydney, Australia

Neuroblastoma, a tumor of the sympathetic nervous tissue, is the most common solid malignancy of childhood outside the central nervous system. Neuroblastomas produce and secrete various neuropeptides, as do other tumors of the neuroendocrine system.[1] Neuropeptides are known to exert both potent trophic and differentiative effects on a cellular level potentially via autocrine and paracrine functions.[2] Measurement of neuropeptide concentrations may be of value for diagnosing and monitoring tumor growth. A number of neuropeptides including bradykinin, bombesin, cholecystokinin, vasopressin, neurotensin, somatostatin, substance P, and galanin have been reported to serve as growth factors for human cancer cells by activating a signal transduction pathway via G-protein–coupled receptors.[3] In the present study we investigated the expression of galanin and galanin receptors in human neuroblastoma tissue.

GALANIN EXPRESSION IN NEUROBLASTOMA

We determined galanin expression in neuroblastoma tissue by reverse transcriptase-polymerase chain reaction (RT-PCR), Northern blot analysis, and immunohistochemistry (TABLE 1). Galanin concentration in neuroblastoma tissue was quantified by radioimmunoassay (RIA). The biological features (N-*myc* amplification, deletion of short arm of chromosome 1, and ploidy) of tumor tissues and results of our studies are summarized in TABLE 1. RT-PCR for the neuroendocrine gene product 9.5 was performed to verify the neuronal origin of the tumor tissues. All three neuroblastoma tissues investigated showed marked expression of galanin, with NB B showing the highest peptide concentration (0.65 ± 0.1 pmol/mg tissue) followed by NB A (0.12 pmol/mg tissue) and NB C (0.03 ± 0.005 pmol/mg tissue). For NB B, the concentration of galanin was 250 times higher than the galanin concentration found in normal adrenal tissue and 30 times higher than the concentration found in pheochromocytoma.[4]

[a]These studies were supported by the Children's Cancer Foundation, Salzburg, Austria.

[e]Address for correspondence: Dr. Barbara Kofler, Children's Hospital, General Hospital Salzburg, Müllner Hauptsr. 48, A-5020 Salzburg, Austria. Phone, 0043 662 4482 2650; fax, 0043 662 4482 4765; e-mail, b.kofler@lkasbg.gv.at

GALANIN RECEPTOR EXPRESSION IN NEUROBLASTOMA

Isolated membranes of all three neuroblastoma tissues investigated showed binding of [^{125}I]galanin and tissue sections (Fig. 1). Two of the three tissues expressed the human GALR1 galanin receptor subtype as shown by RT-PCR (Table 1).

Expression of functional galanin receptors seems to be inversely related to galanin peptide concentration (Table 1). The tumor tissue NB B with the highest galanin concentration expressed less functional galanin receptors. This might indicate a feedback regulation of galanin and its receptors.

TABLE 1. Expression of Galanin and Galanin Receptors in Neuroblastoma

Tumor Tissue	Galanin		Galanin Receptor		PGP 9.5[d,f]
	mRNA[a]	Peptide Concentration[b] (pmol/mg tissue)	[^{125}I]-Binding[c]	GALR1[d]	
NB A stage 4[g] N-*myc* neg 1p not del diploid	++	0.12	+++	Yes	Yes
NB B stage 1-2[g] N-*myc* neg 1p not del triploid	++++	0.65 ± 0.1	+	Yes	Yes
NB C stage 2[g] N-*myc* pos 1p not del triploid	+++	0.03 ± 0.005	++++	No	Yes
HBML[e]	+	nd	+++	Yes	Yes

[a]Relative mRNA levels were determined by Northern blot analysis.
[b]Peptide concentrations were determined by RIA.
[c][^{125}I]galanin binding was performed on membrane preparations.
[d]Expression determined by RT-PCR.
[e]HBML (human Bowes Melanoma cell line) was used as a positive control for GALR1 expression.
[f]PGP 9.5 (neuroendocrine gene product 9.5) was used as a marker for neuroblastoma tissue.
[g]Clinical stage according to INSS.[5]
Abbreviations: del, deleted; nd, not determined.

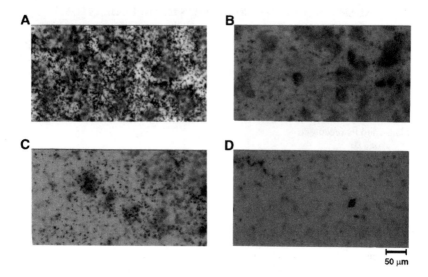

FIGURE 1. Distribution of galanin binding sites in human neuroblastoma tissue. **(A,C)** Total binding sites obtained with human [^{125}I]galanin on 12 μm cryostat sections. **(B,D)** Nonspecific binding in the presence of 100 nM unlabeled galanin; tumor tissue NB A **(A,B)** and NB B **(C,D)**.

CONCLUSION

These studies show for the first time that *in vivo* galanin and functional galanin receptors are expressed in neuroblastoma tissue at varying concentrations. Therefore, we speculate that galanin influences tumor development and/or growth via action on galanin receptors in tumor tissue in an autocrine and/or paracrine fashion; however, further studies are warranted. Investigation of additional tissue samples will show whether there is a correlation in the expression of galanin and galanin receptors in tumor tissue, tumor stage, and outcome.

ACKNOWLEDGMENT

We would like to thank Johann Bauer, Inge Ambros, and Peter Ambros for helpful discussions.

REFERENCES

1. KOGNER, P. 1995. Neuropeptides in neuroblastomas and ganglioneuromas. Prog. Brain Res. **104:** 325–338.
2. ROBBERECHT, P. *et al.* 1992. Structural requirements for the occupancy of pituitary adenylate-cyclase-activating-peptide (PACAP) receptors and adenylate cyclase activation in human neuroblastoma NB-OK-1 cell membranes. Discovery of PACAP (6-38) as a potent antagonist. Eur. J. Biochem. **207:** 239–246.

3. SETHI, T. *et al.* 1992. Growth of small cell lung cancer cells: Stimulation by multiple neuropeptides and inhibition by broad spectrum antagonists *in vitro* and *in vivo*. Cancer Res. **52:** 2737–2742.
4. BAUER, F.E. *et al.* 1986. Localization and molecular forms of galanin in human adrenals: Elevated levels in pheochromocytomas. J. Clin. Endocrinol. Metab. **63:** 1372–1378.
5. BRODEUR, G.M. *et al.* 1993. Revisions of the international criteria for neuroblastoma diagnosis, staging and response to treatment. J. Clin. Oncol. **11:** 1466-1477.

Modulation of a 5-HT$_{1A}$ Receptor-Mediated Behavioral Response by the Neuropeptide Galanin

ILGA MISANE,[a] HALEH RAZANI, FU-HUA WANG, ANDERS JANSSON,
KJELL FUXE, AND SVEN OVE ÖGREN

*Division of Cellular and Molecular Neurochemistry, Department of Neuroscience,
Karolinska Institute, S-171 77 Stockholm, Sweden*

Previous studies have shown that the neuropeptide galanin (GAL) modulates 5-HT$_{1A}$ receptor ([^{3}H]8-OH-DPAT) binding in the rat limbic forebrain membrane preparations.[1] The present study examined whether GAL, when given bilaterally into the lateral ventricle (icv), can modulate brain 5-HT$_{1A}$ receptor-mediated transmission *in vivo* in the

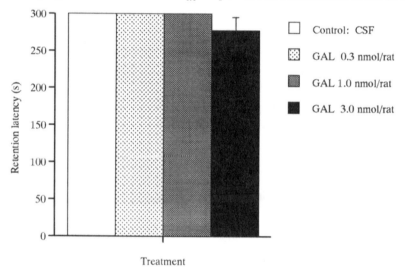

FIGURE 1. Dose-dependent effects of galanin on passive avoidance (PA) retention in the rat. Galanin (0.3, 1.0, or 3.0 nmol/rat) was administered via chronic cannulas bilaterally into the lateral ventricle (icv) 10 minutes before the training session (exposure to inescapable foot-shock). The CSF (icv, bilaterally, 2 μl/side) control group was run concurrently with the galanin-treated groups. The retention test was performed 24 hours later. *Vertical bars* represent means (± SEM) of retention latencies in groups of eight ($n = 8$) animals. Maximal time of latency was set at 300 seconds (cut-off time). Statistical analysis was performed by two-way ANOVA followed by Fisher's PLSD test. GAL, galanin. (Reprinted, with permission, from Blackwell Science Ltd.)

[a]Address for correspondence: Dr. Ilga Misane, Division of Cellular and Molecular Neurochemistry, Department of Neuroscience, Karolinska Institute, S-171 77 Stockholm, Sweden. Phone, +46 8 728 7071; fax, +46 8 302875.

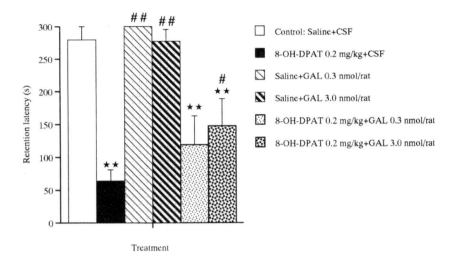

FIGURE 2. The combined effects of galanin and 8-OH-DPAT on passive avoidance (PA) retention in the rat. Rats were injected with 8-OH-DPAT (0.2 mg/kg sc) and/or galanin (0.3 or 3.0 nmol/rat icv, bilaterally) 15 and 10 minutes before the training session, respectively. The CSF (icv, bilaterally, 2 μl/side)+saline (sc 2 ml/kg) control group was run concurrently with the 8-OH-DPAT- and/or galanin-treated groups. The retention test was performed 24 hours later. *Vertical bars* represent means (± SEM) of retention latencies in groups of eight to nine ($n = 8-9$) animals. $\star\star p < 0.01$ versus saline+CSF control group; $^{#}p < 0.05$ versus 8-OH-DPAT+CSF–treated group; $^{##}P < 0.01$ versus 8-OH-DPAT+CSF–treated group. For details of statistical analysis and general information, see legend to FIGURE 1. GAL, galanin. (Reprinted, with permission, from Blackwell Science Ltd.)

rat.[2] For this purpose, we used passive avoidance (PA),[3] an aversive learning model that depends on limbic forebrain structures, particularly, the amygdala. Previous studies showed that administration of selective 5-HT$_{1A}$ agonists, such as 8-OH-DPAT and NDO 008, prior to PA training resulted in a dose-related impairment of PA retention.[4,5] This impairment appeared to be due to stimulation of postsynaptic 5-HT$_{1A}$ receptors.[5]

In the present study, GAL (0.3–3.0 nmol/rat icv) when given 10 minutes before PA training, did not affect PA retention which was tested 24 hours after training (FIG. 1). GAL (3.0 nmol) attenuated the impairment of PA retention induced by 8-OH-DPAT (0.2 mg/kg sc) (FIG. 2). At the 0.2 mg/kg dose, 8-OH-DPAT produced signs of the 5-HT syndrome, indicating postsynaptic 5-HT$_{1A}$ receptor activation. Both impairment of PA and the 5-HT syndrome were completely blocked by the selective 5-HT$_{1A}$ receptor antagonist WAY 100635 (0.1 mg/kg sc) which, by itself, did not affect passive avoidance retention. 8-OH-DPAT given at the low dose of 0.03 mg/kg, which presumably stimulates somatodendritic 5-HT$_{1A}$ autoreceptors *in vivo*, neither altered PA retention nor induced any visually detectable signs of the 5-HT syndrome. GAL (0.3 or 3.0 nmol) in combination with the 0.03-mg/kg dose of 8-OH-DPAT, did not modify PA. The immunohistochemical study of the distribution of icv administered GAL (10 minutes after infusion) showed strong diffuse labeling in the periventricular zone (100–200 μm) of the lateral ventricle. Furthermore, GAL-immunoreactive nerve cells appeared in both the dentate gyrus and the CA1, CA2, and

CA3 layers of the hippocampus as well as in the caudal but not the rostral amygdala. Only endogenous fibers were visualized in the septum. At the level of the dorsal raphe nucleus, a thin periventricular zone of galanin immunoreactivity was seen without labeling of cells. These results suggest that GAL can modulate postsynaptic 5-HT$_{1A}$ receptor transmission *in vivo* in discrete cell populations in the forebrain regions such as the dorsal and ventral hippocampus and parts of the amygdala. The indication that icv GAL may be taken up in certain populations of nerve terminals in the periventricular zone for retrograde transport suggests that this peptide may also affect intracellular events and thereby exert long-term behavioral effects.

REFERENCES

1. HEDLUND, P. & K. FUXE. 1996. Galanin and 5-HT$_{1A}$ receptor interactions as an integrative mechanism in 5-HT neurotransmission in the brain. Ann. N.Y. Acad. Sci. **780:** 193–212.
2. MISANE, I., H. RAZANI, F.H. WANG, A. JANSSON, K. FUXE & S.O. ÖGREN. 1998. Intraventricular galanin modulates a 5-HT$_{1A}$ receptor-mediated behavioural response in the rat. Eur. J. Neurosci. **10:** 1230–1240.
3. ÖGREN, S.O. 1985. Evidence for a role of brain serotonergic neurotransmission in avoidance learning. Acta Physiol. Scand. **544:** 1–71.
4. CARLI, M., S. TRANCHINA & R. SAMANIN. 1992. 8-Hydroxy-2-(di-n-propyloamino)tetralin, a 5-HT$_{1A}$ receptor agonist, impairs performance in a passive avoidance task. Eur. J. Pharmacol. **211:** 227–234.
5. MISANE, I., C. JOHANSSON & S.O. ÖGREN. 1998. Analysis of the 5-HT$_{1A}$ receptor involvement in passive avoidance in the rat. Br. J. Pharmacol. **125:** 499–509.

Distribution of Galanin Immunoreactivity in the Bronchi of Humans with Tuberculosis

M. PILMANE,[a,c] J. SHINE,[b] AND T.P. IISMAA[b]

[a]Latvian Postgraduate and Continuing Medical Education Institute,
Skolas Street 1a, Riga, LV 1010, Latvia

[b]The Garvan Institute of Medical Research, 384 Victoria Street,
Sydney, NSW 2010, Australia

Galanin is a neuropeptide 29-30 amino acids in length.[1] Galanin-containing nerve fibers are widely distributed in the mammalian central and peripheral nervous system[2] and innervate bundles of smooth muscle in the respiratory tract of healthy humans.[3] Generally, galanin localizes to sensory and cholinergic nerve fibers in the airways,[4] suggesting that this peptide might influence airway vascular and secretory function.[5] The aim of the present study was to investigate the distribution of the galanin-immunoreactive elements in the respiratory tract of humans with tuberculosis.

MATERIALS AND METHODS

Patients. Bronchial biopsies from seven patients aged 32–48 years were examined. Three patients exhibited a disseminated form of tuberculosis and four of them had fibrocavernous tuberculosis. All patients were smear positive. The duration of disease varied from 6 months to 10 years. Bronchial biopsies were obtained during bronchoscopy from both lungs.

Immunohistochemistry. Tissue samples were fixed in 10% formalin for 24 hours, embedded in paraffin, and then sectioned at a thickness of 5 μm. After deparaffinization, sections were rehydrated in phosphate-buffered saline solution (PBS) for 10 minutes, incubated in 10% normal goat serum for 20 minutes in a humidified chamber, and then incubated with primary rabbit anti-galanin antiserum[6] (working dilution 1:800) for 1 hour in a humidified chamber. After rinsing in PBS, sections were blocked with 0.3% peroxide for 15 minutes and rinsed in PBS again. A biotinylated goat anti-rabbit secondary antibody (Vector, Burlingame, California, USA; working dilution 1:300) was added for 30 minutes in a humidified chamber. After rinsing in PBS the sections were exposed to an avidin and biotinylated peroxidase macromolecular complex (Vector, Burlingame, California, USA) for 15 minutes in a humidified chamber. Diaminobenzidine was used as a substrate, giving a brown reaction product. Sections were then dehydrated and mounted.

Protein gene peptide 9.5 (PGP 9.5; Ultraclone, Cambridge, UK; working dilution 1:1600) was used to detect neuroendocrine cells and nerve fibers in bronchial biopsies

[c]Address for correspondence: Mara Pilmane, Latvian Postgraduate and Continuing Medical Education Institute, Skolas Street 1a, Riga, LV 1010, Latvia. Phone, 371 7 240 368; fax, 371 7 288 734; e-mail, pilmane@com.latnet.lv

using indirect immunofluorescence.[7] Additionally, sections from each biopsy were stained with hematoxylin and eosin for light microscopy.

RESULTS

Bronchial walls of control lung possessed ciliated epithelium in patients with both forms of disease. Human bronchial wall from affected lung exhibited metaplastic epithelium with intraepithelial white blood cells (FIG. 1a).

PGP 9.5 antiserum stained neuroendocrine cells in the epithelium and nerve fibers around the acini of seromucous glands, among bundles of nonvascular and vascular smooth muscle in the control biopsies of patients (FIG. 1c). No neuroendocrine cells or only a few immunoreactive nerve fibers were found in the bronchi of the tuberculosis-affected lung (FIG. 1b). Large PGP 9.5-positive nerve trunks in the subepithelial layer were detected in three controls and in two patients with affected lungs (FIG. 1d). Galanin-like immunoreactive nerve fibers were seen in both affected and control lung biopsies (FIG. 2a). Some of these fibers were located around secretory parts of seromucous glands and fibrotic tissue among the bundles of collagen and elastin fibres (FIG. 2b). Galanin-like immunoreactivity was also found in large nerve trunks, mainly in lung tissues more significantly affected by tuberculosis (FIG. 2c and d).

DISCUSSION

Few galanin-like nerve fibers were found in the bronchial wall of patients with different forms of tuberculosis. This finding is similar to that of Cheung et al.,[5] who found few galanin-containing nerves in porcine lung. There is a tendency to decreased galanin immunoreactivity in nerves from nasal mucosa towards the major bronchi of mammals.[5] However, specific inflammation, such as tuberculosis, might be a modulator of immunoreactive innervation.[8] Localization of galanin-containing nerve fibers around the seromucous glands may correlate with regulation of glandular secretion, given that an inhibitory effect of this peptide on mucous secretion into airways of rats has been reported.[9] Additionally, galanin has contractile effects on smooth muscle and might participate in the local blood flow to the bronchi.[9]

Prolonged and repeated lung disease in bronchi results in proliferation of substance P-, vasoactive intestinal peptide-, calcitonin gene-related peptide-containing nerve fibers.[10,11] However, we observed no correlation between proliferation of galanin-immunoreactive fibers and either the type of tuberculosis or the duration of disease.

FIGURE 1. Light (**a**) and fluorescence micrographs (**b-d**) of bronchial wall in humans with tuberculosis. (**a**) Metaplastic epithelium in tuberculosis affected lung. Note intraepithelial infiltration with white blood cells. Hematoxylin and eosin, X 400; (**b**) Absence of immunoreactive elements in bronchi of tuberculosis affected lung. X 200; (**c**) Note PGP 9.5-immunoreactive nerve fibers around secretory parts of seromucous glands (*arrows*), X 200; (**d**) PGP 9.5-containing fine nerve fibers and nerve trunks (*arrows*) in bronchi of control lung. X 200.

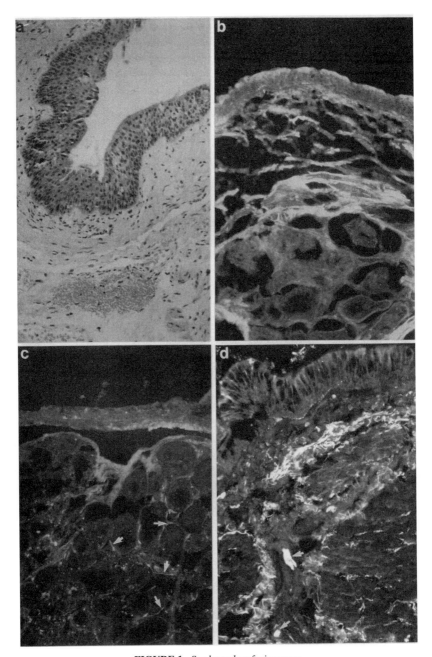

FIGURE 1. *See legend on facing page.*

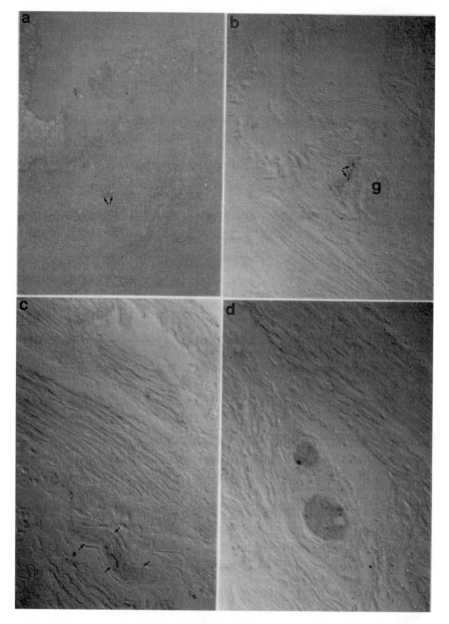

FIGURE 2. Light micrographs of human bronchial wall in patients with tuberculosis. Biotin-avidin histochemistry. Note fine galanin-containing nerve fibers among smooth muscle (**a,** *arrows*) and around the glands (**b,** *arrows*, **g** - glands) in control lung. X 200; Longitudinal (**c,** *arrows*) and transverse (**d**) section of galanin-containing nerve trunk in bronchi of tuberculosis affected lung. X 200.

REFERENCES

1. FATHI, Z., W.B. CHURCH & T.P. IISMAA. 1998. Galanin receptors: recent developments and potential use as therapeutic targets. Ann. Rep. Med. Chem. In press.
2. RÖKAEUS, Å., T. MELANDER, T. HOKFELT, J.M. LUNDBERG, K. TATEMOTO, M. CARLQUIST & V. MUTT. 1984. A galanin-like peptide in the central nervous system and intestine of the rat. Neurosci. Lett. **47:** 161–166.
3. LUTS, A., R. UDDMAN, P. BASTERRA & F. SUNDLER. 1993. Peptide-containing nerve fibres in human airways: distribution and coexistence pattern. Int. Arch. Allergy Immunol. **101:** 52–60.
4. TAKAHASHI, T., M.G. BELVISI & P. BARNES. 1994. Modulation of neurotransmission in guinea-pig airways by galanin and the effect of a new antagonist galantide. Neuropeptides **26:** 245–251.
5. CHEUNG, A., J.M. POLAK, F.E. BAUER, A. CADIEUX, N.D. CHRISTOFIDES, D.R. SPRINGALL & S.R. BLOOM. 1985. Distribution of galanin immunoreactivity in the respiratory tract of pig, guinea pig, rat, and dog. Thorax **40:** 889–896.
6. CAREY, D.G., T.P. IISMAA, K.Y. HO, I.A. RAJKOVIC, J. KELLY, E.W. KRAEGEN, J. FERGUSON, A.S. INGLIS, J. SHINE & D.J. CHISHOLM. 1993. Potent effects of human galanin in man: Growth hormone secretion and vagal blockade. J. Clin. Endocrinol. Metab. **77:** 90–93.
7. COONS, A.D., R.E.H. LEDUC & J.M. CONNOLY. 1955. Studies of antibody production. A method for the histochemical demonstration of specific antibody and its application to a study of the hyperimmune rabbit. J. Exp. Med. **102:** 49–60.
8. PILMANE, M., A. LUTS, F. SUNDLER & R. ZALESKY. 1996. Pulmonary neuroendocrine system in humans with lung tuberculosis. Eur. Respir. J. **9:** 333.
9. WAGNER, U., H.C. FEHMANN, D. BREDENBRÖKER, F. YU & P. VON WICHERT. 1995. Galanin and somatostatin inhibition of substance P-induced airway mucus secretion in the rat. Neuropeptides **28:** 59–64.
10. BARNES, P.J., J.N. BARANIUK & M.G. BELVISI. 1991. Neuropeptides in the respiratory tract. Part I. Am. Rev. Respir. Dis. **144:** 1187–1198.
11. PILMANE, M., A. LUTS & F. SUNDLER. 1995. Changes in neuroendocrine elements in bronchial mucosa in adult diseased lung. Thorax **50:** 551–554.

Galanin-Based Peptides, Galparan and Transportan, with Receptor-Dependent and Independent Activities

MARGUS POOGA,[a,b] MARIA LINDGREN,[a] MATTIAS HÄLLBRINK,[a]
EBBA BRÅKENHIELM,[a] AND ÜLO LANGEL[a,c]

[a]Department of Neurochemistry and Neurotoxicology, Arrheniuslaboratories,
Stockholm University, S-106 91 Stockholm, Sweden

[b]Estonian Biocentre, EE-2400, Tartu, Estonia

GALANIN AND MASTOPARAN

Galanin is a 29/30 amino acid long peptide distributed throughout the nervous system both centrally (CNS) and peripherally. The widespread distribution of galanin and its receptors predicts a number of roles for galanin, and indeed, galanin has been shown to inhibit insulin secretion and acetylcholine release, participate in pain signaling, and modify feeding behavior.[1] Only the NH_2-terminal part of galanin is required for binding to CNS galanin receptors, and in most experimental systems this part exerts agonist properties. The fragment galanin(1-13) is recognized with reasonable affinity by CNS receptors (K_D = 150 nM); the COOH-terminal fragment of galanin contributes only marginally to the binding to these receptors.[2]

The substitution of the COOH-terminal part of galanin with different neuropeptide motifs while preserving the 13 NH_2-terminal amino acids, has given rise to a family of galanin-based chimeric peptides. Some of these peptides, such as M15, M35, and C7, have very high affinity to galanin receptors.[3] Simultaneous binding to two receptors could be the reason for the high affinity, but interaction of the peptide COOH-terminal with the galanin receptor outside the galanin binding pocket or with cellular membranes is generally more probable. Therefore, a chimeric peptide containing the membrane-interacting peptide mastoparan, and galanin(1-13) was designed and synthesized.[4] Mastoparan is a 14 amino acid long peptide originally isolated from wasp venom and it interacts with membranes as an amphipathic helix or at higher concentrations as a bundle of helices.

GALPARAN

The chimeric peptide approach sometimes yields compounds with unpredicted properties, showing features substantially different from those of the parent compounds. Even though galparan can bind avidly to galanin receptors, its effects differ from those of galanin and mastoparan (TABLE 1). Galparan binds to CNS galanin receptors with high affinity, K_D = 6.4 nM. An analog of galparan, galparan 2, has an even higher affinity to galanin

[c]Address for correspondence: Dr. Ülo Langel, Department of Neurochemistry and Neurotoxicology, Arrheniuslaboratories, Stockholm University, S-106 91 Stockholm, Sweden. Phone, +46-8-161 793; fax, +46-8-161 371; e-mail, ulo@neurochem.su.se

TABLE 1. Effects of Galparan (GWTLNSAGYLLGPINLKALAALAKKIL-amide) and Galparan-2 (GWTLNSAGYLLGPINLKA<u>K</u>AALAKK<u>LL</u>-amide; amino acid substitutions in comparison with galparan are underlined)

System	Galanin	Galparan	Galparan-2
Displacement of ^{125}I-galanin[4]	$K_D = 0.74$ nM (in rat frontal cortex)	$K_D = 6.4$ nM (in rat frontal cortex)	$K_D = 0.71$nM (in rat frontal cortex)
	$K_D = 0.4$ nM (in RINm5F cells)[5]	$K_D = 7.1$ nM (in RINm5F cells)[5]	
Insulin secretion[5]	Inhibition by 59%	26-fold stimulation at 10 μM concentration	Twofold stimulation
Acetylcholine release in rat frontal cortex[6]	No effect	Reversible 46–60% induction	Not tested
Na+,K+-ATPase activity[4]	No effect	Activation by 40% at 4 μM concentration	No effect
GTPase activity[7]	No effect	Inhibition by 80% $IC_{50} = 12.1$ μM	Not tested

receptors, $K_D = 0.71$ nM. Galparan 10 μM induces a 26-fold increase in insulin secretion from rat pancreatic islets in a reversible and dose-dependent manner at 3 mM glucose concentration. Depolarization of B cells by KCl does not abolish the galparan-stimulated insulin release, demonstrating that the insulinogenic effect of galparan is mediated at a distal site in the stimulus secretion coupling of the B cell.[5]

Galparan induces *in vivo* acetylcholine release when injected intracerebroventricularly (icv) into the frontal cortex of the rat. These effects are reversible, dose-dependent, and not mediated by galanin receptors or at sites of mastoparan action.[6] On the other hand, galanin inhibits glucose-stimulated insulin release, and icv injections of galanin inhibit acetylcholine release in the ventral hippocampus.

Galparan, furthermore, modulates the activity of GTPases and Na+,K+-ATPase, whereas galanin does not affect these enzymes. A key enzyme in regulating ionic gradient across the membranes, Na+,K+-ATPase, is inhibited by mastoparan. Galparan at micromolar concentrations activates Na+,K+-ATPase and reverses its inhibition by ouabain.[4] Activation of the GTPases is one of the best characterized effects of mastoparan. Galparan, on the contrary, inhibits GTPases and reduces mastoparan-induced activation.[7]

TRANSPORTAN

The complex receptor-independent effects of galparan initiated the studies on its uptake and cellular localization. A derivative of galparan, biotinyl-transportan efficiently translocates from the culture medium into the cells (TABLE 2).[8] Transportan is already detectable in the plasma membrane after 1 minute incubation; penetration into the membranes of the endoplasmic reticulum and Golgi complex proceeds in the next 2–3 minutes. After 15 minutes transportan concentrates in the nuclear membrane and in distinct sub-

TABLE 2. Penetration of Biotinylated Peptides into Human Bowes Melanoma Cells as Determined by Indirect Immunofluorescence

Peptide	0°C	37°C
Transportan GWTLNSAGYLLGK*INLKALAALAKKIL-amide	+ + +	+ + +
Transportan-2 GWTLNSAGYLLGK*INLKAKAALAKKLL-amide**	++	++
Galanin *** GWTLNSAGYLLGPHIDNHRSFHDK*YGLA-amide	–	+
Mastoparan I*NLKALAALAKKIL-amide	+	+

* Biotinylated amino acid.
** Substitutions compared to transportan are underlined.
*** Probably receptor-mediated endocytosis.

compartments of the nuclei. The uptake of transportan is rapid and takes place in all animal cell lines studied so far, which excludes galanin receptor-mediated endocytosis. Lowering the temperature below 18°C, using hyperosmolar culture medium, or cross-linking of proteins on the cell surface does not hamper the internalization of transportan, demonstrating that it is not taken up by endocytosis.[8]

Transportan can deliver medium-sized hydrophilic compounds which can not enter the cells by themselves. The Pro[13] of the parent compound galparan is replaced by Lys in transportan, to enable convenient coupling of cargo molecules to the side chain amino group. So far, transportan has been used as a carrier vector for peptides, oligonucleotides as well as peptide nucleic acid.

The main obstacle to using transportan as a universal carrier vector is its property to inhibit GTPases. Albeit, transportan at concentrations used for delivery does not affect GTPase activity; modified transporting peptides have been synthesized. As compared to galparan-2, transportan-2, which has identical residue changes in the mastoparan part of the molecule, also penetrates the cells, but less efficiently than transportan (TABLE 2).

The properties of galparan and transportan are identical in all experimental setups used so far, which suggests that the properties of galparan-2 could be analogously ascribed to transportan-2. The latter can be considered a less disturbing carrier molecule than transportan, but it is also less efficient.

REFERENCES

1. KASK, K., M. BERTHOLD & T. BARTFAI. 1997. Galanin receptors: Involvement in feeding, pain, depression and Alzheimer's disease. Life Sci. **60:** 1523–1533.
2. LAND, T., Ü. LANGEL, M. LÖW, M. BERTHOLD, A. UNDÉN & T. BARTFAI. 1991. Linear and cyclic N-terminal galanin fragments and analogs as ligands at the hypothalamic galanin receptor. Int. J. Pept. Protein Res. **38:** 267–272.
3. BARTFAI, T., G. FISONE & Ü. LANGEL. 1992. Galanin and galanin antagonists: Molecular and biochemical perspectives. Trends Pharmacol. Sci. **13:** 312–317.

4. LANGEL, Ü., M. POOGA, C. KAIRANE, M. ZILMER & T. BARTFAI. 1996. A galanin-mastoparan chimeric peptide activates the Na+,K+-ATPase and reverses its inhibition by ouabain. Regul. Pept. **62:** 47–52.

5. ÖSTENSON, C.-G., S. ZAITSEV, P.-O. BERGGREN, S. EFENDIC, Ü. LANGEL & T. BARTFAI. 1997. Galparan, a powerful insulin releasing chimeric peptide acting at a novel site. Endocrinology **138:** 3308–3313.

6. CONSOLO, S., G. BALDI, L. NANNINI, M. UBOLDI, M. POOGA, Ü. LANGEL & T. BARTFAI. 1997. Galparan induces in vivo acetylcholine release in the frontal cortex. Brain Res. **756:** 174–178.

7. ZORKO, M., M. POOGA, K. SAAR, K. REZAEI & Ü. LANGEL. 1998. Differential regulation of GTPase activity by mastoparan and galparan. Arch. Biochem. Biophys. **349:** 321–328.

8. POOGA, M., M. HÄLLBRINK, M. ZORKO & Ü. LANGEL. 1998. Cell penetration by transportan. FASEB J. **12:** 67–77.

Time-Dependent Effects of Intrahippocampal Galanin on Spatial Learning

Relationship to Distribution and Kinetics

PÄR A. SCHÖTT,[b] BÖRJE BJELKE,[a] AND SVEN OVE ÖGREN

Department of Neuroscience, Karolinska Institute, S-171 77 Stockholm, Sweden

[a]MR-Center, Karolinska Institute, S-171 76 Stockholm, Sweden

The neuropeptide galanin (GAL), localized in the cholinergic neurons[1,2] of the septo-hippocampal pathway, projecting mainly to the ventral hippocampus (VHPC),[1–3] acts as an inhibitory modulator of basal and evoked acetylcholine (ACh) release.[3,4] There is also evidence that GAL participates in cognitive functions.[4,5] Much of this evidence is based on studies using icv administration of GAL which makes interpretation of neuroanatomic involvement difficult. Another limitation is that the *in vivo* distribution and kinetics of infused GAL are not known. The temporal effect of GAL appears to be important, because the effect on ACh release *in vivo* "disappears" 20 minutes after cessation of GAL perfusion through the probe in the VHPC[4] and the striatum.[6] Therefore, the *in vivo* distribution and kinetics of infused GAL (1.5 nmol/rat, into the ventral hippocampus unilaterally) were compared with the temporal effect of GAL (3 nmol/rat, into the ventral hippocampus bilaterally) on spatial learning in the rat.

In the present study, GAL (3 nmol/rat, into the ventral hippocampus bilaterally via chronic cannulas) was administered 5, 20, or 60 minutes prior to the first trial of each training day. At 5 and 60 minutes, GAL did not produce any significant impairment of acquisition (data at 60 minutes not shown), but at 20 minutes a significant impairment was observed (FIG. 1). The impairment of acquisition seen 20 minutes after administration is consistent with earlier findings showing that GAL (3 nmol/rat) retards acquisition without affecting swim performance.[4]

The distribution of exogenously applied GAL was found (using antibodies for GAL) mainly within the ventral part of the hippocampus and around the infusion site. A very clear diffusion zone with GAL-like immunoreactivity (GAL-like IR) was observed around the site of infusion 5 minutes after exogenously infused GAL (1.5 nmol/rat, into the ventral hippocampus unilaterally) (FIG. 2A). The observation that medium-sized neurons in and around the infusion site displayed GAL-like IR is of particular interest, because the diffusion, internalization, and elimination of GAL are rapid processes and almost no GAL-like immunoreactive cells or GAL-like immunoreactive neuropil could be observed 20 minutes after infusion of GAL into the VHPC (FIG. 2B). However, the behavioral effects do not coincide with the maximal extracellular distribution of infused GAL. This observation suggests that GAL, besides an action at membrane-bound GAL receptors, also affects cellular events, such as regulation of gene transcription, which may contribute to

[b]To whom correspondence should be addressed: Division of Cellular and Molecular Neurochemistry, Department of Neuroscience, Karolinska Institute, S-171 77 Stockholm, Sweden. Phone, +46-8-728 7395; fax, +46-8-302875; e-mail, par.schott@neuro.ki.se

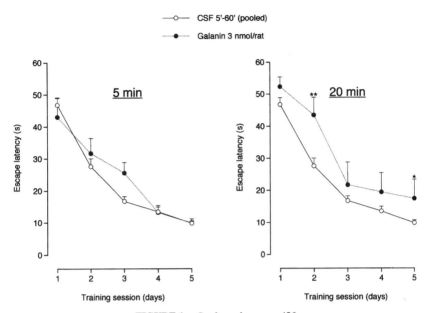

FIGURE 1. *See legend on page 456.*

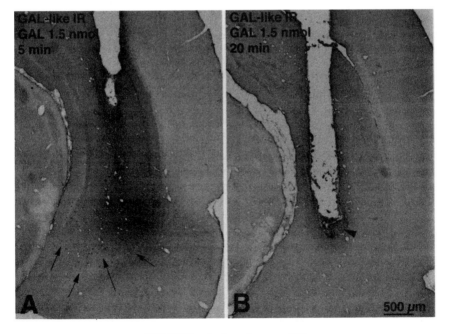

FIGURE 2. *See legend on page 456.*

FIGURE 1. Time-dependent effects of bilateral galanin infusions given 5 or 20 minutes prior to the first trial of acquisition of the spatial learning task. Each value represents the mean ± SEM of the escape latency for each training session (four trials/day) over the 5 days of training. All galanin-treated groups were compared with the CSF control group using a repeated measure of variance (ANOVA) followed by Fisher's PLSD test, galanin versus the CSF control (★★ $p < 0.01$; ★ $p < 0.05$). (Reprinted from Schött et al.[7] with permission from Elsevier Science.)

FIGURE 2. Overview of galanin-like immunoreactivity in the ventral part of the hippocampus (cryostat coronal sections) and the distribution along the track of the cannula at 5 minutes (**A**) and 20 minutes (**B**) after infusion of galanin. The infusion site (*arrowhead*) is well localized within the ventral part of the hippocampus. A minor backflow along the track of the cannula is observed at 5 minutes, but almost nothing at 20 minutes. This indicates that most of the infused galanin is localized in the ventral part of the hippocampus, giving rise to a diffusion zone of galanin-like immunoreactivity. Cells with galanin-like immunoreactivity (*arrows*) can be observed ventromedial to the infusion site at 5 minutes but not at 20 minutes. Scale bar = 500 μm. (Reprinted from Schött et al.[7] with permission from Elsevier Science.)

the *in vivo* action of GAL. Taken together these results further emphasize the importance of the VHPC in the modulatory effect of GAL on cognition in the rat.

REFERENCES

1. MELANDER, T., W.A. STAINES, T. HÖKFELT, Å. RÖKAEUS, F. ECKENSTEIN, P.M. SALVATERRA & B.H. WAINER. 1985. Galanin-like immunoreactivity in cholinergic neurons of the septum-basal forebrain complex projecting to the hippocampus of the rat. Brain Res. **360:** 130–138.
2. MELANDER, T., W.A. STAINES & Å. RÖKAEUS. 1986. Galanin-like immunoreactivity in hippocampal afferents in the rat, with special reference to cholinergic and noradrenergic inputs. Neuroscience **19:** 223–240.
3. FISONE, G., C.F. WU, S. CONSOLO, Ö. NORDSTRÖM, N. BRYNNE, T. BARTFAI, T. MELANDER & T. HÖKFELT. 1987. Galanin inhibits acetylcholine release in the ventral hippocampus of the rat: Histochemical, autoradiographical, *in vivo*, and *in vitro* studies. Proc. Natl. Acad. Sci. USA **84:** 7339–7343.
4. ÖGREN, S.O., J. KEHR & P.A. SCHÖTT. 1996. Effects of ventral hippocampal galanin on spatial learning and on *in vivo* acetylcholine release in the rat. Neuroscience **75:** 1127–1140.
5. CRAWLEY, J.N. 1996. Minireview. Galanin-acetylcholine interactions: Relevance to memory and Alzheimer's disease. Life Sci. **58:** 2186–2199.
6. ANTONIOU, K., J. KEHR, K. SNITT & S.O. ÖGREN. 1997. Differential effects of the neuropeptide galanin on striatal acetylcholine release in anaesthetized and awake rats. Br. J. Pharmacol. **121:** 1180–1186.
7. SCHÖTT, P.A., B. BJELKE & S.O. ÖGREN. 1997. Distribution and kinetics of galanin infused into the ventral hippocampus of the rat: Relationship to spatial learning. Neuroscience **83:** 123–136.

Differential G-Protein–Coupling Profiles of the GalR1 and GalR2 Galanin Receptors

SUKE WANG, TANAZ HASHEMI, STEVEN FRIED, ANTHONY L. CLEMMONS, AND BRIAN E. HAWES

Department of CNS/CV Biological Research, Schering-Plough Research Institute, 2015 Galloping Hill Road, Kenilworth, New Jersey 07033, USA

Since the discovery of the neuropeptide galanin from the bovine digestive system, numerous studies have shown that galanin mediates a variety of physiologic activities by specific galanin receptors. Molecular cloning has identified three galanin receptors (GalRs) that belong to the G-protein–coupled receptor superfamily, characterized by seven transmembrane domains. The amino acid sequences and pharmacologic profiles are significantly different among the GalRs. Although it was reported that GalR1 mediates galanin-stimulated inhibition of forskolin-evoked cAMP production and GalR2 mediates galanin-stimulated inositol phosphate accumulation, this study assesses the ability of GalR1 and GalR2 to couple to various G-protein subtypes.

Several families of G-proteins are regulated by G-protein–coupled receptors. Activation of Gs results in increased adenylyl cyclase I activity and subsequent cAMP production. Activation of Gi inhibits adenylyl cyclase I. Gi activation is also coupled to activation of adenylyl cyclase II, phospholipase A$_2$, K$^+$ channels, phosphoinositide-3-kinase, and specific isoforms of phospholipase C. Activation of Gq results in increased phospholipase C activity and subsequent inositol phosphate (IP) production. Gi, Gq, and Go are also capable of mediating activation of mitogen-activated protein (MAPK). Gi-coupled receptors mediate MAPK activation via a signaling pathway that utilizes the βγ-subunit of Gi, PI-3-kinase γ, the protein kinase Src, a phosphoprotein Shc, an adapter protein Grb2, and Ras-GTP exchange factor Sos. Sos activates the small molecular weight GTP-binding protein Ras which activates a kinase cascade including Raf, mitogen-activated protein kinase/erk kinase (MEK), and finally MAPK. In CHO cells, the Gi-mediated pathway is sensitive to inhibition by pertussis toxin (PTX) and is independent of protein kinase C (PKC) activity. The Gq-mediated MAPK signaling pathway utilizes the α-subunit of Gq, is insensitive to PTX, and is dependent on PKC activity. The Go-mediated MAPK signaling pathway employs the α-subunit of Go, is sensitive to PTX, and is dependent on PKC activity.

In the present study, the effects of galanin or galanin-derived peptides on cAMP production, MAPK activity, and IP accumulation in CHO cell lines expressing the rat GalR1 or GalR2 receptor were determined, thereby assessing the ability of GalR1 and GalR2 to couple to the four major classes of G proteins, Gs, Gi, Go, and Gq.

CHO cells were transfected with plasmids containing cDNAs encoding GalR1 (GalRl/CHO) or GalR2 (GalR2/CHO) receptor and selected by growing the transfected cells in the presence of G418. Saturation binding of ^{125}I-porcine galanin to membrane preparations from the cell lines yielded K$_d$ values of 0.13 ± 0.03 and 0.45 ± 0.12 nM and B$_{max}$ of 339 ± 18 and 55 ± 13 fmol/mg of membrane protein (mean ± SE, *n*= 3) for GalR1 and GalR2, respectively.

Galanin(1-29), galanin(2-29), or galanin(3-29) (3 µM) did not increase the level of intracellular cAMP in GalRl/CHO and GalR2/CHO cells (basal levels 0.6–1.0 pmol/ml) in the presence of cAMP phosphodiesterase inhibitor 3-isobutyl-1-methylxanthene (IBMX, 0.2 mM). Stimulation with 0.1 mM forskolin, by comparison, resulted in a 40- to 60-fold increase in intracellular cAMP. These data suggest a lack of positive coupling of GalR1 and GalR2 to Gs.

In GalRl/CHO cells, galanin(l-29) potently inhibited forskolin-stimulated cAMP production (IC_{50} = 0.46 ± 0.15 nM and I_{max} = 75.3 ± 3.8%). In GalR2/CHO cells, galanin(l-29) inhibited forskolin-stimulated cAMP production (IC_{50} = 1.4 ± 1.2 nM and I_{max} = 32 ± 5%), respectively. These results suggest a strong coupling of GalR1 to Gi and a more modest coupling between GalR2 and Gi.

In GalRl/CHO cells, 100 nM galanin stimulated MAPK activity to nearly three times that of basal levels. Pretreatment of the cells with 100 ng/ml PTX completely blocked the MAPK activity produced by galanin in GalRl/CHO cells. Inhibition of PKC activity, either by pretreatment of the cells with 1 µM bisindolylmaleimide I or by depletion of cellular PKC by an overnight incubation with 1 µM phorbol-12-myristate-13-acetate (PMA), did not affect galanin-stimulated MAPK activity in GalRl/CHO cells. Galanin-stimulated MAPK activity in CHO cells transiently expressing GalR1 was completely inhibited by expression of βARKct (a specific inhibitor of Gβγ signaling). These data indicate that GalR1 mediates MAPK activation via a signaling pathway that utilizes the βγ subunit of a PTX-sensitive G-protein and is independent of PKC which is consistent with Gi-mediated stimulation of MAPK activity.

Galanin also stimulated MAPK activity in GalR2/CHO cells (twofold over control). Pretreatment of the cells with PTX totally inhibited galanin-stimulated MAPK activity. However, unlike GalRl/CHO cells, the galanin-stimulated MAPK activity in GalR2/CHO cells was completely inhibited by bisindolylmaleimide I or PKC depletion. Expression of the Gβγ-inhibitor βARKct did not affect galanin-stimulated MAPK activity in CHO cells transiently expressing GalR2. These data indicate that GalR2-mediates MAPK activation via a signaling pathway that employs the α-subunit of a PTX-sensitive G-protein and PKC, which is consistent with the Go-mediated signaling pathway.

Galanin was unable to stimulate inositol phosphate accumulation in CHO or COS-7 cells expressing GalRl. By contrast, galanin stimulated a sevenfold increase in inositol phosphate production in CHO or COS-7 cells expressing GalR2. The GalR2-mediated inositol phosphate production was not affected by pertussis toxin, suggesting a linkage of GalR2 with Gq/G11.

In summary, GalR1 appears to efficiently couple only to Gi, without activation of Gs, Go, or Gq. GalR2, in contrast, appears more permissive and can pleitropically couple through three distinct G-protein classes, with an approximate rank order of Go = Gq > Gi. The differential signaling profiles and tissue distribution patterns of GalR1 and GalR2 suggest that regulation of galanin action may be mediated at the ligand, receptor, and intracellular levels.

Effects of Three Galanin Analogs on the Outward Current Evoked by Galanin in Locus Coeruleus[a]

ZHI-QING DAVID XU,[b,c] TAMAS BARTFAI,[d] ÜLO LANGEL,[d] AND TOMAS HÖKFELT[c]

[c]Department of Neuroscience, Karolinska Institutet, S-171 77 Stockholm, Sweden

[d]Department of Neurochemistry and Neurotoxicology, Stockholm University, S-106 91 Stockholm, Sweden

Galanin (GAL)[1] has been suggested to be involved in numerous neuronal and endocrine functions as an intercellular messenger molecule/transmitter/modulator/hormone, as summarized in the proceedings of the first galanin meeting in 1990.[2] This has stimulated interest in the search for useful pharmacologic derivatives. Structure activity studies on the effects of GAL fragments and analogs in the central nervous system (CNS) have shown that the NH_2-terminal portion of GAL is important for recognition by the receptor(s).[3,4] A series of chimeric, partly bireceptor-recognizing peptides utilizing the NH_2-terminal GAL-(1-12) fragment and a COOH-terminal portion of another bioactive or nonsense peptide have been synthesized by Bartfai, Langel, and collaborators.[3,4] In particular, three of these, M15 (galantide), M35, and M40, have been shown to act as functional antagonists in several experimental models.

It has been reported that GAL induces a decrease in firing rate and hyperpolarization of locus coeruleus (LC) neurons[5–8] and that M15 reduces this GAL-induced hyperpolarization.[6] In the present study, using the LC slice preparation and voltage-clamp recording, the effects of M15, M35, and M40 on the GAL-induced outward current in LC neurons were investigated.

METHODS

Male Sprague-Dawley rats (150–300 g; ALAB) were used in the experiments. LC slices were prepared as previously described.[9] Briefly, rats were decapitated and LC-containing horizontal slices (300–400 µm thick) were prepared and perfused with oxygenated artificial cerebrospinal fluid. Conventional intracellular recordings were made from LC neurons with sharp microelectrodes filled with 2 M potassium chloride (DC resistance 35–65 MΩ). Whole-cell recordings in brain slices[10] were made with patch pipettes (2–4 MΩ). LC neurons could be identified by their distinctive discharge and membrane properties.[11] All experiments were done under voltage clamp, using the dis-

[a]This study was supported by the Swedish Medical Research Council (04X-2887), Marianne och Marcus Wallenbergs Stiftelse, and Astra Arcus AB.

[b]To whom correspondence should be addressed. Phone, 46 8-7287068; fax, 46 8-331692; e-mail: Zhi-Qing.Xu@neuro.ki.se

continuous single electrode voltage-clamp mode on an Axoclamp 2A amplifier (Axon Instruments). Neurons were routinely held near their resting membrane potential at −60 mV.

M15, M35, and M40 were synthesized as described.[4] GAL was from BACHEM (Bubendorf), idozoxan from RBI, and tetrodotoxin (TTX) from Sigma. Drugs were applied via bath perfusion or by micropipette and pressure injection.

All data are expressed as the mean ± standard error of mean (SEM). Statistical comparisons were performed using Student's t test, and statistical differences were considered significant at $p < 0.05$.

RESULTS

Bath and micropipette applications of GAL inhibited the spontaneous firing of LC neurons and caused hyperpolarization. Under voltage-clamp conditions, superfusion of GAL (1 nM to 3 μM) produced a reversible outward current, which lasted between 3 and 15 minutes in all tested LC neurons ($n = 56$) (FIG. 1) with a peak value within 1–2 minutes. TTX had no consistent effect on the outward current response to GAL (FIG. 1). The peak amplitude of the outward current depended on the concentration of GAL in the range of 1–5,000 nM (FIG. 2). Idazoxan, an alpha-2 adrenoceptor antagonist that blocks the noradrenaline-induced outward current did not reduce GAL-induced outward current (data not shown). In most cells the GAL current did not reverse in the voltage range tested (−40 to −120 mV). These results agree well with our earlier study.[8]

Superfusion with M15 (1–5,000 nM) alone caused a slight inward current (10–50 nA) in 9 of 14 tested LC neurons (FIG. 1). When preincubated with M15 for 3–5 minutes, the GAL-induced current was reduced (FIG. 1), and the dose-response curve for GAL was shifted to the right (FIG. 2). The effect of M15 on GAL-induced current was dose dependent (FIG. 2). However, in most cases M15 did not reverse GAL-induced current completely, even at a high concentration.

Bath application of M35 induced a reversible outward current in all tested neurons ($n = 18$) and was not affected by TTX ($n = 4$) (FIG. 3). The effect was dose dependent

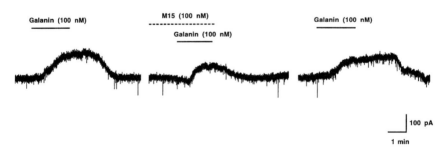

FIGURE 1. Effect of M15 on GAL-induced outward current in the locus coeruleus. In the presence of tetrodotoxin, bath application of GAL (100 nM) induced an outward current (*left panel*). After M15 preincubation, the GAL-induced outward current was reduced (*middle panel*). Note that M15 induced a slight inward current by itself. After washout of M15, the GAL-induced current recovered (*right panel*). The holding potential was −60 mV.

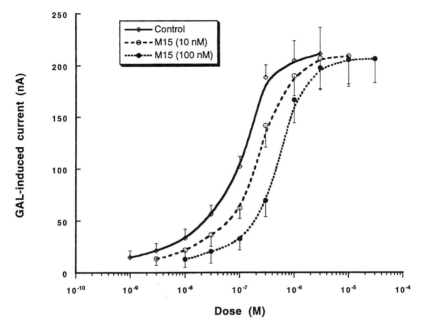

FIGURE 2. Effect of M15 on dose-response to GAL in the locus coeruleus. The amplitude of the outward current was plotted as a function of the concentration of GAL applied by superfusion. The GAL dose response curve was shifted to the right in the presence of M15. In all cells the membrane potential was held at −60 mV.

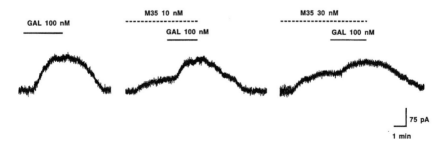

FIGURE 3. Effect of M35 on the GAL-induced outward current in the locus coeruleus. In the presence of tetrodotoxin, GAL (100 nM) induced an outward current (*left panel*). Bath application of M35 (10 nM) induced an outward current by itself and reduced the GAL-induced outward current (*middle panel*), and a higher concentration (30 nM) induced a bigger outward current and further reduced the GAL-induced outward current (*right panel*). The holding potential was −60 mV.

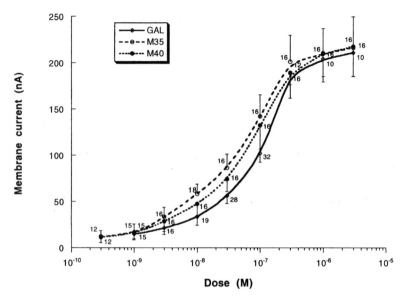

FIGURE 4. Dose-response curve of locus coeruleus neurons to GAL, M35, and M40. The amplitude of the outward current was plotted as a function of the concentration of GAL, M35, and M40 applied by superfusion. The numbers adjacent to each point indicate the number of cells tested at that concentration. In all cells the membrane potential was held at −60 mV.

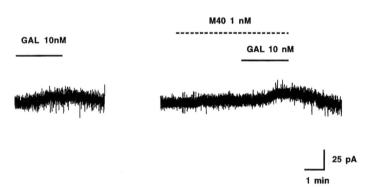

FIGURE 5. Effect of M40 on the GAL-induced outward current in the locus coeruleus. In the presence of tetrodotoxin, GAL (10 nM) induced an outward current (*left panel*). Bath application of M40 (1 nM) induced an outward current. When M40 (1 nM) is co-applied with GAL (10 nM), the recorded outward current was greater than that with M40 or GAL alone (*right panel*). The holding potential was −60 mV.

(FIG. 4). Preincubation of M35 in different concentrations induced an outward current by itself. When co-incubated with GAL, M35 moderately reduced the GAL-induced outward current (FIG. 3).

Similar to M35, M40 alone caused a reversible outward current ($n = 18$), which was TTX resistant ($n = 5$) (FIG. 5). The amplitude of the M40-induced outward current was dependent on the GAL concentration (FIG. 4). Co-incubation of M40 and GAL induced an outward current that was larger than that produced by either M40 or GAL alone (FIG. 5).

DISCUSSION

The present results show that under voltage-clamp conditions GAL induces an outward current in the presence of TTX and that the GAL-induced outward current is dose dependent. Idazoxan, an alpha-2 adrenoceptor antagonist that blocks the noradrenaline-induced outward current in LC neurons does not reduce the GAL-induced outward current, suggesting that the action of GAL is mediated by postsynaptic receptor(s) that are different from alpha-2 receptors. Using *in situ* hybridization a recently cloned GAL receptor, the GAL-R1 receptor, was found in rat LC neurons.[12] All of these results suggest that GAL may activate a GAL receptor(s) located on the membrane of LC neurons.

Of the chimeric GAL peptides tested, M15 attenuated the GAL-induced current in LC neurons, and M35 reduced the GAL-induced current while causing an outward current by itself. M40 caused an outward current but did not significantly block the GAL-induced current; in fact, M40 enlarged GAL-induced current at lower concentrations (1–10 nM).

M15, also termed galantide,[13] is a chimeric peptide composed of GAL (1-12)-Pro-substance P (5-11). M15 displaces ^{125}I-GAL from membranes from the rat ventral hippocampus, midbrain, and spinal cord[6] and insulin-producing Rin M5F cells.[13] M15 fully prevented the inhibitory effect of GAL on hippocampal acetylcholine release in the ventral hippocampus,[6] antagonized the GAL-mediated inhibition of glucose-induced insulin secretion from mouse pancreatic islets in a dose-dependent fashion,[13] and blocked the effects of GAL on the spinal flexor reflex.[6] Here we show that M15, in a dose-dependent fashion, reduces the outward current caused by GAL in the LC, in agreement with the previous study in which M15 reduced GAL-induced hyperpolarization,[6] suggesting that M15 is a GAL antagonist for rat LC neurons. However, M15 did not reverse GAL-induced current completely, even in a high dose, suggesting that M15 is a partial antagonist for GAL receptor in rat LC. Alternatively, there may be several different subtypes of GAL receptor in the rat LC, and M15 is an antagonist only for one of them.

M35, GAL (1-12)-Pro-bradykinin (2-9), has been reported to block GAL effects in the spinal cord[14,15] and on pancreatic islets.[16] M35 also improves acquisition in the Morris swim maze.[17] In the present study M35 caused an outward current while reducing the GAL-induced outward current, suggesting that M35 is a partial antagonist and agonist or an antagonist for one subtype and an agonist for another subtype of GAL receptor. It has been reported that M35 has a GAL-agonist-type effect in rat striatum[18] and hypothalamus.[19,20]

M40, GAL (1-12)-Pro$_3$-(Ala-Leu)$_2$-Ala amide, represents a high affinity GAL receptor ligand and displaces GAL in membranes from the hippocampus, hypothalamus, and rat insulinoma and Rin M5F cells.[21] M40 antagonizes the effect of hypothalamic injection of GAL on feeding behavior.[22] We found that M40 induces an outward current in a dose-dependent fashion. When applied together with GAL, the outward current was greater than that with M40 or GAL alone, indicating a synergistic effect and a GAL-agonist type effect of M40 in rat LC. The GAL-agonist type effect of M40 has also been reported in a variety of models.[19–21,23,24]

Together, these data suggest the existence of multiple GAL receptor subtypes. Recently, three different GAL receptors, GAL-R1,[12,25,26] GAL-R2,[27] and GAL-R3[28] were cloned (see Iismaa *et al.*, Branchek *et al.*, and Walker *et al.*, this volume). The peptide GAL analogs have been helpful in defining GAL subtype receptors while awaiting potent nonpeptide antagonists specific for the different receptors. Such antagonists will improve our understanding of the functional role of GAL and may make it possible to explore therapeutic applications for the treatment of diseases such as chronic pain, neurodegeneration, and depression.

REFERENCES

1. TATEMOTO, K., A. RÖKAEUS, H. JÖRNVALL, T.J. McDONALD & V. MUTT. 1983. Galanin: A novel biologically active peptide from porcine intestine. FEBS Lett. **164:** 124–128.
2. HÖKFELT, T., T. BARTFAI, D. JACOBOWITZ & D. OTTOSON. Eds. 1991. Galanin: A New Multifunctional Peptide in the Neuro-Endocrine System. Wenner-Gren Center International Symposium Series, Vol. 58. MacMillan. London.
3. BARTFAI, T., G. FISONE &, Ü. LANGEL. 1992. Galanin and galanin antagonists: Molecular and biochemical perspectives. Trends Pharmacol. Sci. **13:** 312–317.
4. LANGEL, Ü., T. LAND & T. BARTFAI. 1992. Design of chimeric peptide ligands to galanin receptors and substance P receptors. Int. J. Pept. Protein Res. **39:** 516–522.
5. SEUTIN, V., P. VERBANCK, L. MASSOTTE & A. DRESSE. 1989. Galanin decreases the activity of locus coeruleus neurons in vitro. Eur. J. Pharmacol. **164:** 373–376.
6. BARTFAI, T., K. BEDECS, T. LAND, Ü. LANGEL, R. BERTORELLI, P. GIROTTI, S. CONSOLO, X. XU, Z. WIESENFELD-HALLIN, S. NILSSON, V. PIERIBONE & T. HÖKFELT. 1991. M-15, a high affinity chimeric peptide blocks the neuronal actions of galanin in the hippocampus, locus coeruleus and spinal cord. Proc. Natl. Acad. Sci. USA **88:** 10961–10965.
7. SEVCIK, J., E.P. FINTA & P. ILLES. 1993. Galanin receptors inhibit the spontaneous firing of locus coeruleus neurones and interact with mu-opioid receptors. Eur. J. Pharmacol. **230:** 223–230.
8. PIERIBONE, V.A., Z.Q. XU, X. ZHANG, S. GRILLNER, T. BARTFAI & T. HÖKFELT. 1995. Galanin induces a hyperpolarization of norepinephrine-containing locus coeruleus neurons in the brainstem slice. Neuroscience **64:** 861–874.
9. XU, Z.-Q., V.A. PIERIBONE, X. ZHANG, S. GRILLNER & T. HÖKFELT. 1994. A functional role for nitric oxide in locus coeruleus: Immunohistochemical and electrophysiological studies. Exp. Brain Res. **98:** 75–83.
10. BLANTON, M.G., T.J. LO & A.R. KRIEGSTEIN. 1989. Whole cell recording from neurons in slices of reptilian and mammalian cerebral cortex. J. Neurosci. Meth. **30:** 203–210.
11. WILLIAMS, J.T., R.A. NORTH, S.A. SHEFNER, S. NISHI & T.M. EGAN. 1984. Membrane properties of rat locus coeruleus neurones. Neuroscience **13:** 137–156.
12. PARKER, E.M., D.G. IZZARELLI, H.P. NOWAK, C.D. MAHLE, L.G. IBEN, J. WANG & M.E. GOLDSTEIN. 1995. Cloning and characterization of rat GALR1 galanin receptor from RIN14B insulinoma cells. Mol. Brain Res. **34:** 179–189.
13. LINDSKOG, S., B. AHRÉN, T. LAND, Ü. LANGEL & T. BARTFAI. 1992. The novel high-affinity antagonist, galantide, blocks the galanin-mediated inhibition of glucose-induced insulin secretion. Eur. J. Pharmacol. **210:** 183–188.
14. WIESENFELD-HALLIN, Z., X.J. XU, Ü. LANGEL, K. BEDECS, T. HÖKFELT & T. BARTFAI. 1992. Galanin-mediated control of pain: Enhanced role after nerve injury. Proc. Natl. Acad. Sci. USA **89:** 3334–3337.
15. VERGE, V.M., X.J. XU, Ü. LANGEL, T. HÖKFELT, Z. WIESENFELD-HALLIN & T. BARTFAI. 1993. Evidence for endogenous inhibition of autotomy by galanin in the rat after sciatic nerve section:

Demonstrated by chronic intrathecal infusion of a high affinity galanin receptor antagonist. Neurosci. Lett. **149:** 193–197.

16. GREGERSEN, S., S. LINDSKOG, T. LAND, Ü. LANGEL, T. BARTFAI & B. AHRÉN. 1993. Blockade of galanin-induced inhibition of insulin secretion from isolated mouse islets by the non-methionine containing antagonist M35. Eur. J. Pharmacol. **232:** 35–39.

17. ÖGREN, S.O., T. HÖKFELT, K. KASK, Ü. LANGEL & T. BARTFAI. 1992. Evidence for a role of the neuropeptide galanin in spatial learning. Neuroscience **51:** 1–5.

18. ÖGREN, S.O., A. PRAMANIK, T. LAND & Ü. LANGEL. 1993. Differential effects of the putative galanin receptor antagonists M15 and M35 on striatal acetylcholine release. Eur. J. Pharmacol. **242:** 59–64.

19. PAPAS, S. & C.W. BOURQUE. 1997. Galanin inhibits continuous and phasic firing in rat hypothalamic magnocellular neurosecretory cells. J. Neurosci. **17:** 6048–6056.

20. KINNEY, G.A., P.J. EMMERSON & R.J. MILLER. 1998. Galanin receptor-mediated inhibition of glutamate release in the arcuate nucleus of the hypothalamus. J. Neurosci. **18:** 3489–3500.

21. BARTFAI, T., Ü. LANGEL, K. BEDECS, S. ANDELL, T. LAND, S. GREGERSEN, B. AHRÉN, P. GIROTTI, S. CONSOLO, R. CORWIN, J. CRAWLEY, X. XU, Z. WIESENFELD-HALLIN & T. HÖKFELT. 1993. Galanin-receptor ligand M40 peptide distinguishes between putative galanin-receptor subtypes. Proc. Natl. Acad. Sci. USA **90:** 11287–11291.

22. CRAWLEY, J.N., J.K. ROBINSON, Ü. LANGEL & T. BARTFAI. 1993. Galanin receptor antagonists M40 and C7 block galanin-induced feeding. Brain Res. **600:** 268–272.

23. GU, Z.F., W.J. ROSSOWSKI, D.H. COY, T.K. PRADHAN & R.T. JENSEN. 1993. Chimeric galanin analogs that function as antagonists in the CNS are full agonists in gastrointestinal smooth muscle. J. Pharmacol. Exp. Ther. **266:** 912–918.

24. XU, X.J., Z. WIESENFELD-HALLIN, Ü. LANGEL, K. BEDECS & T. BARTFAI. 1995. New high affinity peptide antagonists to the spinal galanin receptor. Br. J. Pharmacol. **116:** 2076–2080.

25. HABERT-ORTOLI, E., B. AMIRANOFF, I. LOQUET, M. LABURTHE & J.F. MAYAUX. 1994. Molecular cloning of a functional human galanin receptor. Proc. Natl. Acad. Sci. USA **91:** 9780–9783.

26. BURGEVIN, M.C., I. LOQUET, D. QUARTERONET & E. HABERT-ORTOLI. 1995. Cloning, pharmacological characterization, and anatomical distribution of a rat cDNA encoding for a galanin receptor. J. Mol. Neurosci. **6:** 33–41.

27. HOWARD, A.D., C. TAN, L.L. SHIAO, O.C. PALYHA, K.K. MCKEE, D.H. WEINBERG, S.D. FEIGHNER, M.A. CASCIERI, R.G. SMITH, L. VANDERPLOEG & K.A. SULLIVAN. 1997. Molecular cloning and characterization of a new receptor for galanin. FEBS Lett. **405:** 285–290.

28. WANG, S., C. HE, T. HASHEMI & M. BAYNE. 1997. Cloning and expressional characterization of a novel galanin receptor. Identification of different pharmacophores within galanin for the three galanin receptor subtypes. J. Biol. Chem. **272:** 31949–31952.

Index of Contributors